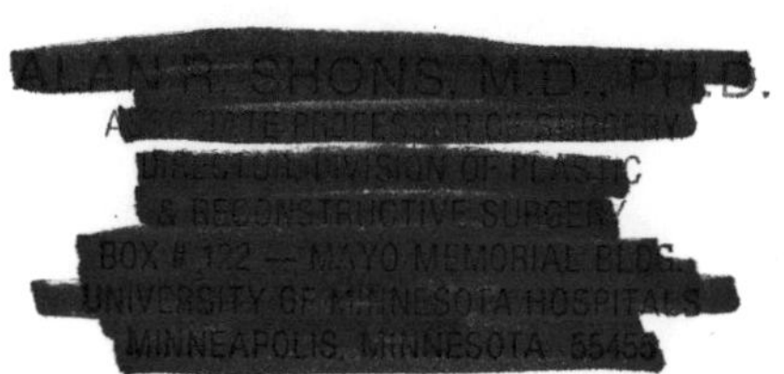

# COMPLICATIONS OF HEAD AND NECK SURGERY

**JOHN J. CONLEY, M.D.**

1979
W. B. SAUNDERS COMPANY
*Philadelphia • London • Toronto*

W. B. Saunders Company: West Washington Square
Philadelphia, PA 19105

1 St. Anne's Road
Eastbourne, East Sussex BN21 3UN, England

1 Goldthorne Avenue
Toronto, Ontario M8Z 5T9, Canada

Complications of Head and Neck Surgery ISBN 0-7216-2649-1



Last digit is the print number: 9 8 7 6 5 4 3 2 1

This book is dedicated to the patients who are anguished by the unsettling phenomena of complications and sequelae that are an immutable part of Man's work and highest intentions. These untoward events, unpredictable and unwanted, lurk in all surgical arenas, in the biological process and in the patient. They give credence to our frailty, from which there is no escape.

# CONTRIBUTORS

ANNE H. ANGERS. Holds a Bachelor of Arts degree in English and does development work and screenings at a children's clinic.
*Management of the Medical Complications of Head and Neck Surgery*

JOHN W. ANGERS, M.D., C.M., F.A.C.A. Clinical Instructor, New York University Medical School; Director, Human Immunology Foundation, New York, New York; Assistant Attending Physician, St. Vincent's Hospital, N.Y., N.Y.; Attending Physician, New York Eye and Ear Hospital.
*Management of the Medical Complications of Head and Neck Surgery*

STEPHAN ARIYAN, M.D. Associate Professor of Surgery, Yale University School of Medicine, New Haven, Connecticut; Attending Physician, Yale-New Haven Medical Center.
*Infection*

DANIEL C. BAKER, M.D. Clinical Instructor of Plastic Surgery, New York University Medical School; Assistant Attending Surgeon, Institute of Reconstructive Plastic Surgery, New York University Medical Center; Resident Instructor, Plastic Surgery Department, Manhattan Eye, Ear and Throat Hospital.
*Complications of Aesthetic Facial Surgery*

OLIVER H. BEAHRS, M.D. Professor of Surgery, Mayo Medical School, Rochester, Minnesota; Consultant, Department of Surgery, Mayo Clinic and Mayo Foundation, Rochester, MN.
*Complications in Thyroid and Parathyroid Surgery*

LESLIE BERNSTEIN, M.D., D.D.S. Professor and Chairman of Otorhinolaryngology, University of California, Davis, School of Medicine; University of California, Davis, Medical Center, Sacramento, California.
*Complications of Cleft Lip and Palate Surgery*

STANLEY M. BLAUGRUND, M.D. Associate Clinical Professor, Mount Sinai School of Medicine, City University of New York; Attending Otolaryngologist, Mount Sinai Hospital; Surgeon Director, New York Eye and Ear Infirmary.
*Complications of Surgery of the Nasal Cavity, Sinuses and Pharynx*

ROBERT L. CAPIZZI, M.D. Professor of Medicine and Pharmacology, School of Medicine, University of North Carolina, Chapel Hill, North Carolina; Chief, Division of Medical Oncology and Attending Physician, North Carolina Memorial Hospital, Chapel Hill, N.C.
*Complications from the Use of Antineoplastic Drugs in the Treatment of Head and Neck Cancer*

JOHN J. CONLEY, M.D. Professor of Clinical Otolaryngology, Emeritus Columbia University College of Physicians and Surgeons, New York, New York; Chief, Head and Neck Service, St. Vincent's Hospital, New York, N.Y.
*Introduction; Operative Complications; Blood Vessel Complications; Carotid Artery Ligation; Oropharyngocutaneous Fistula; Dysphagia; Neural Sequelae; Tracheostomy Complications; Skin Flap and Skin Graft Complications*

EDWARD M. COPELAND, III, M.D. Professor of Surgery, University of Texas Medical School at Houston and University of Texas System Cancer Center M.D. Anderson Hospital and Tumor Institute; Attending Surgeon, M.D. Anderson Hospital and Tumor Institute; Attending Surgeon, Hermann Hospital.
*Prevention of Nutritional Complications*

TERENCE M. DAVIDSON, M.D. Assistant Professor of Otolaryngology, University of California, San Diego, California.
*Treatment of Scars*

REED O. DINGMAN, M.D., F.A.C.S. Professor of Surgery, Emeritus, University of Michigan School of Medicine, Ann Arbor, Michigan; Staff, St. Joseph Mercy Hospital.
*Trauma*

JOHN D. DONALDSON, M.D., F.R.C.S. Assistant Clinical Professor of Otolaryngology, Southern Illinois University, Springfield, Illinois; Attending Physician, Decatur Memorial Hospital, Decatur, IL; Attending Physician, St. Mary's Hospital, Decatur, IL.
*Complications of Tonsillectomy and Adenoidectomy*

STANLEY J. DUDRICK, M.D. Professor and Chairman, Department of Surgery, University of Texas Medical School at Houston; Consultant in Surgery, University of Texas System Cancer Center M.D. Anderson Hospital and Tumor Institute; Chief of Surgery, Hermann Hospital; Consultant, M.D. Anderson Hospital and Tumor Institute.
*Prevention of Nutritional Complications*

JOSEPH L. GOLDMAN, M.D. Professor and Chairman, Emeritus, Mount Sinai School of Medicine, City University of New York; Consultant Otolaryngologist, Mount Sinai Hospital and New York Eye and Ear Infirmary.
*Complications of Surgery of the Nasal Cavity, Sinuses and Pharynx*

OSCAR M. GUILLAMONDEGUI, M.D. Associate Professor of Surgery, University of Texas System Cancer Center M.D. Anderson Hospital and Tumor Institute; Associate Surgeon, M.D. Anderson Hospital and Tumor Institute.
*Prevention of Nutritional Complications*

ROBERT G. HICKS, M.D. Director, Department of Anesthesiology, St. Vincent's Hospital and Medical Center of New York, New York, New York.
*Anesthesia Complications in Head and Neck Surgery*

PAUL H. IZENBERG, M.D. Clinical Instructor, Department of Surgery, Section of Plastic Surgery, University of Michigan School of Medicine, Ann Arbor, Michigan; Staff, St. Joseph Mercy Hospital, Ann Arbor, MI; Attending Staff, Plastic Surgery, Wayne County General Hospital, Eloise, MI.
*Trauma*

HERMAN A. JENKINS, M.D. Assistant Professor-in-Residence of Surgery, University of California at Los Angeles School of Medicine; Staff, University of California at Los Angeles Hospital.
*Complications of Surgery of the Neck*

CHARLES J. KRAUSE, M.D., F.A.C.S. Professor and Head, Department of Otolaryngology, University of Michigan School of Medicine, Ann Arbor, Michigan.
*Complications in Microsurgery in the Head and Neck*

THOMAS J. KRIZEK, M.D. Professor of Surgery, College of Physicians and Surgeons of Columbia University; Attending-Chief of Plastic Surgery, Columbia-Presbyterian Medical Center.
*Infection*

MANUEL LEDERMAN, M.B., D.M.R.E., F.R.C.R. Recognized teacher, University of London and Institute of Cancer Research, Royal Marsden Hospital, London, England; Former Chairman, Division of Radiotherapy and Oncology, Royal Marsden Hospital, London; Former Consultant Radiotherapist, Royal National Throat, Nose and Ear Hospital, London.
*Complications of Radiation Therapy of Cancer of the Head and Neck*

ADOLF K. MIEHLKE, M.D. Professor of Otolaryngology, University of Göttingen, West Germany; Director of Ear, Nose and Throat Department, Göttingen, University, Göttingen, West Germany.
*Complications in Ear Surgery*

JOSEPH H. OGURA, M.D. Professor and Head, Otolaryngology, Washington University School of Medicine, St. Louis, Missouri; Head of Otolaryngology, Barnes and affiliated hospitals, St. Louis, MO.
*Complications of Laryngeal Surgery*

WILLIAM R. PANJE, M.S., M.D. Assistant Professor, University of Iowa, Iowa City, Iowa; Department of Otolaryngology and Maxillofacial Surgery—Director of Division of Head and Neck Surgical Oncology.
*Complications in Microsurgery in the Head and Neck*

IRVING M. POLAYES, M.D., D.D.S., F.A.C.S. Associate Clinical Professor, Plastic and Reconstructive Surgery, Yale University School of Medicine, New Haven, Connecticut; Associate Chief, Section of Plastic and Reconstructive Surgery and Attending Surgeon (Plastic), Yale-New Haven Hospital, New Haven, CT.
*Complications of Surgery of the Salivary Glands*

ROBIN M. RANKOW, M.D., D.D.S., F.A.C.S. Professor of Clinical Otolaryngology, Columbia University College of Physicians and Surgeons; Associate Director, Head and Neck Surgical Service, Columbia-Presbyterian Medical Center.
*Complications of Surgery of the Salivary Glands*

THOMAS D. REES, M.D., F.A.C.S. Clinical Professor of Surgery (Plastic), New York University Medical School; Attending Surgeon, Institute of Reconstructive Plastic Surgery, New York University; Director of Plastic Surgery, Manhattan Eye, Ear and Throat Hospital.
*Complications of Aesthetic Facial Surgery*

RICHARD C. SMITH, M.S. Research Director, Plastic Surgical Associates, Incorporated, Brookline, Massachusetts.
*Treatment of Scars*

SYLVAN E. STOOL, M.D. Professor of Otolaryngology and Pediatrics, University of Pittsburgh School of Medicine, Pittsburgh, Pennsylvania; Director of Education, Department of Otolaryngology, Children's Hospital of Pittsburgh, Pittsburgh, PA.
*Complications of Tonsillectomy and Adenoidectomy*

STANLEY E. THAWLEY, M.D. Associate Professor, Department of Otolaryngology, Washington University School of Medicine, St. Louis, Missouri; Assistant Otolaryngologist, Barnes and affiliated hospitals, St. Louis, MO: Chief of Otolaryngology, Veterans Administration Hospital, St. Louis, MO.
*Complications of Laryngeal Surgery*

GABRIEL F. TUCKER, JR., M.D. Professor of Otolaryngology and Maxillofacial Surgery, Northwestern University Medical School, Chicago, Illinois; Head, Division of Bronchoesophagology/Otolaryngology and Department of Communicative Disorders, Children's Memorial Hospital, Chicago, IL; Attending Physician, Northwestern University Medical Center, Chicago, IL; Consultant,

Cook County Hospital, Chicago, IL; Consultant, Armed Forces Institute of Pathology, Washington, D.C.
*Complications in Endoscopic Procedures*

JOHN ANWYL TUCKER, M.D. Professor of Otorhinolaryngology and Anatomy, Hahnemann Medical College and Hospital, Philadelphia, Pennsylvania; Staff, Hahnemann Hospital, St. Agnes Hospital, Chester-Crozer Hospital, Presbyterian Hospital, Bryn Mawr Hospital, and St. Christopher's Hospital.
*Complications in Endoscopic Procedures*

PAUL H. WARD, M.D. Professor of Surgery, University of California at Los Angeles School of Medicine; Staff, University of California at Los Angeles Hospital.
*Complications of Surgery of the Neck*

RICHARD C. WEBSTER, M.D. Chief, Plastic Surgery Service, Melrose-Wakefield Hospital, Melrose, Massachusetts; Assistant Surgeon (Plastic), Massachusetts Eye and Ear Infirmary, Boston, MA.
*Treatment of Scars*

# PREFACE

Every human endeavor has inherent possibilities of complications. In the excitement attendant on each new step forward in medicine and surgery, the shadow of complexity is always there to add a serious and often unpredictable dimension. Some complications are so severe as to immediately overwhelm a new concept, only to be resolved eventually by other new ideas, instrumentation and technology at a later date. Other complications are so subtle as to lie dormant for decades, allowing a surgical procedure to become relatively acceptable. It is precisely in this milieu of dramatic or delayed misfortune—the by-product of our invention, training and involvement—that we can find the potential for improvement.

Some complications are unpredictable, some are unpreventable and some are incurable. They may be further aggravated by a failure in conscientious reporting. There is a natural disposition to avoid emotional confrontation with all types of disappointment and to emphasize the positive aspect of these encounters. This should never supersede the necessity of the open and frank study of all complications so that their full impact is comprehended on the personal and scientific levels. This scholarly and humanizing experience will make medicine a noble profession.

A book on complications associated with head and neck surgery would help to illuminate the conditions leading to each complication, its prophylaxis and its special treatment. Such a book would cover all organs (with the exception of the eye and the brain) and vital structures in the head and neck. The special sense organs; salivary and metabolic glands; organs associated with chewing, swallowing, breathing and speaking; and vital supportive framework are in the vanguard of assessment. It was soon apparent that the subject was much broader than those sequelae and complications related to major resections. The effects of trauma to the face and the untoward results associated with cosmetic surgery were considered essential, and this began to broaden the concept and added more substance to the book. This led to the adjunctive procedures, such as peroral endoscopy, anesthesia and irradiation. It was felt that these should be included because of their direct association with many head and neck operations and the fact that they contained built-in complications inherent to their own activity and had the potential to add to the complications of the surgical technique. Chemotherapy and immunotherapy have generated great hope and may be of significant assistance in head and neck problems but present both the doctor and the patient with an evoluting projection of complications as they search for their role in therapy. Congenital deformities, such as cleft lip and cleft palate, and basic reconstructive procedures inserted themselves with a list of complications.

Newer techniques associated with microsurgery brought fresh excitement and a new list of complications unique to that craft. The ancient bug-a-boo of infection with its changing pattern of complications had to be dealt with. One of the most serious aspects of surgery in this area deals with the medical complications that can supersede the most successful technical plans and create complications associated with significant morbidity and mortality.

This complex threatening situation from these multiple potential complications can be minimized by a cohesive team of specialists, residents, nurses and paramedical staff. The surgeon assumes fundamental responsibility for all factors that might influence the success of his craft. The anesthesiologist, the internist, the radiotherapist and the oncologist have an involvement that might prove hazardous for the patient beyond the surgical technique itself. The after-care staff is charged with a healing process that might harbor a complication or actually produce a new one. Finally, the major organ systems of the body may themselves fail or contribute indirectly to a complication at the operative site.

Paramount in such a book is the emphasis on prophylaxis and how it may reduce complications. It soon became obvious that perfection is unattainable and that the incidence of complications will depend upon the nature of the biological process, the degree of risk for the patient, the plan of management, the surgeon's expertise and the unpredictables.

All physicians and surgeons who work on the head and neck region appreciate the various complications that may arise in major and minor resections. The otolaryngologist, plastic surgeon, general surgeon and maxillofacial surgeon have faced these problems many times in clinical trials. They have often discussed these puzzling situations over decades at open conferences and have made spectacular advances. It is now time for a gathering and a reassessment of these problems.

This author has found the experience of identifying his complications, along with those of many other surgeons, to be a provocative and educational process. It was evident that the subject matter embraced much more than one surgeon could hope to cover. The final concept of complications in the head and neck included a great variety of biological conditions, specialized organ systems and interdisciplinary operative techniques and consultative support.

The Pack Medical Foundation and the Head and Neck Service of the Columbia-Presbyterian Medical Center have shown interest and support in the publication of this book. The Head and Neck Services of the Columbia-Presbyterian Medical Center and St. Vincent's Hospital, New York, supplied the care for patients with complications by providing head and neck operating room personnel, trained nursing and paramedical personnel, resident staffs and the many consultants. Ida Nathan produced most of the black-and-white prints, working with the difficult task of copying them from 35 mm. color slides. Robert Demarest and John W. Karopelou cooperated with the art work. Patricia Gorman and Lillian Palliser did the heavy and much appreciated job of typing the manuscript. Brian Decker and the staff at W. B. Saunders supplied leadership, organization and production. Mr. Decker, very importantly, persisted with his ideas in the development of the content and style of the text.

JOHN J. CONLEY

# CONTENTS

# 1 INTRODUCTION

*John J. Conley*

Four principal situations govern the possibility of surgical complications in head and neck surgery: (1) obstruction of the airway system, (2) potential for hemorrhage, (3) possibility of infection and (4) failure of a general physiological system (heart, lungs, kidneys, liver or metabolism). The obstruction of the airway system, which is frequently involved in the technique of intubation, tracheostomy and pulmonary toilet, is a major problem. Very young and very old people are particularly susceptible. Serious hemorrhage is related primarily to the great vessels in the region of the neck. Faulty ligature, fistula formation, infection of the wound, local tissue necrosis and previous irradiation are precipitating factors. Serious infection without fistula formation has been markedly reduced but still remains a potential threat. Overall careful medical supervision is needed to analyze and adjust to the range of disabilities in a good- or poor-risk patient. Many head and neck patients are heavy smokers or drinkers, or both, with predictable consequences. Many patients with malignant neoplasms are infirm and undernourished and in the older age groups.

Many of the very serious complications have been significantly reduced. Emergency tracheostomy, tension pneumothorax, soft tissue crepitus, carotid artery hemorrhage, wound infection and cardiac arrest are seen much less frequently than before. In some highly regulated programs, it is possible for a young doctor to complete his residency without having to cope with many of these complications. Improvement in surgical techniques, anesthesia and preparation of the patient have been decisive factors in bettering the success rate of operations.

Where there is surgery, however, there are complications. There is often no single explanation for an unexpected and unwanted development. In some instances, the calculated risk is apparent from the beginning. In other situations, an ideal operation may be carried out on an ideal patient under ideal circumstances and a serious complication may still develop. The precise cause may never be determined.

Some fundamental principles, however, are inviolable. Any transgression of these may have an untoward result. The rules governing hemostasis, wound tension, gentle tissue handling, proper suture material, elimination of infection, recognition of viable tissue and exercise of physiologic control point the way to successful surgery, although they in no way guarantee against complications. Compliance with these principles is axiomatic.

Both patient and surgeon are interested in the highest quality results with the fewest adverse reactions. When the possibility of an adverse turn arises, the surgeon should make every attempt to avoid it. Heroic measures to achieve the impossible have their obvious limitations, which must be assessed preoperatively. Beyond the surgical technique itself, the surgeon is concerned with the quality and availability of the tissue he must deal with. He can temper massive ablation by doing it in stages, combining it with irradiation, or, indeed, may favor irradiation over a serious operation. In precarious situations, he can often avoid infection and wound breakdown by creating a stoma, establishing drainage, using regional flaps, minimizing his technique and using antibiotics.

In the final analysis, the surgeon is obligated to measure the patient's future quality of life against his right to die. The questions to be asked before surgery are limitless and soul-searching, but they are precisely the questions that must be answered.

## DEFINITION

Every operation has a *raison d'etre* and a plan. Every operation also carries with it a predetermined and immutable deficit. Untoward results may be a natural consequence of the operation. Under these circumstances, certain sequelae should be expected and accepted. There are always scarring, fibrotic induration, some edema. stiffness and discomfort. This is a part of the natural healing process. If the surgical procedure is extended to include the larynx, mandible, tongue or facial nerve, there is a much more severe aesthetic and physiological deficit, but it is still an expected and natural consequence of the operation. This situation may be misunderstood or misinterpreted by the patient or by members of the legal profession, and it could be declared a complication for which the doctor is responsible. What they fail to recognize is the fact that the surgeon performed the operation in accordance with the patient's wishes and in order to correct or ameliorate a condition that was found to be unacceptable by or life-threatening to the patient. The patient was apprised of the condition, the operation, the deficit and the possible complications and was assured that no guarantee whatsoever could be given under any circumstances. He requested that the operation be done and gave specific permission for it. He may be depressed and hostile about the expected sequelae of the operation, yet they could not be classified as a "complication," since they are not unexpected and certainly are not the fault of any person. In spite of this, natural sequelae are frequently called "complications" rather than sequelae of the treatment of the disease the doctor tried to cure. This is a strategic and pivotal point in the philosophy of treatment for all parties concerned.

There is another situation that requires discussion. This concerns the "perfect" operation, which is planned and carried out on the ideal patient without a flaw. An unexpected and inexplicable development may enter the postoperative picture. It may represent an unrecognized weakness in the original plan or an inefficient technique, or it may defy rational explanation. The healing process is altered and a new situation is inserted into the postoperative course that requires medical or surgical remedial action. This is usually identified as a complication, but again, it may be intimately associated with the original disease process.

Hopefully, every operation will correct a disease state, a congenital or acquired deformity or a malfunctioning organ. Not every operation, however, guarantees a good result. The operation may fail in its fundamental purpose without overt complications. This is the hardest disappointment to bear, but it is part of the surgical process and may often be more difficult to handle, and ultimately to correct, than the unexpected and unexplained overt complication arising from a new surgical procedure. This failure does not condemn the procedure itself but emphasizes the broad scope of potential results and variables, ranging from gross failure of the technique to solve the problem to serious permanent deficit or death. All of these consequences are implicit in all types of surgery and must be accepted by both patient and surgeon. Indeed, in the final analysis, the patient may equate a sequela with a complication, and the surgeon may recognize a relationship between and an overlapping of these results. Because of this potential interrelation and coexistence, this book will deal with both of these undesired and unhappy situations in a general way without severe distinction or categorization.

## GENERAL PROGRESS

Over the past 20 years, there has been a steady decline in the incidence of serious complications associated with surgery of the head and neck. The advent of tracheostomy; prophylactic antibiotics; improved general anesthesia; careful medical supervision; a better understanding of blood chemistry, electrolyte balance and blood replacement; and the skillful use of the nasogastric feeding tube have established some safeguards. The development of the team, consisting of the chief surgeon, advanced fellows, specialized residents, interns and skilled anesthesiologists; the constant attention of medical consultants, highly trained nurses and paramedical assistants; and the judicious use of ancillary surgical specialties have now made extensive and complicated surgery possible for almost 95 per cent of the patients presenting.

There has been a dramatic reduction in infection after ear operations owing to antibiotics and the development of microsurgical techniques. The surgical treatment of sinusitis has been limited to those cases due to intractable infections. Allergic management now plays a significant role. Specific and nonspecific abscesses and infections in the neck and throat are managed medically and surgically.

The death rate due to tracheostomy has been reduced to 0.2 per cent. The death rate associated with carotid artery hemorrhage and elective common carotid artery ligation is still around 12 per cent, and the incidence of stroke is approximately 30 per cent. Out of 1000 radical neck dissections, the carotid artery was exposed in only 15 instances. It was electively ligated five times and ruptured twice. This striking improvement in wound control was attained by (1) the use of the most efficient incisions during the operation, (2) the use of regional flaps when neck skin was considered to be unreliable, (3) the creation of an intentional oro- or pharyngostoma in high-risk individuals and (4) the consideration of carotid artery protection, either by dermograph or transposed muscle flap, when fistulization or wound breakdown was considered a possibility. No carotid arteries ruptured when the skin and mucous membrane covering were intact. Only two patients formed a false aneurysm and only one formed a true aneurysm. The prime purpose in every wound then is to attain mucous membrane and skin approximation. In the past 10 years, none of the some 3000 head and neck patients in our personal experience have died from tension pneumothorax, operative hemorrhage or postoperative hemorrhage, and only two have died of airway obstruction. This record, of course, is influenced by the quality of the case load, the extent of the disease being treated, the age group, the expertise of the operating staff and anesthesiologists and the quality of postoperative care.

In spite of all the experience and all of the precautions, one must contend with a persistent, irreducible, unpredictable, small incidence of hematoma, seroma, loss of tissue flaps and skin grafts, localized fistula, poor nutritional and healing states, tissue anoxia, irradiation necrosis, exposed carotid arteries, airway complications, infections and dysphagia. "High-risk cases" double the incidence of complications. One must therefore accept the premise that there will always be complications in surgery but that they can and should be reduced to the lowest incidence that is compatible with good medical practice. Good medical practice contains such variables as the nature and severity of the disease process, the general condition of the patient, the skill of the surgeon and his supporting staff and then the effects of the unknown and unsolved mysteries in disease and wound healing.

## WOUND CARE

The vast majority of external surgical wounds in the area of the head and neck are clean. Ninety-five per cent heal *per primam* under proper preparation, management and control. The principal causes of infected wounds are contamination from the oral or pharyngeal cavities, hematoma, dehiscence or gross external or internal contamination. Approximately five per cent of postoperative wounds require treatment for gross infection. This is anticipated in high-risk cases by beginning antibiotics preoperatively. High-risk cases include those requiring surgery in areas that are grossly contaminated or have a high incidence of potential contamination, extensive resections that enter the oral or pharyngeal cavities and extensive resections in individuals who are poorly nourished or who have a physiological or metabolic abnormality and those situations in which surgical intervention would increase the risk to the surrounding structures, such as the brain, the orbit, the ear and associated soft tissues. Hematoma is a precipitating cause of many wound complications. This is managed by aspiration, milking the hematoma from the wound or, in major cases, reopening the wound for evacuation and control of the clot. Dehiscences are either resutured or marsupialized. The potential of infection is obviously present in ulcerating cancers of the oral, pharyngeal and laryngeal cavities and in wounds due to industrial, automobile and street accidents.

Tetanus toxoid is administered routinely for all grossly contaminated wounds that were inflicted in the street or a factory. I have never seen either a tetanus or gas gangrene infection that was due to a surgical wound made in the head and neck region in an operating room theater.

The prophylaxis against wound complications begins with proper preparation of the patient and his skin. The hair in the area of the operation is carefully shaved. The skin itself is washed with soap and water. The mechanical washing, bathing and rinsing of the regional area contributes significantly to its cleanliness. Local skin antiseptics are used to further reduce the residual bacterial population. Povidone-iodine and pHiso-Hex are used currently for this purpose. Povidone-iodine discolors the skin about the head and neck, and this may be considered a deterrent by some patients and physicians. The pHisoHex may be used by the patient on the day prior to and the morning of the operation in a general wash, including the hair, face and neck and upper chest. The skin is prepped again in the operating room with Povidone-iodine or pHisoHex.

Emphasis should also be placed on surgical technique; it should be relatively atraumatic and carried out expeditiously. Dehydration and drying of the open wound should be prevented by the use of moist saline sponges. Obviously, one of the most important aspects of surgery is the absolute control of bleeding. Fine catgut is used for small bleeders and silk is used for the more significant arteries and veins. Cautery is also very effective against small vessel bleeding and oozing. All major wounds are drained either by the hemovac system or Penrose drains.

The optimal closing of the wound enhances the healing process. The approximated tissue must be vital and should be closed without undue tension. Accurate layer approximation is ideal. The rules governing the type of suture material to be used relate to tissue acceptability, strength and durability of the suture material and tissue reaction to different types of suture material. The nonabsorbable sutures, such as silk, cotton and nylon, have the advantages of permanency and limited tissue reactivity. Some of the individual's tissues will react to this type of foreign body and ultimately will reject it. This creates a small suture sinus from which the suture material will be either discharged or removed with a small forceps. Once the suture material is out, the wound heals promptly. Absorbable suture material, such as plain catgut, chromic catgut and synthetics (Vicryl, Dexon), usually cause an increased local tissue reaction, are somewhat bulkier and are absorbed after an interval of several weeks to six months. The physical, technological and biological qualities of modern suture material offer a surgeon a great range of possibilities for approximating the wound under favorable circumstances.

## THE OPERATING ROOM

Over 95 per cent of patients who enter the operating theater for surgery in the head and neck have the operation and return to their rooms without a serious complication. Occasionally, untoward events may occur before or during the course of the operation. Rarely, a patient may have an unexpected reaction to the preoperative medication: He shows a drop in blood pressure, urticaria and extreme apprehension or lethargy. The surgeon must analyze these symptoms carefully to rule out serious pathology and apply appropriate corrective treatment before proceeding.

Conditions occurring during induction of anesthesia are associated with the administration of various combinations of drugs and inhalants to put the patient to sleep and permit introduction of an endotracheal tube. When this is complicated by laryngospasm or airway obstruction, it can lead directly to cardiac arrest. An inexperienced anesthesiologist who cannot promptly correct this situation seriously compounds the problem. Under these circumstances, an endotracheal tube must be inserted immediately or an emergency tracheostomy must be performed. If successful, this action forestalls cardiac arrest and in most instances permits the operation to proceed.

It is prudent to assess all local physical distortions the patient might present to the anesthesiologist prior to the induction phase and to consider alternate methods of intubation. Trismus, previous surgery in the oral and pharyngeal cavities, distortion of the normal anatomy and displacement of the glottis are all warning signs that a patient requires special attention and expert management. The surgeon or his representative should be present during this period to advise, assist and, if necessary, take over in the event of an emergency. It is obvious that an inexperienced trainee in anesthesia is not the ideal person to cope with this situation. If the consequences of this complication are harmful or difficult to evaluate, the operation should be rescheduled after the situation has stabilized.

Once the endotracheal tube has been introduced, it is essential to check five conditions relative to the tube and airway system. (1) The bevel of the tube should be positioned away from the posterior wall of the trachea to prevent obstruction. (2) The balloon on the tube should never be overdistended and should not obstruct the beveled opening. (3) The tube should be in the trachea and not in the main bronchus and should not cause pressure against the lower portion of the vocal cords. (4) The adapters on the tube should not come apart during the operation or kink the tube at its point of attachment. (5) The tube should be secured to the cheek by sutures or with adhesive tape so that it will not come out during the operation. A nasoendotracheal tube is usually directed toward the head of the table; an oral endotracheal tube is directed laterally so that the anesthesiologist will be in contact with one of the patient's arms. Right angle "trees" are helpful in holding the connecting tubes during the operation. Appropriate monitoring equipment for the cardiac system, temperature, intra-arterial and venous pressure readings and gas exchange is set up. the surgeon is now ready to position, prep and drape the patient.

Many patients remain throughout surgery where the anesthesiologist puts them on the table, which may be an inconvenient spot for the surgeon and his assistants. The head and neck should be slightly toward the side of the surgeon. It should be possible to move and shift the head in order to gain extension or flexion, if desired. The head should be encased in a sterile towel, with a sheet and towel underneath the shoulders, neck and head. The area about the head and neck should be open. Sheets used by the anesthesiologist to "tent off" his equipment are frequently cumbersome and may interfere with the territory in which an assistant may have to stand. Some anesthesiologists like to see their equipment as it enters the mouth, and some like to touch it from time to time. This should not be necessary if everything is secured in place and the anesthesiologist is trained in his craft.

## GENERAL FACTORS

### Biological

A preoperative survey of the patient will help to identify many of the predictable biological factors that might contribute to complications. The history is usually quite revealing and illuminates the general status of the patient: (1) Age is a definite factor since most malignant tumors in the head and neck develop after the age of 50 and are therefore often associated with degenerative diseases common in old age, arteriosclerotic changes and possibly a history of pulmonary disease or coronary insufficiency. (2) The social habits of this high-risk group often indicate clinical or subclinical pulmonary disturbances associated with chronic bronchitis, emphysema, asthma and poor pulmonary toilet. These may be aggravated by excessive smoking. (3) The liver may be affected by heavy alcoholic intake or a history of previous liver infection, thus predisposing the patient to liver insufficiency. (4) Ultimately, kidney insufficiency may develop. (5) Many of these patients have had difficulty eating or swallowing and admit that they have lost 10 to 20 pounds. This insufficiency may reach proportions that require hyperalimentation preoperatively and, in some instances, modification of the treatment program to a less aggressive form. (6) This dietary deficiency may be associated with secondary anemia. (7) This entire picture may have an overlay of organic disease or debilitating conditions associated with diabetes or congenital abnormalities. (8) Primary cancer in the area of the head and neck may become locally infected, causing another postoperative complication. (9) Many of these patients are already on some type of medication to control organic disease, to relieve pain, to supplement an inadequate diet or to assist a faltering vital organ. Each drug must be identified and evaluated for its effect on the human organism, necessity, relationship to the planned operative technique and long-range value.

In addition, if there is a distinct possibility that the patient has already been treated with radiotherapy, considering its debilitating effect, there is no question that the dangers of complications during and after the operation are increased. It is imperative that a careful assay of all these biological factors be done preoperatively; it may mean the difference between success and failure of the entire program. Consultations and the team approach are the most rational solution to these complex biological problems.

### Technical

An analysis of specific technical factors may significantly reduce complications. The first step in this analysis is the determination of the patient's operability, which depends on the size and position of the primary cancer, its known or potential capacity for metastasis and the general psychological and physiological status of the patient. This preoperative plan, the type of anesthesia, the possibility of blood replacement, the need for tracheostomy and nasogastric feeding tubes as well as other types of physiological support are routine considerations.

There are certain *sine qua non*'s in surgical technique that can never be taken for granted. Hemostasis should be absolute. All mucous membrane closures should be "spit-tight." Undermining should never be excessive. All flaps should be viable, and tissue should not be closed with undue tension. The type and size of the suture material should be appropriate for the job it has to do. Compliance with these fundamental principles establishes the groundwork for healing *per primam* with a minimum of wound complication. When an attempt is made to deviate from these criteria, the incidence of complications will develop in direct proportion to the violation of the principles.

## PREPARATION OF THE PATIENT

Each patient is scheduled to wash his hair, face, neck and upper chest with pHisoHex the night before surgery and then again on the morning of surgery. After the patient has been anesthetized, the area to be operated on is washed again with pHisoHex. If the endotracheal tube has to be in the active surgical field, the anesthesiologist is requested to position it under sterile conditions, using gloves and a clean endoscopic blade. The tube is prepared with pHisoHex and sutured to the chest or cheek with sterile 0 silk. It is, of course, more desirable to have the anesthetic equipment placed out of the surgical field, but this is not always possible in head and neck surgery. If it is anticipated that a regional flap will be used during the operation, the potential donor area is also prepped. Most of the regional flaps are transposed from the anterior chest, presenting no particular problem in preparation. when the flaps are taken from the posterior cervical area, however, the patient must be elevated somewhat on the table, with a rolled sheet under his shoulders and several folded sheets or a neurosurgical head-rest under his occiput. This gives a surgical approach to a somewhat inaccessible region. For advanced cases in which free skin grafting is anticipated, the lateral leg is prepared simultaneously with the head and neck area. Hair on the chest, axilla and leg is shaved off. Hair on the scalp is selectively cut, parted or shaved off.

### Drapes

Most head and neck patients are draped with a standard head drape consisting of a sheet and one towel under the shoulders, neck and head and one towel wrapped about the head (Fig. 1–1). The towel about the head is positioned above the ears and eyes, usually going around the upper part of the forehead. The eyes are taped shut, since they are frequently in the surgical field. The towel about the head should not be draped and tightened over the eyes. In most instances, the drapes should be sutured to the skin or scalp to prevent shifting.

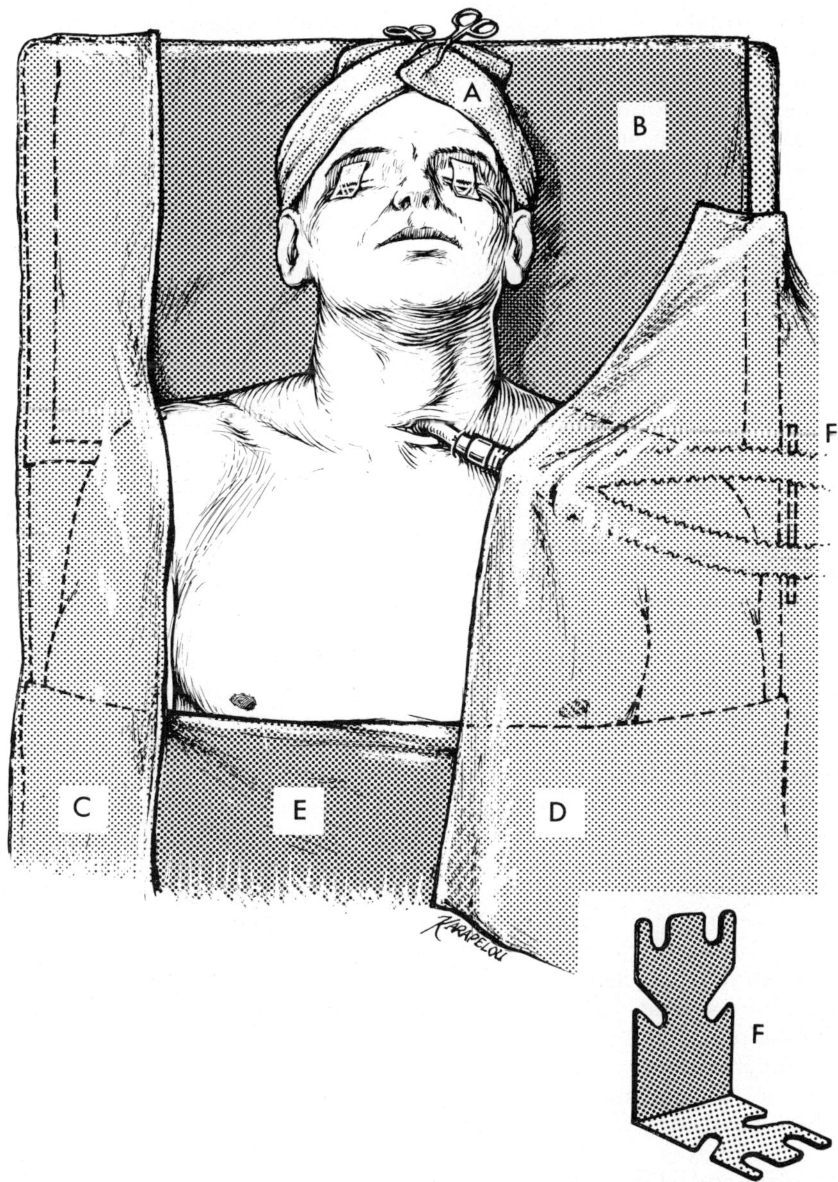


**Figure 1–1.** Standardized draping for major head and neck operation. *A,* Head drape. *B,* Towel and sheet under the head. *C,* Side drapes. *D,* Lateral sheet. *E,* Chest drape. *F,* "Fork" to hold anesthetic tubes. Note that the eyes are taped and an endotracheal tube is sewed to the chest.

Towels are used for lateral draping, and then the perimeter of the field is overdraped with small sheets. Only the area under active surgical involvement need be exposed; all other regions may be covered with towels that can be easily removed for extension of the surgery or the development of the flaps. The drapes should lie flat. "Tenting" of the drapes is undesirable. This exposure of the patient should accommodate space for three or four surgeons around the upper portion of the table.

## ANESTHESIA — THE SURGEON'S VIEW

The vast majority of operations in the area of the head and neck are done under general anesthesia. The anesthesiologist is, therefore, the surgeon's most important collaborator. He must put the patient to sleep, intubate him, sustain and protect him during the operation, awaken him and put him in the best condition for postoperative recovery. He must understand all aspects of gas concentration and exchange, drugs, electrolyte agents, the pharmacology of the major organ systems and monitoring systems. He must be expert enough to intubate the patient under the most difficult emergency conditions. He must position the tube correctly in the trachea, after establishing that it is not in the pharynx, esophagus or main bronchus. The gas must pass freely, without interference from kinking or occlusion of the tube or obstruction from its beveled end. The tube must be fixed to the patient's cheek or forehead with tape or sutures. His lungs should be clear, and the anesthetic machine should be properly equipped. The balloon making the system somewhat air-tight should not be overinflated in order to avoid causing inordinate pressure on the cricoid, trachea or inferior aspect of the vocal cords.

The type of anesthetic selected is based on the general condition of the patient, the nature of the operation and the experience of the anesthesiologist. The technique and instrumentation should be relatively sterile. In cases of large cancers of the oral, pharyngeal and laryngeal regions, it is desirable to place an endotracheal tube in the trachea by a preoperative tracheostomy and then proceed with the ablation. This eliminates the problem of operating with anesthetic equipment blocking the way. In all other situations, the endotracheal tube is inserted through the oral or nasal cavity. Most anesthesiologists oxygenate the patient first, apply a topical anesthetic to the pharynx and larynx, paralyze the patient and then insert the endotracheal tube. There are a variety of exceptions to this basic routine, however. Modifications include blind intubation under local anesthesia, the use of the curved or straight blade, circumvention of various degrees of trismus by passing the tube through the side of the mouth in edentulous patients or by using the nasal route and the accommodations and precautions required when the anatomy of the oral and pharyngeal cavities is distorted by previous treatment in the neck or gullet. When there is doubt as to whether the tube can be passed orally, an elective tracheostomy should be done immediately before the surgery.

The general anesthetic is frequently balanced with a combination of gases, oxygen, relaxants and narcotics. Controlled hypotension may be used to shorten the operating time, improve the quality and precision of the technique and reduce the need for blood replacement. The most important criterion for its use is the patient's physiological status. Approximately half the candidates for radical surgery in the head and neck do not qualify because of their age or because their cardiovascular, pulmonary, kidney or liver conditions do not warrant the risk. The anesthesiologist should never use hypotensive anesthesia on a patient who does not qualify merely to please the surgeon.

In controlled hypotension, the blood pressure is lowered to around 70 to 80 mm Hg and maintained at that level during the operation. Hypovolemia or hypoxia should not be allowed to complicate this technique, as they may lead directly to cardiac arrest. The blood pressure should be permitted to return to normal at the end of the operation.

Of paramount importance is the position of the endotracheal tube. This is determined before starting the operation by listening for breath sounds in both lungs and noting equal excursion of movement when the lungs are expanded by positive pressure. The most satisfactory type of endotracheal tube in head and neck surgery is the "anode tube" with the coiled spiral spring, which provides flexibility without the risk of collapse or kinking. The use of the firm plastic tube is quite satisfactory for general surgical procedures in which the anesthesiologist does not have to compete in the actual operative field and has the entire head and neck region under direct visualization. When the endotracheal tube lies in the field of surgery, however, it must be made to curve and turn to accommodate the movements of the surgeon and his assistants. The firm plastic tube cannot be used to accomplish this without danger of kinking.

In many head and neck operations, it is necessary to move the head during the procedure to gain better exposure. This means that the oroendotracheal tube will also be moved. It is essential, therefore, that the tube be secured in such a way that it will not be displaced by this movement. Suturing it to the lateral cheek, under sterile conditions, is perhaps the cleanest and most secure method of fixation. Many anesthesiologists use tincture of benzoin and adhesive tape, which is completely satisfactory if the tube is out of the field of surgery.

Movement of the tube may cause it to come out, become impacted against the inferior aspect of the vocal cords and cricoid cartilage or be pushed inadvertently into a main bronchus. When the tube comes out, it must be quickly reinserted. This can be a very tense situation for an inexperienced anesthesiologist who finds himself in a bloody operative field with a patient in a superficial plane of anesthesia, gagging or coughing and threatening laryngospasm. Suction, relaxation and good visibility are indispensable during this interval. In the meantime, the surgeon should be prepared for an emergency tracheostomy.

When the endotracheal tube is incorrectly positioned in a main bronchus and this is unrecognized, the patient will manifest some degree of mild hypoxia. This condition may be suggested by poorly aerated blood in the operative field. The tube usually enters the right main bronchus. Most patients can be sustained for varying periods of time with only one side of the lung in use. When the anesthesiologist is not aware of this situation, however, and it occurs in an elderly patient with chronic lung disease, it puts a prolonged extra strain on the cardiopulmonary system that could lead to heart failure and cardiac arrest. The surgeon, aware of this condition mainly because of the dark color of the blood in the wound, is obligated to alert the anesthesiologist, who should then check all features of the anesthetic system and correct any deficiencies. Blood gas evaluation at this time is essential.

In rare cases, the tube will descend deeply into a main bronchus and lead directly to a single lobe bronchus. Gas exchange may appear correct, and even auscultation and feeling the movements of the chest may not reveal the precise condition. This malpositioning of the tube leads directly to severe cyanosis, progressive bradycardia and hypotension. At this point, cardiac arrest is imminent. All drapes should be removed immediately, the cuff of the endotracheal tube deflated and the position of the tube evaluated. Gradually, the tube should be withdrawn to its correct position in the trachea, which should cause an immediate improvement. Repositioning of the tube usually rectifies the condition by the time the blood gas concentrations are determined. It is then the responsibility of the anesthesiologist and the surgeon to determine whether the operation should be continued.

## ARCHITECTURE OF THE OPERATION

Every operation has its own unique basic architecture of excision and reconstruction. This framework is based on the surgical anatomy of the wound and the physical functions of the affected part. The architectural "product" is developed with lines, angles, curves and planes. These factors are applied to the skin, subcutaneous tissue, muscle, bone, nerves, blood vessels and mucous membrane with the intention of excising them and establishing a void requiring reconstruction. A system of tools is used for entrance, exposure, testing, analysis and surgical movement.

The preparation of the shape and contour of the excision is a highly controlled exercise in the craft of measurement and planned removal. The design is based on the biological determinants of the operation, and it often determines the fate of the patient. The design of a wound mirrors the perimeters of the monobloc.

The process of reconstruction embodies another concept of architecture. Here the designs incorporate principles of building, molding, augmenting and stabilizing. They are the precise reversal of the excisional phase, and it is the incorporation of these two stages almost simultaneously that adds a special dynamics to the operative experience.

### Rhythm of the Operation

All the architectural activities are controlled by the concept of surgical rhythm. A surgeon's physical movement through an operative procedure exhibits a great deal of his character and style and reveals the graceful interplay of the human hand and its instruments with open flesh. It seems superfluous to discuss the position of the surgeon as he addresses the operative field, because each surgeon ultimately assumes a posture that suits him. Some prefer the table high, some low. Some operate sitting down; most like to stand. Some shift excessively, some are quiet and some even lean on the patient. This variety of postures is reflected in the use of the arms, wrists and fingers and contributes to the rhythm of the procedure. The rhythm is full of personal expression, improvisation and confidence, moving at tempos that reflect either familiarity with a condition or the threat of an uncomfortable encounter. The quality of the rhythm is influenced by the length of the operation, the surgical anatomy of the territory that is to be cut and the emotional and technical caliber of the surgeon. When all the factors are optimally balanced, the operation should represent the highest level of surgical endeavor.

## GENERAL REMEDIAL PRINCIPLES

There is an integral system of responsibility and priorities during the course of all head and neck surgery and its postoperative period. The basic authority rests with the responsible surgeon, but the success of the endeavor ultimately depends on the cooperative efforts of the resident and the nursing staff as well. It is obvious that a trained team of informed people offers the best advantages for the patient. Unfortunately, this is not always available. Inexperienced private-duty nurses may prove to be a hazard, even though their presence is reassuring to the patient and his family. This deficiency is usually more than compensated for by a competent resident staff. The surgeon and resident should explain to the nurse the importance of a patent airway, adequate suction and control of the hemovacs and the functioning of a nasogastric feeding tube for nourishment. It is attention to these fundamentals that reduces morbidity and insures the best opportunity for healing without complication.

Postoperative complications fall into two general categories — those specifically related to the healing of the wound and those related to the general physiological condition of the patient. Early recognition of an impending complication may help avoid its serious effects.

(1) Complications of operations on the *scalp* generally take the form of infection or loss of tissue, which is remedied by appropriate antibiotics, debridement and regrafting. (2) Wounds about the *orbits, sinuses, ears,* and *temporal bone* may become complicated by local infection, loss of skin graft or regional flap or separation of the wound, or they may cause blindness. A decision must be made about debridement, regrafting or allowing the wound to heal by secondary intention. When these wounds are close to the dura or intracranial cavity, any complication portends the possibility of much more serious intracranial consequences.

(3) A complication associated with *parotid gland* surgery may be an unexpected, severe paresis of the face. This paresis is usually secondary to inadvertent stretching or clamping of the facial nerve. If the surgeon

is not aware of this condition of the nerve, re-entry and exploration is indicated. Hematoma of the parotid wound is not uncommon. (4) Complications about the *nose, face* and *lips* are associated with wounds that are closed with undue tension, twisting or kinking of a regional flap, hematoma, loss of part of a skin graft or wound distortion or separation. Hopefully, most of these complications can be avoided by appropriate operative measures during the closure of the wound.

(5) *Oral cavity* complications concerning the *tongue, buccal mucosa, alveolus, floor of the mouth* and *palate* are associated with tissue loss, infection, hematoma and distortion. Oral flaps can become necrotic from distortion, twisting, kinking, inadequate basic blood supply, postirradiation status and movement. Most of these flaps are permitted to heal by secondary intention, or they are dressed with an onlay skin graft after the wound has been cleaned. (6) Complications in the *pharynx* and *larynx* consist of wound infection, fistula formation, localized edema, regional paralysis, stenosis and distortion. When these complications are severe, it may be necessary to debride the wound and dress it with a split skin graft in an open style or by transposing a regional flap. (7) *Thyroid* and *parathyroid* complications relate to hemorrhage, airway obstruction, vocal cord paralysis and metabolic disorders.

## PSYCHOLOGICAL COMPLICATIONS

Every person confronted with the diagnosis of cancer and with the need for a major ablative procedure in his head and neck experiences a significant emotional reaction to the threat to his life and the inevitable alterations in his appearance and ability to carry on. This reaction is characterized by depression, anxiety, fear and insecurity. Ideally, these rather natural immediate responses are counterbalanced by a stabilizing reaction that is derived from his lifelong reservoir of self-esteem, competence, ability to cope and adjust, healthy relationships with spouse and friends, successful employment and religious beliefs. There is no doubt that the patient needs all the support he can get from these sources, but in many cases today — particularly in urban life — many of these sources are lacking. Support is then sought from the social structure of the community and government. These latter resources are often limited, impersonal or only theoretical. They can never replace or match human kindness. This complex framework of support supplies emotional reassurance, a barrier against apathy and a direction toward resumption of an active life with new perimeters.

Each patient is different in his response to a threat to his life and in the way he tries to overcome the affliction. A procession of fantasies, symbols, hope and fears continues throughout his first consultation, entry into the hospital, the operation, the healing process and then return to life's routines. The patient is never the same after this, but his adaptive capacity is what will lead him back to a life that has some meaning for himself and his family. The meaning in his new life that he will trust and understand is the one closest to his original life pattern or his identity through his work and social existence. The more closely and quickly he can return to that pattern, or some modification of it, the better he will be. The more he misses this target, the more adaptation will be required and the more stress he will have to endure.

Ablation of certain organs and physiological systems causes inordinate stress because of irretrievable losses. The deprivation of an eye, hearing or speech is a permanent disadvantage requiring permanent adaptation of profound proportions. When there is serious disfigurement of the face, the patient still hopes that, although his body image is permanently changed, it can be repaired and reconstructed to various degrees. Interference with the functions of eating and swallowing are depressing and frustrating. Nature has provided that adaptation without undue stress is feasible even when 50 per cent of an organ system has been ablated. Some of the modern excisional techniques, however, go beyond this 50 per cent perimeter and may even encompass other organs, compounding the crippling and altered physiology. The patient's condition may be ameliorated to a certain extent by reconstructive procedures. but he lives with a constant deficit that requires emotional and physical adaptation.

Psychiatric help is not usually needed with these problems unless the patient has had previous psychological problems or is overwhelmed by the therapeutic program. Panic, apathy, obstructive neuroses, psychoses and contemplated suicide understandably require special management. The isolated individual needs more support than someone with a strong family orientation does. The patient has proved capable of hoping for a useful life once he was confronted with the knowledge of his tumor, what must be done about it and what effect it will have on his life. His adversary is beyond his control, his treatment is recommended by a person he does not know and his salvation cannot be guaranteed. In spite of this formidable array, adaptation is relatively successful in the vast majority of cases. Suicide occurs in fewer than 0.05 per cent of cases and is associated with either a "death wish" or a misconception about the prognosis. It is a fact that among patients who are not suffering from constant and inordinate pain only a minuscule number are willing to depart from this life.

# 2 ANESTHESIA COMPLICATIONS IN HEAD AND NECK SURGERY

*Robert G. Hicks*

It has not been said unwittingly that anesthesia may be the most dangerous aspect of surgery in the head and neck, and this bold statement is derived from the fact that the anesthesiologist must put the patient to sleep, maintain this somnolent, relaxed state, control respiration and monitor electrolytes, blood volume, cardiac status and physiologic response. After this, he is responsible for the patient's recovery to consciousness and for the proper functioning of his organ systems. In addition, he must be a superior intubation craftsman because he may be dealing with an infant or a distorted or crippled upper airway system. Many of the patients are in the older age groups and suffer from cancer in the head and neck or other serious physiologic or organ deficiencies. He must be well versed in the use of a variety of drugs and in physiologic reactions. All of his techniques and positions are in the immediate vicinity of the operative field, often creating crowding and decreased accessibility. He has a special relationship with the chief surgeon and must also function in the role of instructor to the resident staff in anesthesiology. There is little doubt that this very responsible position requires the highest vigilance and adaptability.

By and large, the speed, smoothness and quiet of an operative team exemplifies its members' knowledge, understanding and confidence in each other and their function. This is the hallmark of good service and high professionalism. When this structure is disorganized by any of the possible misadventures that exist in the real world of surgery, one is confronted with deviations that could lead to disaster. It is for this reason that all the factors that are operative in developing complications must be analyzed for a complete understanding of this subject and development of a prophylactic approach.

## SURGICAL CONCERNS

### The Surgery

Adequately planned anesthesia begins with knowledge of the surgical purpose and scope. To this is added the patient's physical and psychological conditions and the selection of premedication, primary agents and technique. Then, strategy for anesthesia management evolves.

The first decision the anesthesiologist must make is whether the patient and the operation are suitable for regional or for general anesthesia. Many of the technically simpler procedures up to and including rhytidectomies are often performed with most satisfactory regional anesthesia. The difficulties arise when the surgeon determines the anesthesia according to the operation rather than the patient. Patients filled with anxieties are rarely good candidates for regional anesthesia. Sedatives selected for basal hypnosis to allay their fears are sometimes used in excess in order to accomplish control. Occasionally, the amount of drug necessary to provide a manageable patient leads to inadequate ventilation or airway obstruction. These are just as important with regional anesthesia as they are with general anesthesia. All too often, surgeons remove head and neck towels and drapes and discover that the patient has been seriously compromised from lack of attention to these strict rules.

On the other hand, it is important to remember that good regional anesthesia is a science and not an art. Its purpose is to provide the minimal amount and concentration of the anesthetic agent in the proper place. Systemic toxicity levels vary with each regional anesthetic, but it is quite obvious that blood-brain concentrations are higher when any specific amount is delivered to the head and neck rather than to a more peripheral extremity, where circulatory gradients may diminish what would otherwise be a toxic level.

Sedation of the patient under regional anesthesia is axiomatic. It is as important to select the proper sedative as it is the regional agent. When regional agents are imperfectly delivered and pain occurs, barbiturate sedation invariably produces a degree of delirium and an unmanageable patient. This is not the time to add more sedative. It is the time to discontinue or to convert to general anesthesia.

The anesthesiologist must have a knowledge of the nature of the defects to be repaired or the disease being treated and the influence these aberrations may have on the anesthetic and physiologic course he plans for the patient. Essential to this is a complete understanding of the critical anatomy of the head and neck and of the vital role of the structures therein. With such familiarity, technical and pharmacologic difficulties may be anticipated and avoided. Needless to say, this spells out one concept — control. Control of respiration, both external and internal, through proper airway management on the one hand and neutralizing the untoward effects of disease states such as thyrotoxicosis or fever on the other are essential to the survival of the organism. This survival in turn is dependent on the continual provision of the most satisfactory environment for the cells of the body.

### The Surgeon

Above all else the head and neck surgeon must possess two essential qualities:

1. He must be fully equipped by training and temperament to provide for the flexibility necessary in the event of sudden emergencies or unanticipated patient responses.
2. The head and neck surgeon must respect and respond to the absolute rule of a good airway.

### The Operating Team

Equally shared responsibility for the safety of the patient is essential between the surgeon and the anesthesiologist. Each must have a mutually concerned, cooperative understanding of the difficulties and problems encountered by the other. Nursing and assistant personnel must be fully informed and as attentive to details as the principals. The circulating personnel must be able to provide for the needs of the scrub nurse, the surgeon and the anesthesiologist. All specialized equipment must be arranged for, prepared and in proper working condition prior to its use. A failure in any of these aspects of team effort directly affects operative risk as much as the impaired physical status of the patient does.

### Pre-existing Physical Defects

Congenital defects of the head and neck are significant only when they create airway problems. Although endotracheal anesthesia is, by and large, the effective remedy for this type of malady, congenital anomalies often impair the establishment of a satisfactory airway. Hare lip and cleft palate are of little importance except for drying and clearing copious secretions that accumulate in the oropharynx. Occasionally, the defect may be large enough to inhibit proper placement of an oropharyngeal airway during the induction phase of anesthesia prior to intubation. When this occurs, induction with inhalation agents may become prolonged owing to a partially obstructed airway.

Macroglossia, which is most often associated with some retarded children — especially gargoylism — can be a difficult problem in airway management. Not only is it a problem in selection of oropharyngeal airway size, so that several sizes must be immediately available, but also it is difficult to establish proper placement since the natural curvature of the tongue and pharynx might be altered and not correspond to airway curvatures. Gargoylism can also be particularly troublesome in laryngoscopy because of the macroglossia and the misshapen mandible. A flat-bladed laryngoscope can add to these difficulties because of inadequate tongue guards. Should this become too difficult technically, a fiberoptic laryngoscope can be of help in securing tracheal placement. Unlike fiberoptic laryngoscopy and intubation in the adult, for which the endotracheal tube is placed over the fiberoptic coil and slid into position over it, the small lumina of infant- and child-sized endotracheal tubes precludes this option. In these cases, one must follow a course parallel to the fiberoptic strand. A conventional laryngoscope blade may be helpful in visualizing this strand as it courses in the oropharynx.

Congenital laryngeal stridor is a term applied to myriad airway defects involving the laryngeal doorway. Some of these are serious enough to challenge the most technically proficient anesthesiologist, so that tracheotomy as a route of endotracheal intubation is mandatory. The least difficult laryngeal anomaly to deal with is one in which there is overdevelopment of the aryepiglottic folds, which are flabby and sometimes invaginate between the vocal cords, causing airway obstruction. Webbing of the vocal cords may occur to such an extent that passage of an endotracheal tube is prohibitive, except at the cost of inflicting unnecessary trauma. Proper surgical correction prior to intubation is preferable. Subglottically, atresia of the trachea, especially in the region of the cricoid, may present an impassable channel and tracheotomy is mandatory. Tracheoesophageal fistula must be diagnosed as to the type. Where significant patency between these organs is present, a preoperative plan for feasibility of orotracheal versus direct tracheotomy intubation and sealing for airway control must be developed.

### The Small Child or Infant

The natural anatomic differences in the airway between the small child or infant and the adult must be appreciated to facilitate laryngoscopy and intubation. These differences primarily concern the infant larynx. Not only is the structure much smaller but also it must be remembered that the tissues are exceptionally delicate and unnecessary or rough instrumentation will result in edema and trauma. An infant's larynx is more anterior and displaced more cephalad than an adult's larynx. The epiglottis may appear less developed and short and often assumes an omega shape rather than an ellipse, making the arytenoid cartilage and vocal cords more difficult to visualize. The vocal cords are usually at more of a right angle to the sagittal plane than in the adult, where they are at more of an acute angle to the sagittal plane with the anterior cords more cephalad than the posterior section. The narrowest portion of an infant's larynx is just subglottic at the level of the cricoid and not at the vocal cords as it is in the adult. The operator is sometimes tempted to place too large an endotracheal tube when it easily passes the vocal cords. If it does not pass the cricoid with ease, it should not be forced. To do so would inevitably result in subglottic edema and laryngeal stridor post extubation. The shorter length of the larynx and trachea in the infant must be kept in mind so that too long a tube or a tube placed too far will not become lodged in one or another bronchus. The tracheal length in infants is rarely more than two centimeters. The angle of bronchial take-off is equal on the right and the left in the infant, with the result that an endobronchial intubation can be produced as frequently on either side. The adult bronchi angulate more acutely on the right side than on the left with a higher incidence of endobronchial intubation resulting on the right side.

The short larynx of the infant is a problem when sealing the airway with a cuff. Although infant cuffs are available, these are all too long. Consequently, the cuffs invariably are in opposition to the vocal cords and arytenoid cartilage as well as to the trachea. The consequence is edema and trauma to these structures. Pharyngeal packing around an uncuffed endotracheal tube is preferable. This also serves to inhibit inspissating esophagogastric contents that may otherwise drain and pool about the glottic fissure.

## Diseases, Tumors and Trauma of the Head and Neck

The two main concerns in planning anesthesia for this category of patient are the ability to establish a satisfactory airway and the ability to prevent foreign material from being carried into the lower airway system. Whenever the pre-existing condition has distorted the anatomy, a judgment must be made as to whether orotracheal intubation via laryngoscopy can be satisfactorily and safely performed or whether one must elect a preliminary tracheostomy. Too often, surgeons find patients under general anesthesia and muscle relaxants employed to facilitate laryngoscopy impossible to intubate. In the unconscious and paralyzed patients, this leads to hectic and avoidable moments, with the patient's life or cerebral function at stake. Should any doubts arise in the evaluation of the patient prior to surgery, an indirect laryngoscopy may provide sufficient information to select the safest approach. In the same regard, one can often establish whether trismus might be severe enough to necessitate tracheotomy. Occasionally, one is faced with the dual difficulty of an enormous tumor of the anterior neck and oral structures vitiating the possibility of direct laryngoscopy. In all such cases, intubation must be planned with the patient awake and topically anesthetized. Whether this can be accomplished nasotracheally or by manual oral technique, it is a blind method. Techniques of a serious and potentially complicating nature should be attended by both anesthesiologist and surgeon. When serious trauma has produced hemorrhage and danger of asphyxia from inhalation of blood or tissue, tracheotomy is the immediate choice for airway control. Noncollapsable endotracheal tubes, such as the spiral wire latex type, are most satisfactory since they can assume very sharp angles and contours without kinking and compressing the interior lumen and thus impairing ventilation.

In some cases of laryngeal cancer in which the tumor surfaces on the route of the endotracheal tube, discretion is often the better part of valor. It is wiser to perform a preliminary tracheotomy on such patients rather than risk fragmentation of the tumor, which could move the mitotic cells down the trachea for later implantation and extension of the disease into the trachea or bronchi.

## Diseases of Other Organ Systems

Maximal control of physiologic defects due to diseases of other organ systems is essential prior to safe anesthesia. All of our commonly used general anesthetics are biologically active agents chosen for their ability to depress the sedative and analgesic elements of the central nervous system. They also affect the vital centers of the central nervous system that deal with respiration and cardiac functions. These agents invariably mimic either the cholinergic or adrenergic pathway of the autonomic nervous system. In this way, they can alter the function of all vital organs both directly and indirectly. Diseases of the nervous system itself as well as those of the heart, lungs, liver, kidneys and glandular and muscular systems may have seriously impaired one or more organs, with the result that a superimposed anesthetic might be a risk to life. Such conditions as epilepsy, increased intracranial pressure or parkinsonism can be profoundly influenced by anesthesia. Cardiac arrhythmias, coronary perfusion and congestive failure along with pulmonary ventilation must be maximally controlled to effect satisfactory oxygen and carbon dioxide diffusion and transport. Metabolic hepatic defects, renal filtration and excretion and blood volume are essential to the satisfactory detoxification and excretion of all of the intravenous anesthetics and of a part of the inhalation anesthetics. Imbalance of thyroid and insulin levels as well as pituitary and adrenal activity can produce fatal responses from anesthetics or anesthetic stress. Once impairment of such a vital organ has been determined, it is important that the extent of disease be assayed by the internist and the patient, who should be brought to the optimal physiologic status by medication prior to surgery. When immediate surgery is necessary to save a life, the anesthesiologist must be prepared to treat these conditions during the surgery, if it is at all within the realm of a calculated risk.

### Physical Status and Operative Risk

In attempting to classify physical status for purposes of anesthesia and stress, the American Society of Anesthesiologists has adopted numerical values from 1 to 5. Class 1 covers that patient who has no impairment of any vital organ system. Class 2 includes that patient who has slight impairment. Class 3 represents moderate impairment. Class 4 patients have severe impairment. Class 5 is used for a moribund patient. If the patient is a surgical emergency, a letter "E" precedes the numerical denotation. The physical status is not itself the operative risk of the patient. It is only one of the contributions to operative risk. The quality of the surgical facility, the surgeon, the anesthesiologist and the supporting personnel all contribute to operative risk. Where any factor is impaired, the risk to the patient is increased.

## SURGICAL COMPLICATIONS

### Anatomic Defects Produced by Surgery

Not infrequently, complications of surgery affect the course of anesthesia. This is particularly true when the surgery involves structures of the head and neck. Unique to this area is the upper airway control, which is mutually the concern of both surgeon and anesthesiologist. Misadventure can be precipitately disastrous or subtly disarming, with difficulties following surgery. Should the surgeon require a momentary displacement of the endotracheal tube in order to facilitate the procedure, it is imperative that he make his needs known to the anesthesiologist, who must decide whether the patient's physical control can withstand interruption of ventilation and if so, for how long. Any indication by monitoring that physiologic systems are showing deterioration must be attended to instantly. Damage to the recurrent laryngeal nerve corrupts the airway after extubation. The patient will exhibit signs of upper airway obstruction, including noisy respirations, retraction of the sternal notch and sternum and flaring of the lower rib cage on inspiration. Should there be any concern, immediate reintubation must be performed and a decision must be made concerning tracheotomy. When both recurrent laryngeal nerves are involved, the tracheotomy must remain for several weeks while wallerian degeneration of the nerves takes place. The vocal cords move from complete adduction to a midposition and ventilation becomes satisfactory through the larynx. These changes are referred to as Semon's law.[6]

Should deep cervical fascial tissues tear or rend, in the absence of a major resection when release of air from these tissue spaces is unimpaired, mediastinal and subcutaneous emphysema may occur. This is sometimes referred to as the Bowden-Schweizer syndrome[2] and is due to a valvelike effect at the tear, with inspiration sucking air into the deep cervical fascial planes. As respiration continues, the air moves into the mediastinal area and the subcutaneous spaces. Expansion of this emphysema may compress intrapleural spaces sufficiently to embarrass pulmonary function. Indeed, it may even continue toward rupture of the pleurae and development of tension pneumothorax. Pneumothorax during surgical dissection at the root of the neck can follow puncture of the parietal pleura, which is somewhat higher on the right side.

Unnoticed open venous vessels can draw in unwanted air in quantities sufficient to cause air embolism. A large embolus of 50 to 60 cubic centimeters or the accumulation of smaller bubbles in the right atrium may be sufficient to interfere with cardiac function. Should this occur, a typical millwheel murmur can be heard over the precordium. In such cases, the patient must be immediately turned so that his left side is down and his right side is up to trap the air in the right atrium and prevent it all from entering the lung as an air embolus. Should this happen, the vagovagal reflex could produce cardiac arrest. Central nervous system damage may result if sufficient air passes through the cardiopulmonary circulation and finds its way into the cerebral circulation. If air persists in the atrium, it may be necessary to remove it with a syringe and needle. Previously placed central venous pressure lines may also be helpful in removing such air emboli. The more the patient's head is elevated on the operating table, the more likely is such an accident.

Ligation of major vessels of the neck during surgery may damage the central nervous system. When it becomes necessary to ligate carotid arteries, an attempt should be made to temporarily compress the artery to determine whether collateral cross-over cerebral circulation is adequate. There is a controversy as to whether increasing carbon dioxide tension will protect the cerebral cortical areas during such a procedure. It is more likely that large doses of barbiturates or cooling or a combination of the two will be far more effective in preserving cerebral cortical cells.

Ligation of an internal jugular vein on one side appears more frightening than it usually is. The patient's head becomes edematous and cyanotic. It is preferable to stage the ligation of both internal jugular veins. Usually, it is only when the second jugular is sacrificed that one must follow the patient for signs of cerebral edema. Adequate vertebral vessel circulation will gradually take up the overload from compromised jugular drainage. Postoperatively, such patients should be placed with their heads up, and vital signs, including temperature, should be monitored frequently for at least 24 hours. Fluid intake must be limited. In some patients, the use of diuretics, such as mannitol, to slightly dehydrate the patient may be desirable. Any sudden temperature elevation around 12 hours after ligation may signal serious edema and attendant cerebral anoxia from compression. In order to preserve cortical cells, it may be necessary to employ hypothermia and/or large doses of phenobarbital or sodium thiopental (Pentothal). Large doses of barbiturates may depress ventilation sufficiently to require artificial ventilation and the employment of curare to prevent straining. Cerebrospinal fluid decompression can be effected by an indwelling subarachnoid catheter or a neurosurgically placed Richmond's cranial screw. Such a decompression vehicle also serves the purpose of monitoring intracranial pressure vacillations. Only when measured cranial pressures have returned to normal and pressure vacillations have ceased should artificial ventilation and cooling be discontinued. Such efforts as these may be necessary to prevent cortical damage, which is as likely from severe cerebral edema as it is from direct anoxia.

Large, bulky, compression dressings, which are used following extensive head and neck surgery, must be carefully placed to prevent compression of the airway or impaired circulation of the head. Their presence alone is rarely an indication for elective tracheotomy at the end of surgery. The endotracheal tubes should never be removed until the patient is awake and the dressing has been applied. The comfort of the patient and the observance of smooth ventilation indicate that all is well and the dressing is satisfactory. Notwithstanding this, all such patients should have a tracheotomy set at their bedsides in the event of unforeseen complications.

## Physiologic Defects Produced by Surgery

Severe blood loss during surgery in this region is rarely a cause of shock, since the major vessels of supply are usually exposed during resections or are immediately available for compression. Sometimes, however, one encounters almost uncontrollable bleeding when resections involve the base of the skull. Prevention of excessive blood loss during surgery by the use of sufficient intravenous catheters with large enough bores is essential. At least one 16 gauge catheter must be used for fluid or blood replacement and must be independent of the line kept open for intravenous anesthesia drug control. Adequate supplies of blood must be available preoperatively for any planned procedure. When the patient is in physical status 1 or 2 (p. 17) and physiologically is age sixty or less, controlled hypotension might be considered to prevent excessive blood loss. More frequently than during surgery, blood loss sufficient to induce oligemic shock may occur in the immediate postoperative period, when a ligature may come loose or more remotely when a stripped carotid artery may blow out. The sudden or gradual hypotension from sudden blood loss cannot be considered shock. Rapid replacement of fluids can sustain blood volume sufficiently to prevent the clinical signs of shock. When fluid replacement is insufficient or too slow, the patient's peripheral or capillary circulation fails and the resultant clinical picture is called shock. The blood pressure is very low, the pulse is rapid and the skin is cold, diaphoretic and cyanotic. The respirations become more rapid and deep. If awake, the patient is anxious. Capillary refill, as determined by finger pressure on the skin, is exceptionally sluggish and may not be perceptible. Urinary output fails from inadequate renal flow. Should shock continue for any length of time, the treatment becomes less effective and eventually death ensues. Of paramount importance in the treatment is fluid replacement to maintain adequate circulating volume. Eventually, whole blood must be replaced, but Blalock[1] has shown that it is more important to replace circulating volume rapidly than to maintain the carrying capacity of the hemoglobin. Simple fluid solutions will remain in the circulation only a few hours. In order to nourish cellular structures, they must contain sufficient electrolytes to move between the extracellular and cellular compartments. Shires[7] and Jenkins[4] have advocated the use of lactated Ringer's solution for sudden blood loss and have demonstrated its efficacy. Volume expanders such as dextran solutions have proved to be effective in maintaining circulating volume while permitting autoinfusion of fluid from the extravascular spaces because of their high osmotic pressure. The amount of infusion beyond the volume of the original expander is predictable in amount and duration. Eventually, blood must be used to replace that lost, but when electrolytes and expanders have been used, the blood must not be administered too quickly or overhydration will result. It should be used to replace the electrolytes or expanders as they leave the circulation.

In treating shock, one is often tempted to employ vasopressors in order to maintain cardiac output and increase peripheral blood pressure to maintain perfusion of vital organs. It is better to accomplish this through adequate circulating volume. Vasopressors prevent the perfusion of the capillary bed by further constriction of capillary arteriolar structures. These arterioles are sufficiently constricted from the shock state, with resultant sluggish stagnant capillary blood flow. The capillary unit in shock, with its trapped circulation, has impaired internal cellular respiration, with resultant cellular hypoxia and elevated carbon dioxide tension. Some have advocated the use of peripheral vasodilators in shock in order to improve capillary perfusion.

Sarnoff[5] has demonstrated a cardiac component of shock with impaired contractility and output due to poor coronary perfusion. A vasopressor would be ideal if it were active primarily on the heart and minimally active peripherally. Metaraminol bitartrate (Aramine) has proved to be of value in this state since it markedly dilates the coronary vessels while being minimally active at peripheral sites.

Any decrease in renal flow and nourishment can adversely affect the kidney. This organ is very sensitive to insult and responds with varying degrees of shutdown. Prolonged shock can result in severe damage to tubular structures. Urinary output and concentration must be continuously followed during and after the shock state in order to determine to what degree renal function has been impaired and when it may recover function. When treatment of shock has been effective, it is necessary to follow kidney function to ensure adequacy of recovery. Shock produces acidosis, and it may become necessary to alkalinize the patient. Damage to the kidney can seriously alter systemic electrolytes, with a resultant hyperkalemia. Ion-exchange resins or even renal dialysis might be necessary until the kidney recovers sufficiently to maintain a reasonably balanced function.

Cerebral perfusion may become impaired, as it is with other vital organs. Resulting damage to the cortex must be treated, as we have described elsewhere (p. 18). It is important to commence such treatment as quickly as the damage is discerned. To delay treatment is to increase damage accordingly. In treating shock, it is essential to remember that the blood is pooled in the splanchnic bed as a defense mechanism. Blood is lacking in the systemic circulation. When the shock has been successfully treated, there remains a total fluid overload, and a redistribution of fluid occurs. This redistribution can be greatly altered by the ability of the kidney to function well.

Reflexes can be elicited around the carotid bulb during surgery. These were first described by Heymans[3] in his classic cross-carotid circulation experiment in dogs. Pressure or manipulation of the carotid stimulates impulses over the sinus nerve, a branch of the glossopharyngeal nerve. Following central integration, efferent impulses travel over the vagus nerve to produce cardiac and respiratory disturbance. Hypotension, bradycardia and hypoventilation, or even apnea, may occur. If noticed and untreated, cardiac arrest may occur. As soon as a carotid reflex is diagnosed, surgical manipulation must stop until treatment is given. The surgeon can treat this most effectively with a simple injection of procaine in the adventitia at the bifurcation of the carotid artery. This injection blocks the afferent impulse over the sinus nerve, with the signs of efferent arc stimulation disappearing. The anesthesiologist can also treat this reflex by intravenous injection of atropine to block cholinergic responses or by injection of small doses of ephedrine, a centrally and peripherally effective vasopressor, to augment adrenergic vegetative response.

Hormonal responses that can complicate anesthetic management during surgical intervention are limited to the thyroid gland. In some cases of thyrotoxicosis that appear to be medically euthyroid after treatment, the glands may demonstrate significant activity when manipulated. The infusion of excess thyroxine into the circulation may precipitate hypertension, tachycardia and arrhythmias. It will also increase oxygen consumption abruptly and produce hyperpyrexia. Adrenergic blocking agents are effective remedies for the cardiac disturbances. High ventilatory oxygen concentrations are important in providing the critical environment for adequate cellular oxygen tension. Morphine is an ideal anesthetic agent in such cases because it effectively conserves oxygen need by reducing cellular metabolism. Parathyroid surgery for active tumors does not of itself produce anesthetic difficulties during the surgery. Anesthetic complications during parathyroid surgery are due to the effects of the tumor prior to surgical intervention. Hypercalcemia can have a serious effect by increasing cardiac contractility and bradycardia. Effective treatment can be readily provided by pharmacologic means.

### Anatomic Defects Produced by Anesthesia Technique

More common complications produced by the anesthesiologist include damage to the lips and oropharyngeal structures by improperly or traumatically placed oropharyngeal airways and laryngoscopes. These structures are all relatively delicate, and technical care must be exercised to avoid tissue damage and bleeding. Complications with the endotracheal tube very often are the result of inadequate masseter muscle relaxation during laryngoscopy with inadequate visualization of the structures. Occasionally, lightening of the anesthesia and relaxation can produce the awkward complication of the patient biting the endotracheal tube and completely occluding his own airway. This simply requires more anesthesia or relaxation, or both, if a bite-block is not present during surgery to re-establish patency. It can be more difficult, however, at the end of surgery and anesthesia when the patient is awakening and is being disconnected from anesthesia control prior to extubation. The bite-block should never be removed prior to extubation and placement of an oropharyngeal airway. If the complication does occur, one can simply cut the endotracheal tube flush with the teeth and allow it to slip behind them, restoring patency.

Endotracheal tube placement must be carefully checked to be sure that it is not in the esophagus, where perforations can occur from too much pressure or from too long a stylet. The distance an endotracheal tube extends into the trachea is important in preventing endobronchial intubation. Consequences of this include hypoxia, hypercarbia and the gradual collapse of the nonventilated lung, where considerable shunting of pulmonary circulation occurs. It is equally important that an endotracheal tube be securely fixed in position, so that accidental removal from the trachea does not occur during manipulation of the head and neck. Proper taping and wrapping the tube in gauze and fixing it to the face or the skin with collodion are suitable methods for most procedures. When extensive resection of the face and neck are involved, the most satisfactory method of fixing an endotracheal tube has been to sew it to a corner of the mouth at the circumoral fold. The suture must not be so fine as to pull through a one centimeter subcutaneously placed entry. Number 2 silk is the most advisable and does not scar the face. Too deeply placed a suture will engage muscle and some of the smaller tendrils of nerves controlling the lips, with resultant palsies.

Nasotracheal tubes are adequate for relatively short procedures lasting one or two hours at most. After this time, edema of the turbinates is not uncommon, so that gradual compression of these soft rubber tubes occurs. Impairment of ventilation is most commonly limited to the increased resistance of the compressed lumen. This results in increased physiologic dead space and increased work of respiration. Occasionally, the lumen of an adult-sized endotracheal tube can become so compressed that it is impossible to pass a 12 French suction catheter through. With a nasotracheal tube, if the head is too sharply flexed, kinking of the tube may develop at the nasopharynx. Placement of a nasotracheal tube must be performed as carefully as with an orotracheal tube. The beveled side of the tube must face the midline so that the point of the tube does not create a submucous resection as it is passed back through the nose. These tubes are made with bevels cut right or left for use in either nostril. Again, the passage of the tube must be delicately performed to avoid eliciting nasal mucosal tears and copious nosebleed. The tip of most endotracheal tubes is unsatisfactory for nasotracheal use. The tip must be rounded and smooth to prevent these mucosal tears. The tube must also be soft and sufficiently flexible to prevent tearing through the posterior pharyngeal mucosa and dissecting downward in the posterior pharyngeal space.

Endotracheal tube cuffs have been involved in many complications. The cuff has to be properly positioned almost at the end of the tube to engage the tracheal wall and not the laryngeal structures, where ulcer granulomas can form. Unexpected rupture of the cuff during controlled ventilation with a respirator can produce ineffective ventilation, hypoxia and acidosis. A cuff can sometimes develop a bubble and deviate the direction of the endotracheal tube bevel, with the result that it lies flush against the wall of the trachea, completely blocking the lumen. An overinflated cuff may sometimes balloon beyond the tip of the endotracheal tube and block the lumen. When one is sure of good endotracheal tube placement in the trachea and airway obstruction develops, the first thing to do is decompress the cuff. Most often the obstruction immediately disappears. Soft, high volume, low pressure cuffs have become available in recent years to prevent tracheal erosion ulceration with eventual atresia sometimes requiring surgical tracheoplasty. These are essential when the endotracheal tube will remain in place more than a few hours. They are advisable when there is any question of the adequacy of circulation to the trachea or when that circulation may become compromised by hypotension or shock.

Pharyngeal packs placed in lieu of endotracheal cuffs or to supplement their seal must be counted and removed at the end of endotracheal anesthesia.

Careless positioning and padding of the patient on the operating table can result in peripheral nerve injury and palsy. All bony prominences must be well protected with arm boards and towels or sheets. Hyperextension of an upper extremity can result in brachial plexus injuries.

Eyes must be protected with inactive ointments during anesthesia. The anesthetized patient may not maintain completely closed eyelids. This, together with absent lacrimation, may produce conjunctival or corneal burns from drying. When there is any question of surgical contact near the eye, the lid should be closed with tape or a suture.

All prosthetic devices, such as false teeth and glass eyes, must be removed prior to surgery. Fixed bridges and capped teeth must be fully protected by padding with gauze during laryngoscopy and intubation.

Moving the unconscious patient from table to stretcher at the end of a surgical procedure must be done with great care to prevent injury to the extremities or the neck. Cervical fractures can result from too rough handling at this point.

## Physiologic Defects Produced by Anesthesia

Complications produced by the anesthesia or anesthesiologist in this area can be prevented by attention to a detailed checklist. One must be constantly aware of the fluid and electrolyte requirements of sensible and insensible losses as well as of replacement of all lost blood volumes. A central venous catheter may be of significant help in this regard. Adequacy of ventilation can be checked by monitoring vital signs. When prolonged artificial ventilation is employed, an intra-arterial line or heparin lock is essential to secure arterial blood gas samples. Positioning of the patient is important in maintaining a level and satisfactory plane of circulatory hemodynamics. The anesthetized patient has some degree of suppression of the compensatory sympathetic peripheral vascular mechanisms. He is not as adaptable to the influence of posture and gravity as his awake counterpart is. This must be taken into account when head-up positions are requested by the surgeon. When blood volume is decreased, it may interfere with venous return to the heart, and a decrease in cardiac output and mean arterial blood pressure can ensue. An often overlooked concern is temperature control. A massively opened neck exposed for long periods of time can allow great loss of body heat. Cold blood should be warmed to body temperature. Unless hypothermia is elected and its complications and idiosyncrasies watched for, inattention to central body temperature can result in accidental hypothermia. Lowering of peripheral blood pressure due to vasoconstriction, peripheral cyanosis and cold acidosis can result from hypothermia. Drugs such as curare are inactivated by hypothermia so that relative overdoses may occur, giving rise to prolonged and severe neuromuscular block as the patient rewarms.

Needless to say, it is also essential to maintain a constant watch of the cardiovascular system. Blood pressure, pulse and continuous electrocardiographic monitoring are essential. When controlled hypotension is employed, peripheral blood pressure may sometimes be inaudible during auscultation. An oscillometer or Doppler may be required to measure blood pressure.

Muscle twitch response measurements are essential when muscle relaxants are used in controlled ventilation. The degree of moment-to-moment muscle block may indicate the drug requirements for adequate relaxation. Conversely, the twitch response return indicates the adequacy of decurarization so that the patient will be able to sustain adequate spontaneous ventilation once the procedure has terminated and he has been extubated.

Urine sampling via an indwelling catheter is a must when there is any concern for urinary output or when one is dealing with diabetic patients. Frequent urine sampling in the diabetic patient can determine the amount of insulin requirements.

## Pharmacologic Defects Produced by Anesthesia

Complications in this category begin with the appropriateness and adequacy of premedication. An undersedated, anxious patient has higher oxygen consumption and a higher level of circulating catecholamines. The latter can precipitate hazardous cardiac arrhythmias. An overmedicated patient may have inadequate ventilation and hypotension. Both of these should be treated prior to induction of general anesthesia. Proper selection of premedicants is also important. The use of a cholinergic drug, such as morphine, in an asthmatic patient can produce a serious asthmatic crisis. The use of an adrenergic type premedicant, such as meperidine hydrochloride (Demerol), in a patient with tachycardia can produce an even greater tachycardia with decreased cardiac output and hypotension.

Proper selection of an anesthetic agent for the patient and his surgery must be guided with a pharmacologic balance directed toward suppressing untoward physiologic responses in any disease state. For the patient with angina or with metabolic hepatic disease, agents must be selected to provide the best possible coronary or hepatic perfusion.

The use of adjunct agents, such as muscle relaxants, in patients with myasthenia gravis or of hypotensive agents in patients who are not in the best physical status or within an acceptable physiologic age range must be avoided. Trimethaphan camphorsulfonate (Arfonad) should not be used if a trial dose produces little response or if relatively continuous, large doses are required for maintenance. Using nitroprusside should also be abandoned in cases of patients requiring very large maintenance doses or when blood lost has not been replaced sufficiently. In these latter cases, an accumulation of cyanmethemoglobin may interfere with the oxygen-carrying capacity and result in tissue asphyxia.

Pharmacologic attention must be paid to the treatment of other organ system deficiencies that may exist previously or occur during induction of anesthesia. Of particular attention in this regard are the use of insulin in patients with diabetes and the use of cardiac drugs in patients with any of the cardiac-type disturbances associated with contractility and rhythm. In the diabetic patient, increasing urine sugar and ketone levels, associated with a narrowing pulse pressure, usually indicate hyperglycemia and the need for covering insulin. Intraoperative insulin requirements are best handled intravenously. The reason for this is that any hypotension may interfere with the uptake of subcutaneously deposited insulin. Repeated doses may all be picked up simultaneously when normotension recurs, and the result may be insulin shock.

Certain pharmacologic incompatibilities occur, such as the synergistic neuromuscular blocking effect of muscle relaxants and some antibiotics. When the patient is under treatment with antibiotics prior to and during surgery, care must be taken in the use and amounts of relaxants.

Regional anesthesia for the head and neck, as in other body areas, may produce three types of complications. There may be hypersensitive responses that are not necessarily dose-related. There might be cardiovascular or central nervous system responses that are dose-related. The proximity of the central nervous system and the heart to regional anesthesia depots in the head and neck permits a high and rapid blood-brain and blood-cardiac dose ratio. Hence, equal doses of a regional agent deposited distal and proximal to these organs respectively would exhibit different blood concentrations at the organ interface due to diffusion dilution. Hypersensitive reactions must be treated with antihistamines. Cerebral responses are the product of overstimulation. Convulsions may be treated with a barbiturate, an airway and oxygenation. The stimulatory phase may be so fleeting that convulsions are not seen, the only evidence being syncope and respiratory depression. In such situations, only airway establishment and artificial ventilation, with whatever cardiovascular support is necessary, are indicated. The cardiovascular responses can run the gamut from hypotension treated with vasopressors to cardiac arrhythmias treated with cardiac sedatives to cardiac arrest requiring artificial massage or defibrillation.

The use of antagonist compounds requires mention. Narcan is an effective but fleeting antagonist for narcotics. Careful attention to dose response may reveal a subsequent dose indicated in ten to fifteen minutes to maintain recovery from any narcotic depression. Corresponding care must be provided when muscle relaxants are reversed with neostigmine (Prostigmin) and atropine.

## IMMEDIATE POSTOPERATIVE CARE

Certain precautions must be restated concerning postoperative care. Serious attention must be given to avoiding serious trauma when moving the unconscious patient. Vital functions must be continuously monitored until full recovery of all vital functions is established and physiologic stability is ascertained. Pain must be adequately treated not only for patient comfort but also because of the hypotensive influence it provokes. Surgeons and anesthesiologists must be near the recovery area until recovery is complete in case of any complications. Attention to bandages and checking for bleeding and anything that may compress the airway or essential circulation is mandatory.

## CHARACTERISTICS OF SAFE AND SUCCESSFUL ANESTHETIC MANAGEMENT

1. The anesthesiologist is familiar with the patient and his condition.
2. The anesthesiologist is familiar with the operation planned and has discussed any problems with the surgeon when outlining his anesthetic management.
3. The patient understands the procedures to be performed and has been effectively sedated with premedicants, having perhaps some degree of retrograde amnesia, without a disturbance of his physiologic balance.
4. The anesthetic induction is swift and

sure, and the maintenance is smooth and unruffled.

5. Problems are treated quickly by both surgeon and anesthesiologist after rapid assessment and without flustering or argument.

6. The emergence from the anesthetic and surgical states is smooth and uncomplicated.

## Bibliography


1. Blalock, A.: A consideration of the present status of the shock problem. Surgery, *14*:487–508, 1943.
2. Bowden, L., and Schweizer, O.: Pneumothorax and mediastinal emphysema complicating neck surgery. Surg. Gynecol. Obstet., *91*:81–88, 1950.
3. Heymans, C.: Role of the cardioaortic and carotid-sinus nerves in reflex control of respiratory center. N. Engl. J. Med., *219*:157–159, 1938.
4. Jenkins, M. T.: Common and Uncommon Problems in Anesthesiology. Philadelphia, F. A. Davis Co., 1968, pp. 212–225.
5. Sarnoff, S. J., et al.: Ventricular function; circulatory effects of aramine; mechanism of action of "vasopressor" drugs in cardiogenic shock. Circulation, *10*:84–93, 1954.
6. Semon F.: On the proclivity of the abductor fibers of the recurrent laryngeal nerve to become affected sooner than the adductor fibers, for even exclusively in cases of undoubted central or peripheral injury or disease of the roots or trunks of the pneumogastric, spinal accessory, or recurrent nerve. Arch. Laryngol., *2*:197–222, 1881.
7. Shires, T., Coln, D., Carrico, J., and Lightfoot, S.: Fluid therapy in hemorrhagic shock. Arch. Surg., *88*:688–693, 1964.

# 3 OPERATIVE COMPLICATIONS

*John J. Conley*

## COMPLICATIONS OF BIOPSY TECHNIQUES

Histologic documentation is an absolute concomitant of all radical tumor resections. Excisional biopsy or the atraumatic removal of a small section of an exposed ulcerating cancer causes the least disturbance of the cancer and the patient. *Aspiration biopsy* is extremely effective in helping diagnose metastatic squamous cell carcinoma of the cervical nodes and somewhat less effective with other neoplasms in the head and neck. Most of the dangers associated with aspiration biopsy are theoretical. The technique can, unfortunately, cause dissemination or implantation of tumor tissue in the needle track. If it is cancer, inadvertent implantation is corrected by the ablation. There is, of course, the remote possibility that a hemorrhage will be caused by puncturing a great vessel or entering a hemorrhagic tumor, but this has always been controlled by localized pressure. Air embolus is not considered a likely development.

*Formal incisional biopsy* is, understandably, more traumatic since it opens tissue spaces and fascial planes and directly violates the integrity of the tumor or the metastasis by cutting with knife or scissors. The surgeon, when reoperating in these areas, always tries to include the biopsy site, but spillage may be a hazard owing to the proximity of vital structures that should remain inviolate. The complications of open biopsy can be further compounded by inadvertent injury to major blood vessels and nerves.

There is a danger of causing facial paralysis when biopsying tumors of the deep lobe of the parotid gland that have stretched and pushed the facial nerve to the surface of the specimen, thus exposing it to injury. Large metastatic tumors may involve the hypoglossal and the vagus and spinal accessory nerves, which could conceivably be injured during the open biopsy. This danger can be minimized by aspiration biopsy in most instances.

When the cancerous mass has compromised these nerves, they should be resected with the specimen. Their rehabilitation under these circumstances is not necessary or warranted. To diagnose and treat primary tumors of these nerves, such as neurilemoma, it is usually necessary to resect both nerve and tumor. If the proximal and distal stumps of the nerves are available, they can be grafted with a free autogenous nerve graft. The recurrent laryngeal nerve may be injured or resected during a thyroidectomy, with resultant hoarseness and reduction in vocal range, quality and force. This deficit may be improved by free nerve grafting, nerve crossover from the laryngeal fascicle of the vagus nerve, neuromuscular pedicle implantation or Teflon injection.

One of the unexpected complications of biopsying a posterior cervical lymph node may be paralysis of the spinal accessory nerve. This nerve is intimately intermingled with blood vessels, fibrofatty tissue and lymph nodes in the posterior triangle of the neck. The lymph nodes may be matted together or may envelop the spinal nerve; they may cause bleeding when they are removed. Management of these conditions may lead to inadvertent injury of the nerve. If this occurs, the nerve should be reconstructed by direct approximation or free nerve grafting.

When an open biopsy is performed on

certain vascular tumors, the surgeon must be prepared to control brisk bleeding. He should be alert to the fact that the chemodectomas (carotid body tumor, glomus jugulare tumor), juvenile nasopharyngeal angiofibroma and hemangiomatous tumors are subject to excessive bleeding during a biopsy or an operation. Preliminary study of these tumors with angiography may reveal them to be pathognomonic. If these tumors must be biopsied, it will probably be necessary to use numerous ties, transfixions, a cautery and packing with an absorbable cellulose gauze (Surgicel). It is conceivable, and unfortunate, that excessive bleeding under some of these circumstances requires multiple transfusions and, occasionally, ligation of the great vessels.

## CAROTID SINUS REFLEX

Every head and neck surgeon is occasionally confronted with a carotid sinus reflex. This reflex derives from the carotid sinus and the nerve of Herring, which is a division of the glossopharyngeal nerve. The carotid sinus nerve descends into the connective tissue between the internal and external carotid arteries to innervate the carotid sinus and the carotid body. Connections with the vagus, hypoglossal and sympathetic nerves are frequently present, but their role is still obscure.

The carotid sinus is a pressoreceptor. Stimulation of this sinus causes the slowing of the pulse and a precipitate drop in blood pressure. The focus of sensitivity for this reflex is the proximal segment of the internal carotid artery, just above the bifurcation.

The carotid sinus may be affected by internal or external pressure, twisting, touching or manipulation. It is more sensitive in older patients and in those with atheromatous disease in this blood vessel. A tight-fitting dressing, palpation of this area or even turning the patient's head may precipitate faintness, syncope and collapse in certain individuals.

The anesthesiologist should always be alerted when the surgeon approaches the carotid bulb. A reflex reaction may be triggered by manipulation of a large tumor in the neck when the surgical activity is quite distant from the carotid bulb. Approximately 15 per cent of patients having a radical neck dissection will manifest this reflex reaction to some degree. A patient's blood pressure may drop below 60 mm. Hg, or even to zero for short intervals. When the surgeon is alerted by the anesthesiologist to an abrupt drop in blood pressure, bradycardia or arrhythmia, he should stop stimulating the carotid sinus and immediately infiltrate 1 per cent lidocaine, without adrenalin, into the adventitia around the carotid sinus and along the nerve of Herring. A return to normal blood pressure and pulse is usually apparent within a minute. If it is not, additional infiltration should be carried out. The head should be turned to the upright position, all clamps should be removed from pressure on the artery and the area should not be stimulated in any way. The anesthesiologist should check on the physiological, chemical and anesthetic status of his patient to rule out more serious cardiac complications. After the physiological signs have returned to normal, the surgeon may continue with the dissection.

## PERSISTENT LYMPHEDEMA OF THE FACE

This condition stems from a critical reduction in the number and volume of venules and lymphatic vessels draining the tissues in the face and neck. The etiologic factor is a direct result of the extension and combination of radical neck dissection and irradiation. Bilateral radical neck dissection removes the majority of the essential venous and lymph systems in the anterior and lateral cervical regions. Preoperative and postoperative irradiation increases this deficit by local destruction of these conduit systems in the regional flaps and the associated tissue beds. This combination of aggressive composite therapies is capable of producing varying degrees of edema about the face.

There is a direct ratio between the extent of obliteration of the cervical lymph nodes, lymph vessels and veins and the amount of edema produced in all structures above the level of the neck. A simple surgical entry into the neck permits reconstitution of the regional lymph system within several months. In contrast to this, a unilateral radical neck dissection causes complete postoperative lymph blockage in the neck. This blockage causes a temporary swelling of the ipsilateral cheek, orbit and intraoral cavity that may persist for a year or longer. There is a graduated ongoing reconstitution of lymph flow extending from a postoperative period of a few weeks to five years. A superficial lymphatic system in the dermal and subdermal tissues of the regional neck flaps makes the first connection for lymph digression. Subsequently, collateral connections are made with the opposite side of the neck through the submental and submandibular lymph nodes and their connecting vessels. Fisch (1968)[4] demonstrated the pernicious effects of radical surgery and irradiation on the cervical lymph system, and his publication deserves special review. It is logical that the more obliterating factors that are applied to the cervical lymph system, the greater the possibility of postoperative facial edema. When bilateral radical neck dissection is carried out, the possibility of contralateral connections and assistance is eliminated, with resultant increased obstruction and back flow. The intralymphatic pressure distal to the sites of obstruction causes marked dilatation of the lymph vessels and may destroy the effectiveness of the lymph valves. When irradiation is applied to the neck through large ports as preoperative or postoperative treatment, there is further obliteration and obstruction of the lymph flow at all levels. Fisch has shown that therapeutic irradiation reduces the number and size of the cervical lymph nodes significantly, and obliterates most of the lymph vessels over an interval of five weeks to 19 months. In addition, the scar pattern of the skin incisions will obstruct the superior lymph flow if the incisions are horizontal and encompass the anterior and lateral cervical areas. This is precisely the position of the upper scar in the majority of neck dissections. Resection of the oral and pharyngeal mucosa adds another obstruction by removing these potentially compensatory lymph channels. The escalation of the obliteration of one region of lymph drainage after the other, compounded by destructive ionizing irradiation, presents the background for permanent lymphedema.

This edema may involve the scalp, face, eyelids, ears, cheek, lips, tongue, buccal area, palate, pharynx and larynx. The swelling causes a sense of stiffness, a deterioration in the function of these organs and a predisposition to localized infection and may interfere with the upper airway system. The eyelids may be swollen shut, the lips may balloon and the tongue may swell to fill the major portion of the oral cavity. The swelling in the skin creates a brawny stiffness. Once the edema has

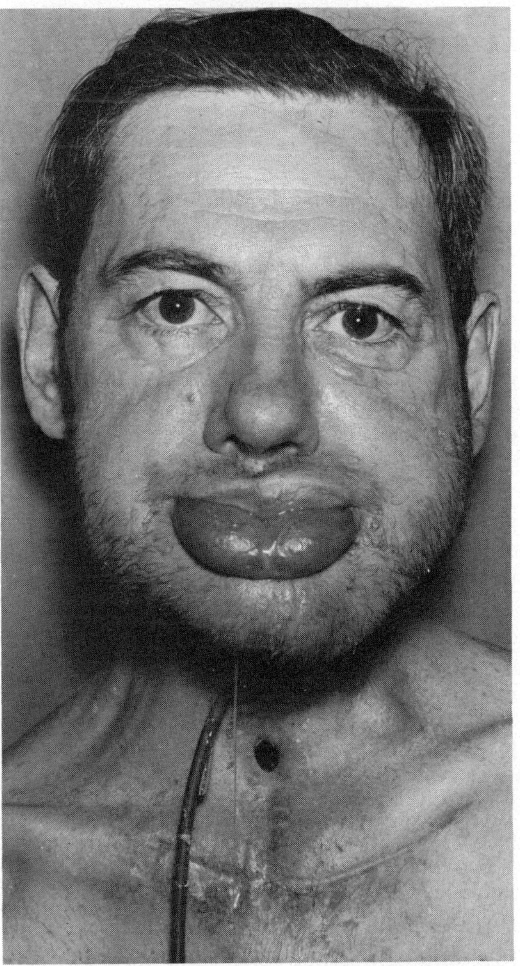

**Figure 3–1** This patient had a vertical midline incision with two large lateral flaps opened along the lower border of the mandible for access to the neck and oral cavity. He also had an intentional submental stoma to facilitate healing of the wound. The wound healed per primam, but the edema of the lips persisted for 12 months.

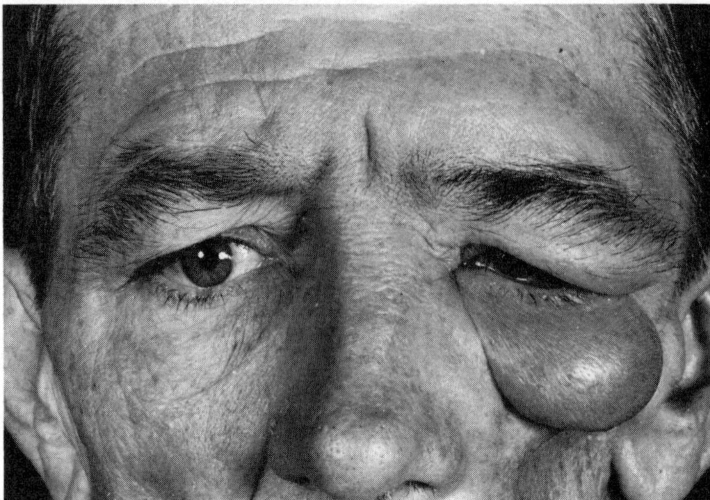

**Figure 3–2** Severe persistent lymphedema in lower eyelid following resection of maxilla, parotid and neck.

reached this stage, regeneration and reconstitution of the lymph and venous elements in the neck flaps are reduced to a minimum owing to persistent and permanent fibrosis and atrophy. There is meager evidence that islands of lymphoreticular tissue develop in these desolate areas but do not truly form a lymph system.

It is essential to use prophylactic antibiotics in the early stages to minimize regional cellulitis and localized infection. Elevation of the head and neck assists the gravitational laws of drainage and prevents an exaggeration of the edematous phenomenon where gravity is not favored. The possibility of resultant persistent facial edema should be considered in all extensive treatment plans, and attempts should be made to preserve a rerouting facility. The use of heavily irradiated regional flaps for repair or resurfacing should be avoided, as this will only add to the obstructive edema. In certain circumstances, however, this may be unavoidable. Rerouting of the lymphatics into the subcutaneous dermal lymphatics in the neck flaps provides one of the potential means of improvement of this condition. The position of the scars and the presence of the platysmal muscle in the absence of irradiation may be used to advantage. The use of large nonirradiated regional flaps to supply a fresh venous and lymph vessel system in the cervical region is advantageous when carried out at the time of the primary resection. The substitution as a secondary method of treatment for persistent lymphedema one or two years after the primary operation may be helpful but is a hazardous technical undertaking because of the fibrosis and scarring about the carotid artery system. These flaps keep their new and nonirradiated vascular and lymph vessels intact and can be used as a diversionary system for the obstructed fibrotic and obliterated tissues of the neck. They must be in continuity with the low levels of obstruction and edema, so that they can supply the potential for reconnection of the drainage elements of the face. The dilated obstructed lymph vessels, often having ruptured valves, seek new conduits for drainage through a normal regional flap. Wedge resections of edematous tissues about the face, oral cavity and pharynx are not practical. O'Brien and associates (1977)[8] reported that 55 per cent of 22 cases of lymphedema of an obstructive nature in the upper and lower limbs averaged a 38 per cent reduction in volume with microlymphaticovenous anastomosis. This sophisticated technique of lymphatic anastomosis requires highly experienced microvascular surgery. Microlymphaticovenous anastomosis for the relief of facial edema has not been reported, but it is not beyond the realm of imagination with the abundance of regional blood vessels and dilated lymph channels and the availability of healthy regional flaps.[1, 2, 3, 5, 6, 7, 9, 10]

## AIR EMBOLUS

Air embolus as a serious complication in head and neck surgery is extremely rare. This author has not once documented that complication out of 3000 radical neck dissections. This rarity, however, does not eliminate the possibility of its occurrence, and one should be prepared to carry out immediate remedial action. It is highly probable that the phenomenon is much more common than is recognized, that it exists on a subclinical level and that in mild to moderate instances of air entrapment it is self-correcting. Relatively large volumes of air can be injected into the venous system, slowly over a period of time, without critical effect. On the other hand, large volumes of air entering the large veins of the neck pass into the right auricle. This can produce critical symptomatology leading to tamponade of the heart and death if not recognized and treated properly. In all large wounds in the head and neck, there is an extensive exposure of the cut ends of the small veins and lymph vessels. During the course of an operation, large veins may be inadvertently opened. Owing to the negative pressure in the veins, there is a potential for air to pass directly through their openings into the main venous collecting channels. When this occurs in a massive and sudden manner on the basis of an opening in a large vein at the root of the neck that is not controlled and is sucking in large volumes of air, the patient develops cyanosis, a drop in blood pressure, a loud churning noise over the precordial area and a gradual weakening and then disappearance of the peripheral pulse. Cardiopulmonary collapse is imminent and leads directly to cardiac arrest. The site that is permitting the aspiration of air should be immediately controlled by clamping or tamponade. The patient should be turned on his left side with the head slightly down, and the right auricle should be aspirated through the chest. The patient's circulation is supported by external cardiac massage, oxygen, controlled endotracheal anesthesia (if that is not already in effect) and blood or fluid replacement. The best prophylaxis for air embolus is meticulous identification and clamping of all major venous systems in the neck and their securement with a ligature or transfixion.

An air embolus and the air frequently seen in large- and medium-sized veins in the neck during the course of an operation are separate occurrences. The latter is almost always associated with nitrous oxide anesthesia. When a small vein is cut, several bubbles may be released. It is much more striking to see a large accumulation of bubbles in the inferior segment of the internal jugular vein moving back and forth with respiration. This curious phenomenon may occur in 20 per cent of the radical neck dissections. It is believed to be associated more with the nitrous oxide mixture than with the accumulation of air from the tiny feeding venules that are open in the wound. Some of these bubbles must enter the right heart, but they have never caused a serious complication. The situation is resolved by the ligation of the inferior portion of the jugular vein in the classic neck dissection. In other circumstances, it does not require specific treatment.

The phenomenon of air embolus has increased considerably in the extensions of operations on the cardiovascular and pulmonary systems, in craniotomies, in deep-sea diving and, occasionally, in air inflation in the external auditory canal. The use of hyperbaric treatment has proved to be extremely helpful in the management of some of these problems.

Longenecker (1965)[8] reported on a classic case of air embolus from an apparent rent in a tributary to the internal jugular vein during radical neck dissection. There was a loud crunchy sound over the precordium, carotid artery pulsations disappeared and the patient became cyanotic. The patient was immediatley placed on his left side, the operating table was tilted to a head-down position, 100 per cent oxygen was administered, external cardiac massage was begun and the patient was transfused. The condition improved within one minute and a half, and the patient had an uneventful convalescence. James (1961)[6] described the mechanism of air entering the venous system on the basis of relative negative venous pressure. The air travels to the right side of the heart and the pulmonary circulation. It is trapped in the right ventricle by an increase in the pulmonary arterial pressure. The beating of the right ventricle against this trapped air produces the loud churning sound over the precordium. If the condition is not corrected, right-sided heart failure and cardiovascular collapse ensue. Durant and Oppenheimer (1963)[3] stated that 50 milliliters of air injected intravenously into an 80 kilogram man lying on his back would prove fatal. They reduced the fatality in dogs by placing them on their left side. Shivpuri and coworkers (1959)[10] emphasized the loud churning noise over the precordium as a presymptomatic diagnostic sign of air embolus. Bailey (1956)[2] reported that the meticulous control of venous bleeding and venous aspiration by clamping would eliminate air embolus.

Ericsson and associates (1964)[4] reviewed 93 cases of air embolus that had been published in the world literature and stated that there was an overall fatality of 73 per cent. They advocated placing the patient on the left side in the head-down position and closed chest cardiac massage. Ahren and Thulin (1965)[1] reported a case of air embolus following inflation of the external auditory canal for the treatment of serous otitis. The air passed along defects in the roof of the bone of the middle ear, along the dura, toward the middle fossa. There was a rupture of a branch of the middle meningeal artery with a massive extradural hematoma, resulting in death. Fairman and his colleagues (1968)[5] reported on a fatal case of air embolus following inflation of the middle ear via the external auditory meatus. The air traveled, in their case, along the pericarotid connective tissue and entered the thin-walled venous sinuses in this area to the cavernous sinuses and then traveled via this venous drainage route to the right side of the heart. They proposed several alternate theories as to how the air traveled from the middle ear toward the brain. Kindwall (1973)[7] states that the only definitive treatment of cerebral air embolus is compression of the patient in a recompression or hyperbaric chamber at 6 atmospheres absolute as soon as possible after the occurrence of the embolus. He stated that the use of the cardiopulmonary bypass has increased the relative incidence of air embolus in the brain. Waite and Mazzone (1967)[13] reported on basic studies on cerebral air embolus in respect to physiological changes, hyperbaric effects and decompression in respect to submarine activity. Takita and associates (1968)[11], Van Genderen and Waite (1968)[12] and Winter and Alvis (1971)[14] have supported the principle of hyperbaric treatment in the management of cerebral air embolus.

## CHYLOUS FISTULA

Chylous fistula in the neck complicates 1 to 2 per cent of the radical neck dissections. Although it occurs predominantly in the left side of the neck in association with the thoracic duct, approximately 25 per cent appear on the right side. Variations on the anatomy of the thoracic duct, including multiple channels and feeders, certainly increase the possibility of chylous leak.

All fresh radical neck wounds contain small quantities of lymph and, in some instances, of chyle. This is due to the cutting of afferent and efferent lymph vessels and to the manipulation of the chyle ducts.[6, 7] At this stage, chyle is impossible to identify clinically, since it is mixed with blood and serum. After an interval of two to seven days, chyle can usually be identified by its milky appearance in the hemovac tubes. It may be differentiated from standard wound effusions by an analysis of the fat content, by the presence of fat droplets and by the separation of a fat layer. The specific gravity is higher and the protein content is lower.[3] As it accumulates in the wound, it causes redness of the flap and a bulge underneath the flap with marked induration of the tissue. This condition may be exaggerated by continuing the nasogastric feedings.

Chyle is composed of lymph and emulsified fat from the lymph system draining the intestinal tract. It contains from 2 to 4.5 per cent protein and 1 to 3 per cent fat. The main liquid component is triglyceride. From 2 to 4 liters of chyle are transported daily.[3]

The management of this complication falls into two categories, namely, the minimal leak, which is controlled by aspiration and pressure, and the extensive leak, which requires exploration and ligation. Leaks are reduced to a minimum by the identification and ligation in every radical neck dissection of the chyle duct, its auxiliary duct on the right side and their tributaries. They are ligated with #4-0 silk. This does not guarantee that a chylous complication will not occur because of the variations in chyle drainage. A chyle leak may be immediately recognized intraoperatively while working in the area of the thoracic duct. The leak should be effectively ligated immediately. During the progress of the surgical development, this area should be reinspected upon occasion to ascertain whether there is any puddling of chyle in the region of the thoracic duct. If there is, a search should be made for its source, and it should be ligated or transfixed with #4-0 silk. When the surgeon is suspicious, he should put the patient in Trendelenberg's position and have the anesthesiologist apply prolonged positive pressure as he searches for an occult leak.

If chylous leak is suspected postoperatively, the patient should be carried on intravenous feedings. This significantly decreases the volume of chyle produced in the intestinal tract. The aspirant should be sent to the laboratory for analysis for triglycerides and fat. A pressure dressing should be placed over the site of the leak, and the patient's electrolytes should be carefully monitored. The patient's physiology can adapt to losses of up to 1000 cc. for short periods of time, but chronic losses greater than that amount will disturb both the electrolyte and the protein balance. Approximately half of the patients will respond to this conservative treatment. If the patient has leaked over 500 cc. daily for five days and is showing no sign of responding to conservative treatment, the leak should be exposed and transfixed. The patient should be given a high fat nasogastric feeding. This causes a marked increase in the quantity of chyle and gives it a thick, creamy consistency. The lower part of the wound is opened under local anesthetic, and the patient is placed in Trendelenberg's position. The chyle previously in the wound may have created a coagulant that can be removed with a blunt instrument. The leak is usually discovered in the region of the thoracic duct as it comes up out of the thorax into the neck. It is ligated with #4-0 silk. A small Penrose drain is placed in the wound, and then a pressure dressing is applied. The patient is then placed on the conservative regime of no nasogastric tube feedings for two or three days.

In a review by Allen and Briggs in 1901,[1] they stated that Cheever had reported on chyle leak as early as 1875. They made a specific analysis of two of their cases and a résumé of 17 additional cases. In 1907, Stuart[8] reported on 40 cases culled from the world literature and stated that chylous fistula was associated with a 12.5 per cent mortality. More recent reports by Rufino and MacComb (1966)[7], Fitz-Hugh and Cowgill (1970)[4] and Crumley and Smith (1975)[3] have brought the subject up to date. Frazell and Harrold (1951)[5] and Cavallo and his coworkers (1975)[2] have reported on the rare condition of chylothorax associated with radical neck dissection.

Crumley and Smith (1976)[3] reviewed 12 cases of chylous fistula following radical neck dissection. They reported an incidence of 1 to 2 per cent. Twenty-five per cent of their cases occurred on the right side. In 75 per cent of their cases, a chylous leak was noted during the operation, was treated and subsequently developed a postoperative fistula.

There are three case reports of chylothorax complicating radical neck dissection: Frazell and Harrold (1951)[5], Fitz-Hugh and Cowgill (1970)[4] and Cavallo and associates (1975)[2]. The mechanism of how the chyle enters the thorax is a source of speculation. None of these patients had a pneumothorax. All had a considerable amount of drainage of chyle in the neck. Operative ligation of the chyle duct does not appear to be contributory. When this is associated with neck dissection, the reduction of tube feedings and control of the chylous leak in the neck is the first step. The chest is managed by thoracentesis or underwater tube drainage. The outlook is favorable.

## WOUND CLOSURE

The complications associated with the closure of a wound relate to the biologic situation of the wound and the suture material used to close it. Potential infection, hemorrhage and foreign body implantation are the predominant etiologic factors in complications. Metabolic deficiencies and postirradiation effects with atrophy and fibrosis also predispose to wound complications. All of the wounds that communicate with the oral and pharyngeal cavities are potentially infected. These three situations are controlled by optimal preparation of the patient, closure of the wound without stress, absolute hemostasis and the use of antibiotics.

Suture material in the wound is essential to wound management but adds the increment of stress and foreign body implantation. The assessment of the effects of suture material is gained by clinical trial and by the investigation of implantation of these materials in laboratory animals. There is obviously no single suture material that is ideal for all surgical situations. It is necessary, therefore, to combine the requirements for wound closure with the suture material that will accomplish this in the most efficient physical and biologic manner. Van Winkle, Jr., Salthouse, Hastings and Matlaga[1, 2, 3] have presented comprehensive reports on the biologic effects of suture absorption and have outlined the principles of suture selection. Studies on silk, nylon, polyester, polypropaline, polyglactin 910, polyglycolic acid and chromic surgical gut have been reported. The nonabsorbable synthetic suture material created the least reaction and had improved strength and great durability. The synthetic absorbable suture material caused less reaction, gave additional strength and remained effective in the wound for a longer interval of time than corresponding chromic catgut. The absorption of the synthetic fibers was a slow hydrolytic process in the presence of tissue fluids, whereas, with surgical catgut, absorption was mediated through cellular and tissue proteases.[2]

The surgeon today must understand all principles of wound closure and, indeed, the physiological characteristics of the wound he is dealing with before he makes a selection of materials. He may select from absorbable and nonabsorbable materials in a monofilament or multifilament fabrication. The organic absorbable materials are different varieties of catgut that are usually manufactured from sheep submucosa or beef serosa. The synthetic absorbable sutures, either single or braided, are polyglactin 910 and polyglycolic acid. Some of the nonabsorbable sutures are listed as silk, cotton, nylon, polypropaline, polyesters and steel. Although silk is classified as a nonabsorbable suture material, studies have indicated that it loses almost all of its tensile strength in a period of a year and frequently cannot be identified in the wound after two years.[3]

The closure of wounds in the area of the head and neck often requires the use of multiple types of suture material. Three-O chromic catgut has been found satisfactory for the uncomplicated mucosal closures. It has a variable period of absorption but usually persists for a minimum of two weeks. In high-risk wounds, where there is the danger of delayed separation and additional stress, Vicryl or Dexon offers prolonged security and is preferred. Major blood vessels in the soft tissues are ligated with #3-0 or #4-0 silk. Smaller blood vessels are ligated with chromic catgut or with absorbable synthetic material. Subcutaneous tissue, fascia and muscle are closed with absorbable material in most instances. In high-risk cases, slowly absorbable material or nonabsorbable material may be used. Subcutaneous tissues are closed with absorbable material, and the skin is closed with #4-0 to #6-0 nonabsorbable material. Stainless steel wire is rarely used in soft tissue closures but is routinely used to approximate bones. Nonabsorbable material placed in the submucosal layer is used for the repair of the trachea. The approximation of all tissue is accomplished by square knots of silk and cotton. These knots have a tendency to remain tied, whereas a synthetic nonabsorbable material has a tendency to slip and become untied. It is therefore important with monofilament material that each knot be set and meticulously tied and that three to five loops be used. These wound are then further stabilized with sterile strips externally.

## WOUND DRAINAGE

### *Penrose Drains*

Penrose drains are a reliable method of draining any type of wound. They permit accumulated blood and serum to move along the channel created by the drain to a dependent exit. These drains are placed in strategic positions in the wound to accommodate the movement of free blood and serum in compliance with gravity. They are identified externally with either a safety pin or a suture so that they cannot be lost inside the wound. If they should become lost inside the wound, they will predispose to infection with a chronic draining sinus. A search of this sinus with a hemostat permits the removal of the drain. The wound heals promptly.

The Penrose drain will not precipitate bleeding, creates a controlled open wound that is more susceptible to secondary infection and will not prevent a hematoma if the bleeding is excessive. The drains are removed after they have accomplished their purpose of permitting the serum and blood to drain off prior to the healing process. When the drainage has stopped, the drains are removed. A Penrose drain will not erode a major vessel and may remain in the wound from two days to two weeks. They require less attention than the hemovac system and, in this respect, may prove to be superior when constant supervision is not available. In most instances, however, they have been replaced by the hemovac system.

### *Hemovac System*

Hemovac drainage (suction drainage) has proved to be a significant advance in the control of healing wounds about the head and neck. It assists in the coaptation of the tissues of the wound, reduces the incidence of hematoma and lessens the possibility of internal and external contamination. These suction tubes are placed strategically in the wound in order to gain the greatest advantage for drainage. They are never placed directly over great vessels because of the danger of compression necrosis. They are positioned near a deficient mucosal repair in order to cause the immediate suctioning of any mucus that might pass through this opening into the suction tubes, thus permitting the remainder of the wound to heal in a normal fashion. Internal suction reduces the importance of an external pressure dressing, but it does not eliminate the necessity of a supportive dressing. These drains will not prevent a hematoma if there is excessive bleeding or if they are malpositioned in the wound or are nonfunctioning. It is a fallacy to believe that these tubes will function automatically. They require inspection by a resident doctor or trained nurse every hour in the immediate postoperative phase and then at least four times a day once the wound has stabilized. If there is any doubt about their functioning, they should be tested with aspiration or the injection of 1 cc. of air or sterile saline solution. The "bellows" provided with the hemovac system permits the patient to be mobile but is not as satisfactory as a connection to wall suction with the gauge set at 120 mm. Hg. The principal complication is failure to function, and this, in most instances, is due to a failure on the part of the supervising attendants.

Hemovac drainage provides important information. The amount and character of the drainage should be recorded each day. The amount may vary from as little as 30 cc. to 1000 cc. and above in a 24 hour period. A minimal amount of drainage indicates that either the wound is exceptionally dry or the hemovacs are not functioning properly. Under the latter circumstance, the existence of a hematoma is obvious. A maximal amount of drainage indicates excessive bleeding, which requires reopening of the wound to control the bleeding.

The character of the drainage is revealing. In the beginning, it is almost entirely sanguinous; later in the postoperative course, within two to seven days, it becomes serous. Mucus, pus and chyle are readily discernible in the tubes because of their color and thick consistency. The specific tubes draining this type of material should not be removed until the major part of the wound is healed. After the wound is well-healed, the tube associated with the abnormal drainage may be removed. Occasionally, one of the tubes will develop a hissing sound, indicating that it is exposed in the oral cavity owing to a breakdown in the mucosal repair. This tube is permitted to remain in position while the remainder of the wound continues healing in an almost normal fashion.

There is no specific deadline for the removal of hemovac tubes. In an uncomplicated dissection, they may be required for three to five days; in a composite resection, they may be needed for seven to 10 days. With heavily irradiated wounds, the hemovacs usually stay in position for an additional two or three days. The basic rule is that it is appropriate to remove the hemovac once it has accomplished its purpose and the wound has healed. If it is removed prematurely, an accumulation will occur in the wound, and this may cause disruption or secondary infection. The wound should then be aspirated or drained with a Penrose drain. If there is any doubt about hemovac removal, the tubes may be disconnected from the suction system and placed on gravitational drainage for a day.

## PNEUMOMEDIASTINUM AND PNEUMOTHORAX

The condition of pneumomediastinum and pneumothorax was first reported by Champneys in 1884.[6] He reported on 82 cases of pneumothorax associated with tracheostomy and documented a gross association with mediastinal emphysema in five cases. Pneumothorax was found to be one of the most serious complications in the developing technique of tracheostomy at that time. In 1918, Buford[5] recognized this complication in association with thyroidectomy. Subsequently, Keis (1934)[8] and Barrie (1940)[2] further documented the increase of pneumothorax and pneumomediastinum in association with the increased surgical activity on the thyroid gland. In 1950, Bowden and Schweizer,[4] and subsequently Aiken and Smith (1952)[1] and Schweizer and Howland (1956)[10] reported on this complication in association with radical neck dissection. The introduction of these three separate sequential types of surgical operations carried with them some of the etiologic factors for the production of pneumomediastinum and pneumothorax. Operations in the region of the trachea, the upper mediastinum and airway system and the root of the neck are a factor.[9] These techniques may or may not be associated with struggling, straining, gasping, coughing and stressful anesthetic experiences for the patient.

The causes of pneumomediastinum and pneumothorax may be direct or remote.[10] Operations in the root of the neck open the deep cervical fascia.[11] Alteration in the ventilatory exchange by obstruction, secretions or lightness with bucking on the tube may create a sucking wound in the root of the neck. The imbalance in air pressure sucks the air through these potential fascial spaces into the superior mediastinum. It is important to establish a free exchange of air at this moment and, more importantly, to alert the anesthesiologist to optimally regulate the entire anesthesia system. Hopefully, this will resolve the problem. If the alarming sucking sound persists and a ball type valve situation is created by the soft tissues, the intramediastinal pressure is increased and there is a possibility that the air will rupture into the pleural space. Remedial action on the part of the anesthesiologist is the key to success.

Certainly, not all pneumomediastinum or pneumothorax situations are attributable to mechanical failure.[9] The rupture of an alveolar bleb permits air to escape into the mediastinum, with potential extension via perivascular and fascial spaces into the thoracic cavity, neck and soft tissues. Emphysema, atelectasis with hyperventilation and overinflation of the lung are predisposing factors. Smooth anesthesia induction will contribute greatly to the reduction of these possibilities. Rarely, a direct injury to the apex of the pleura during a radical neck dissection can occur if dissection is carried too deeply into the root of the neck.[14] By far, the highest incidence of pneumothorax occurs following tracheostomy in children and neonates. Reported incidence has varied between 13 and 17 per cent.[14] Mediastinal emphysema has been demonstrated in 15 to 43 per cent of children and infants following tracheostomy.[14] Routine postoperative x-ray is advised.

A small pleural leak intraoperatively can

often be treated by inflating the lungs to provide expansion and eliminate trapped air. If the wound can be closed to provide an airtight seal, a small residual pneumothorax of 10 to 15 per cent, in an otherwide healthy patient, should cause little compromise and resolves without sequelae. Careful postoperative x-ray follow-up is mandatory.

A large pleural leak with tension pneumothorax is a surgical emergency that requires immediate decompression. If this condition is not diagnosed and treated promptly, the patient may die. It is quickly apparent that there is respiratory and circulatory embarrassment. There is labored breathing, frequently of the asthmatic type, and a severe reduction in the movement of intrapulmonary air. Pressure on the anesthetic bag does not cause normal expansion of the thoracic cage. There are diminished breath sounds on the side of the atelectasis, a mediastinal shift, a crunching systolic noise and hyperresonance. Subcutaneous emphysema may be present. Emergency x-rays confirm the diagnosis. Under severe circumstances, immediate needle aspiration with a #14 to 16 needle into the upper anterior thorax will confirm the diagnosis and improve the condition of the patient. In the vast majority of instances this should not be considered definitive treatment.

The best overall treatment is thoracentesis and underwater drainage. A #14 to 16 soft rubber urethral catheter is immediately placed through the second anterior intercostal space and connected to underwater drainage.[11] This causes immediate improvement. When the bubbling has stopped and the subsequent x-ray indicates the lung is adequately expanded, the tube may be removed in two or three days. Although needle aspiration is very effective as an emergency measure, the definitive treatment should be supported with a catheter and underwater drainage. The vast majority of cases of emphysema in the mediastinum resolve spontaneously. In rare circumstances, pneumomediastinum may have to be treated by underwater drainage if there is any serious sign of respiratory or cardiac embarrassment. Tracheostomy is ordinarily not indicated for this condition. If, however, there is a need to improve airway passage or pulmonary toilet and to effect overall respiratory control, the technique should be carried out.

Pneumothorax and pneumomediastinum requiring definitive treatment as a complication in head and neck surgery today is very rare. In a series of 5000 head and neck cases seen by the author over the past 10 years, only two patients developed pneumothorax requiring definitive treatment. It has by no means diminished, however, as a general hospital emergency. Steier and his colleagues (1974) reviewed 544 patients with pneumothorax over a seven-year interval. Although the yearly incidence of traumatic and spontaneous pneumothorax has been quite constant, there was a precipitous increase in the incidence of iatrogenic pneumothorax in the past five years. Treatments, including external cardiac massage, percutaneous subclavian cannulation and continuous ventilatory support accounted for the vast majority of the iatrogenic increases. Patients with chronic obstructive lung disease were particularly susceptible. Steier and his coworkers emphasize that this is an acute surgical emergency that demands immediate decompression. The overall mortality was 16 per cent. In a group of 29 patients, there was a delay in decompression while awaiting confirmation by chest roentgenogram, and, in this group, there was a 31 per cent mortality. The mortality in the group receiving prompt treatment was 7 per cent. All of the patients in this series had subcutaneous emphysema. These data indicate the increase in the survival rate of those patients who were promptly diagnosed and treated and also emphasize new procedures that are increasing the incidence of pneumothorax in new categories. Neffson (1949) reported a 25 per cent mortality for unilateral pneumothorax and an 80 per cent mortality for bilateral pneumothorax. The diminution of this threatening and often catastrophic complication over the past 20 years is attributed to improvements in basic surgical techniques for the area at the root of the neck, to the smooth regulation of anesthetic techniques and to the prompt recognition and definitive management.

## RECURRENT CANCER

The most serious of all complications is recurrent cancer. There is no guaranteed prophylaxis for it. According to reports in the literature, recurrence rates range from 5 to 50 per cent at the primary site and from 20 to 40 per cent in the regional lymph bed in the lateral neck. These broad variations in recurrence rates can be attributed to the nature of the tumor, its aggressive behavior, the existence of undifferentiated tumors without a capsule, vein and nerve invasion, extension along fascial spaces and into muscles and soft tissues, and a high penetrability of lymph vessels.

The possibility of local recurrence may be readily apparent or veiled. There are five different warning signs to be considered:

### *Granulation Tissue*

Granulation tissue may appear in any open, healing wound and responds to local treatment. Any granulation tissue that does not improve within one or two weeks should be biopsied.

### *Persistent Edema*

Persistent edema is usually generalized. It frequently fluctuates from day to day or week to week. In the beginning, it is rather soft; then, it gradually fibroses and becomes firmer. It is the result of lymph and venous stasis. Recurrent cancer, which can contribute to persistent edema, must be ruled out. Postirradiation status always exaggerates the edema. When recurrent cancer is seriously suspected, tomography and deep biopsy are indicated.

### *Neuroma*

Neuromas have telltale signs and symptoms that usually separate them from recurrent cancer. They are located at the site of a nerve plexus, most commonly at the level of C-3 or C-2. Tying the stump of the sensory cervical roots with a silk ligature can lead to neuromas.

Neuromas may occur in other regions of the head and neck, such as in a cut nerve in the alveolar canal, in the region of the occiput and along the facial, trigeminal and hypoglossal nerves. When the neuroma is available for examination, as in the lateral neck, there is usually mild to moderate pain and a sensation of tingling when it is touched. It is rarely more than 2 cm. in diameter. It is not resected unless it is unusually painful or there is a high suspicion of recurrent cancer.

### *Lump*

The presence of a specific lump in an area of major ablation is strongly suggestive of recurrent cancer. This lump is usually asymptomatic. It expands gradually as the weeks go by. It may be situated in an organ system in the head and neck, such as the tongue, palate or parotid region, or it may develop in a lymph node. These lumps al-

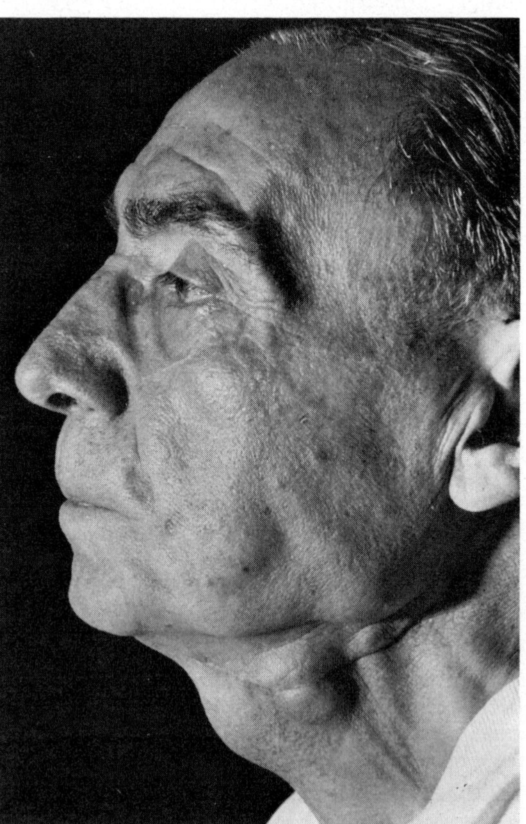

**Figure 3–3** Recurrent cancer following irradiation and radical neck dissection.

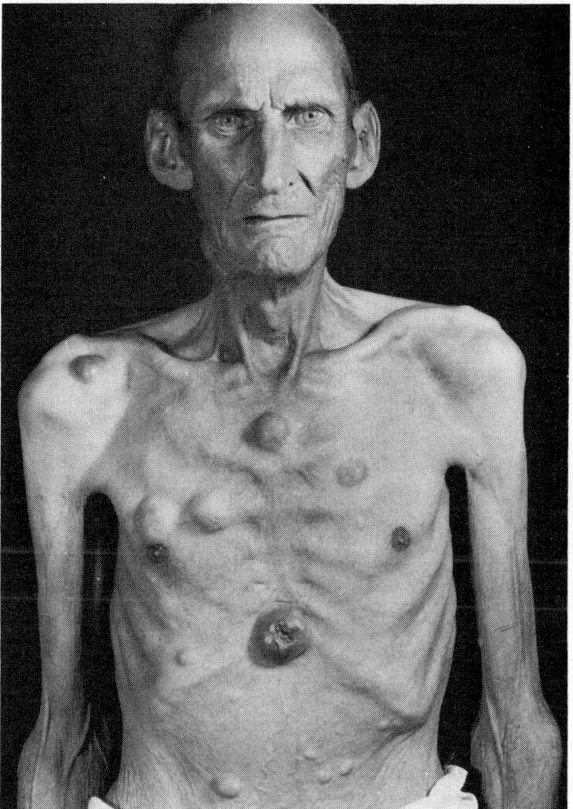

**Figure 3–4** Widespread hematogenous dermal metastasis from cancer of the tongue in the absence of deep jugular metastasis.

most always represent recurrent cancer and are to be biopsied without delay.

### *Ulceration*

Ulceration in a postoperative site may represent localized infection or stitch abscess. Most ulcerations in the head and neck respond to local treatment and heal within several weeks. If the ulcer persists, a biopsy is done.

The treatment of recurrent cancer in the head and neck is a serious challenge — with a poor prognosis. Ordinarily, the best opportunity to cure cancer is the first opportunity, and all efforts from that point yield diminished dividends. When the recurrence is well-entrenched, one cannot expect it to be more than 20 per cent curable, even with the most aggressive treatment.

If the recurrent cancer is accessible, then surgical excision and postoperative irradiation are indicated. If it is inaccessible, surgery is not done and the palliative tools of irradiation, electrodesiccation, cryosurgery and chemotherapy are applied. Efforts at palliation may be temporarily helpful, but uncontrolled cancer in the head and neck with ulceration of the skin, fistulization, local necrosis, interference with function, airway obstruction and hemorrhage are distressing problems for the patient, the patient's family and the surgeon to cope with.

## Bibliography

**Persistent Lymphedema of Face**

1. Baxter, T. J.: The histopathology of small vessels following microvascular repair. Br. J. Surg. *59*:617, 1972.
2. Clodius, L., and Wirth, W.: A new experimental model for chronic lymphedema of the extremities (with clinical considerations). Chir. Plastica (Berlin) *2*:115, 1974.
3. Cockett, A. T. K., and Goodwin, W. K.: Chyluria: attempted surgical treatment by lymphaticovenous anastomosis. Urology *88*:566, 1962.
4. Fisch, U.: Lymphography of the Cervical Lym-

phatic System. Philadelphia, W. B. Saunders Company, 1968.
5. Gilbert, A.: Lymphaticovenous anastomosis by microvascular technique. Br. J. Plast. Surg. (in press).
6. Handley, W. S.: Lymphangioplasty. Lancet *1*:783, 1908.
7. Laine, J. B., and Howard, J. M.: Experimental lymphaticovenous anastomosis. Surg. Forum *14*:111, 1963.
8. O'Brien, B. M., Sykes, P. J., Threlfall, G. N., and Browning, F. S. C.: Microlymphaticovenous anastomoses for obstructive lymphedema. Plast. Reconstr. Surg. *60*:197, 1977.
9. Thompson, N.: Surgical treatment of chronic lymphedema of the lower limb with preliminary report of new operation. Br. Med. J. *2*:1566, 1966.
10. Yamada, Y.: Studies on lymphatic venous anastomosis in lymphedema. Nagoya J. Med. Sci. *32*:1, 1969.

### Air Embolus

1. Ahren, C., and Thulin, C. A.: Lethal intracranial complications following inflation in the external auditory canal in treatment of serous otitis media and due to defects in the petrous bone. Acta Otolaryngol. (Stockh.) *60*:407, 1965.
2. Bailey, H.: Air embolism. J. Internat. Coll. Surgeons *25*:675, 1956.
3. Durant, T. M., and Oppenheimer, M. J.: Embolism caused by air and other gases. Heart Bull. *12*:66, 1963.
4. Ericsson, J. A., Gottlieb, J. D., and Sweet, R. B.: Closed-chest cardiac massage in the treatment of venous air embolism. N. Engl. J. Med. *270*:1353, 1964.
5. Fairman, H. D., Brown, N. J., and Hallpike, C. S.: Air embolism as a complication of inflation of the tympanum through the external auditory meatus. A clinicopathological study of a fatal case. Acta Otolaryngol. *66*:65, 1968.
6. James, T. N.: Air embolism. Am. Heart J. *61*:423, 1961.
7. Kindwall, E. P.: Massive surgical air embolism treated with brief recompression to six atmospheres followed by hyperbaric oxygen. Aerospace Med. *44*:663, 1973.
8. Longenecker, C. G.: Venous air embolism during operations on the head and neck. Report of a case. Plast. Reconstr. Surg. *36*:619, 1965.
9. Oppenheimer, M. J., Durant, T. M., and Lynch, P.: Body position in relation to venous air embolism and associated cardiovascular-respiratory changes. Am. J. Med. Sci. *225*:362, 1953.
10. Shivpuri, D. N., Viswanathan, R., and Sharma, M. L.: A presymptomatic diagnostic sign of venous air embolism. J. Indian Med. Assoc. *33*:86, 1959.
11. Takita, H. W., Olszewski, W., Schimert, G., and Lanphier, E. H.: Hyperbaric treatment of cerebral air embolism as a result of open heart surgery: report of a case. J. Thorac. Cardiovasc. Surg. *55*:682, 1968.
12. Van Genderen, L., and Waite, C. L.: Evaluation of the rapid recompression high pressure oxygenation approach to the treatment of traumatic cerebral embolism. Aerospace Med. *39*:709, 1968.
13. Waite, C. L., and Mazzone, W. F.: Cerebral air embolism. I. Basic studies. U.S. Naval Submarine Medical Center Research Report No. 493, April, 1967.
14. Winter, P. M., Alvis, H. J., and Gage, A. A.: Hyperbaric treatment of cerebral air embolism during cardiopulmonary bypass. J.A.M.A. *215*:1786, 1971.

### Chylous Fistula

1. Allen, D. P., and Griggs, C. E.: Wounds of the thoracic duct occurring in the neck: report of two cases. Resumé of 17 cases. Am. Med. 401–404, 1901.
2. Cavallo, C. A., Hirata, R. M., and Jaques, D. A.: Chylothorax complicating radical neck dissection. Am. Surg. *41*:266–268, 1975.
3. Crumley, R. L., and Smith, J. D.: Postoperative chylous fistula prevention and management. Laryngoscope *86*:804–813, 1976.
4. Fitz-Hugh, S. G., and Cowgill, R.: Chylous fistula. Arch. Otolaryngol. *91*:543, 1970.
5. Frazell, E. L., Harrold, C. C., and Rasmussen, L.: Bilateral chylothorax. Ann. Surg. *134*:5, 1951.
6. Royster, H. P.: Complications of surgery for cancer of the head and neck. *In* Artz, C. P., and Hardy, J. P. (eds.): Complications in Surgery and Their Management. Philadelphia, W. B. Saunders Company, 1967, pp. 290–306.
7. Rufino, C. D., and MacComb, W. S.: Bilateral neck dissections. Cancer *19*:1503, 1966.
8. Stuart, W. J.: Operative injury of thoracic duct in the neck. Edinb. Med. J. *22*:301, 1907.

### Wound Closure

1. Salthouse, T. N., and Matlaga, B. F.: Polyglactin 910 suture absorption and the role of cellular enzymes. Surg. Gynecol. Obstet. *142*:544, 1976.
2. Van Winkle, W., Jr., and Salthouse, T. N.: Biological response to sutures and principles of suture selection. Ethicon Research Foundation, pp. 1–20, 1976.
3. Van Winkle, W., Jr., and Hastings, J. C.: Consideration in the choice of suture materials for various tissues. Surg. Gynecol. Obstet. *135*:113, 1972.

### Pneumomediastinum and Pneumothorax

1. Aiken, D., and Smith, H. F.: Pneumomediastinum and pneumothorax following block dissection of the neck. Br. J. Surg. *40*:325, 1953.
2. Barrie, H. J.: Interstitial emphysema and pneumothorax after operation on the neck. Lancet *1*:996, 1940.
3. Beahrs, O. H.: Complications of surgery of the head and neck. Surg. Clin. North Am. *57*:823, 1977.

4. Bowden, L., and Schweizer, O.: Pneumothorax and mediastinal emphysema complicating neck surgery. Surg. Gynecol. Obstet. *91*:81, 1950.
5. Buford, C. G.: The entrance of air into the mediastinum during operations on the base of the neck. Surg. Gynecol. Obstet. *26*:540, 1918.
6. Champneys, F. H.: Addendum to third communication on artificial respiration in stillborn children — Mediastinal emphysema and pneumothorax in connection with tracheostomy: An experimental inquiry. Med. Chir. Tr. London *67*:101, 1884.
7. Forbes, G. B., Salmon, G. W., and Herwig, J. C.: Further observations on post-tracheotomy mediastinal emphysema and pneumothorax. J. Pediatr. *31*:172, 1947.
8. Keis, J.: Studies on the cause of mediastinal emphysema and pneumothorax in goiter operations. Munch. Med. Wochenschr. *81*:669, 1934.
9. Madan, S. C., Rosenthal, S. P., and Bochetto, J. F.: Pneumomediastinum and pneumothorax following lower neck surgery. Arch. Surg. *98*:153, 1969.
10. Schweizer, O., and Howland, W.: Diagnosis and treatment of tension pneumothorax complicating radical surgery about the lower neck and thorax. Anesth. Analg. *35*:375, 1956.
11. Marchetta, F. C., and Sake, K.: Pneumothorax—frequency following radical neck surgery. Paper delivered at meeting of Society of Head and Neck Surgeons, Washington, D.C., March 30, 1959.
12. Montgomery, W. W.: Surgery of the Upper Respiratory System. Vol. 2, Philadelphia, Lea & Febiger, 1973, p. 108.
13. Neffson, A. H.: Acute Laryngotracheobronchitis. New York, Grune and Stratton, 1949.
14. Salmon, L. F. W.: Tracheostomy. Proc. R. Soc. Med. *68*:11, 1975.
15. Steier, M., Ching, N., Roberts, E. B., and Nealon, T. F.: Pneumothorax complicating continuous ventilatory support. J. Thorac. Cardiovasc. Surg. *67*:17, 1974.

# MANAGEMENT OF THE MEDICAL COMPLICATIONS OF HEAD AND NECK SURGERY

4

*John W. Angers*
*Anne H. Angers*

*We are grateful to Nancy S. Reid for her help in carrying out this chapter*

## INTRODUCTION

Medical treatment of complications following head and neck surgery is a poor substitute for prevention, and prevention begins with observation. It has been said that "Careful observation is the basis for the art of medicine." One program for carrying this out most effectively is that used at St. Vincent's Hospital and Medical Center in New York City, where all head and neck patients are admitted to one floor. This procedure facilitates the observation of the patients by the nurses and other medical personnel. Their knowledge and reporting of the early signs and symptoms of complications have often prevented major medical emergencies. The nursing personnel report to the head nurse, or her assistant, any problems or such observations as a patient's nervousness, shakiness or cold extremities or any changes in the vital signs.

The following is an example of a very helpful and observant statement: "Mr. Jones is not doing well. He has tachycardia and is cold and sweating preoperatively although he was jovial the night before." Questioning of the patient might lead to the discovery of a severe alcohol withdrawal syndrome of 24 to 48 hour duration.

A preoperative medical consultation should be ordered even if there are only minor indications, since these early observations lead to rapid management of complications postoperatively. In addition to a medical consultation, the patient should undergo a physical examination, appropriate laboratory work-up (SMA-19), chest x-ray as well as specialized x-rays when needed, electrocardiogram and pulmonary function tests, when indicated. Of course, a detailed medical history should always be obtained at the time of the patient's admission to the hospital.

It is a paradox that while medicine and surgery are taking gigantic steps forward in areas such as organ transplantation and radical head and neck surgery, with massive reconstruction of the head, neck and face being performed, there is an increased morbidity and mortality in the postoperative period. With major surgery come equally major medical problems. In light of the increase in surgery-related problems, the preoperative work-up becomes invaluable.

The following are examples of postoperative medical problems that demonstrate the importance of prevention:

Pulmonary embolism can be averted by using simple preoperative measures, such as assessing the lower extremities and using an elastic stocking when indicated. There are approximately 142,000 deaths due to pulmonary embolism in American hospitals each year.[5] Unrecognized and untreated pulmonary emboli are fatal in 25 per cent of the cases. Early diagnosis and immediate effective therapy can reduce the death rate to 10 per cent.[13]

Postoperative arrhythmias can often be prevented before surgery by inserting a temporary demand pacemaker the morning of the operation.

The electrocardiogram is a must preoperatively for patients of all ages. In young people, for example, it can be used in the diagnosis of Wolff-Parkinson-White syndrome, which predisposes the patient to tachycardia during or after surgery. A preoperative electrocardiogram will warn and prepare the doctor.

## CARDIOVASCULAR STATUS

If the patient has cancer that will kill unless removed, the seriousness of any underlying cardiovascular disease is relative, and surgery should be viewed from this position. The patient's cardiovascular situation must be assessed from a functional point of view for proper management. The modified version of the New York Heart Association's classification of assessment is as follows:[1]

| *Cardiac Functional Status* | *Prognosis* |
|---|---|
| Uncompromised | Good |
| Slightly compromised | Good with therapy |
| Moderately compromised | Fair with therapy |
| Severely compromised | Guarded despite therapy |

Preoperative clinical assessment for patients with cardiovascular problems includes a complete history with a physical examination. The breathing pattern, pulse rate and rhythm and strength are noted. The jugular venous pressure is noted, since it is an excellent indicator of the overall cardiac status except in cases of acute left ventricular failure, when it may be normal. Ventricular enlargement and apical impulse are noted. A chest x-ray and an electrocardiogram are required. A vector cardiogram and an echocardiogram are done when indicated.

The basic principles of improving cardiac function consist of correcting overweight and edema. The patient is advised to stop smoking two weeks preoperatively and to take adequate rest and exercise.

### Heart Failure

Heart failure is usually manifested by low oxygen delivery to the tissues. A mild failure may only show up under stress of surgery or postoperatively. All heart failure should be corrected preoperatively, when at all possible, even at the expense of delaying surgery.

#### *High Output Heart Failure*

High output heart failure with a low arterial to venous oxygen differential lowers the oxygen supply to the tissues, thus putting a greater demand on the heart. In thyrotoxicosis and chronic alcoholism, the myocardial metabolism is impaired, and thus it mimics the high output heart failure state. This type of heart failure often goes unrecognized until a stress period. It is seen in anemia, hyperthyroidism, atrioventricular fistula, beriberi, Paget's disease, alcohol-induced heart disease and pulmonary emphysema. Most cases are successfully managed by correcting the underlying disease.

#### *Low Output Heart Failure*

Chronic low output heart failure is seen more often as congestive heart failure, with fluid and salt retention and overload. Dependent edema, hepatomegaly, protodiastolic and presystolic gallop and pulsus alternans are manifested. A more advanced stage would also manifest basilar rales with expiratory wheezes.[11] This advanced failure must be corrected preoperatively.

The management of low output heart failure consists of digoxin by mouth or intravenously but never intramuscularly. Diuresis is obtained with furosemide or ethacrynic acid. Potassium replacement is a necessity. Sodium restriction is also employed in advanced cases. Oxygen is given, using 40 per cent Puritan face mask. Strict attention should be given to fluid intake and output.

Cardiac cachexia is often mistaken for cancerous cachexia but is not as ominous. It may be corrected by managing the heart failure.[15]

### *Resistant Heart Failure*

Thyrotoxicosis, beriberi, chronic alcoholism and pulmonary embolism immediately suggest themselves here. In this type of heart failure, the underlying cause must be corrected before surgery.

Hypothyroidism must be searched for carefully, since it predisposes patients who have had head and neck surgery previously to cardiac arrest during surgery. Care should always be taken with a patient who has partial or total thyroid removal, and the hypothyroid state must be corrected preoperatively.

## Ischemic Heart Disease

### *Angina Pectoris*

When a patient has angina pectoris, the head and neck surgery is not absolutely contraindicated if the angina is manageable. Nitroglycerine is left at bedside in order to maintain the patient's confidence. Angina patients are treated with propranolol unless there is an element of congestive heart failure, asthma or insulin-dependent diabetes mellitus. If there is an accompanying mild or moderate congestive heart failure, the patient is digitalized and then given propranolol. Propranolol is discontinued 24 to 48 hours before surgery. If the patient is on large doses of propranolol (over 120 mg. per day), it must be tapered off slowly over a span of two to four days. Arrhythmias are corrected or brought under control preoperatively. Five milligrams of diazepam (Valium) four times a day with an analgesic are helpful for the patient with chronic heart disease.

### *Myocardial Infarction*

Myocardial infarction has a high operative mortality, depending on the time between the heart attack and the surgery. Infarction within three months of surgery has a 40 per cent mortality, according to one group.[1] Surgery between three and six months after myocardial infarction has a 15 per cent mortality. If more than six months have elapsed, the mortality is approximately 6 per cent.[15] Surgery in patients with remote infarction — more than one year from the time of surgery — is tolerated well.[25]

All patients with a history of myocardial infarction should have complete enzyme studies done, not only preoperatively but also for four days postoperatively. The highest incidence of myocardial infarction occurs on the third postoperative day. The creatinine phosphokinase (CPK) and its isoenzymes (MB-type) are helpful in monitoring the postoperative patient, since the MB-type is elevated during myocardial injury. Additional monitoring of blood pressure, heart rate, serial electrocardiograms, central venous pressure and urine output is necessary. If any cardiac embarassments occur, these patients are taken to the surgical intensive care unit, and the following additional monitoring is done: arterial blood gases, intra-arterial blood pressure, pulmonary artery pressure and pulmonary arterial wedge pressure. The last two are measured by means of a Swan-Ganz catheter. Oxygen 40 per cent with a Puritan face mask is used postoperatively with high humidity on all patients with a history of myocardial infarction[1] to prevent arrhythmias and mucus plugging.

## Cardiac Arrhythmias

Cardiac arrhythmias are serious, life-threatening episodes that occur during the operative and postoperative periods, especially in patients with a history of cardiac disease. The etiological factors that play a role in arrhythmias are hypomagnesemia, hypokalemia, hyperkalemia, digitalis excess, alkalosis, acidosis, hypotension, hyperemia and ventricular overload secondary to overzealous fluid therapy.[15] Occasionally, cardiomyopathy of ethanol origin or septicemia might be the cause. Below are listed the types of important arrhythmias and their methods of management.

#### SINUS TACHYCARDIA

A heart rate of 100 to 190 is seen in the postsurgical period. It may be secondary to fever, hypovolemia, pain or anxiety. This arrhythmia usually terminates when causative factors are removed. If it is secondary to congestive heart failure, the patient is digitalized immediately. In an emergency, propranolol may be given slowly intravenously. If it is associated with acute myocardial infarction, pulmonary embolism, pneumonia, hyperthyroidism or anemia, treat the underlying disease. Administer oxygen. Propranolol may be used in emergency situations and is given in doses of 10 to 80 mg. every 6 hours by mouth or it is slowly given intravenously as 1 mg. in 10 ml. saline, repeated if necessary.

#### PAROXYSMAL ATRIAL TACHYCARDIA

P.A.T. is usually due to premature atrial beats with a re-entry phenomenon. It has an abrupt onset, with a heart rate of 140 to 240 beats per minute. Treatment consists of carotid sinus massage for 10 to 20 seconds on one side at the time. This will terminate half of the attacks in a sedated and digitalized patient, if they are not due to digitalis excess. The first drug to use is edrophonium chloride (Tensilon) 5 to 10 mg. intravenously, which enhances the AV conduction delay. Carotid massage should be tried again. The next step is rapid digitalization intravenously. Finally, and most effective, if no heart failure is present, propranolol is slowly given 1 mg. in 10 ml. saline intravenously and may be repeated, or it may be given by mouth in a dose of 10 to 80 mg. every 6 hours. Procainamide and quinidine are tried.

When P.A.T. is seen with heart block, it is due to digitalis toxicity in two thirds of the cases. The digitalis should be discontinued and hypokalemia, if present, should be corrected. Propranolol intravenously 1 mg. in 10 ml. of saline is given over 3 to 5 minutes. This may be repeated twice, first checking the blood pressure.

Nonparoxysmal junctional tachycardia has a gradual onset with a rate of 50 to 100 per minute with irregular P–R interval if seen with digitalis toxicity. Then, digoxin is discontinued and diphenylhydantoin (Dilantin) is given along with potassium chloride.

#### ATRIAL FIBRILLATION

This is seen in ischemic heart disease or in patients with chronic lung disease. Digitalization and adequate oxygenation are often sufficient to control the ventricular rate. Occasionally, cardioversion is necessary. If rapid and immediate control of the ventricular rate is necessary, propranolol is given at the rate of 1 mg. every 3 to 5 minutes up to 15 mg.

#### ATRIAL FLUTTER

The ventricular rate varies with the degree of atrioventricular (AV) heart block. Digitalization followed by administration of quinidine or procainamide is the therapy of choice. Propranolol is also effective after digitalization.

#### AV NODAL (JUNCTIONAL) RHYTHM

The heart rate is 40 to 60 per minute. Always consider the possibility of digitalis toxicity or the sick sinus syndrome.

### *Bradycardias*

Bradycardias are those having an atrial or ventricular rate of less than 60 beats per minute.

#### SINUS BRADYCARDIA

This is seen postoperatively owing to high vagal activity and sedation or anesthesia plus surgery. Certain vagal stimulation drugs will also bring this about. This bradycardia responds well to atropine 0.4 mg. to 1 mg. intravenously. Occasionally, it is due to the sick sinus syndrome.

#### HIGH-GRADE AV BLOCK

This occurs when few of the regular atrial impulses are not conducted owing to a state of refractoriness in the conduction system, atrium, AV node or bundle of His. If symptomatic, a temporary pacemaker may be necessary.

#### MULTIFOCAL ATRIAL TACHYCARDIA

This is not uncommonly seen in elderly postoperative patients. Atrial rate is 100 to 250 per minute. It responds to better oxygenation plus administration of quinidine or propranolol.

#### VENTRICULAR PREMATURE BEATS

This is the most frequently seen arrhythmia. It usually has the least hemodynamic changes. Establishing proper oxygenation and ventilation is often sufficient to correct it. Shifts of potassium postoperatively are among the most common causes of ventricular irritability after hypoxia. This responds well to 75 mg. lidocaine intravenously. Other therapy is usually instituted if an organic heart disease exists, there are more than 6 beats per minute, the ventricular premature systole interrupts the T waves or a combination of these. If congestive heart failure exists, administer digitalis first and then add an antiarrhythmic, such as quinidine, procainamide hydrochloride (Pronestyl), diphenylhydantoin (Dilantin) or propranolol hydrochloride (Inderal).

#### SICK SINUS SYNDROME

This syndrome presents itself as a bradycardia with or without episodic tachycardia after a stressful period. The heart rate is 25 to 55 beats per minute. It rarely responds to drugs. If symptomatic, a transvenous demand pacemaker is inserted preoperatively. If the idioventricular rhythm rate is 40 beats per minute or less, or if the EKG shows no visible P wave with a wide QRS complex, a pacemaker insertion is mandatory.

### *Heart Block*

#### FIRST DEGREE HEART BLOCK

This means a prolonged P–R interval in excess of 0.2 second on the EKG. It is of no significance *per se*.

#### SECOND DEGREE HEART BLOCK

Type I (Wenckebach period) has an increasing P–R interval with a missed QRS complex, and thus a dropped beat. This type may respond to atropine. Otherwise, it is handled like a Type II (Mobitz) block. Type II has a fixed P–R interval with a dropped QRS complex. Preoperatively, a temporary transvenous demand pacemaker is inserted to prevent arrhythmia. If this is functional in the second week postoperatively, a permanent pacemaker should then be inserted.

#### THIRD DEGREE (COMPLETE) HEART BLOCK

This means a failure to conduct any impulse from atrium to ventricle. A transvenous demand pacemaker is necessary preoperatively, and a permanent pacemaker must be installed postoperatively.

#### HEMIBLOCK

Hemiblocks or bifascicular blocks, as reported on the EKG, are often indicators of relatively severe disease in the conduction system of the heart and more often than not require a transvenous demand pacemaker. The morning of and after surgery, the pacemaker is often found to be functional, thus averting a catastrophe. Temporary or permanent transvenous pacemakers are of demand-type and are only functional when they are necessary.

### *Temporary Cardiac Pacemaker Insertion*[15]

Transvenous demand pacemakers are inserted for the following conditions:

1. Severe bradycardia
2. Adams-Stokes syndrome
3. Sick sinus syndrome with bradycardia
4. Atrial fibrillation with a very slow ventricular response
5. Symptomatic heart block
6. Arrhythmias arising in a patient with recent myocardial infarction
7. Suppression of refractory recurrent ventricular tachycardia

### *Effects of Drugs and Anesthetics on the Cardiovascular System*

Most anesthetic agents have a depressant effect on the heart, brought about by direct depression of myocardial contractility. This results in a decreased cardiac output that may produce hypotension, thus causing a further decrease in coronary perfusion. The end result is myocardial ischemia. Hence, this vicious cycle leads to circulatory failure. Cyclopropane, ethyl ether and halogenated agents excite the sympathetic nervous system and the cardiac contractility and irritability, so that arrhythmias are more likely to occur when these agents are used. The prolonged intraoperative periods of myocardial depression, ischemia and irritability often result in myocardial infarction, arrhythmias or left ventricular failure.[15] This results in a very stormy postoperative course with higher morbidity and mortality. Reserpine and propranolol have a depressant effect on the myocardium. Reserpine depletes the myocardial catecholamine stores. It may take up to two weeks to restore the catechols to normal. *Propranolol* — a $\beta$-adrenergic blocking agent — exerts its effect by decreasing cardiac contractility and by reducing the heart rate. If emergency surgery is contemplated, isoproteronol is the drug of choice if the heart rate or myocardial contractility is depressed secondary to propranolol. The positive inotropic effect of ionic calcium is effective in improving cardiac contractility in the presence of propranolol. Calcium is given as a bolus, 100 to 200 mg. calcium chloride intravenously, or it is administered as an intravenous drip of 1 gm. calcium chloride in 250 ml. fluid.[15]

### *Management of Cardiogenic Shock*

Cardiogenic shock may be divided into (1) coronary shock with acute myocardial infarction and pump failure due to loss of more than 40 per cent of myocardial muscles or (2) noncoronary shock due to postoperative arrhythmias, cardiomyopathies, pulmonary emboli or cardiac tamponade.

Both shock states are recognized by a systolic pressure of less than 90 mm. Hg in a normotensive individual or by a decrease in the blood pressure amounting to 80 mm. Hg less than the usual systolic pressure in a hypertensive individual. Most important to watch for is an oliguric state with a urine output of less than 30 ml. per hour.

It is necessary to continously monitor the EKG, the CVP and the pulmonary artery end diastolic pressure and pulmonary wedge pressure (left ventricular filling pressure) by means of a Swan-Ganz catheter. Intravascular catheters are also inserted to measure systemic arterial pressure. Most of all, the urine output must be monitored. Arterial blood gases and electrolytes should be monitored frequently. Change in the central venous pressure (CVP) is a valuable guide to fluid replacement.

A good and reliable airway is established. Any patient in shock — except hypovolemic shock — must be intubated and placed on a volume cycle respirator. The $F_{IO_2}$ is increased as needed, usually starting at 40 per cent oxygen in the inspired flow rate.

Analgesia is obtained by using morphine — 5 mg. intravenously — over 1 to 2 minutes, with a second dose of 5 mg. after 10 minutes have elapsed. If respiratory distress occurs, 2.5 to 5 mg. nalorphine are given intravenously. Meperidine hydrochloride, 25 mg. intravenously, is often used instead of morphine. Diazepam (Valium), 5 mg. intravenously, is also often used to correct agitation. If $PaO_2$ is lowered, 40 per cent oxygen by Puritan face mask is used. One hundred per cent oxygen at 5 to 7 liters by face mask is effective in more severe cases.

Acidosis, i.e., severe lactic acidemia, should be corrected, for this leads to arrhythmia, autolysis and intravascular coagulation. Intravenous sodium bicarbonate is given, adjusting the apparent deficit of the base by monitoring the pH. Minor changes in the pH are better left untreated, however.

Oliguria (low urine output) is treated as follows: (1) if the CVP is less than 10 mm. or the pulmonary wedge pressure (PWP) is less than 18, a challenge dose of 250 cc. of 5 per cent glucose and water is given with mannitol; (2) if the CVP is greater than 12 or the PWP is greater than 20, loop diuretics such as furosemide or ethacrynic acid are given. They are effective even with low renal perfusion and pulmonary edema.

Bradycardia is often due to vagotonia

and is corrected by giving atropine sulfate, 0.4 to 2.0 mg. intravenously by push. Dopamine, 200 mg. in 500 cc. of 5 per cent dextrose in water (D/W), is administered at the rate of 1 to 5 $\mu$g. or more per kg. per minute to restore pressure and cardiac output.[12] Isoproterenol by intravenous infusion — 1 to 2 mg. per 500 ml. of fluid — is often effective in accelerating the rate of a sinus, a junctional or an infranodal pacemaker. Transvenous pacemakers are occasionally effective in restoring cardiac output.

In summary, the management of cardiogenic shock is as follows: (1) the cause of shock must be established, (2) pain and anxiety must be relieved, (3) hypovolemia must be corrected, (4) the physiological heart rate must be re-established, (5) the patient is digitalized, more often than not, and (6) the acidosis is corrected.

## THE RESPIRATORY SYSTEM

For most of the patients undergoing head and neck surgery, a great deal of attention is paid to the basic lesson of humidification, so elegantly worked out by Walker in 1961.[27, 28] A high humidity–heated Puritan face mask, its many connections allowing for the appropriate oxygen:air ratio, is readied preoperatively by every bed on the head and neck floor. Thus, the postoperative program to maintain the integrity of the cardiopulmonary system is begun preoperatively.

### Preoperative Evaluation

The preoperative evaluation is aimed at the discovery of pulmonary abnormalities, especially those of borderline cases that have gone undetected previously. Careful observation and a thorough history, focusing on the respiratory system when indicated, should uncover subtle problems that the patient either denies or is unaware of. For instance, smokers often minimize their history of coughing and are untruthful about the number of cigarettes they smoke. Since tobacco inhibits ciliary action, all patients are urged to discontinue smoking two weeks prior to surgery. Nicotine increases the heart rate, blood pressure and cardiac output. Carboxyhemoglobin concentration in smokers varies from 5 to 10 per cent and thus interferes with oxygen transport.[25] Smoking also leads to an abnormal ventilation perfusion ratio.

Hoarseness usually implies carcinoma of the larynx, but it also may mean bronchogenic carcinoma involving the left recurrent laryngeal nerve. Hemoptysis may be confused with bleeding from higher up in the respiratory tract.

Dyspnea with fatigue at rest usually is a sign of an obstructive lung disease, such as emphysema or chronic bronchitis. If dyspnea is seen in restrictive lung disease, it is in a very advanced state.[5] On examination, one should be aware that patients with restrictive lung disease usually have a rapid, shallow respiration with fine rales; the patient with obstructive lung disease has prolonged expiration of three to five seconds.

Pulmonary function tests are usually done preoperatively. Those tests that should at least be performed are as follows: a vital capacity (VC), one second forced expiratory volume ($FEV_1$) and arterial blood gases.[3]

Alveolar hypoventilation is most commonly seen postoperatively owing to anesthetics, sedatives or analgesics that depress the respiratory center. The *sine qua non* of alveolar hypoventilation is an elevated $PaCo_2$ with a decreased $PaO_2$, unless the patient is on high $FiO_2$ (fraction inspired oxygen concentration).

Clinical ventilation-perfusion abnormalities are as follows: (1) a low ventilation-perfusion ratio is seen in diffuse interstitial fibrosis, obstructive lung disease and pneumonia, in which arterial blood gases show a decreased $PaO_2$ and an elevated $PaCo_2$; (2) a high ventilation-perfusion ratio has a higher $PaO_2$ and a lower $PaCO_2$.

Right-to-left shunt is due to ventilation-perfusion imbalance. The imbalance is established by the demonstration of little change in the $PaO_2$ while the patient is receiving 100 per cent oxygen. This is seen in bronchial plugging, pneumonia, respiratory distress syndrome and shock lung.[3]

Diffusion block is seen in pulmonary fibrosis.[5] In head and neck cancer, this is now seen more often due to the greater use of bleomycin, which causes pulmonary fibrosis. The pneumonitis due to bleomycin responds to steroid therapy, hence steroids may be tried in the preoperative period to assess the reversibility of the lung changes. Actually, diffusion block responds well to oxygen therapy.

## Respiratory Problems Seen in Patients with Head and Neck Disease

In the head and neck patients, the upper airway is often bypassed with an endotracheal or tracheostomy tube. All inspired gases should, therefore, be delivered to the patient fully saturated with water vapor at body temperature.[2] Thus, a heated Puritan face mask is used on all postoperative patients to maintain the integrity of the ciliated mucosa in the tracheobronchial tree. Up to 500 cc. of water can be absorbed in this way and must be taken into account when calculating fluid intake. Reduced ciliary activity is seen with dry air; this slows the transport of mucus and allows it to become viscous, thus slowing the transport even more. This is followed by accumulation of inspissated secretions, leading to airway obstruction — an added insult to an already compromised airway.

### *Restrictive Lung Disease*

In restrictive lung disease, there is a diminished vital capacity and functional residual capacity. The $PaO_2$ may be normal or diminished. In severe cases, the $PaCO_2$ may be normal or elevated. The extrathoracic causes include restrictive dressings around the chest, crushed chest, kyphoscoliosis and others. The intrathoracic causes include pleural effusion, healed lung disease, diffuse pulmonary fibrosis and adult respiratory distress syndrome.

In restrictive lung disease postoperatively, the patient develops hypoventilation, ineffectual cough resulting in retained secretions and atelectasis and lung infections. Endotracheal intubation or tracheostomy allows the prevention of many of these problems. A chest physiotherapist is called upon to increase postural drainage and to help prevent further atelectasis. Hydration is essential. Rest, sitting in a chair at bedside and early ambulation are also prescribed. Oxygen therapy is given after arterial blood gases are assayed. Antibiotics are given, depending upon the culture and sensitivity. An incentive spirometer is also used to encourage deep breathing.

### *Obstructive Lung Disease*

Obstructive lung disease is usually manifested as a normal vital capacity except when very severe obstructive phenomena exist. The $FEV_1$ is reduced, as is the $FEV_3$. The arterial blood gases show decreased $PaCO_2$ with a low pH in the acute phase. The acute phase includes asthma, bronchitis, emphysema and bronchitis with bronchospasms. Obstructive lung disease needs more support postoperatively. Humidified warm air plus endotracheal tube or tracheostomy helps in removal of bronchial secretions. Antibiotics are often given, depending upon culture and sensitivity.

Patients with advanced obstructive lung disease preoperatively, are given intermittent positive pressure with a bronchodilator when indicated, i.e., if the response to the bronchodilator is positive on trial. Asthmatic or chronic bronchitis with bronchospasm responds well to bronchodilators. Isoproterenol, ½ cc. of 1/200 solution in 2 cc. saline, is added to a nebulizer. Occasionally, when secretions are tenacious, isoetharine (Bronkosol) is used. Chronic asthmatics are often administered cromolyn sodium for a long time preoperatively, for this inhibits the release of mediators of type I immediate hypersensitivity from mast cells.[23] A chest physiotherapist should be consulted preoperatively. On the morning of surgery, postural drainage is also given. Steroid therapy is reserved for the severe, allergic, bronchial asthma or for the patient having severe bronchitis with bronchospasm.

## The Postoperative Period

Antibiotics are often given, usually ampicillin or erythromycin, when sensitivity to penicillin exists because they are bactericidal. Occasionally, other types are used, depending upon the sensitivity of the organism involved. Adequate hydration — 2000 to 3000 cc. of fluid per 24-hour period — and aminophylline are used in severe obstructive disease.

The patient should be encouraged to ambulate within 24 hours of surgery in most head and neck cases. Deep breathing is encouraged. Often, the mucus plugs are postoperatively loosened this way. Ten cc. of sterile saline are introduced into the bronchial tree when a tracheostostomy is present in order to promote coughing and loosen the secretions.

### *Cell-mediated Immunity*

Cell-mediated immunity and chemotaxis are often impaired in chronic obstructive lung disease. Anesthetic agents are also known to depress cell-mediated immunity. Macrophage phagocytosis accounts for 80 per cent of clearance of organisms from the respiratory tract, and thus it is very important to restore macrophage phagocytosis and chemotaxis. Thus far, only two drugs are known to restore these functions: levamisole hydrochloride, which is an antihelminthic agent available only in England, and thiabendazol (Mintezol), also an antihelminthic agent that is available in this country. Thiabendazol is known to be a safe, nontoxic stimulator of cell-mediated immunity. Both also restore chemotaxis of leukocytes and macrophages.

### *Laryngectomy*

Laryngectomy and other surgery on the head and neck surgical patient, who more often than not is a heavy smoker with severely compromised lung cilia functions, are best handled by high humidity with 20 to 40 per cent oxygen ($FIO_2$) with a Puritan face mask. A cuffed tracheal tube should be inserted, and the secretions suctioned by aspiration every 30 to 60 minutes by the nurses. Drying of secretions is prevented by high humidity. Five to 10 cc. saline are injected into the tracheal area, which promotes coughing of mucus plugs. Intermittent positive-pressure breathing (IPPB) is used with a cuffed tube quite effectively; it is advisable to suction around the tube before releasing the pressure. The patient is repositioned frequently to prevent complications.

### *Atelectasis*

Atelectasis is seen in the elderly and the obese. Incipient atelectasis is detected by the presence of moist rales, usually localized posteriorly. There may also be diminished breath sounds with bronchial breathing over a localized segment. This is followed by a sudden fever and a rapid pulse. Inspection reveals an inspiratory lag. This should not be a frequent occurrence if all preventive measures are taken.

A chest physiotherapist is called in for consultation preoperatively. In the nontracheostomized patient, nasotracheal suction can be performed by insertion of a sterile catheter. More than half of the time, the catheter will fall into the trachea and suction can be performed.[5]

Bronchoscopy is occasionally used to remove mucus plugs and wash the tracheobronchial tree. At present, IPPB is used more often in atelectasis. The active inflation of the lungs and effective nebulizing aerosols reduce the incidence of postoperative complications. This is possible because the peak instantaneous expiratory flow velocity is greater than the peak instantaneous inspiratory flow velocity.

## Acute Respiratory Insufficiency

The *sine qua non* of acute pulmonary insufficiency is a decrease in $PaO_2$ in arterial blood gases, although the $PaCO_2$ may be low, normal or elevated. A low $PaO_2$ and an elevated $PaCO_2$ are often seen in head and neck surgical patients. The presence of underlying chronic lung disease is the usual cause; an inadequate tracheal-bronchial toilet that allows for accumulation of secretions may also be a factor. In emphysema, the mechanism is mostly due to trapped air, in addition to carbon dioxide retention and decreased alveolar ventilation. The heavy sedation plus the anesthetic contribute to the patient's hypoventilation, which leads to a decrease in $PaO_2$ and an elevation of $PaCO_2$. It must be remembered that a $PaCO_2$ above 40 torr (mm. Hg) indicates underventilation and that below 40 torr it means overventilation, whether primary or compensatory.[25]

Acute respiratory insufficiency with a low $PaO_2$ and a low or normal $PaCO_2$ is seen most often with atelectasis, pulmonary edema, pneumonia and pulmonary emboli. This is also seen in respiratory distress syndrome, which shall be discussed later. Atelectasis, very frequently due to mucus plugging, has been discussed previously.

### *Pulmonary Embolism*[13]

Despite the recent advances in medicine, venous thrombosis and pulmonary embolism remain major problems in the postoperative period. Bed rest, with its accompanying venous stasis and immobilization, is certainly a predisposing factor of thrombophlebitis. Surgery itself causes an elevation in concentration of plasma procoagulants, an increased fibrinogen level, thrombocytosis, increased platelet activity and defective fibrinolysis.[5, 13]

At one time, pulmonary embolus often went unrecognized and undiagnosed, but it is now known to occur frequently in the postoperative period. Prophylaxis by identifying high-risk individuals with such predisposing factors as history of previous emboli, advanced age, bed rest and obesity is the only rational approach. The common sources of emboli are the veins in the lower limbs, from which 75 per cent arise. Others arise from the deep pelvic veins and the inferior vena cava.[22]

The best ways of preventing the thromboembolic phenomenon are early ambulation, active leg exercise and elastic stockings. Occasionally, in high-risk patients, a small dose of heparin is administered on the following schedule: 5000 units subcutaneously 2 hours before surgery and 5000 units subcutaneously every 12 hours until the patient is fully ambulatory. This schedule alters the coagulation tests only minimally, if at all, but a low dose of heparin is known to potentiate the naturally occurring plasma inhibitor of activated Factor X.[13, 22]

Two other approaches to preventing thrombophlebitis are worth mentioning. One is the administration of aspirin to prevent platelet adhesiveness, and the other is sulfinpyrazone (Anturane); both have antithrombotic properties.[5]

The best technique for detecting pulmonary emboli is a lung scan plus an evaluation of arterial blood gases. This should be done when the following symptoms are present: tachypnea and dyspnea, tachycardia, hemoptysis and pleuritic-type chest pain of sudden onset. The probability of massive pulmonary embolization is less than 2 per cent if the $PaO_2$ is greater than 90 mm. Hg.

The management of pulmonary emboli should be done in the following manner. An analgesic (either meperidine hydrochloride [Demerol] or morphine) should be given to relieve pain. Oxygen should be administered. Heparinize with an immediate dose of 10,000 units of heparin for the normal individual. This is followed by 5000 to 8000 units of heparin every 4 to 6 hours for 10 days.[13] Anticoagulants like sodium warfarin (Coumadin) can be given from the 4th or 5th day on. Remember that there is a disparity in the rate of suppression of vitamin K–dependent factors, that is, factors VII, IX, X and prothrombin, by sodium warfarin (Coumadin). Heparin is discontinued between the 7th and 10th days.

In conclusion, close observation and supervision in the preoperative period and early ambulation postoperatively have reduced the incidence of pulmonary embolization.

### *Adult Respiratory Distress Syndrome*

This syndrome encompasses a number of clinical conditions whose seriousness is unrecognized by many. During the war, it was called post-traumatic pulmonary insufficiency or "shock lung." Apparently, approximately one third to one half of the patients who die in the intensive care units throughout the country do so with such pulmonary derangement.[5] Actually, this syndrome does resemble progressive acute pulmonary insufficiency. The clinical course starts with shortness of breath, tachypnea, hypotension and cyanosis that does not respond to oxygen. The arterial blood gases show a decreased $PaO_2$. The etiologic factors are varied. Trauma, blast syndrome, overinfusion of crystalloids or colloids, overtransfusion, oxygen and circulating vasoactive peptides have all been implicated in its origin.

The lung in shock is the first target organ to come into contact with the vasoactive peptides, to which it responds. The lung acts as a microfilter for infused blood. If any aggregates are infused, the lung traps them. In the head and neck surgical patient, aspiration with hypervolemia or hypovolemia can lead to a shock lung state.

The shock lung state presents itself as follows: some hours after the shock syndrome has been corrected, it may recur insidiously, when the patient is only slightly hypotensive and may appear stable; the patient will suddenly appear to be suffering from dyspnea and tachycardia, and refractory cyanosis ensues. Rales are variable in consistency. The $PaO_2$ on room air or on supplemental oxygen is greatly reduced to 40 to 60 mm. Hg. (Remember that in the normal older patient, the $PaO_2$ may be 70 mm. Hg.) To the surprise of the physician, the administering of 100 per cent $O_2$ does not result in improved $PaO_2$. This is due to right-to-left shunting caused by areas of the lung that are perfused but not ventilated. The x-ray of the chest reveals bilateral alveolar fluffy infiltrate that is much more peripheral than in pulmonary edema.

#### MANAGEMENT OF RESPIRATORY DISTRESS SYNDROME

Keep the airway patent at all times with humidity from a heated Puritan face mask running at 40 per cent oxygen. The patient with respiratory distress syndrome or shock lung requires endotracheal intubation with mechanical ventilation. Monitor arterial blood gases and keep the $PaO_2$ above 60 mm. Hg. Keep inspired air ($FIO_2$) at 40 per cent oxygen except for short periods of time when higher concentrations may be used. Be aware that high oxygen concentrations cause a toxic state in the lungs.

Steroids are administered next; methylprednisolone, 15 mg./per kg. every 6 hours for 72 hours intravenously, as a bolus, reduces the lung alveoli and cerebral edema.[5]

If these steps fail, a positive end expiratory pressure (PEEP) of 5 to 16 cm. of water is used on a mechanical ventilator after intubating or putting in a cuffed tracheal tube. The rationale for PEEP is that it reduces hypoxemia (increases functional reserve capacity [FRC] and alveolar recruitment) by re-expanding the collapsed alveoli and pushing oxygen through those in the lung. The surfactant integrity also needs high oxygen, which is necessary to prevent alveolar collapse, the primary defect in shock lung. Diffuse microatelectasis and a large right-to-left shunt is corrected by PEEP in many cases now. Otherwise, this condition has a dismal prognosis.

In summary, PEEP is believed to counteract the tendency of the alveoli to collapse by keeping a constant pressure in the airway and returning the normal properties to the surfactant.

## SHOCK

For ease of discussion, the shock syndrome shall be divided by the three types: hypovolemic, septic and cardiogenic.

### Hypovolemic Shock

Hypovolemic shock is the end result of a decrease in circulating blood volume, caused by such factors as pooling in certain areas of the body (i.e., third spacing), hemorrhage and insufficient replacement of fluid loss during the surgery or early postoperative period. Because hypovolemic shock is sequential, it can be followed and interrupted, or possibly reversed, in its early phase more easily than the other two shock states can.

Hypovolemic shock is characterized by inadequate tissue perfusion. There is decreased cardiac output (CO), hypotension and a decrease in the central venous pressure (CVP). The body attempts to compensate by increasing the heart rate and by systemic periarteriolar vasoconstriction. The increase in autonomic system activity and in circulating catecholamines results in increased cardiac contractility. The end result is that a greater proportion of the blood goes to liver, heart and brain, with a lesser amount of blood going to the kidneys, gut, muscles and skin.[23] There is, therefore, a decrease in urine output. Hence, in a patient with a normal kidney, the urine output is used as a guideline in diagnosing hypovolemia and inadequate hydration. The reduction in cerebral blood flow is often manifested by confusion, agitation and insensibility in some; others remain alert for a much longer time.

Hypoxemia with inadequate tissue perfusion results in metabolic acidosis because of anaerobic metabolism. This is compensated for by respiratory alkalosis. A continuing hypoxemia in certain areas of the body results in a failure of the microcirulation, which is a further step toward a nonreversible shock state.[21]

## Cardiogenic Shock

Cardiogenic shock is more thoroughly reviewed in the cardiology section. Its main cause is pump failure, either primary or secondary. (Pump failure is also seen in the end stage of septic shock.) It must be remembered that, in the elderly patient with some degree of heart failure, there is a degree of tissue hypoxia contributing to sepsis and septicemia.

## Septic Shock

Septic shock is hypotension associated with septicemia and hypovolemia. The mechanisms involved in the hypotension of sepsis are a decreased peripheral resistance and constriction of precapillary and postcapillary sphincters with fluid loss to tissues. The central blood volume is also decreased, with a myocardial ischemia leading to myocardial failure. The final outcome is poor tissue perfusion with anoxia, acidosis and fluid and plasma losses into interstitial space. The septicemia is usually of gram-negative bacteria origin, but more and more it is due to gram-positive organisms.[23]

Both pre- and postoperatively, hypovolemia is corrected as soon as detected, or even suspected, since overhydration is easily correctable with today's loop diuretics. Manifestations of septic shock are hypotension, tachycardia and tachypnea, with a normal or high cardiac output.

The patient may be surprisingly alert, although agitation with confusion finally results and the patient becomes obtunded. The extremities may be warm and dry at the onset, but they later become very cold and clammy. The skin may have a mottled appearance. The extremity pulses are weak and thready.

Unfortunately, the patient has usually been heavily sedated and given analgesics, has been anesthetized and, more often than not, has been given steroids. Hence, the early signs of septic shock will not appear until hypotension and hypovolemia appear. The decrease in blood volume and cardiac output are manifested by low urine output.

### *Prevention of Septic Shock*

A rational approach to making a diagnosis is to be highly suspicious, that is, determining rapidly whether there is an obstruction or loculated pus that must be drained surgically. Reversal of the infectious and hemodynamic processes can not be achieved satisfactorily if the source of infection is left undrained.

Prevention of septic shock begins when a patient first enters the hospital through adequate administration of fluids preoperatively and adequate culture and sensitivity studies of all areas that could be a source of sepsis postoperatively.[24] Special attention is paid to the individual with chronic lung disease. The incentive spirometer is used preoperatively in patients with lung disease. Intermittent positive pressure breathing with saline plus isoproterenol (Isuprel) or isoetharine (Bronkosol) are also used frequently. The dehydration, hypertensive state and heart failure are corrected preoperatively.

Airway obstruction occurs quite quickly, and ventilation fails rapidly unless precautions are taken. Thus, careful observations for dyspnea, restlessness, agitation, cyanosis, stupor and sternal retraction are made.

A short, spasmodic cough is often a warning of mucus plugs with atelectasis. The inner cannula of the tracheostomy tube is cleaned frequently, for it easily becomes encrusted with secretions. The oropharynx is aspirated before releasing the endotracheal cuff, which is inserted at time of surgery when necessary.

A few complications of endotracheal and tracheostomy tubes are as follows: massive atelectasis due to improper insertion into one of the main stem bronchi, usually the right; dislodging and obstruction of the tube, which can be obviated or corrected by properly anchoring the tubes; and kinking.

### *Therapy for Septic Shock*

Insert a central venous pressure (CVP) line or a Swan-Ganz catheter if heart disease is suspected and constantly monitor during therapy. If hypovolemia with a low hematocrit exists, correct by giving whole blood. If hypovolemia with a close to normal hematocrit occurs, give up to 2000 cc. of fluid with sodium chloride or colloids. Fluid challenge with 200 to 250 ml. of 5 per cent dextrose in water is administered over half an hour. If CVP increases by more than 5 cm. of water per 100 ml. of infused fluid, the patient is not fluid-depleted. As the CVP comes up, the colloids and isotonic crystalloids are administered more slowly. Remember that a significantly elevated CVP in the face of continued hypotension suggests cardiac tamponade, myocardial infarction or congestive heart failure; it also often relates to chronic lung disease.

As the CVP rises, the cardiac output may increase the shock state. Twenty to 40 gm. of salt-poor albumin should be given. Plasma and plasma protein factor (Plasmanate) are often used. If there is any evidence of bleeding diathesis, fresh frozen plasma is given; however, there is a greater risk of hepatitis with its use.

The patient with underlying chronic pulmonary hypertension of inappropriate response should have a floating, balloon-tipped catheter (Swan-Ganz) inserted into the pulmonary artery.[11] The pulmonary artery and pulmonary wedge pressure can be measured. Venous blood gases are also noted; this measures the arteriovenous oxygen difference and roughly indicates the cardiac output.

Arterial blood gases should be measured at the onset and throughout therapy. The patient in shock must be intubated or tracheostomized, and oxygen should be administered through a heated Puritan face mask. A Foley catheter is inserted to monitor the urine (greater than 30 cc. per hour). The patient is digitalized (not in cases of acute myocardial infarction) with 0.5 to 0.75 mg. intravenous digoxin; 0.25 mg. is given at 4-hour intervals two times for a total dose of 0.02 mg. per kg.[1]

Blood cultures are done and bactericidal drugs, such as gentamycin and methicillin are given. Give 3 gm. methicillin intravenously every 6 hours. Gentamycin, 1.7 mg. per kg., is given as the initial loading dose, followed by 1 to 1.5 mg. per kg. according to the serum creatinine. The creatinine level in milligrams per cent multiplied by eight equals the interval in hours.

Occasionally, clindamycin is used against anaerobic bacteria, and chloramphenicol is used against other types of bacteria. Steroids are used, e.g., methylprednisolone (Solu-Medrol), 30 mg. per kg. by intravenous bolus by two doses, or dexamethasone, 100 mg. intravenously over 5 minutes and repeated every 6 hours for the first 24 to 48 hours. The rationale is that it improves capillary perfusion, facilitates oxygen transport and protects cellular and subcellular structures.[1]

Acidosis is corrected by giving sodium bicarbonate. The amount of base needed is estimated by multiplying the base deficit by the volume of the extracellular fluid (ECF). For example, a base deficit of 15 mEq. per liter multiplied by 20 liters (70 kg. man's ECF) equals 300 mEq. One half of the deficit is corrected at 1 mEq. per minute while monitoring the pH.[23] The remainder is gradually corrected in the next 24 hours.[6] Compensation is made for potassium loss. Slow loading of fluid will often prevent the overloading of a shock lung. Fluid overload and renal failure are corrected by giving furosemide, if the CVP is greater than 10 cm. of water or PW pressure is greater than 18 cm. of water, or by giving mannitol, if the CVP is less than 10 cm. or the PW is less than 18 cm. Urine output is monitored throughout and kept at greater than 30 ml. per hour by using diuretics.

Occasionally, disseminated intravascular coagulation (DIC) develops and is treated with fresh frozen plasma or with heparin, as mentioned previously.

If hypotension persists despite the fact that antibiotics have been given, adequate left ventricular filling pressure has been achieved and hypoxemia and its acidosis have been corrected, it is time to consider vasoactive drugs. Dopamine is administered by slow infusion, approximately 1 to 5 $\mu$g. per kg. per minute (200 mg. are added to 500 cc. of fluid).[12] This is adjusted until the correct level of urine output and adequate arterial pressure are achieved, since it increases kidney perfusion.[12] At lower doses, dopamine has both $\alpha$- and $\beta$-adrenergic effect. Increasing the dosage may result in an $\alpha$-adrenergic vasoconstrictive effect. This is blocked either by phentolamine (Regitine) intravenously or, occasionally, by 5 mg. chlorpromazine (Thorazine) intravenously.[5,18]

If dopamine fails, norepinephrine is tried, for it has a $\beta$-adrenergic effect on the heart and mainly an $\alpha$-adrenergic effect on the peripheral circulation (vasoconstriction). Continued titration is a must with this drug. Occasionally, it works when all else fails. The tachycardia plus hypoxemia and acidosis often lead to arrhythmias that must be quickly corrected.

In conclusion, the incidence of septic shock has markedly decreased because sepsis and early warning signs of shock are treated early.

## DIABETES MELLITUS

Anesthesia imposes a stress state on the diabetic's glucose metabolism. Surgery also increases glucose intolerance. Initially, there are four basic principles to be kept in mind when considering glucose metabolism:

First, the body needs 200 gm. of carbohydrates per day to maintain a glucose level without gluconeogenesis, thus preventing hypoglycemia and ketoacidosis.

Second, it is better to err toward hyperglycemia, thus preventing ketosis.

Third, get the patient out of ketoacidosis, correct any electrolyte imbalance and rehydrate well before surgery.

Fourth, infectious agents grow well in sugar. Therefore, a hyperglycemic state leads to susceptibility to infections.

The diabetic management shall be discussed in regard to the fasting state (starvation), the surgical state and hyperosmolar nonketotic diabetes.

### The Fasting State

The brain has priority over glucose, which it utilizes for energy. The remainder of its energy is derived from lactates and glycerol. Actually, the bodily need for glucose is decreased during starvation because glycogen is broken down. By the 16th hour of starvation, glycogen stores are depleted, and gluconeogenesis becomes the source of glucose. Therefore, ketoacidosis results because of beta-hydroxybutyric acid and acetoacetic acid, formed from fats and proteins.

#### *Insulin*

There are 8 to 15 microunits per milliliter of insulin in the blood. This increases to 100 microunits under stimulation by protein, lipids, sugar ingestion and surgery.[6] Insulin accelerates the cell membrane permeability to glucose and is necessary for glycogen and triglyceride storage. It suppresses glycogenolysis, lipolysis, and proteolysis, thus preventing ketosis.

Glucagon secreted by the alpha cells of the pancreas opposes insulin and serves in a catabolic way. It activates glycogen breakdown. Glucagon is a rapid counterregulator of insulin; it attempts to maintain normal glucose levels. Ketoacidosis is thus promoted by low insulin with high glucagon, which usually is also being seen.

The pituitary growth hormone is an insulin antagonist and also increases the sensitivity of adipose tissue to catabolism.[6]

### The Surgical State

Surgery combined with anesthetic agents causes a 70 per cent increase in blood sugar. Infection causes an increase in glucagon secretion, thus promoting tissue breakdown with cachexia and muscle wasting. The drugs used preoperatively are discontinued on the day of surgery. Sulfonylurea seems to cause the beta cells to secrete more endogenous insulin and is not effective under surgical stress. Thus, it can not be relied upon. Because of the variability of the diabetic status, each case must be reviewed individually at the time of surgery.

#### *Diabetics Well-controlled with Oral Agents*

Well-controlled individuals lack the symptoms and signs of diabetes mellitus, such as polyuria and polydipsia. Their urine sugar is 1+ to 2+ after meals, and the post prandial sugar is less than 250 mg. per 100 ml. Severe ketosis does not result from stressful situations in the mild diabetic who is controlled by diet alone. He is not treated unless sugar goes over 250 mg. per 100 ml. and signs and symptoms of diabetes appear. During the preoperative fasting stage, glucose levels will fall and prevent severe hyperglycemia. On the day of surgery, in the postoperative period, a urinalysis for sugar and ketones is routinely done on all diabetics.

Insulin coverage is used with regular insulin postoperatively; urinalysis results serve as a guideline. Fifteen units of insulin are given for a 4+ sugar in the urine, 10 units are given for 3+ sugar and 5 units are given for 2+ sugar. No insulin is required below the last level. Careful observations are made for vascular and renal complications, and a search for infectious foci is made.

#### *Diabetics Moderately Controlled with NPH Insulin*

Urinalysis for sugar and acetone will dictate the insulin coverage.

The moderate diabetic who has not been on insulin is often started on it preoperatively for better control. This is especially so if a long surgical procedure is contemplated. Parenteral 5 per cent glucose with solute is also started, and at least one fourth to one third of the solute should be 5 per cent glucose with physiologic saline. Between 100 to 200 grams of dextrose are also given each day. Remember that the stress of surgery and anesthetic factors, plus parenteral glucose, lead to increased insulin requirements. Gluconeogenesis is, therefore, averted if enough glucose is given, but it must be covered by insulin in sufficient dosage.[8]

If the patient has been on insulin and has had problems with control, a regimen to prevent peaks in sugar levels is used. A very satisfactory regime is to give a half dosage of a moderate-acting insulin (NPH) — 10 to 15 units or more every 12 hours plus 75 to 100 gm. of glucose — to prevent ketosis. Serum sugar levels are determined twice a day, and urine is closely monitored. Intake and output of fluid are also carefully monitored, especially if there is any evidence of vascular disease. Sufficient potassium must be added to the solute.

The fact remains that the surgical mortality rate of the adequately controlled diabetic is scarcely above that of the nondiabetic.[8]

#### *The Severe Diabetic*

He absolutely depends on the exogenous insulin for support. Without it, he becomes ketotic; that is, he develops metabolic ketoacidosis with compensating respiratory alkalosis. Severe ketoacidosis below 15 mEq. of $CO_2$ combining power and a high anion gap are contraindications of surgery.[8] One must correct acidosis and the acid–base balance before surgery.

Preoperatively, the morning of surgery, starting the patient on 5 to 10 per cent glucose solution will give him 100 to 200 gm. of carbohydrates, hence turning off gluconeogenesis. This will prevent the ketosis of diabetes. The patient should be given one half to a full dose on insulin, making sure that 50 to 100 gm. of glucose and solutes are given each 8-hour period. Measure urine for sugar and acetone preoperatively and measure blood sugar and electrolytes every 12 hours. In the recovery room, blood sugar and electrolytes should also be measured. Follow the urine for sugar and acetone and monitor accordingly the dose of regular-acting insulin given four times a day. Fifteen units of regular insulin is given for 4+ sugar, 10 units for 3+ sugar and 5 units for 2+. No insulin is given for 1+ or less sugar.

Davidoff reports that the managment of these patients requires meticulous care because glycosuria may ensue in the truly insulin-dependent diabetics receiving small to moderate doses of insulin plus rapid glucose infusion. The glycosuria may be sufficiently heavy to constitute a significant drain on the total body glucose stores, and gluconeogenesis will follow with its accompanying ketoacidosis.[2] In other words, carbohydrate starvation and ketoacidosis may occur in the midst of plenty, masquerading as diabetic ketoacidosis postoperatively.[8] Careful following of these basic rules will prevent catastrophe.

### Hyperosmolar Nonketotic Diabetes Syndrome

This syndrome is a catastrophic situation that must be corrected before surgery is even contemplated. The patient is hyperosmolar and hyperglycemic, has extremely high sugar and is severely dehydrated. The plasma, insulin, cortisol and growth hormones are low. Water and salt deprivation are contributing factors. Small doses of insulin (5 to 10 units) plus a massive fluid load with saline or one-half normal saline is the therapy of choice.

In conclusion, careful monitoring will result in a normal postoperative course if the numbers are corrected.[16]

## RENAL PROBLEMS COMPLICATING HEAD AND NECK SURGERY

Oliguria is decreased urine output amounting to less than 400 ml. per 24 hours. The kidney is very sensitive to hypotension, hypovolemia and hypoxia. The glomerular capillary pressure must be in excess of the plasma oncotic pressure of 25 mm. Hg and the renal venous pressure of 12 mm. Hg, or the urine output will drop and ischemic renal disease will result. Surgery and anesthesia increase catecholamine output, and thus afferent arteriolar vasoconstriction, resulting in further decrease in kidney perfusion and further ischemia. The effective renal blood flow determines the glomerular filtration. Circulatory impairment leads to increased release of renin, which leads to increased angiotensin formation, resulting in a decreased glomerular filtration. This leads to tubular dysfunction with oliguria of less than 400 ml. per day and azotemia.

### Prevention of Ischemic Renal Failure

In the preoperative, operative and postoperative periods, ischemic renal failure prevention is as follows:

1. providing adequate preoperative hydration
2. avoiding nausea and vomiting with high fluid loss or correcting as soon as possible
3. avoiding hemorrhaging and replacing blood and fluid loss
4. correcting poor cardiac output by digitalization
5. correcting any hypoxemia with oxygen and any anemia with transfusions
6. correcting severe liver disease preoperatively (Patients with severe liver disease have marked impairment in renal functioning that leads to the hepatorenal syndrome, a severe form of prerenal azotemia.)
7. correcting decreased plasma oncotic pressure by restoring plasma volume with plasma or albumin

### Prerenal Azotemia or Ischemic Renal Failure

Prerenal azotemia results from persistent underperfusion of the renal vasculature. There is, therefore, some sodium retention in order to restore volume. As a result, the urine sodium and chloride will be low (less than 200 mEq. per liter). Potassium loss is high, reflecting a high aldosterone output. Occasionally, the urine sodium will be high while the chloride is low. The urine osmolality is nearly always greater than that of the plasma. The urea rises out of proportion to creatinine because the kidney reabsorbs the cleared urea.

### *Management of Prerenal Azotemia*

Decreased urine output must be corrected by counteracting the underperfusion and contracted volume. If no heart failure exists, 500 ml. of isotonic saline may be given when there is a falling urine output.[19] It has been shown that there is a preoperative increase of the urine output. It has also been shown that preoperative expansion of the extracellular fluid volume will protect the kidney. Treat cardiac failure, if it exists, thus mobilizing the edematous state. Use diuretics judiciously and only when indicated. Furosemide and ethacrynic acid inhibit tubular reabsorption in the loop and are now known as, and may be used as, loop diuretics. They will cause diuresis even in the underperfused kidney. Mannitol is occasionally used to restore urine output.

## Acute Parenchymal Renal Failure[19]

Acute parenchymal renal failure is due to glomerulonephritis, acute cortical necrosis and allergic nephropathies. The pathophysiology involves volume contraction secondary to shock, cardiovascular disease, massive hemorrhage, drug allergies and nephrotoxins. Hemolytic reaction may result in acute tubular necrosis (ATN). Urine may show casts plus renal tubular epithelial cells. The urine osmolality is equal to that of the plasma, and there is an elevated urine sodium concentration greater than 40 mEq. per liter. Occasionally, there is a high output renal failure due to toxins and antibiotics. The oliguric phase lasts from days to weeks. Anuria is rare.

The diuretic phase of this failure advances gradually until the urine output is greater than the fluid intake, which leads to dehydration and collapse of the vascular system. Strict intake and output of fluids plus weighing may be a helpful guide. Measure the CVP if signs of failure exist. Observe carefully for sepsis. Electrolytes and creatinine are the guidelines for assessing the need for dialysis. Hyperkalemia is corrected with enemas of a brand of sodium polystyrene sulfonate (Kayexalate) until dialysis is performed.

## Postrenal Azotemia or Obstructive Uropathy

Obstructive uropathy actually means acute renal failure due to obstruction. Therefore, any obstruction to urine flow must be corrected quickly. For instance, an indwelling catheter should be inserted when prostatic obstruction is suspected. Infusion intravenous pyelogram or retrograde pyelography will demonstrate the block, and it may be easily correctable.

## Acute Renal Failure

Most patients with acute renal failure (ARF), especially when seen postoperatively, will be managed conservatively for a short period. Then, the nephrologist is called to make an assessment for hemodialysis. Occasionally, peritoneal dialysis is used.

### *Management of Acute Renal Failure*

Protein in the patient's diet should be limited. Prudent replacement of the fluid lost in the urine and stools plus an additional 5 to 7 ml. per kg. per day are necessary. More fluid should be added if the patient is febrile. Weigh the patient daily to assess hydration. Electrolytes should be measured daily; sodium intake should equal sodium lost in the urine and elsewhere. Be careful not to overhydrate.

### *Hyperkalemia*

If any evidence of renal failure exists, do not administer potassium. When the serum potassium reaches 5.5 mEq. per liter, sodium polystyrene sulfonate exchange resin (Kayexalate) should be given. Fifteen to 30 gm. are given up to four times daily, either by mouth or by means of retention enemas. An EKG is often a helpful tool in following the potassium level. An elevated potassium concentration of 6.5 mEq. per liter or more is an emergency situation. Rapid infusion of 25 gm. of glucose combined with 10 to 15 units of regular insulin will lower the serum potassium concentration in 30 to 60 minutes and keep it there for at least six hours. Five to 10 ml. of 10 per cent calcium chloride given intravenously in 5 to 10 minutes while observing the EKG will counteract the effect of excess potassium on the heart.

Magnesium intake, especially antacid preparations, should be restricted in patients with ARF. When the serum bicarbonate falls below 15 mEq. per liter, metabolic acidosis is corrected by administering sodium bicarbonate intravenously.

### *Convulsions*

Convulsions are prevented by avoiding water overload and hypertension. Short-acting barbiturates, diazepam (Valium) or diphenylhydantoin (Dilantin), are used.

### *Congestion*

Congestion of the body is serious and requires prompt dialysis to remove excess fluid and electrolytes. Drugs excreted by the kidney must be monitored carefully.[15]

### *Hypertension*

Hypertension is treated with 300 mg. diazoxide intravenously by push to be followed by dialysis. Sodium nitroprusside, 100 mg. per liter, will do the same.

## GENERAL PHYSIOLOGICAL SUPPORT

### Fluid and Electrolyte Therapy

The basic concept behind fluid and electrolyte therapy is that the body needs 600 to 800 ml. of water per 24 hours to replace the insensible water loss. The kidneys' fluid requirement is about 40 ml. per hour for optimal function, i.e., a urine output of 40 ml. per hour. The kidneys also excrete 40 mEq. of potassium per day. Postoperatively, a patient is given 75 to 100 ml. of solute per hour. This may be given as 5 per cent dextrose with one-half normal saline. Forty mEq. of potassium is administered per day, the obligatory loss per 24 hours.

For the sake of simplicity, two assumptions shall be made: (1) we are dealing with a patient weighing 70 kg., and (2) he has adequate kidney function; that is, the specific gravity of the urine is 1.016 or higher with a pH of 5.8 or lower. Weighing the patient daily, plus keeping an intake and output sheet, gives a fair idea of the state of hydration.

### *Water Depletion*

Water depletion is due to low intake of water or high water loss. There is a decrease in body fluid volume with hyperosmolarity. Thirst, apathy, weakness, anorexia, nausea, thin weak pulse, postural hypotension, low urine volume and hypernatremia occur. Dry mouth with an increase in urine specific gravity is also seen. The serum urea nitrogen creatinine ratio is probably the best clinical guide to volume depletion. In its severe form, this goes on to apathy, stupor and hyperosmolarity. Three mEq. above normal of sodium means a water deficit of one liter. This should be replaced over a 12-hour period of giving glucose and water.[24]

### *Water Excess*

Water excess is often iatrogenic, owing to loading a patient with electrolyte-free water. This is also seen when there is an excess secretion of antidiuretic hormone. There is an increase in body weight and urine volume with a decrease in serum sodium. More severe forms of water excess lead to nausea, vomiting and convulsions due to brain edema. Withholding of water is the therapy of choice, giving only 650 ml. per day. Mannitol diuresis is indicated in cerebral edema. If this fails, then 100 to 200 cc. of 5 per cent sodium chloride are given.[16]

### *Hyponatremia*

Hyponatremia of less than 135 mEq. per liter is the most common electrolyte problem seen. There are several types but only three will be discussed here.

#### DILUTIONAL HYPONATREMIA

Dilutional hyponatremia is due to water excess and leads to poor mentation, backache, apathy and nausea. Vomiting is rare. In the head and neck trauma or postsurgical patient, there may be an inappropriate antidiuretic hormone (IADH) secretion with water retention and inhibition of aldosterone secretion. Depression is often the only symptom with a sodium of less than 125 mEq. per l. and with a high urine sodium. Water should be restricted to 650 ml. per day.

#### HYPONATREMIA WITH CIRCULATORY INSUFFICIENCY AND DEHYDRATION

This form of hyponatremia is due to loss of isotonic fluid, such as in diarrhea, sweating, adrenal insufficiency and diabetic ketoacidosis. There is a reduced glomerular filtration rate often seen when too much water with too little salt is given. Hypokalemia exists. Therapy consists of replacing the sodium and potassium deficit.[24]

#### HYPONATREMIA WITH CIRCULATORY INSUFFICIENCY AND EDEMA

Congestive heart failure, cirrhosis and nephrosis are the main causes. Three factors involved are the intrinsic renal factors, with decreased glomerular filtration rate, increased antidiuretic hormones and, finally, resetting of the osmostat. Therapy consists of restricting water to 500 ml. per day. Occasionally, 25 to 50 gm. of salt-poor albumin will help in restoring the plasma volume. Rarely, peritoneal dialysis is used. Actually, correcting the primary disease will correct this low sodium without decreasing the edema.

### *Hypernatremia*

The sodium is greater than 148 mEq. per l., which is caused by an abnormal renal retention of sodium. Edema and weight gain result. Occasionally, this is seen in tube-fed patients when hyperosmolar high-protein solutions are used. This syndrome develops from lack of water and osmotic diuresis of urea. Therapy consists of diluting the tube feeding. Sodium restriction with judicious use of diuretics will correct the edema and weight gain. Loop diuretics such as furosemide are excellent.

### *Hypokalemia*

This is caused by diuretics and prolonged administration of potassium-free fluid. Systemic alkalosis is both the reason for and result of potassium depletion because the renal tubules exchange sodium for potassium ions. Metabolic alkalosis produced by chloride loss will lead to more sodium exchange for potassium. The deficit may be severe, with as much as 3 to 10 mEq. per kg. body weight. Remembering that more than 8 mEq. per l. of potassium is lethal, potassium replacement is given in a 40 to 60 mEq. per l. solution. The daily need for potassium is 40 mEq. per day.

#### ACIDOSIS

Potassium depletion is seen in diabetic ketoacidosis and renal tubular acidosis. Acidosis makes the potassium leave the cells. Signs of potassium depletion are malaise and weakness with muscle paresis. The EKG shows ectopic atrial beats. Therapy consists of giving potassium chloride solution. Never give more than 20 mEq. of potassium per hour. Potassium depletion can usually be corrected in three or four days.

### *Magnesium Deficiency*

The symptoms and signs for this deficiency are the same as those of calcium deficiency, that is, agitation, hyperactive tendon reflexes, muscle tremor and, eventually, generalized tremors. The serum magnesium is less than 1.5 mEq. per liter. Magnesium deficiency is seen in patients with diarrhea, malabsorption, malnutrition, prolonged intravenous feeding, alcoholism, certain renal diseases, diuretic therapy, hyperaldosteronism, hyperparathyroidism and diabetic ketoacidosis. It is also seen in patients on hyperalimentation. When tetany due to magnesium sulfate occurs, a 10 to 20 per cent solution of magnesium sulfate is given intravenously at a rate not to exceed 1.5 ml. of a 10 per cent solution. With malabsorption, 60 mEq. (20 ml.) of magnesium hydroxide is given daily by mouth.

### *Calcium and Phosphate*

Sixty per cent of serum calcium is bound to albumin. Hypercalcemia affects the kidneys, the central nervous system and the gastrointestinal tract. Severe hypercalcemia with a calcium greater than 15 mg. per cent results in polyuria, dehydration, anorexia, lethargy and stupor.[24] One of the principles of therapy is to hydrate with 3 to 6 l. per day with a large amount of sodium. Hyperphos solution, 15 ml. every 6 hours, should be used. This will lower the calcium. The parathyroid adenoma removal will lower calcium and lead to hypocalcemia.

Hypocalcemia is treated postoperatively by giving 20 to 50 ml. of 10 per cent calcium gluconate intravenously over 10 to 30 minutes. The long range therapy consists of giving up to 4 gm. of calcium gluconate or lactate three times a day. If this does not control the hypocalcemia, 50,000 units of Vitamin D are given two times a day.

Hypophosphatemia is seen in patients on hyperalimentation or long-term intravenous feeding and in chronically ill patients. A phosphate level below 2.5 mg. per 100 ml. may be significant and can be corrected, as mentioned previously. Lethargy and a slurred speech may go on to an hypophosphatemic coma.

## Nutrition

The immediate labile energy reserves found in extracellular fluid amounts to 1000 calories, whereas the daily fasting energy requirement is 2000 calories. It must be remembered that the labile reserves of amino acids and glucose from glycogen last less than 24 hours; the fat reserve can last for 25 to 35 days.

When first seen, the head and neck surgery patient is often in a state of chronic subnutrition with a fall in the ratio of essential amino acids to the total plasma acids. This poor or inappropriate intake is a result of obstruction, pain or anxiety. After surgery, the demand for amino acid release is great, for new protein synthesis is needed for repair of injured tissue and for energy.

Hypoxia, with its increase of cell membrane permeability and its interference with the cell's sodium pump, is seen at surgery. Potassium, of which there are 32,000 mEq. in the body, diffuses out of cells into the circulation. The osmolality is maintained by cell leak. The loss of cell integrity leads to normosmolar hyponatremia, which predisposes to gram-negative sepsis and shock states. Cellular integrity is much more easily preserved if there is adequate glucose and insulin along with proper oxygenation. It reduces protein catabolism and potassium loss and promotes sodium diuresis.[24]

Four separate ways of modifying the catabolic response to surgery are as follows: (1) preserve the nitrogen balance by a generous intake of calories and protein; (2) increase environmental temperature; (3) use blood transfusion; and (4) administer glucose with insulin for proper utilization of glucose in the very malnourished patient.

### *Tube Feeding*

In many head and neck surgery patients, proper nutrition is maintained with tube feeding. It (or feeding by mouth) is often started 24 to 48 hours after surgery. The basal requirements for nutrition are supplied in 30 calories per kg. per day as follows: 50 per cent as carbohydrates (4 calories per gm.); 35 per cent as fat (9 calories per gm.); and 15 per cent as protein (4 calories per gm.). This is diluted with 2400 ml. water with an osmolarity of 500 mOsm per liter. Blenderized feedings made from baby food or table food are often used. All mixtures used contain the eight essential amino acids plus nonessential ones.

On the first day of tube feeding, clear fluids are given in addition to some intravenous solutions. The next day, total tube feeding is used.

#### CORRECTIONS AND COMPLICATIONS OF TUBE FEEDING

Aspiration is prevented by feeding the patient when he is sitting up. Diarrhea, dehydration and azotemia are due to the hypertonicity of the feeding mixture. Adding water and decreasing fats will stop this. Fluid retention may be corrected with the administration of diuretics. Diarrhea and bloating may be due to lactose intolerance, which occurs in 25 per cent of the patients. A lactose-free diet will correct the problem.

### *Minerals and Vitamins*

Hypomagnesemia is often seen in poorly nourished persons and in heavy users of alcohol or after prolonged intravenous feeding. Neuromuscular irritability with tremors and jerkiness will result. Tachycardia may be seen, and it may be the only manifestation. Magnesium gluconate, 500 to 1500 mg., is given by mouth. Magnesium should not be given in renal disease without close monitoring.

Trace elements are usually present in the multivitamins administered. Iron is added when indicated. If trace elements are low, a unit of plasma protein fraction (Plasmanate) or plasma will take care of the problem.

For proper utilization of food and energy production, 5 ml. of multivitamins are added to the intravenous feeding or a high potency vitamin formula (Theragran Liquid) is added to the tube feeding. Fat-soluble vitamins A, D, E and K are added to the diet but only as set by maximum daily requirement standards. Water-soluble vitamins, such as the B's and C's, are also administered in amounts of 5 to 10 times the daily requirement. Folic acid, 1 to 2 mg., is added daily, since in 25 per cent of head and neck surgery patients there is a folate deficiency. Vitamin $B_{12}$, 1000 $\mu$gm. per week is also given if its level is low. Hyperalimentation with tube feeding is complex, and intravenous or parenteral feeding is usually discouraged because of the many complications. It is also rarely indicated.

## LIVER DISEASE

Preoperatively, any patient with a history of heavy intake of alcohol or an enlarged liver should have a complete liver profile done plus a prothrombin time (PT) and an activated partial thromboplastin time (APTT). A serum electrophoresis is often also done. Since 80 per cent of heavy users of alcohol have a palpable liver, liver and spleen scans are done to check for hepatocellular damage and evidence of hypersplenism. If previous infectious liver disease is suspected, a test for serum hepatitis should be done. Jaundice, ascites, edema, palmar erythema and spider nevi suggest significant liver disease. Occasionally, direct and indirect Coombs tests are indicated if hemolysis is suspected.

### Hepatitis

Hepatitis is known to be due to the infectious hepatitis virus (Type A) and the serum hepatitis virus (Type B). Only 50 per cent of transfusion-transmitted hepatitis, however, is due to hepatitis virus B.

Serum hepatitis occurs in 0.1 to 0.3 per cent of patients receiving blood.[10] The mortality rate in transfusion recipients at one time was 12 per cent, but now, owing to better management, it is much lower.[13] The majority of those succumbing are under the age of 5 or over the age of 65. The incubation period for Type B hepatitis is 35 to 120 days. The use of hyperimmune globulin may modify the disease in susceptible individuals.[17]

In acute infectious hepatitis (Type A), one to two months should lapse between a normal liver test and surgery. Recovery from acute infectious hepatitis is slow. Immune serum globulin (ISG), 2 ml., is said to protect those in close contact and is now being used in a prophylactic program. It is effective against the development of clinical hepatitis in approximately 90 per cent of cases.

Serum hepatitis (Type B or Australia antigen–positive hepatitis) is not affected by immune serum globulin (ISG) innoculations, and hyperimmune serum globulin (HSG) is presently used in prophylaxis. HSG is not readily available as yet.

Although all donor blood is screened, there is no absolute guarantee against the possible transmission of the disease. There is a high rate of serum hepatitis seen when fibrinogen or Factor IX preparations are given, and therefore these must be used judiciously.

Approximately 5 to 7 per cent of acute hepatitis becomes chronic persistent hepatitis. These patients should have their laboratory tests repeated every two months until they go into remission. If elective surgery is contemplated, the patient should have been in remission for three months.[17]

Acute alcoholic hepatitis is discussed further under "Alcoholism." The major point to be noted here is that alcoholism does lead to a fatty liver with or without necrosis. These changes are due to the alcohol itself and not to some undefined toxin. The fatty degeneration can be reversed at this stage by removal of alcohol from the diet plus the addition of a high protein, high carbohydrate diet. The liver returns to normal in 75 per cent of the cases. Others go on to steatonecrosis.

Jaundice or ascites in a cirrhotic patient increases the risks with abdominal surgery, but most head and neck surgery can be done safely if extra attention is paid to proper hydration and replacement of albumin. Encephalopathy is carefully watched for and is corrected quickly by giving 500 mg. kanamycin by mouth three times a day. Additionally, the diet should be free from proteins. Hypoprothrombinemia, if present, is treated with Vitamin $K_1$ parenterally.

Viral hepatitis has a 10 per cent mortality rate with major surgery. If enzyme changes are indicative of an acute or a chronic active hepatitis, surgery should be postponed. The chronic persistent hepatitis (nonactive) has a better prognosis and tolerates surgery well. Percutaneous needle biopsy of the liver is a good diagnostic tool if viral activity is suspected and cannot be assessed by laboratory studies.[28]

### Prevention of Problems in Liver Disease

The problems in liver disease are avoided if dehydration, salt overload, hypokalemia, hyperkalemia, hypoxia and hypotensive states are prevented. Often, gut-sterilizing antibiotics are used. Kanamycin (Kantrex) is preferred because it is not toxic to hepatocytes. The prothrombin time and activated partial thromboplastin time are assayed. If albumin is low or low normal, fresh whole blood should be transfused. Meperidine hydrochloride (Demerol) and morphine are used judiciously.

### Postoperative Jaundice

Postoperative jaundice is seen in a patient whose surgical procedure has lasted more than four hours. Hypotension is also a predisposing factor. If seen within six hours after surgery, it should be considered a hemolytic jaundice, for a maximum bilirubin level occurs three to six hours after surgery with hemolysis. Liver chemistries and a retyping and cross match are done, and a check is made for incompatible transfusion reaction. Blood is checked for red cell agglutinins. Both direct and indirect Coombs test are done. If a high indirect bilirubin reaction, an elevated reticulocyte or a falling hematocrit is noted, the urine is checked for bile and urobilinogen.[28]

A large hematoma causes only a small rise in the bilirubin. When the bilirubin is over 5 mg. per cent, hemolysis is usually accompanied by liver disease, passive congestion or shock. Patients with chronic congestive heart failure often develop a low-grade jaundice postoperatively.

### Benign Postoperative Intrahepatic Cholestasis

Benign postoperative intrahepatic cholestasis is a syndrome that occurs after a long surgical procedure and in conjunction with a bout of hypotension or prolonged hypotension with hypovolemia and multiple transfusions. The bilirubin level goes up to between 15 and 40 mg. per cent in 2 to 10 days. The alkaline phosphatase level rises, and the enzymes may be slightly elevated. The liver biopsy shows dilute canaliculi with bile casts and inspissated bile. Thus, this is mostly an obstructive phenomenon. It clears up slowly if left alone.

### Other Postoperative Problems

The occurrence of jaundice following halothane-induced hepatitis is seen. Jaundice with fever, elevated transaminase level and eosinophilia and monocytosis are the presenting signs.

Hepatic encephalopathy is rarely seen with head and neck surgery patients. Early signs are often subtle, with personality changes and changes of mentation, clonus and asterixis and increased reflexes, including Babinski's. Later, the patient becomes confused and drowsy. This proceeds to stupor and coma. Azotemia, hypokalemia and dehydration preoperatively with bleeding are predisposing factors.

## ALCOHOLISM

Heavy drinking combined with heavy smoking predisposes an individual to head and neck cancer. Over 50 per cent of these head and neck patients have chronic lung disease, which poses the problem of respiratory disease because of ciliated mucosa.[15] In addition, since alcohol is a liver toxin, it causes hepatitis of various grades. Anorexia, fever, hepatomegaly, abdominal pain and tenderness and ascites and encephalopathy are all manifestations of the alcoholic liver.[14] This is reviewed under "Liver Disease" (see p. 60).

Alcohol causes a decrease in the cardiac indices.[13] The cardiac contractility and the left ventricular function are diminished, and there is a diminished stroke volume. More advanced cases go into cardiomyopathy with nutritional deficiency—especially of thiamine. The beriberi heart will develop.

A number of patients are nervous when admitted and are given diazepam (Valium) to help correct this. Most patients do not disclose the full extent of their alcoholic intake and diazepam is thus given to help lessen the postoperative withdrawal syndrome.

Postoperatively, a tremulous patient with a history of drinking must be handled differently from other patients. Diazepam, 5 to 10 mg., is given intramuscularly or by mouth every 2 to 4 hours to prevent full-blown delirium tremens (DT's). In the past, when delirium tremens went unrecognized, there was up to an 8 per cent mortality. If they do occur, 5 mg. of diazepam is given parenterally every 15 minutes for up to 10 doses. Diazepam has the least detrimental effects on the alcoholic, and it does have antiseizure properties as well.

In addition to the administering of diazepam, there are other differences in handling the postoperative alcoholic patient. He is given more fluid with a higher carbohydrate content, for a hypoglycemic state often exists, with low adenosine triphosphate (ATP) and a low nicotinamide-adenine dinucleotide (NAD). Ten cc. of multivitamins are added to the intravenous solution.[14] One hundred mg. of thiamine is given intramuscularly four times a day. Serum magnesium is given intramuscularly, and 2 cc. of 50 per cent magnesium sulfate is given twice a day until the correct serum magnesium level is obtained, and then it is adjusted accordingly. A 10 per cent glucose solution is often added instead of the usual 5 per cent.[14]

Often, these individuals are low in other trace elements, such as zinc, and these are added to bring the levels up to normal.

Forty per cent oxygen is administered by heated Puritan face mask.

Occasionally, antibiotics are used if moist rales and fever are present. A dose of 100 mg. of hydrocortisone sodium succinate (Solu-Cortef) is sometimes added to the solute to decrease inflammatory edema in the brain, liver, kidneys and heart—thus reducing the symptomatology of the alcoholic. As soon as feeding by tube is possible, a high carbohydrate, high protein and low fat diet is essential.

## BLOOD DYSCRASIA

The head and neck surgeon sees the entire range of blood dyscrasia, for he is often asked to see patients with bleeding from the nose and the mouth that is often associated with various abnormalities of the blood. The anemias seen in these patients are often due to multiple causes.

On admission, anemic patients are tested as follows: complete blood count with indices, stool for occult blood, serum iron and iron-binding capacity. Serum folate and serum $B_{12}$ levels are determined for many head and neck surgery patients, since poor papillation of tongue and leukoplakia are often associated with cancer and pathologic conditions of the oral mucosa cavity. Twenty-five per cent of our patients had a folate deficiency in a small series, and a low grade of anemia ensued. Folic acid is necessary for immune competence and integrity of mucus membranes. Gastric achlorhydria is seen in about 25 per cent of a small series we tested when cancer of the oropharynx was present.

## Anemias

*Microcytic anemias* are usually due to blood loss and iron deficiency. *Normocytic anemia* is seen in chronic diseases, such as cancer and liver and renal disease. *Hemolytic anemias* are usually related to or due to systemic disease. *Megaloblastic anemias* are related to folate, vitamin $B_{12}$ or pyridoxine deficiencies. A chronic disease may also cause this type of anemia.

## Transfusions

Preoperative evaluation of anemias can also lead to transfusion of a patient who has a hemoglobin of less than 10 gm. or a hematocrit of less than 30, especially if a lengthy procedure is contemplated. Most of these patients receive multiple transfusions at the time of surgery.

Transfusions are usually of packed red cells unless the albumin is low, in which case whole blood is used. It must be remembered, however, that transfusion reactions are seen more often when whole blood is given. Remember that one unit of packed cells brings the hematocrit up approximately 3 per cent.[7]

### Transfusion Reactions

1. Febrile reactions are common and are generally due to antibodies to white cell and platelet antigens. A hemolytic reaction must always be ruled out in febrile episodes. Severe reactions are then given washed buffy coat–poor red cells, from which plasma, white cells and platelets have been removed.

2. In cases of hyperkalemia, storage of blood causes an increase of potassium by 1 mEq. per l. of plasma daily. If the patient is hyperkalemic, he should be given only fresh blood.

3. When urticaria is seen alone, it can be handled by giving 50 mg. of diphenhydramine hydrochloride (Benadryl) or another antihistamine. Occasionally, steroids must be given.

4. Hypocalcemia is very rare and is easily corrected by giving 10 cc. of 10 per cent calcium gluconate. This reaction is due to an excess of citrate ions in the blood given. It is only seen in advanced liver disease, since the citrate of the transfused blood would be metabolized by a normal liver.

5. Post-transfusion hepatitis occurs in 0.1 to 1.0 per cent of transfused blood. The blood used is screened by means of the Australia antigen test for hepatitis, but this test has reduced the occurrence rate by only 25 per cent, since it does not screen for hepatitis A or C. Furthermore, it does not pick up all of hepatitis B. At present, hyperimmune gamma globulin should be given if hepatitis is suspected. Pooled gamma globulin is indicated if hyperimmune gamma globulin is not available.

6. Hemolytic reactions, when due to red blood cell incompatibility, are serious. They should be considered a possibility whenever anxiety, chills, fever, shock, flushed face pain or findings of disseminated intravascular coagulation or hemoglobinuria are present. A reaction may occur after 50 ml. of blood are given but, under anesthesia, may go unrecognized. Hemoglobinemia and hemoglobinuria, and occasionally jaundice, occur a short time after transfusion. Later, oliguria and anuria appear. If not managed properly, acute renal failure ensues.

The first step in management of a hemolytic reaction is to stop the transfusion. Maintain the intravenous line and infuse mannitol (925 gm.) over a 5 minute period as soon as possible. Urine flow is maintained at 100 ml. per hour or more with high infusion. If urine output falls, repeat mannitol but do not give more than 100 gm. per 24 hours. Correct hypotension and hypovolemia with saline and plasma protein factor (Plasmanate). Correct disseminated intravascular reaction if it occurs.

### Bleeding Disorders

Hemorrhagic diathesis may be prevented in most surgical cases. A good history, with clues such as bleeding from dental extraction or at previous surgery, is the most helpful. Nose bleeds suggest platelet or capillary abnormalities, such as in hereditary hemorrhagic telangiectasia. Purpura hemorrhagica is seen in von Willebrand's disease and in decreased or poorly functioning platelets. Hemophilia is suggested by hemarthrosis and deep muscle hematoma. A history of drug ingestion must be taken, because aspirin may be a predisposing factor to bleeding diathesis.[21]

A preoperative work-up consists of a complete blood count and platelet estimate or count. Prothrombin time (PT) and activated partial thromboplastin time (APTT) are done. When the above tests are normal but bleeding exists, one should then think of platelet dysfunction. An abnormally quick PT means liver disease, anticoagulant therapy by sodium warfarin (Coumadin) or similar drugs or, possibly, an extrinsic system defect. These are Factors V, VII and X or fibrinogen deficiencies. The plasma Factors XII, XI, IX, VIII and V are measured by the APTT. If prolonged PT exists, the patient is given 50 mg. of vitamin $K_1$ intravenously to return it to normal. A prolonged PT often means liver disease.[21]

### Disseminated Intravascular Coagulation

Disseminated intravascular coagulation (DIC) occurs because of thromboplastic substances that are released into the circulation. Shock and hemolytic transfusion reactions cause DIC, the mechanism of which is unknown. Thromboplastic material activates fibrinolysis. Intravascular coagulation results in hypofibrinogen in the circulation plus fibrinogen (Fi) breakdown product. The latter interferes with the functions of platelets and fibrinogen. Therefore, fibrinogen and thrombin levels fall, with a decrease in Factors V, VII, VIII, IX and X. Platelets also are decreased.

DIC is a syndrome of thrombocytopenia, multiple plasma coagulation deficiencies and secondary fibrinolysis due to activation of the coagulation systems and platelet aggregation within the vascular tree. This is best handled by stopping coagulation with heparin and transfusion with whole blood. Occasionally, it is necessary to administer fibrinogen. DIC, during or after surgery, is most frequently the result of an incompatible blood transfusion, often presented as oozing.

### Fibrinolysis

Fibrinolysis is the result of a continuation of the fibrinolytic activity when it is no longer needed to stop fibrin formation on vessel walls. This is seen in DIC and liver disease with hypofibrinogenemia.

Fibrinolysis is managed by giving $\epsilon$-aminocaproic acid orally or intravenously. Five grams are given first, and repeated every 4 to 6 hours. Thus, plasma plasminogen activating factor will cease, and the hemorrhagic diathesis will subside. Heparinize the patient first.

### Other Diathesis

Occasionally, a patient on sodium warfarin (Coumadin) anticoagulant needs surgery. The drug is discontinued and, usually, no excessive bleeding occurs. The patient is transfused if bleeding does occur.

High risk thrombotic patients are given 5000 units of heparin subcutaneously 2 hours before surgery and every 12 hours throughout the postoperative period. Apparently, this reduces thrombosis and embolization. The peak effect obtained is one tenth that of the usual, but it still prevents thrombosis.

## Bibliography


1. Basta, L. L., Bruce, T. A., Elkins, R. D., et al.: The cardiovascular system. *In* Papper, S. (ed.): Medical Care of the Surgical Patient. Boston, Little, Brown & Co., 1976, pp. 19–52.
2. Bendixen, H. H., Egbert, L. D., Hedley-White, J., et al.: Respiratory Care. St. Louis, The C. V. Mosby Co., 1965.
3. Beahrs, O. H.: Complications of surgery for cancer of the head and neck. *In* Artz, C. P., and Hardy, J. D. (eds.): Management of Surgical Complications. Philadelphia, W. B. Saunders Co., 1975, pp. 277–290.
4. Bushnell, L. S.: Acute respiratory failure in the surgical patient. *In* Skillman, J. J. (ed.): Intensive Care. Boston, Little, Brown & Co., 1975, pp. 203–228.
5. Chalon, N., Lowe, D. A., and Malebranche, J.: Effect of dry anesthetic gases on tracheobronchial ciliated epithelium. Anesthesiology, *37*:338, 1972.
6. Chatton, M. J., and Ullman, P. M.: Nutritional and metabolic disorders. *In* Krupp, M. A., and Chatton, M. J. (eds.): Current Medical Diagnosis and Treatment. Los Altos, California, Lange Medical Pubns., 1976, pp. 754–782.
7. Condon, R. E.: Fluid and electrolyte therapy. *In* Condon, R. E., and Nyhus, L. M. (eds.): Manual of Surgical Therapeutics. 2nd ed. Boston, Little, Brown & Co., 1975.
8. Davidoff, F.: Rational metabolic management of diabetic patients undergoing surgery. *In* Skillman, J. J. (ed.): Intensive Care. Boston, Little, Brown & Co., 1975, pp. 353–385.
9. Frazier, H. S.: Pathogenesis of renal impairment in surgical patients. *In* Skillman, J. J. (ed.): Intensive Care. Boston, Little, Brown & Co., 1975, pp. 277–292.
10. Grady, G. F., and Lee, V. A.: Hepatitis B immune globulin — prevention of hepatitis from accidental exposure among medical workers. N. Engl. J. Med., *293*:1067–1069, 1975.
11. Grossman, R. F., and Aberman, A.: Editorial: Emergency management of acute pulmonary edema. Ann. Intern. Med., *84*:488, 1976.
12. Holzner, J., Karginer, J. S., O'Rourke, R. A., et al.: Effectiveness of dopamine in patients with cardiogenic shock. Am. J. Cardiol., *32*:79, 1973.
13. Kakkar, V. V., Corrigan, T. P., and Fassaed, D. P.: Prevention of postoperative pulmonary embolism by low dose heparin: An international multicentre trial. Lancet, *2*:45, 1975.
14. Mundth, E. D., Shine, K. I., and Austen, W. G.: Physiological response of the cardiovascular system to surgery and surgical disease. *In* Skillman, J. J. (ed.): Intensive Care. Boston, Little, Brown & Co., 1975, pp. 129–202.
15. Munro, H. N.: General aspect of the regulation of protein metabolism by diet and by hormones. *In* Munro, H. N., and Allison, J. B. (eds.): Mammalian Protein Metabolism. Vol. 1. New York, Academic Press, 1964, pp. 381–481.
16. Prince, A. M., Szmuness, W., Manu, M. K., et al.: Hepatitis B "immune" globulin: Effectiveness in prevention of dialysis-associated hepatitis. N. Engl. J. Med., *293*:1063–1067, 1975.
17. Reid, P. R., and Thompson, W. L.: The clinical use of dopamine in the treatment of shock. John Hopkins Med. J., *137*:276–279, 1975.
18. Robson, J. S.: Acute renal failure. *In* Walker, W. F., and Taylor, D. E. (eds.): Intensive Care. Edinburgh, Churchill Livingstone, 1975, pp. 144–159.
19. Salzman, E. W.: Hemostatic disturbance and thrombosis. *In* Skillman, J. J. (ed.): Intensive Care. Boston, Little, Brown & Co., 1975, pp. 387–416.
20. Shafer, A. W., and Hampton, J. W.: The hematologic system. *In* Papper, S. (ed.): Medical Care of the Surgical Patient. Boston, Little, Brown & Co., 1976, pp. 123–146.
21. Sherry, S.: Editorial: Low-dose heparin prophylaxis for postoperative venous thromboembolism. N. Engl. J. Med., *293*:6, 1975.
22. Shoemaker, W. C.: Pathophysiology of shock. *In* Walker, W. F., and Taylor, D. E. (eds.): Intensive Care. Edinburgh, Churchill Livingstone, 1975.
23. Skillman, J. J.: Disturbance of body fluids, ions and acid-balance. *In* Skillman, J. J. (ed.): Intensive Care. Boston, Little, Brown & Co., 1975, pp. 63–127.
24. Skillman, J. J.: Respiratory insufficiency. *In* Skillman, J. J. (ed.): Intensive Care. Boston, Little, Brown & Co., 1975, pp. 513–528.
25. Thompson, W. L., Johnson, A. D., and Maddery, W. L.: Diazepam and paraldehyde for treatment of severe delirium tremens. Ann. Intern. Med., *82*:175, 1975.
26. Walker, J. E., Wells, R. E., and Merrill, E. W.: Heat and water exchange in the respiratory tract. Am. J. Med., *30*:259, 1961.
27. Wells, J. D., and Hall, W. D.: The Liver. *In* Papper, S. (ed.): Medical Care of the Surgical Patient. Boston, Little, Brown & Co., 1976, pp. 183–194.

# BLOOD VESSEL COMPLICATIONS

5

*John J. Conley*

## PREOPERATIVE PROPHYLAXIS

A thorough knowledge of all of the factors that could lead to hemorrhage is essential in prophylaxis. In the preoperative phase, a history relating to blood dyscrasia, excessive bruising, previous hemorrhages, cardiovascular disease, diabetes and degenerative disease of the lungs, liver and kidneys and a previous history of irradiation or the inclusion of irradiation in the postoperative plan can exaggerate the bleeding phenomena that lead directly to serious complications.

Laboratory data leading to the documentation of anemia, infection, abnormal blood components, lowered platelets and prolonged bleeding and clotting time require additional investigation before proceeding with an elective resection. These laboratory and physiological data are evaluated in relation to the extent of the planned resection, since there is a direct correlation between the extent of resection and the volume of bleeding. The patient's blood should be typed and cross-matched to ensure the availability of blood for replacement. In all high-risk cases, attention should be given to the elective protection of the carotid artery system. It is axiomatic that the patient be put in the most favorable physiological condition prior to surgery. The dangers attendant with physiological abnormalities should be reduced to a minimum preoperatively, and the control of any abnormalities during and after surgery should be part of the management program. The consulting internist is often invaluable under these circumstances (see Chapter 4).

## INTRAOPERATIVE BLEEDING

Bleeding is inevitable in every operative procedure. Every healing wound generates an organized blood clot, which is the beginning of the recovery process. In a general sense, bleeding occurs in direct proportion to the size of the operation. The general principles that support the various surgical techniques in the area of the face and neck are standardized within certain flexible perimeters, and even the most experienced surgeon can be surprised and challenged by the bleeding phenomena. Alterations in the surgical anatomy, extensive and composite problems, previous irradiation and surgical intervention pose specific hazards for bleeding. The most experienced surgeon has the best opportunity of coping with this, but he is engaged more frequently with difficult and dangerous situations, and, consequently, there is a higher possibility for an inadvertent complication. On the other hand, the more often any complication occurs, the greater the opportunity for the surgeon to develop expertise in coping with its consequences.

Controlled hypotensive anesthesia will reduce the blood loss and expedite the surgical technique. It can only be applied when the patient is in the proper physical condition. Out of a group of 100 major resections in the area of the head and neck, only 50 of the candidates would qualify. It is a serious mistake to voluntarily use it if the patient's physiological resources are incompetent. Its advantages are that it may reduce the volume of blood loss by half and may shorten the length of the operation by one third.

When patients do not qualify for hypotensive anesthesia, one may use the elevation of the head of the table. The angle of elevation is between 15° and 30° and is monitored with respect to the patient's vital signs. This reduces venous congestion and also reduces small vessel oozing.

The technique of coping with bleeding has several aspects. The rhythm of the technique can progress in many open wounds in the neck by smothering the small bleeders with lap pads and gauze. This is often more effective than attempting to apply individual hemostats to each small bleeder. All vessels named in an anatomical textbook should be identified, clamped and ligated specifically. Smaller vessels are ligated with #3-0 chromic catgut or #4-0 silk. Major blood vessels are ligated with #3-0 silk. The internal jugular vein and carotid artery system are ligated and then transfixed with #3-0 silk. Coagulation is used on all small blood vessels in the wound. Bleeding is effectively controlled as the operation progresses. At the termination of surgery, all wounds are carefully inspected and all bleeding points are controlled to the maximum degree. This may require additional coagulation, ligature or transfixion or packing of an inaccessible recess with Surgicel (an absorbable cellulose gauze). Compliance with these statements is the best prophylaxis against hematoma. In rare instances, bleeding may be inordinate during the operation. In an extreme case, 10 to 20 units of blood may be required for replacement. When the hazards of excessive bleeding transcend the rationale of proceeding with the operation, the wound should be packed and the operation stopped. The surgeon may re-enter a relatively dry wound in a period of seven days for completion of the technique.

A precaution should be taken to avoid placing a hemostat or ligature on a major vessel or a tributary of a major vessel that may contain an atheromatous plaque. The walls of these degenerate vessels are ligated with an adequate stump, a soft square knot and a distal transfixion suture of #2-0 or #3-0 silk. The common sites of atheromatous degeneration are at the carotid bulb and internal carotid artery and in the region of the thyrocervical trunk.

There are specific areas where intraoperative bleeding is excessive owing to the high vascularity of those regions. The pterygoid region represents high and persistent vascularity due to the large and numerous venous connections of the pterygoid plexus. The internal maxillary artery is the principal arterial contributor. Clamping of the pterygoid muscles and their associated venous and arterial structures prior to cutting them gives the best opportunity for control. The surgeon, however, is almost routinely compelled to repeatedly tie off bleeding points and to carry out broad transfixions in this area, using #2-0 or #3-0 chromic catgut on small Mayo needles. Coagulation may be helpful but will not control this type of bleeding. In some instances, bleeding persists in spite of all technical efforts, and, under these circumstances, the bleeding areas are packed with Surgicel. The area of the temporal bone is laced with large and important vascular structures. The internal carotid artery passes through it anteriorly, the sigmoid blood sinus posteriorly, the jugular bulb inferiorly and the superior and inferior petrosal blood sinuses medially. Special attention is given to maintaining the integrity of the internal carotid artery, but the other proximal blood sinuses are frequently involved in resections in this area. Bleeding is controlled by general packing and tamponade. This is accomplished by gauze strip packing, cotton rolls or pledgets, Surgicel or temporal or sternocleidomastoid muscle transposition. The internal jugular vein and transverse sigmoid sinus may be transfixed with #2-0 silk after an appropriate amount of bone has been removed to permit the dura to be transfixed. There is one set of pharyngeal veins at the level of the upper section of the thyroid cartilage draining the pharynx and another connecting set associated with the hypoglossal nerve at this level that require special identification and ligature. There are multiple intravenous connections at this site and they must be handled on an individual basis in order to prevent injury to the hypoglossal or superior laryngeal nerves. They are ligated with #3-0 silk. The area of the thyrocervical trunk in the root of the neck may prove troublesome. The thyroid, transverse scapula and cervical branches from this vessel require individualization and specific ligature

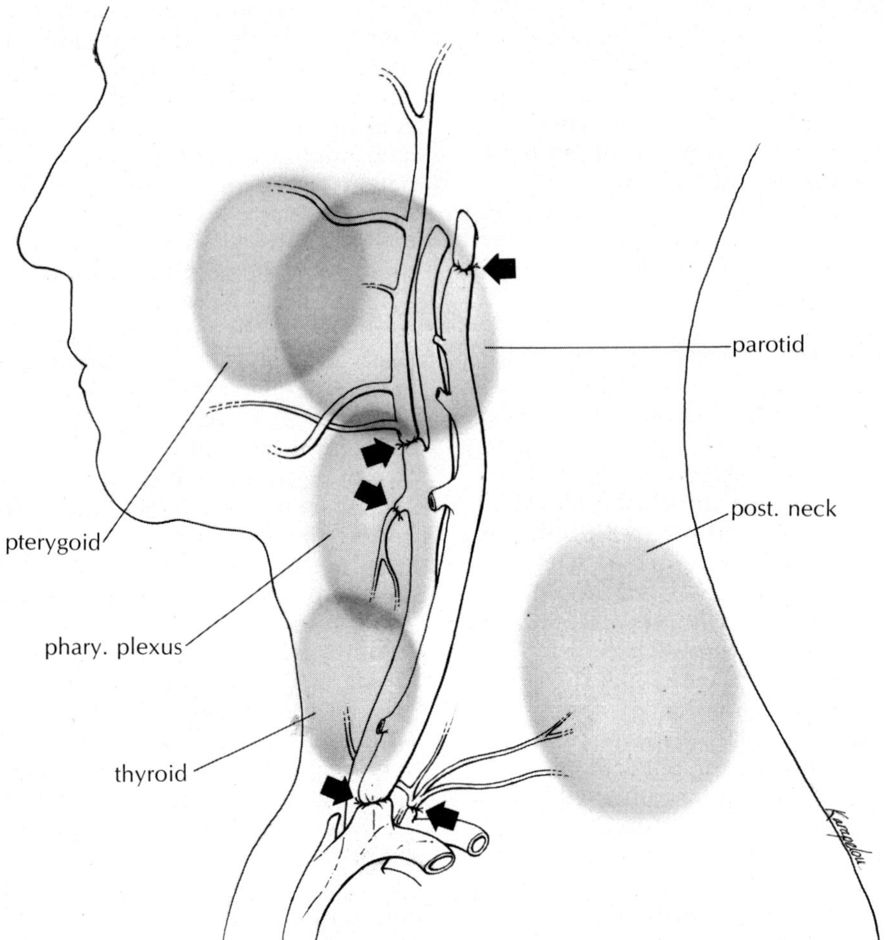


**Figure 5–1** Regions of high vascular concentration subject to bleeding.

with # 3-0 silk. Additional precautions must be taken if there is atheromatous disease in the major vessels at this site.

## Highly Vascularized Neoplasms

There are specific neoplasms in the area of the head and neck that are recognized to be exceptionally bloody.

### *Juvenile Nasopharnygeal Angiofibroma*

The pertinent features of this rare tumor that lead to complications are its inaccessibility, its tendency to bleed profusely and its high recurrence rate. Over 90 per cent occur in teen-age males. The original treatment of this tumor consisted of evulsion through the nasopharynx, which was always bloody and usually consisted of a gross subtotal resection with a high recurrence rate. The use of radiotherapy has been found to be effective in many instances, but the late pernicious effects of dryness, arrested local development and possible osteomyelitis and, in some instances, its role as an etiologic factor in the production of cancer have greatly curtailed its use.

This tumor has been known to bleed excessively from a biopsy performed in an office. This is due to a deficiency in the contractile properties of its blood vessels. When this tumor is suspected clinically in a teenage male, a careful study by carotid angiography is indicated. This will identify the essential feeder vessels, which are primarily derivatives of the internal maxillary artery; the size, position and occult extensions of the tumor; and its involvement with such contiguous structures as the orbit, the base of the skull and the sinuses. The subtraction modification of angiography will aid in the identification of the more subtle extensions. This study may be pathognomonic and eliminate the necessity for open biopsy. When open biopsy is indicated, it should be done in the operating theatre. Preoperative trial use of steroids, stilbestrol and combinations of hormones has not eliminated the necessity for surgical intervention.

The surgical approach through the palate is adequate for tumors that are localized over the sphenoid. The reuse of this approach for recurrences, however, may result in permanent perforation of the palate. Lateral rhinotomy affords a more adequate exposure and the possibility of coping with extensions into the sinuses, orbit, buccal region and infratemporal space. The majority of these tumors lead into the pterygoid region, which contributes to excessive bleeding as the tumor is being isolated and mobilized. There is also persistent bleeding from any laceration or tearing of the tumor itself. Attempts at ligation or transfixion of these bleeding points frequently cause additional bleeding. They are better controlled by surgical packing.

Once the perimeter and the extensions of the tumor have been mobilized and isolated, it can be removed from its origin in the tendons and muscles at the base of the sphenoids or in the region of the pterygoid process. Bleeding is increased at that precise moment, and the anesthesiologist should be advised accordingly so that he may maintain an adequate blood volume. Once the tumor has been removed, excessive bleeding diminishes and may be easily controlled with gauze packing. One to 3000 cc. of blood may be required for replacement.

If surgical removal is contraindicated or rejected, one may consider the selective em-

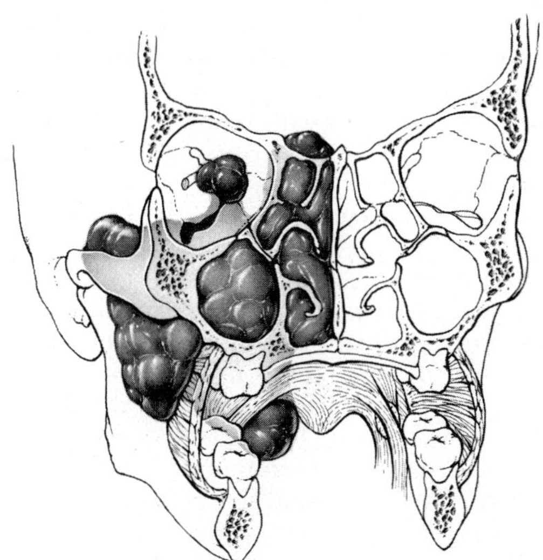

**Figure 5–2** Large juvenile nasopharyngeal angiofibroma extending into the orbit, sinuses, infratemporal area, nasopharynx and pterygoids.

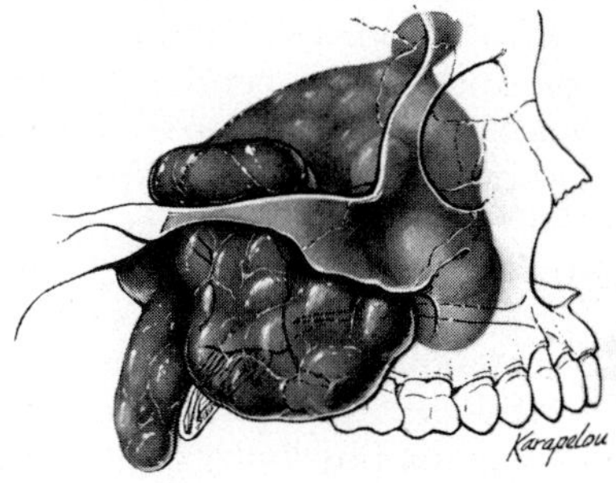

bolization of this neoplasm. Considerable improvement has been made in the area of embolization over the past 10 years. Luessenhop and his associates (1962)[5] first introduced the concept of embolization of arteriovenous malformations with radiopaque Silastic (polymeric silicone) spheres in 1962. Much of the original work was done on intracranial arteriovenous malformations, and then the concept was gradually adapted to other vascular abnormalities.[1, 2, 3, 4, 6, 7, 8] The prime investigations were associated with inaccessible vascular lesions located in the spinal cord and brain and then dealt with highly vascularized tumors.

The technique has proved effective as a palliative tool, as an adjunct to surgery and as a treatment unto itself. It may be associated with neurologic complications in about 5 per cent of the cases. This evolution has progressed from the use of embolic muscle, Gelfoam (absorbable gelatin sponge) and silicone spheres to the use of silicone glue.[3] The basic concept was to regionalize the embolic phenomenon and its ramifications in the neoplasm, thus reducing its size, cellular content and vascular system. In certain instances, embolization may be used as the total method of treatment or in conjunction with surgery, which is carried out within one week so as to precede any attempt at revascularization of the neoplasm.

This technique was not devoid of accidents; the embolic material occasionally escaped into the brain, with resultant hemiplegia, partial blindness or death. The incidence of complications with this technique still remains at about 5 per cent, even though elaborate preparations are taken to prevent the escape of the emboli. The selective injection of silicone glue has eliminated some of these hazards. The glue solidifies in the neoplasm, thus reducing its mass and bleeding capabilities.

Pletcher, Dedo, Newton and Norman (1975)[7] reported on the preoperative embolization of juvenile angiofibroma with Gelfoam. They compared 16 patients who had not been embolized preoperatively with 7 cases who had had preoperative embolization and documented a significant reduction in bleeding and ease of surgical excision in the embolized cases. Although they had no neurologic complications, they caution against the possibility of entering the central nervous system by reflux or misplacement of the catheter or aberrant vascular channels.

The complications and sequelae of juvenile nasopharyngeal angiofibroma occur in the region of the base of the skull and at the apex of the orbit. Blindness, meningitis, cerebrospinal fluid leak and exsanguination may be associated with extensive tumors. Special attention is therefore paid to the optic system, the dura and the bleeding potential. The incidence of local recurrence is approximately 30 per cent. Fortunately, most of these recurrences appear in the nasopharynx and are limited in growth and extension. They should be observed for growth determination. If they are stabilized, small and asymptomatic, they may continue to be observed. If they show a tendency to increase in size, they should be either operated on again or treated with cryosurgery. It is fortuitous that, in an exceptional instance, these tumors may undergo spontaneous regression as the teen-age male approaches maturity.

### *Paragangliomas*

This rare group of chemodectomas is characterized by a high vascular pattern and intimate association with the major regional blood vessels. The carotid body tumor is associated with the carotid bulb and internal and external carotid arteries. It is also associated with the vagus, hypoglossal, glossopharyngeal and, to a lesser extent, spinal accessory and sympathetic chain. Those chemodectomas arising at the base of the skull and in the region of the middle ear are associated, primarily, with the jugular bulb. Since the base of the skull is involved, the facial, auditory, spinal accessory, vagus, glossopharyngeal and hypoglossal nerves may be involved. They may also compromise the internal carotid artery. All of these tumors are composed of a very rich arcade of interlacing blood vessels and, in many instances, are surrounded by a vast interlacing network of vessels. All of these factors are conducive to excessive bleeding.

A carotid arteriogram reveals the size, shape and extent of these neoplasms and their relationship to the great vessels. Angiography may be pathognomonic for this

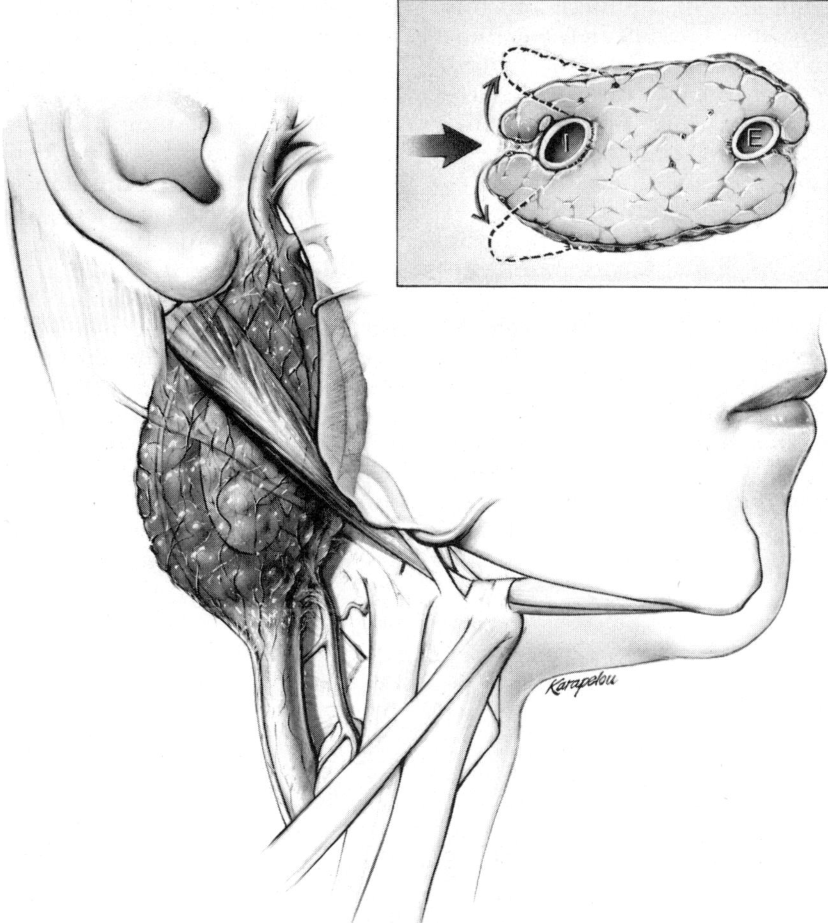


**Figure 5–3** Large carotid body tumor extending to the base of the skull.

neoplasm and, in the vast majority of instances, has replaced open biopsy. Indeed, attempts to remove or biopsy these neoplasms are often fraught with severe hemorrhage, necessitating carotid ligation in some instances and risking death. These tumors receive their blood supply primarily from the external carotid artery and thyrocervical trunk.

There are two main aspects to the surgical approach to these neoplasms. The overriding consideration is the preservation of the carotid artery system, and the secondary consideration is the maintenance of blood volume. The paragangliomas in the neck consist of carotid body tumors, glomus jugulare and chemodectomas associated with the external carotid artery frequently present in the nasopharynx. An approach through a lateral neck incision encounters the rich interlacing network of arteries and veins about the periphery of the tumor. These vessels are selectively ligated. The tumor is specifically identified as a brownish-red, bulging mass at the level of the carotid bifurcation. It is intimately attached to the adventitia. The plane of dissection on these tumors is between the adventitia and the media. They are approached over the lateral portion of the internal carotid artery, where they are the thinnest, thus permitting this thin margin of closure to be split, opened and delicately peeled from the vessel. The ascending pharyngeal artery enters this neoplasm just above the internal aspect of the bifurcation of the bulb. Care must be taken that it is not ripped from the carotid bulb. The external carotid artery is transfixed at the level of the bulb, and this latter vessel is used as a handle in the manipulation of the neoplasm.

Fifteen per cent of these cases have preoperative paresis of one of the cranial nerves. Eighty-five per cent of these cases have a cranial nerve enmeshed in the neoplasm. Special care is therefore required to dissect these neoplasms carefully from the vagus, hypoglossal, spinal accessory and superior laryngeal nerves as the dissection progresses. The internal jugular vein is usually preserved.

The carotid artery system is secured throughout this technique by identification and mobilization inferiorly. An untied tape is placed above it. If there is an inadvertent cut in the vessel, the vessel is temporarily compressed in its proximal and distal portions, and the rent is repaired by direct approximation with #4-0 arterial silk. The operation then progresses. If the internal carotid artery is compromised by the neoplasm, and this is recognized preoperatively, one would hesitate to proceed with an elective surgical procedure. If one did proceed under these circumstances, owing to the pernicious behavior of the neoplasm, then reconstitution of the vessel would be considered as part of the operative technique. If the internal carotid artery is inadvertently destroyed during the operation, every effort should be made to rehabilitate it by patching, vein grafting or the substitution of a dacron prosthesis.

The nerves at the base of the skull are in serious jeopardy in glomus jugulare. These tumors may enter the foramina at the base of the skull, compress the internal carotid artery and internal jugular veins at this high

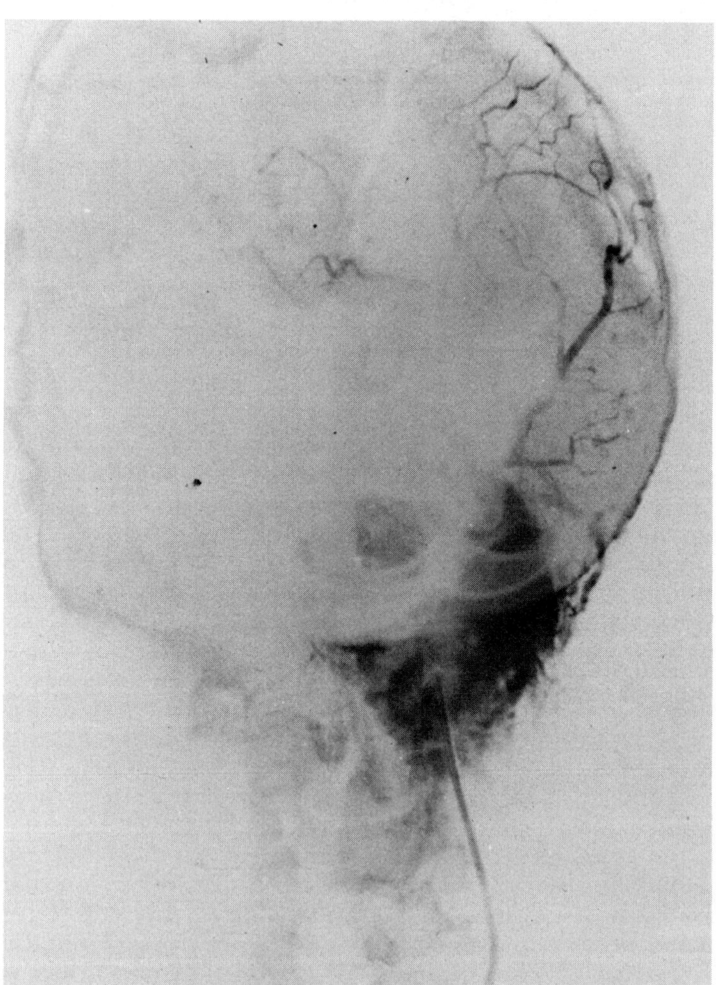

**Figure 5–4** Extremely vascular carotid body tumor at the base of the skull.

level and compromise the vagus nerve. Some of these neoplasms are relatively inaccessible and may require lysis of the hypoglossal nerve and digastric muscle and even osteotomy of the ascending ramus of the mandible for adequate exposure. These structures are routinely repaired at the termination of the resection. Injury to or resection of the vagus nerve at this high level usually prohibits reapproximation or autogenous nerve grafting. All of these patients have hoarseness and marked difficulty in swallowing postoperatively. They must be nourished with a nasogastric feeding tube for an interval of three to four weeks. Swallowing gradually improves over a period of 12 months but never becomes normal.

Chemodectomas arising in the middle ear are usually detected in an early phase owing to the symptoms produced in the ear. Small glomus tympanicus and glomus jugulare tumors confined to the middle ear are removed by microsurgical technique with a minimum of complications or sequelae. As these tumors enlarge, however, facial nerve paralysis, deafness and labyrinthine signs may enter the picture. Chemodectomas arising in the area of the petrous bone and at the base of the skull may attain a very large size before being recognized. Involvement of the IX, X, XI and XII cranial nerves is frequently present prior to the operation. The patient may also have preoperative deafness and facial paralysis. Tumors of this magnitude in this position have frequently entered the cranial cavity and are only rarely amenable to monobloc resection. The combination of an otologic surgeon with a neurosurgeon offers the best chance for the removal of these tumors along the base of the skull. The complications include cerebrospinal fluid leak, extensive hemorrhage, herniation of the brain, permanent disability to cranial nerves and extended morbidity. Many of these tumors are therefore treated palliatively by irradiation, selective blood vessel obliteration, decompression, silicone glue injection and gross subtotal resection.

### *Nonencapsulated Hemangiomas and Lymphangiomas*

Small lesions in this category do not present sequelae or complications since they are usually handled expeditiously by simple excision. Large nonencapsulated hemangiomas and lymphangiomas may have serious complications and sequelae. They are capable of distorting and destroying large portions of the ear, eyelid, nose and cheek and of causing grotesque swellings about the lips, tongue, parotid gland and face. Fortunately, the vast majority of hemangiomas have a limited growth span and undergo some type of spontaneous regression before the age of 2 or 3 years.[26] They have been assisted in this pattern of regression by injections of sclerosing agents,[22] application of dry ice and, more recently, by the administration of prednisone. Although these tumors have proved to be quite sensitive to irradiation, the late, pernicious effects of this modality have almost eliminated its applicability except in heroic problems.

When the tumor has regressed spontaneously or as a result of prednisone treatment, there frequently are sequelae, consisting of discoloration of the skin or regional deformity. The majority of these cases require multiple-stage reconstructive operations ex-

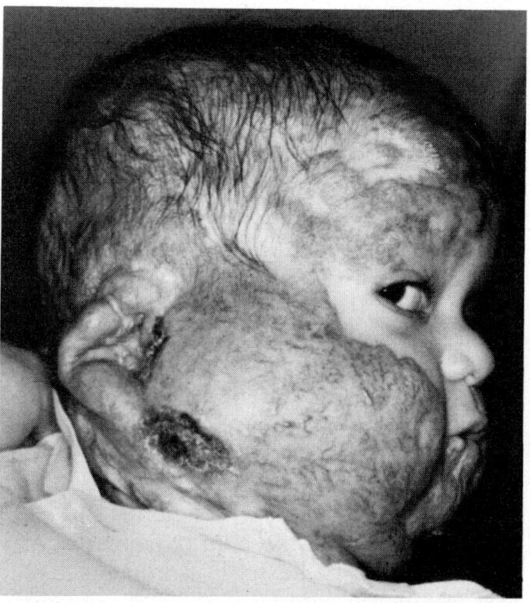

**Figure 5–5** A 6-month-old baby presents with a massive capillary and cavernous hemangioma involving the face and neck. He is beginning to undergo spontaneous resolution. Fortunately, it has not affected the oral cavity, pharynx or larynx. It has already caused great deformity about the ears. There is no surgical or radiation therapy that is indicated on this lesion at this time. At a later date, multiple reconstructions will be carried out.

tending over a period of years. Surgical resection should never create a greater defect than the neoplasm represents. The treatment is therefore usually conservative. As a rule, it consists of a subtotal resection of the residuum of the neoplasm with preservation of the physiognomy and function. Operative bleeding is the primary complication in resection of these large tumors. It is best controlled by packs, pressure, selective ligation of feeder vessels and then minute attention to the smaller bleeding points. Innumerable ligatures, transfixions and cauterizations are employed. There are always some residual swelling, scar contraction, regional paresis and functional deficiencies, which are natural sequelae to the management of these difficult problems.

Lister (1938),[16] Wallace (1953)[26] and Bowers, Graham and Tomlinson (1960)[4] have described the natural history of the strawberry nevus and other types of hemangiomas and have emphasized the overriding consideration for conservative treatment, since a large percentage of these nevi will improve or disappear spontaneously within the first two years of life. A variety of treatments have come into vogue for the management of these problems, such as the use of irradiation, surgical excision, injection of sclerosing agents and cautery. None of the treatments were completely satisfactory because of the unpredictable nature of the hemangioma, the resultant mutilation and scarring and the late pernicious effects from irradiation. Brooks (1931)[5] attempted to embolize arteriovenous fistulae with muscle fragments. These fragments measured approximately 0.5 cm. in diameter and were injected through the feeder vessel into the abnormality. This frequently causes some temporary improvement.

Luessenhop (1969),[21] Cunningham and Paletta (1970)[7] and Bennett and Zook (1972)[3] further reported on the use of embolization with muscle fragments and were successful in attaining improvement, usually temporary. Luessenhop and his associates (1960, 1962 and 1965)[18,19,20] continued with his investigations on embolization. Hilal, Michelsen and Mount,[14] in 1970, and Hilal, Michelsen and Driller, in 1969 and 1974,[13] added significantly to the embolization technique by introducing Gelfoam, Silastic spheres and, more recently, liquid silicone. Hilal and Michelsen (1975)[12] consider liquid silicone to be an improvement over previous modalities. Doppman, Zapol and Pierce (1971)[9] reported on the use of the silicone rubber preparation in 1971.[8] Other workers have used arterial embolization in a selective manner to control gastrointestinal hemorrhage,[1] epistaxis[25] and inoperable and inaccessible tumors[17] in the intracranial cavity, the base of the skull and the spinal cord.[15,23] Bean and his colleagues (1949)[2] documented the vascular changes of the skin during pregnancy. Zarem and Edgerton (1966)[27] reported on the induced resolution of cavernous hemangioma following prednisone therapy with a review of 11 patients who have responded favorably. Edgerton (1975)[10] made a comprehensive review of the treatment of hemangiomas and further emphasized the favorable results obtained with prednisone. Brown, Neerhout and Fonkalsrud (1972),[6] Fost and Esterly (1968)[11] and Prensky and Gado (1973)[24] have reported on the value of steroids in the management of hemangiomas in infancy and childhood. Although the effects of steroid treatment can be profound, and even unpredictable, it certainly is worthy of consideration in all large hemangiomas about the head and neck—those interfering with breathing, swallowing and talking, those that threaten a vital organ such as the eye, ear, nose or lips and those that are increasing in size—before considering any other type of management program.

### *Arteriovenous Fistulae*

Arteriovenous fistulae are divided into three categories. They may be congenital or associated with penetrating wounds, or, only very rarely, they may follow a surgical resection. The congenital variety consists of literally hundreds of small communications. Those that occur in the area of the head and neck rarely produce heart failure in the early stages. Although they are not common in the head and neck, they can afflict the scalp, lip and jaw. They form a firm, pulsatile mass, usually with a thrill or bruit. The complications encountered in treating the congenital variety of arteriovenous fistulae are excessive bleeding, disfigurement and local recurrence. Arteriography is helpful in establishing the number and position of the small shunting vascular system but will not reveal the dormant or inactive shunts about the periphery of the active lesion. There is no satisfactory treatment for this lesion unless one is fortunate enough to encompass the entire system in a surgical resection. Ordinarily, none of these lesions can be cured by a simple excisional technique. The vessels implicated in the area of the head and neck are the temporal artery and vein in the scalp, the alveolar artery and vein in the mandible, branches of the external maxillary artery and vein in the maxilla, branches of the internal maxillary artery and vein in the pterygoid and mesenteric regions, and branches of the external maxillary artery and vein in the upper neck, and, in the superior portion of the neck, the internal carotid artery and the internal jugular vein. The magnitude of this problem in certain instances equals that of the circulatory system itself at that site. Ligations of the feeder vessels, embolization, irradiation, silicone glue and gross subtotal resection often end with gradual, slow, local recurrence.[1, 2, 3, 4, 5, 6, 7, 8, 9, 10, 11, 12]

Hilal and Michelsen (1975)[5] have made a special report on 27 patients with extra-axial vascular tumors and arteriovenous malformations about the head and neck. Their total vascular experience is with more than 100 cases involving the brain and spinal cord. They describe their therapeutic and percutaneous embolization management programs for vascular tumors of the base of the skull, arteriovenous abnormalities in the subtemporal area and pterygoid fossa, vascular lesions of the vertebral bodies, glomus jugulare tumors and dural arteriovenous malformations. They state that Gelfoam as an embolization material was not completely satisfactory. Silastic spheres offered an improvement in the technique, but now they have developed a liquid Silastic material that is heavily impregnated with tantalum powder for x-ray visualization. This Silastic adhesive technique has proved to be very satisfactory in their hands and may be used as a therapeutic technique unto itself or in preparation for surgical resection. These workers report 2 per cent serious complications in 100 consecutive cases. They reported a 78 per cent improvement in the embolization of their extra-axial vascular lesions and emphasize the importance of long-term follow-up, since many of these cases have a tendency to recur.

Traumatic arteriovenous fistulae are usually the result of a penetrating wound in the neck or in the deep part of the face. They are identified on angiography as a single or double communication between the regional vessels. When they are accessible, they are best treated by surgical excision, which usually affords a cure without any complication. If they are associated with the common or internal carotid artery system, it is important that the integrity of this system be maintained. It is striking that arteriovenous fistulae are extremely rare as a complication of head and neck surgery. This is due to the fact that most of the major surgery in this area is extirpative, and the vessels that might ordinarily participate in an arteriovenous connection are either resected or ligated along with their supporting soft tissue structures. This author has seen only two in his professional career, one in the pterygoid region between the branches of the internal maxillary artery and the pterygoid plexus and one high in the neck after a radical neck dissection between the internal jugular vein and the internal carotid artery. The one in the pterygoid area was managed successfully by excision; the one in the neck was managed by separation of the vessels with higher ligation of the internal jugular vein and preservation of the continuity of the internal carotid artery.

It is obvious that the bleeding phenomenon can present a serious and complex problem under certain circumstances in surgery of the head and neck. It is essential to monitor the blood loss accurately, to maintain close contact with the anesthesiologist, to estimate the quantity of blood loss by measurement in the suction bottle and to quantitate the amount of blood on the sponges and lap pads. Blood replacement is an ongoing and inevitable factor. Intraoperative evaluation of the hematocrit readings and blood gas levels will add specific information in an area that often has wide variations when estimating the blood loss.

## Aneurysm

Aneurysm formation as a complication following head and neck surgery is extremely rare. This author has seen only three in 3000 extensive resections. They were associated with vessel trauma, low-grade infection or intrinsic atheromatous abnormality. In the first of these cases, a large pseudoaneurysm developed two months after radical neck dissection. A large metastatic papillary adenocarcinoma of the thyroid had encircled the lower portion of the common carotid artery. The neoplasm was split and carefully dissected from the wall of the vessel by including the adventitia in the specimen. The wound was treated with suction drainage and one of the tubes was in contact with the artery at this site. There was a low-grade infection in the wound that lasted five days. Angiogram confirmed the diagnosis of pseudoaneurysm of the common carotid artery two months later. The surgeon performed a bypass on this vessel connecting the subclavian artery with the upper portion of the internal carotid and then ligating the aneurysm. The patient has been living free of tumor and free of complications for 16 years. In this instance, one must assume that the pseudoaneurysm was secondary to the stripping of adventitia from the artery, low-grade infection and pressure from a suction tube. Another patient (age 69) developed a pseudoaneurysm of the internal carotid artery one month after a radical neck dissection. It was associated with atheromatous disease and diagnosed by angiography. The internal carotid artery was kinked and redundant in length, with the result that the pseudoaneurysm could be excised and the vessel directly anastomosed. There was no complication. In the third case, an aneurysm was formed after temporal bone resection in an extremely thin-walled internal carotid artery at its entrance into the petrous bone. The aneurysm occurred one month after surgery; it was small and ruptured while under observation. This complication was managed with compression of the vessel by packing. There were no sequelae.

The predisposing factors to aneurysm, therefore, are the stripping a major vessel of its adventitia, and consequently its blood supply; the presence of degenerative disease in the vessel; the presence of infection or postirradiation atrophy of the vessel wall; and the effects of suction tube pressure directly over the major artery. The essential difference between a pseudoaneurysm and a carotid artery "blow-out" is that the bleeding in a pseudoaneurysm is entrapped and contained within the supportive tissues of a vessel wall and a carotid artery "blow-out" occurs when the surface of the artery is exposed to the open by a necrotizing process.

Beall and his coworkers (1962)[1] document the rarity of aneurysm of the common carotid artery with only seven cases appearing out of 2300 operations performed for peripheral aneurysm. Raphael and associates (1963)[7] reported 13 aneurysms involving the common carotid artery from a group of 221 peripheral aneurysms that were traumatic in origin. Carotid artery aneurysms following the subintimal injection of the contrast media in carotid angiography were reported by Braunstein[2] in 1964. Aneurysms after rehabilitation of the carotid artery and endarterectomy and with the use of a prosthesis and venous patches also have been reported to occur by Buscaglia, Moore and Hall (1969),[3] Cohen, Brief and Mathewson (1970),[4] McLaughlin and Flotte (1969),[5] Rainer and his colleagues (1968),[6] Raphael and his associates (1963)[7] and Smith and his coworkers (1970).[8]

The carotid aneurysm usually presents as an asymptomatic pulsatile lateral cervical mass with a systolic bruit. Aneurysm in all of the tributaries of the carotid artery system, including the intracranial branches, should be accurately documented by angiography. Because of the critical importance and unpredictability associated with carotid artery ligation, it is desirable to maintain flow continuity by an internal or external shunt, when it is possible.

## POSTOPERATIVE BLEEDING

### Immediately Postoperative Bleeding

There are three principal causes for excessive bleeding in the immediate postoperative phase. (1) Generalized oozing can produce over 500 cc. of blood in a hemovac system within a period of several hours. There is interference with contractility and in the clotting mechanism, permitting blood to escape from vessels that would ordinarily have formed a clot. The specific causes are

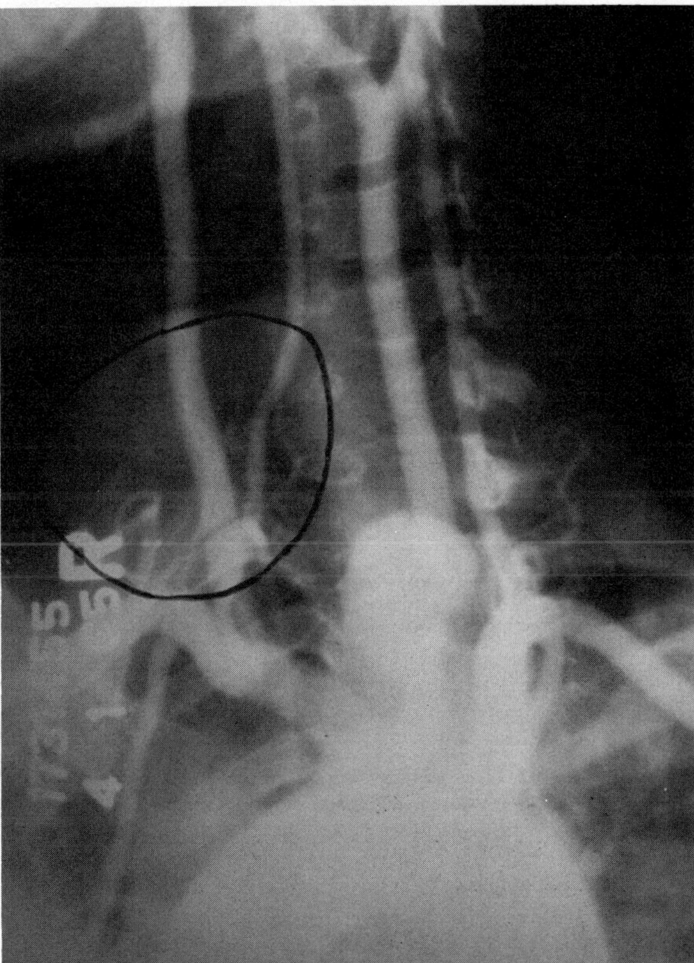

**Figure 5–6** Pseudoaneurysm of the common carotid artery secondary to pressure of hemovac tube and minimal infection. This was corrected by prosthetic bypass from subclavial to internal carotid artery by Dr. Frederick McAllister.

rarely identified, but it may be associated with chronic hypoxia, small changes in the pH of the blood and chemical changes affecting contractility and blood clotting. All of these factors are checked, and any abnormalities are corrected. The condition of the neck flap, the airway system and the vital signs are evaluated. All of these patients require blood replacement. The patient is returned to the operating room and reanesthetized and the wound is opened. The clots are removed and the wound is watched; all discernible bleeding points are coagulated or ligated. When the bleeding is rapid and sudden, it indicates either (2) reopening of an untied major vessel or (3) the slippage of a ligature on a major vessel. The patient may lose 500 cc. of blood in five minutes. Supportive and corrective measures are begun on an emergency basis in the operating room. The major arteries that may contribute to this bleeding are the external carotid artery or any of its primary branches, the superior thyroid artery and the thyrocervical trunk. The venous structures that may be involved are the ligatures on the internal jugular vein, the veins in the pterygoid and pharyngeal plexus and, to a lesser extent, the posterior facial and external jugular veins. If one is fortunate enough to find the bleeding vessel, it is immediately clamped and ligated or transfixed with # 3-0 silk. If suturing is impractical, such as at the base of the skull or in the temporal bone region, tamponade with surgical gauze, dental rolls or regional muscle flaps may prove to be lifesaving. The gauze packs are not removed for one to two weeks. The patient is placed on broad-spectrum antibiotics. Surgicel has a specific applicability to bleeding in areas that are inaccessible from a technical point of view.

These measures are lifesaving measures to be carried out expeditiously, with all emphasis on the immediate control of bleeding by whatever means are necessary, supported by adequate blood replacement and the maintenance of an adequate airway, either by endotracheal intubation or tracheostomy. These factors have priority over all other situations. Some of these wounds may be reclosed immediately. Others will have to remain partially open until the packing is removed, the bleeding condition stabilized and the general condition of the patient justifies wound management.

### Delayed Postoperative Bleeding

The principal complications causing delayed postoperative bleeding relate to wound infection, fistula formation and radiation necrosis. It may occur from one to six weeks following the operation. It is not to be expected in cases in which the mucosa and skin repair heal per primam. The bleeding usually comes from a specific vessel, the most common being the carotid artery. The common site on the carotid artery is in the region of the bulb or at the ligated external carotid artery stump. When there is a major "blow-out," the patient may exsanguinate within a matter of a few minutes or may die either from asphyxiation caused by aspirating the blood or from shock with cardiac arrest. All of these cases are preceded by localized infection associated with fistula formation, ulceration and radiation necrosis. There is an extension of the ulcerating and necrotizing process until the wall of a major vessel is destroyed, with a resulting hemorrhage. Any of the branches of the external carotid artery may be involved in this process, along with the superior thyroid artery and thyrocervical trunk. The veins are much less likely to rupture because the internal and external jugular veins have been resected; they do not maintain as high an intraluminal pressure as arteries, and they are more prone to thrombus formation. Specific complications predisposing to postoperative hemorrhage are discussed in the sections dealing with those complications (fistula and carotid artery ligation). Suffice it to say that this triad of wound complications is the primary cause of delayed postoperative bleeding, and one can never feel secure against the possibility of bleeding that presents these complications.

## DEEP VEIN THROMBOSIS

Head and neck surgery may be associated with deep vein thrombosis and its potential complications of localized pain, edema, claudication, restricted movement and pulmonary emboli. Graham and his colleagues (1976)[1] reviewed 103 patients undergoing head and neck and ear operations by screening them for deep vein thrombosis using I-125-labelled fibrinogen. Sixteen per cent of the patients undergoing head and neck operations developed deep vein thrombosis. In addition to this, 12 per cent of these patients developed thrombosis in the leg when the ankle vein was used as a drip site. It is obvious from the data that deep vein thrombosis is more common in head and neck surgery than has been suspected, since most of it is asymptomatic. Joffe (1976)[2] investigated the incidence of deep vein thrombosis in otolaryngologic surgery, using clinical examination, I-125-labelled fibrinogen and the Doppler ultrasound technique to establish the diagnosis. He found 11 per cent with deep vein thrombosis. The incidence in general surgical patients varies from 28 to 51 per cent. The lower incidence in head and neck cases is likely to be associated with minimal tissue trauma and early mobilization. Elderly people with vascular disease, diabetes or hypertension should have an active prophylactic program, using elastic stockings, elevation, active and passive movement in bed postoperatively and early ambulation. Symptomatic venous thrombosis associated with embolus is an extremely serious situation requiring medical evaluation for anticoagulation (see Chapter 4).

## Bibliography

#### Juvenile Nasopharyngeal Angiofibroma

1. Baum, S., and Nusbaum, M.: Control of gastrointestinal hemorrhage by selective mesenteric arterial infusion of vasopressin. Radiology, *98*:497–505, 1971.

2. Doppman, J. L., Zapol, W., and Pierce, J.: Transcatheter embolization with a silicone rubber preparation. Invest. Radiol., *6*:304–309, 1971.
3. Hilal, S. K., and Michelsen, J. W.: Therapeutic percutaneous embolization for extra-axial vascular lesions of the head, neck, and spine. J. Neurosurg., *43*:275–287, 1975.
4. Kricheff, I. I., Madayag, M., and Braunstein, P.: Transfemoral catheter embolization of cerebral and posterior fossa arteriovenous malformations. Radiology, *103*:107–111, 1972.
5. Luessenhop, A. J., Gibbs, M., and Velasquez, A. C.: Cerebrovascular response to emboli. Observations in patients with arteriovenous malformations. Arch. Neurol., 7:264–274, 1962.
6. Luessenhop, A. J., Kachmann, R., Jr., Shevlin, W., et al.: Clinical evaluation of artificial embolization in the management of large cerebral arteriovenous malformations. J. Neurosurg., *23*:400–417, 1965.
7. Pletcher, J. D., Dedo, H. H., Newton, T. H., and Norman, D.: Preoperative embolization of juvenile angiofibromas of the nasopharynx. Ann. Otol. Rhinol. Laryngol., *84*:740–746, 1975.
8. Sokoloff, J., Wickbom, I., McDonald, D., et al.: Therapeutic percutaneous embolization in intractable epistaxis. Radiology, *111*:285–287, 1974.

### Nonencapsulated Hemangiomas and Lymphangiomas

1. Baum, S., and Nusbaum, M.: Control of gastrointestinal hemorrhage by selective mesenteric arterial infusion of Vasopressin. Radiology, *98*:497, 1971.
2. Bean, W. D., Cogswell, R., Dexter, M., and Embick, J. F.: Vascular changes of the skin during pregnancy. Surg. Gynecol. Obstet., *88*:739, 1949.
3. Bennett, J. E., and Zook, E. G.: Treatment of arteriovenous fistulas in cavernous hemangiomas of face by muscle embolization. Plast. Reconstr. Surg., *50*:84, 1972.
4. Bowers, R. E., Graham, E. A., and Tomlinson, K. M.: The natural history of the strawberry nevus. A.M.A. Arch. Derm., *82*:667, 1960.
5. Brooks, B.: Discussion of Noland and Taylor. Trans. South. Surg. Assoc., *43*:176, 1931.
6. Brown, S. H., Neerhout, R. C., and Fonkalsrud, E. W.: Prednisone therapy in the management of large hemangiomas in infants and children. Surgery, *71*:168, 1972.
7. Cunningham, D. S., and Paletta, F. X.: Control of arteriovenous fistulae in massive facial hemangioma by muscle emboli. Plast. Reconstr. Surg., *46*:305, 1970.
8. Doppman, J. L., DiChiro, G., and Ommaya, A. K.: Percutaneous embolization of spinal cord arteriovenous malformations. J. Neurosurg., *34*:48, 1971.
9. Doppman, J. L., Zapol, W., and Pierce, J.: Transcatheter embolization with a silicone rubber preparation. Invest. Radiol., *6*:304, 1971.
10. Edgerton, M. T.: The treatment of hemangiomas: With special reference to the role of steroid therapy. Ann. Surg., *183*:516, 1976.
11. Fost, N. C., and Esterly, N. B.: Successful treatment of juvenile hemangiomas with Prednisone. J. Pediatr., *72*:351, 1968.
12. Hilal, S. K., and Michelsen, J. W.: Therapeutic percutaneous embolization for extra-axial vascular lesions of the head, neck, and spine. J. Neurosurg., *43*:275, 1975.
13. Hilal, S. K., Michelsen, J. W., and Driller, J.: Magnetically guided devices for vascular exploration and treatment. Radiology, *113*:529, 1974.
14. Hilal, S. K., Michelsen, J. W., and Mount, L.: Therapeutic embolizations of vascular malformations of the external carotid circulations: Clinical and experimental results. Presented at the 11th Symposium Neuroradiologicum, Göteborg, Sweden, 1970.
15. Kricheff, I. I., Madayag, M., and Braunstein, P.: Transfemoral catheter embolization of cerebral and posterior fossa arteriovenous malformations. Radiology, *103*:107, 1972.
16. Lister, W. A.: Natural history of strawberry nevi. Lancet, *1*:1428, 1938.
17. Longacre, J. J., Benton, C., and Unterthiner, R. A.: Treatment of facial hemangioma by intravascular embolization with silicone spheres. Case report. Plast. Reconstr. Surg., *50*:618, 1972.
18. Luessenhop, A. J., Gibbs, M., and Velasquez, A. C.: Cerebrovascular response to emboli. Observations in patients with arteriovenous malformations. Arch. Neurol., 7:264, 1962.
19. Luessenhop, A. J., Kachmann, R., Jr., and Shevlin, W.: Clinical evaluation of artificial embolization in the management of large cerebral arteriovenous malformations. J. Neurosurg., *23*:400, 1965.
20. Luessenhop, A. J., and Spence, W. T.: Artificial embolization of the cerebral arteries. Report of use in a case of arteriovenous malformation. J.A.M.A., *172*:1153, 1960.
21. Luessenhop, A. J.: Artificial embolization for cerebral arteriovenous malformations. Prog. Neurosurg., *3*:320, 1969.
22. Morgan, J. F.: Use of Sodium Morrhuate in the management of hemangiomas. J. Oral Surg., *32*:363, 1974.
23. Olcott, C., IV, Newton, T. H., Stoney, R. J., and Ehrenfeld, W. K.: Intra-arterial embolization in the management of arteriovenous malformations. Surgery, *79*:3, 1976.
24. Prensky, A. L., and Gado, M.: Angiographic resolution of a neonatal intracranial cavernous hemangioma coincident with steroid therapy. J. Neurosurg., *39*:99, 1973.
25. Sokoloff, J., Wickbom, I., and McDonald, D.: Therapeutic percutaneous embolization in intractable epistaxis. Radiology, *111*:285, 1974.
26. Wallace, H. J.: The conservative treatment of hemangiomatous nevi. Br. J. Plast. Surg., *6*:78, 1953.
27. Zarem, H. A., and Edgerton, M. T.: Induced resolution of cavernous hemagiomas following Prednisone therapy. Plast. Reconstr. Surg., *39*:76, 1967.

### Arteriovenous Fistulae

1. Bookstein, J. J., and Goldstein, H. M.: Selective arterial embolization in the management of post-biopsied arterio-venous fistula. Radiology, *109*:535, 1973.
2. Coursley, G., Ivins, J. C., and Barker, N. W.: Analysis of 69 cases of congenital arteriovenous fistulas. Angiology, 7:201, 1956.
3. Doppman, J. L., DiChiro, G., and Ommaya, A. K.: Spinal cord arteriovenous fistulas. J. Neurosurg., *34*:48, 1971.
4. Gomes, M. M. R., and Bernatz, P. E.: A review of arteriovenous fistulas. Mayo Clin. Proc., *45*:81, 1971.
5. Hilal, S. K., and Michelsen, J. W.: Therapeutic percutaneous embolization for extra-axial lesions in the head, neck and spine. J. Neurosurg. *43*:275–287, 1975.
6. Luessenhop, A. J., Kachmann, R., and Shevlin, W.: Artificial embolization of cerebral arteriovenous malformations. J. Neurosurg., *23*:400, 1965.
7. Meaney, T. F., and Chicatelli, P. D.: Transcatheter clot embolization for arteriovenous fistula. Cleve. Clin. Q., *41*:33, 1974.
8. Moberg, P. J., Dahlgran, S., and Raabe, N.: Arteriovenous fistula: A case report. Acta Obstet. Gynecol. Scand., *53*:91, 1974.
9. Olcott, C., IV., Newton, T. H., Stoney, R. J., and Ehrenfeld, W. K.: Intra-arterial embolization in the management of arteriovenous malformations. Surgery, *79*:3, 1976.
10. Rizk, G. K., Atallah, N. K., and Dridl, G. I.: Arteriovenous fistula managed by catheter embolization. Br. J. Radiol., *46*:222, 1973.
11. Stewart, I. A., and Gardner, A. M. N.: Endarterial electro-coagulation in treating arteriovenous fistulas. Br. J. Surg., *59*:146, 1972.
12. Szilagyi, D. E., Elliott, J. P., and De Russo, F. J.: Congenital peripheral arteriovenous fistula. Surgery, *57*:61, 1965.

### Aneurysms

1. Beall, A. C., Jr., Crawford, E. S., Cooley, D. A., et al.: Extracranial aneurysms of the carotid artery: Report of seven cases. Postgrad. Med., *32*:93, 1962.
2. Braunstein, H.: Dissecting aneurysm of the carotid artery and aorta after carotid angiography. Am. Heart J., *67*:545, 1964.
3. Buscaglia, L. C., Moore, W. S., and Hall, A.: False aneurysm after carotid endarterectomy. J.A.M.A., *209*:1529, 1969.
4. Cohen, A., Brief, D., and Mathewson, C.: Carotid artery injuries. An analysis of 85 cases. Am. J. Surg., *120*:210, 1970.
5. McLaughlin, J. S., and Flotte, T.: Carotid artery surgery. Am. Surg., *35*:676, 1969.
6. Rainer, W. G., Guillen, J. O., Bloomquist, C. D., et al.: Carotid artery surgery. Morbidity and mortality in 257 operations. Am. J. Surg., *116*:678, 1968.
7. Raphael, H. A., Bernatz, P. E., Spittell, J. A., Jr., et al.: Cervical carotid aneurysms: Treatment by excision and restoration of arterial continuity. Am. J. Surg., *105*:771, 1963.
8. Smith, R. B., Perdue, G. D., Collier, R. H., et al.: Postoperative false aneurysms of the carotid artery. Am. Surg., *36*:335, 1970.

### Deep Vein Thrombosis

1. Graham, J. M., Robinson, J. M., Ashcroft, P. B., and Glennie, R.: Deep vein thrombosis in ear, nose and throat surgery. J. Laryngol. Otol., *90*:427, 1976.
2. Joffe, S. N.: Postoperative deep vein thrombosis in otolaryngologic surgery. Arch. Otolaryngol., *102*:135, 1976.

# 6

# CAROTID ARTERY LIGATION

*John J. Conley*

## PREDISPOSING FACTORS IN HIGH-RISK CASES

There is a group of patients identified as "high risk" because the complications in this group are more than twice those in the individual with normal physiology. Any patient with primary or secondary anemia or a hemoglobin below 10 should be studied and prepared before proceeding with the major operation. Diabetics are prone to wound infection, poor healing quality and vascular disease; in many instances, there is difficulty in controlling the diabetes. Individuals with cardiovascular disease and chronic obstructive pulmonary disease present the surgeon with the most fundamental of both medical and surgical complications. Any patient who has lost more than 20 pounds and any patient with a total protein below 3.5 does not heal well and is prone to complications. In a series of 19 patients in this category, conducted by this author, 53 per cent developed complications postoperatively and 22 per cent developed cutaneous fistulas.

### Scope of Operation

There is a direct relationship between the type and scope of the resection and the incidence of complications. The uncomplicated neck dissection is rarely associated with a carotid artery complication. Once the surgery is augmented into a composite resection, however, the incidence of fistula formation, wound infection and slough of the flaps dramatically increases.[1, 3, 4] Individuals with extensive atheromatous disease in the main artery system or its tributaries are more prone to artery and wound complications because of relative ischemia. When it is necessary to remove the adventitia from the vessel wall because of the proximity of tumor or because of scar formation, one deprives the vessel of a major part of its nourishment and places it in an unfavorable situation if it must combat other wound complications. Another escalation in serious complications occurs when bilateral radical neck surgery is done simultaneously. This has been emphasized by Moore and Smith (1951),[6] Morfit (1952),[7] Perzik (1952)[8] and Moore and Frazell (1964).[5] Frazell and Moore (1961)[2] present data to support a significantly reduced rate of complications when bilateral radical neck surgery is done in stages. Stell (1969)[9] reported a 3 per cent carotid artery rupture in 280 patients undergoing major surgery in the head and neck. Seventy-seven per cent of these died, and 11 per cent had neurologic complications. He felt that the two overriding predisposing factors were preoperative irradiation and chronic upper respiratory infection. In order to protect the artery, Stell advocates the double horizontal incision, staging the procedures, transposition of the carotid arteries, protection of the carotid artery with muscle flaps and free grafts. Eighty-eight per cent of his patients who ruptured had a prodromal bleed within 48 hours of the rupture. This ominous sign indicates elective ligation in most instances. He also emphasizes the importance of an adequate airway and immediate blood replacement.

### Irradiation

Preoperative irradiation is one of the most serious handicaps one can impose on a healing wound. A dosage over 4000 rads, large portals involving the entire cervical area and a postirradiation time interval of over six months are the specific hazardous features associated with irradiation. This combination of factors frequently permits fibrosis, atrophy and endarteritis to reach a critical level.

Ninety-two per cent of the 12 cases of carotid artery rupture analyzed by Dibbel, Gowen and Shedd (1965)[4] were patients who had had previous irradiation. Curutchet, Terz and Lawrence (1972),[3] in their evaluation of the autogenous dermal graft for carotid artery protection, reported a 6 per cent incidence of carotid artery rupture. It escalated from 1 per cent in patients undergoing primary resection and unilateral neck dissection to 11 per cent in those having bilateral neck dissection following irradiation. MacComb (1968)[9] reported a 3.2 per cent incidence of carotid artery rupture in a review of 1498 radical neck dissections. Ketcham and Hoye (1965)[7] reported an incidence of 3 per cent of carotid artery hemorrhage associated with head and neck surgery in a review of 574 operations in the head and neck. Marchetta, Sako and Maxwell (1967)[10] made a significant comparison between the complications associated with irradiated wounds and those in nonirradiated wounds. Eighty-three patients who had had irradiation presented a 7 per cent incidence of carotid artery rupture and a 43 per cent incidence of wound complications, in comparison with no carotid artery ruptures and a 22 per cent incidence of wound complications in a comparable group of patients who had not had irradiation. Krause, Smith and McCabe (1972)[8] have documented the increased complications associated with irradiation of oral and pharyngeal neoplasms. Gall, Sessions and Ogura (1977)[5] made a comprehensive retrospective report on complications in major surgery in the head and neck. There was a 49 per cent incidence of complications in the inferior hypopharynx, 42 per cent in the superior hypopharynx, 28 per cent in the supraglottic and 24 per cent in the glottic. The complications they analyzed were wound infection, wound necrosis, salivary fistula, hematoma and carotid artery rupture in the immediate and postoperative stages. They did not find any correlation between complications and low-dose preoperative irradiation, various forms of carotid artery protection and surgical pathological findings, including the size of the tumor, the number of positive nodes and the cellular characteristics. Their incidence of carotid artery blow-outs ranged from 2.5 per cent for well-differentiated tumors to 5.2 per cent for the undifferentiated ones. Only 1 per cent of their patients developed a wound infection, 4.2 per cent developed a wound slough, 3.9 per cent had an incidence of salivary fistula, 1 per cent showed hematoma and 3.5 per cent had carotid artery rupture. The operative mortality was 1 per cent, the incidence of those dying of delayed complications was 2.1 per cent.

Yarington, Yonkers and Beddoe (1973)[14] reported on the complications of radical neck dissection and stated that irradiation had a higher incidence of complications in direct proportion to the amount of irradiation used. They had a mortality rate of 1.3 per cent. The total incidence of complications was 25 per cent, and the incidence of major complications was 17 per cent. Joseph and Shumrick (1972)[6] stated they had a 77 per cent incidence of dehiscence, 73 per cent incidence of fistula and 50 per cent incidence of carotid artery necrosis in 105 patients who had unplanned preoperative irradiation. When the irradiation was planned, the incidence of dehiscence fell to 35 per cent, that of fistula dropped to 23 per cent and that of carotid artery necrosis fell to 2 per cent. In nonirradiated cases, there was a 15 per cent incidence of dehiscence, 8 per cent incidence of fistula and no carotid artery necrosis. Sellars and Jarvis (1975)[12] reported a 0.7 per cent operative mortality rate and a 24 per cent incidence of complications in a group of 147 laryngectomies, 49 of which had radical neck dissections. Fifteen per cent developed a pharyngeal fistula, 8 per cent had a chylous leak and 1 per cent had a carotid artery rupture. Briant (1975)[2] emphasized the increased danger of complication in individuals who had had a high dose of radiation, unplanned, uncoordinated and at intervals exceeding six months prior to the operation. He also emphasized that when neck dissection was added to the resection of the primary cancer, the incidence of fistulization was markedly increased. He felt that in irradiated wounds the nasogastric tube should probably not be removed before three weeks after surgery.

Bresson, Rasmussen and Rasmussen (1974)[1] found fistulas in 65 per cent of 148 patients undergoing total laryngectomy. The incidence of fistulization in individuals who have had conventional irradiation doubles that in nonirradiated cases and quadruples if they have had high-voltage irradiation. Streptococcus and staphylococcus were the predominant organisms in infections associated with early fistulization, whereas *Pseudomonas* and *Escherichia coli* were the common pathogens after an interval of 48 hours. He found *Pseudomonas* to be the most common organism infecting these wounds and recommended adequate drainage, .25 per cent acetic acid soaks and dressing changes three times a day. He also found hematoma and great vessel rupture to be relatively common in the early trials in these cases. Fistulization was of primary concern, and that has been remedied by creating a controlled externalized stoma. Tucker and his associates (1974)[13] reported no major wound complications in the 33 patients who were treated with high-dose irradiation in the region of the tonsils and then subjected to major surgical excision. Their minor complication rate was 3 per cent. They felt that close cooperation between the radiotherapy and surgical services contributed to their favorable results. Robins and his coworkers (1975)[11] reported no major complications in 24 cases of head and neck cancer undergoing first high-dose irradiation and then radical resection in a period of from four to six weeks. There was a 21 per cent incidence of minor complications, however, consisting of peristomal tissue loss, seroma, infection, fistula and hematoma.

### Fistulas

The presence of a cutaneous fistula may critically affect the carotid artery and lead to either elective ligation or exsanguinating hemorrhage. If the fistula is small in size and situated anteriorly in the neck, it will not ordinarily affect the carotid artery. If it is large and positioned in the lateral portion of the neck, in proximity to the carotid artery, one must recognize the threat to the carotid artery. The vast majority of fistulas appear within the first two weeks, and this is almost always due to leakage of saliva at the pharyngeal closure. These factors will be discussed in Chapter 7.

### Wound Infection

Wound infection is a serious threat to the carotid artery. Primary infection is fortunately not common, but secondary infection resulting from mucosal stitch dehiscence or necrosis of the tissue flaps is a serious biologic problem. The majority of these wounds are contaminated by *Staphylococcus aureus,* but one must be prepared to combat *Pseudomonas, Escherichia coli,* pathogenic organisms from the mouth and anaerobic organisms (see Chapters 7 and 8).

### Incisions

Flap necrosis is a direct threat to the carotid artery system. The lines of incision may be of critical importance in borderline flaps. Extensive undermining certainly deprives the flap of a certain amount of nourishment. Thinning of the flap may interfere with the subdermal vascular arcade, with an extensive loss of tissue as a result. Ischemia may also result from irradiation fibrosis, wound infection, hematoma, nutritional depletion, tension on the flap during closure and external pressure. There is hardly an imaginary line in the cervical area that has not been used as an incision for surgical entry.[1, 2, 3, 4, 5, 6, 7] Horizontal incisions are cosmetically acceptable when they are placed in the natural lines of the neck. They cut across the longitudinal axis of the vessels that penetrate to the dermis and epidermis; however, interconnections are so rich that this is rarely a factor.

Crile (1906)[4] used the "Y" incision in the lateral cervical area and reported his experience with 132 cases. Attie (1957)[1] presented an extended single transverse incision in the neck for the accomplishment of radical neck dissection. MacFee (1960)[5] advocated bilateral horizontal incisions in the cervical area to accomplish neck dissection. Martin (1953)[6] favored the double "Y" incision with the inferior one inverted. This provided excellent exposure, but localized necrosis did occur in some instances, just at the connection of the flaps in the upper "Y" over the carotid artery bulb, and this increased the risk of carotid artery complication. Moore (1967)[7] presented modifications of these incisions that were applicable in bilateral neck dissection. Bocca and Pignataro (1967)[2] presented their vast experience with a combination of various types of cervical flaps.

The most secure incision in the lateral cervical area is the single vertical incision that runs in harmony with the ascending vessels. The next most secure is the horizontal cervical incision. When modifications of these are adapted for the purposes of exposure or extension into the oropharynx or oral cavity, one must always calculate a reduction in the available nutrient vessels. This reduction in nourishment is exaggerated by the extent of the undermining, the level of the undermining, the nutrient factors of the flap and the presence of postirradiation fibrosis and atrophy. It is therefore imperative to assess all of these features in the design of any flap intended to protect the carotid artery system.

## PROPHYLAXIS

The most significant factor in the preservation of the carotid artery system is an awareness and applicability of all of the prophylactic features that will enhance its integrity. The patient should be in the optimal physiological condition. If he has had intensive irradiation with severe skin changes in the cervical area, it may be wiser not to depend on this skin to heal per primam and to use a regional flap. The incisions and undermining of the cervical flaps should not go beyond the flap's capacity to survive. The mucous membrane should be closed without tension, be everted and be spit tight. Individual sutures or a running horizontal mattress (Connell) of #3-0 chromic catgut is adequate for the uncomplicated wound. If there is a tendency for the mucosa to invert, an everting mattress suture should be placed to accomplish eversion. These may be alternated with the standard individual suture. In high-risk patients who have had irradiation, #3-0 Vicryl or #3-0 Dexon is substituted for the catgut in order to have extended approximation. Every attempt is made to have at least a double layer closure. When this is not possible in a high-risk case, one should consider either a reinforcement suture line with a regional muscle flap or the creation of a pharyngostome.

### Dermal Grafts

Dermal skin grafts should be considered in all cases in which there is a high risk of carotid artery exposure. These grafts can be procured readily from the lateral thigh by elevating an epidermal layer that is ten to twelve thousandths of an inch in thickness and by removing a layer of dermis beneath this, which is 16 to 18 thousandths of an inch in thickness. The epidermal layer is then approximated to the thigh and the dermal graft is transposed into the neck. If a fistula forms, the flaps become necrotic and the artery becomes exposed with the dermal graft over it, then it will epithelialize in most instances and protect the artery from ulceration. If the wound heals without complication, the dermal graft becomes a fibrous blanket over the artery. It is somewhat paradoxical that one expects the dermal graft, which is a free transplant, to survive in an infected and devitalized tissue bed and thus afford protection, whereas the wound itself does not have the capability of duplicating this performance. These grafts have, however, proved themselves effective in many instances.

Loewe (1913),[2] Peer and Paddock (1937)[3] and Thompson (1960)[8] did the original investigative work on buried dermal and epidermal grafts. They established the original practicality of their use.

Corso and Gerald (1963)[1] first reported on the use of buried dermis for the protection of carotid arteries. They experienced no carotid artery ruptures in 28 instances of breakdown of the wound with exposure of the graft. Reed and Harrington (1969)[6] reported on 12 instances of skin breakdown with exposure of the dermal graft and no complicating hemorrhage in irradiated patients. These grafts epithelialized. Reed and Halsey (1974)[5] reported on 100 major resections in the head and neck area; 93 per cent of the patients had previous irradiation. The graft became exposed in 16 per cent of the cases, and there were no carotid artery hemorrhages. The exposed dermal grafts epithelialized. They emphasized the advantages of the dermal graft and the necessity for covering the entire carotid artery system with it.

Smithdeal, Corso and Strong (1974)[7] reported the protection of the carotid arteries in a group of 69 patients who had had preoperative irradiation and compared them with a group of 82 patients who had had preoperative irradiation but no carotid artery protection. They state that there is a definite advantage in those individuals who had the autogenous graft and that this was particularly striking in individuals who had postoperative wound breakdown with exposure of the carotid arteries and salivary fistula. Reed, Zafra and Ghyselen (1968)[4] proved the capacity of dermal grafts for self-epithelialization and their value as protection to a threatened carotid artery system.

### Regional Flaps

There has been full recognition of the necessity of protecting the carotid artery in the development of regional muscle and skin flaps. Even a pedicle of omentum has been used. These flaps represent the surgeon's awareness of the dangers of exposing the carotid artery and his response in attempting to protect it.

Mutter (1842)[8] presented a posterior cervical flap that was used to relieve burn deformities. Berger (1889)[1] developed a posterior cervical flap for repair of neck deformities. Zovickian (1957)[12] emphasized the importance of using a posterior cervical flap in dressing a large pharyngeal wound, in protecting the carotid artery and in repairing the pharyngeal fistula. Staley (1961)[11] was one of the early investigators to advocate muscle flaps. Conley (1960, 1962)[2, 3] presented a variety of regional flaps and muscles to protect the carotid artery. Corso, Gerold and Frazell (1963)[4] advocated a posterior shoulder flap to close large salivary fistulas. Schweitzer (1962)[10] introduced the use of the levator scapula muscle to protect the artery. Jaques (1971)[7] described the trapezius muscle flap. Goldsmith and Beattie (1970)[6] transposed a pedicle of omentum into the neck to protect the artery. Foote and Chandler (1972)[5] used fascia lata, and Schuler and Horton (1976)[9] de-epithelialized a lateral cervical flap that was based superiorly.

The levator scapula muscle may be rotated or inverted after an inferior release in order to cover the major portion of the carotid artery. It is conveniently positioned and is the most popular muscle flap. Its transposition increases shoulder drop, however. It will not reach from the base of the skull to the clavicle. The indication for using this muscle flap would be primarily in a high-risk case, and special care must be taken to preserve its blood supply before transposition. Usually, the factors that threaten wound healing also threaten this muscle. The sternocleidomastoid muscle is ideal for carotid artery protection, but, unfortunately, it is usually removed in the classic composite resection. A large portion of the trapezius muscle may be moved over to protect the artery. Certain portions of the artery may be buried in the constrictor muscles of the pharynx, but care must be exercised that the artery is not constricted.

The greatest advance in reducing the necessity for carotid artery ligation is the establishment of a planned pharyngostome. When the ablation is extensive, when the irradiation is excessive, when the tissue remaining in the wound is minimal and when the general physiological condition of the patient is borderline, one should develop a controlled pharyngostome in every instance at the time of the primary operation. This will reduce the incidence of carotid artery exposure and hemorrhage more than any other single technique or concept. When the regional tissue is absent or unsatisfactory for coverage, a regional flap should be substituted.

Food ingestion should be delayed for two to three weeks in all high-risk cases. This is evaluated by the condition of the flaps, which may represent thickening, hyperemia, edema and cellulitis. If the hemovac is draining saliva or purulent material, feeding is delayed.

## CAROTID ARTERY LIGATION

The most critical blood vessels in the head and neck are the common and the internal carotid arteries. There is little question about the dangers of electively ligating these vessels or of encountering a rupture. Watson and Silverstone (1939)[23] reported that the first recorded carotid artery ligation by Andre Paré in France in 1552 resulted in hemiplegia and aphasia. Since that time, numerous authors have attested to the dangers of ligation. Moore and Baker (1955)[17] reported 17 per cent mortality and 28 per cent neurologic complications in elective ligation. Gandhi and Oppenheimer (1962)[12] had 20 per cent complications; Ketcham and Hoye (1965)[14] had no complications in elective ligation in 16 patients. Shumrick (1973)[20] reported only 16 per cent neurologic complications and no deaths from elective ligation.

Ligation of these vessels after rupture and exsanguination is understandably a much more serious situation because of the effects of hypovolemia and hypotension on the cerebral and vital organ circulation. Moore, Karlan and Sigler (1969)[18] reported 50 per cent mortality following ligation after hemorrhage; Shumrick (1973)[20] reported a mortality of 61 per cent and 25 per cent neurologic complications with ligation following rupture of the carotid arteries. Only 16 per cent of his patients survived the ordeal without complication. Martinez and his coworkers (1975)[15] have reported a 14 per cent mortality in seven patients undergoing elective ligation and resection of the carotid artery and a 64 per cent mortality in 11 patients who had compulsory ligation because of an acute rupture. Conley and associates (1952, 1953, 1957, 1959, 1962 and 1964)[2–10] have written extensively regarding the hazards of ligation and measures to evaluate and reduce these hazards and emphasize the essentiality of this vessel.

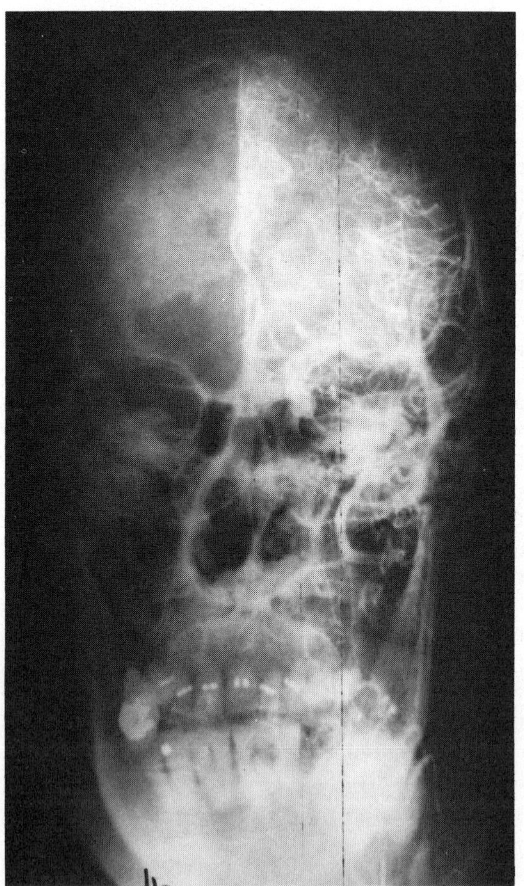

**Figure 6–1** Angiogram demonstrating failure of cross circulation. This case would certainly have a complication from carotid artery ligation.

These data support the fact that the preservation of these arteries is paramount to any surgical program on the neck. This objective is attained in great measure by recognizing the complications that can compromise these vessels and taking all of the precautions to prevent them. When carotid artery hemorrhage is threatened, it is to the patient's advantage to have this vessel ligated electively under normal physiological circumstances.

## Elective Ligation

The adventitia of the carotid artery is an effective barrier against invasion by cancer. One can frequently find a delicate plane between the desmoplastic reaction in the adventitia and the media of the artery. If the wall of the artery is invaded by cancer, the surgeon must decide whether to resect the artery or to leave cancer on its wall. The consequences of carotid artery resection will be discussed later in this chapter and must be weighted against the possibility of helping the patient against the malignant biologic process and the dangers attendant with carotid artery surgery.

When the cervical flaps become necrotic, when the carotid artery becomes exposed in the presence of a fistula and when the patient is in a postoperative status, the pos-

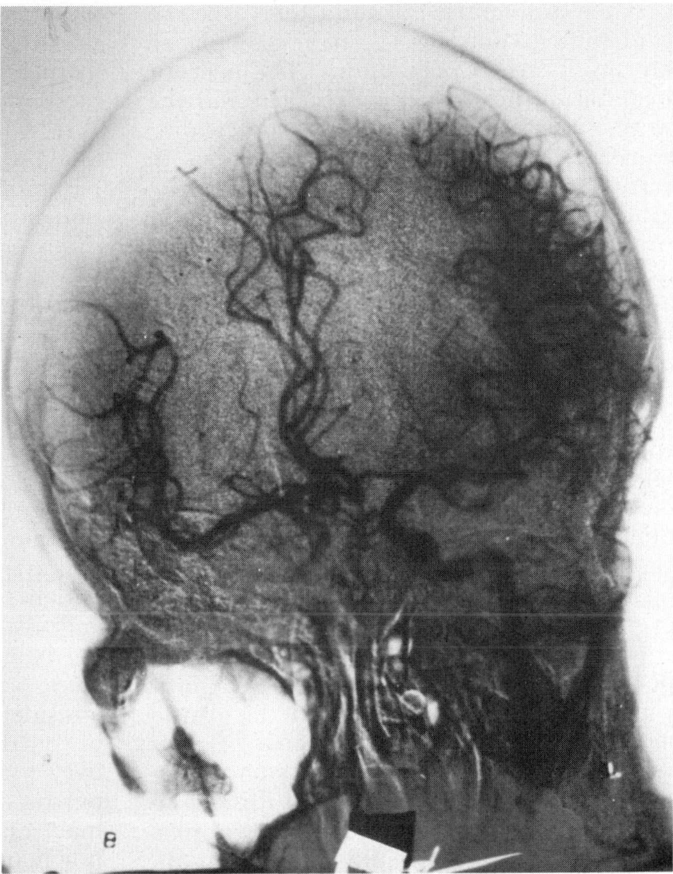

**Figure 6–2** Angiogram showing abundant vascular crossover via the anterior and posterior cerebral communicating vessels. This patient tolerated carotid artery ligation without complication.

sibilities of that artery rupturing are significant. As the necrotic slough extends into the artery itself, there is a formation of a "blister" on the wall of the artery that may be discernible clinically. The "blister" is a clear area where the wall of the artery has been critically thinned and the blood flow in the internal part of the lumen is discernible. There is no question but that this vessel will rupture.

Another significant clinical sign is slight bleeding or oozing from the wall of the artery or from one of its tributaries during this necrotic process. This preliminary bleeding, which is often disregarded, may be the precursor of artery rupture, and these vessels should also be considered for elective ligation. The incidence of carotid artery rupture in the presence of wound complications varies from 1 to 10 per cent. The threat depends upon the etiologic factors causing the exposure of the artery, upon the ability of the wound to limit and reverse the process of necrosis and also upon the response to local treatment.

Pertinent to elective ligation of the carotid artery is the exposure of the artery in a healthy portion of the neck not affected by the necrotic slough. The superior and inferior segments of the artery are prepared for ligation. Enough of the artery is removed to permit secure burying of the stumps in healthy tissue. The artery is ligated with # 2-0 silk and then transfixed distal to this ligation with # 3-0 silk.

The necrotic process that caused the destruction of the artery concomitantly destroys tissue flaps, mucous membrane and intervening tissue. Under these circumstances, it is necessary to transpose a regional flap over the stumps of the artery. Simultaneously with this, all of the necrotic tissue in the lateral portion of the neck is debrided and the same regional flap is used to resurface the entire lateral neck in an externalization procedure.

When a potential carotid artery problem is identified clinically, the patient is placed on carotid artery precautions. The necrotic material in the wound is debrided and the wound is externalized and protected against constant contamination by saliva with rerouting or the application of a split skin graft. The best method of preparing these wounds for skin grafting is the application of saline dressings every hour. This not only assists in cleaning the wound but also permits determination of whether the wound is improving or deteriorating. If the wound is deteriorating, the staff should be alerted, a special nurse should be in attendance and specifically instructed concerning the possibility of hemorrhage, four units of matched blood should be in the icebox on the patient's floor and a set of surgical instruments should be at the patient's bedside. Elective ligation will be determined on the basis of events that occur during this regime.

Ketchem and Hoye (1965)[14] reported a 3 per cent incidence of carotid artery hemorrhage in a group of 574 major head and neck operations. The vast majority of their cases had been previously treated with radiotherapy, and they considered this a contributing factor. They advocated appropriate positioning of the skin incisions, protection of all carotid arteries in high-risk cases with muscle flaps and prophylactic antibiotic therapy. Another contributing cause of carotid artery blow-out was direct invasion of the artery by neoplasm. Their anticipation of a possible blow-out, and preparation for it with all members of the nursing and hospital staff, with immediate control of the bleeding and rapid blood replacement prevented any deaths or neurologic complications. This is indeed a remarkable record.

## Emergency Ligation for and Consequences of Carotid Artery Hemorrhage

When this event occurs, firm pressure is applied to the cervical area with anything that is available. The patient is placed in the Trendelenberg position and a large bore needle, #15 to #18, is inserted intravenously immediately or an intravenous catheter is inserted by a cut-down technique. Fluid replacement is begun immediately. Matched blood is ideal, but saline, packed cells, plasma or even "O−" blood may be substituted in dire circumstances. Four to six units of blood may be necessary for replacement.

It is imperative that the airway be adequate and stabilized. The majority of these patients have a tracheostomy tube in position, and this is kept patent by active suction in order to prevent the aspiration of blood, which could lead to asphyxia. It can also be used for ventilatory purposes, since the administration of oxygen is essential. If the patient is not wearing a tracheostomy tube, an oral endotracheal tube should be inserted immediately. It can be converted to a tracheostomy after the crisis is past. Immediate blood replacement, adequate oxygenation and a controlled airway system are of paramount importance. The longer these aids are denied, the greater is the risk to the patient.

Pressure over the bleeding point, which has been applied by the first person on the scene (an attendant, a technician, a nurse or a resident doctor), may prove to be effective in controlling the bleeding. If it is not effective, finger pressure by a knowledgeable person applied at precisely the critical point may solve the problem. If neither packing nor manual pressure controls the bleeding, the vessel should be boldly exposed and clamped. When the patient is in satisfactory condition, he is moved to the operating room for definitive treatment. The stumps of the vessels are exposed back into healthy tissue and ligated and transfixed with #2-0 and #3-0 silk sutures. They are either buried in regional healthy tissue or covered with a healthy regional flap after appropriate debridement. All of these wounds associated with fistula formation are externalized.

It is important to attempt to keep accurate records during this emergent period relating to vital signs, central venous pressure, medications administered, emergency hematocrit, pH, $PO_2$, $PCO_2$ and electrocardiographic tracings, but all of these tests are secondary to the heroic measures necessary for the physical control of bleeding, the maintenance of an adequate airway and fluid replacement.

Moore and Baker (1955)[17] outlined the etiology, hazards and clinical factors relating to shock. Moore, Karlan and Siglar

(1969)[18] presented the factors influencing the safety of carotid artery ligation in 151 cases. Their presentation documented the fact that if a patient went into shock associated with carotid artery ligation his chances of suffering a stroke or dying were doubled. Twenty-three per cent of the patients undergoing elective ligation suffered strokes and 17 per cent died. Fifty per cent of those undergoing compulsory ligation suffered strokes and 38 per cent died. Two patients out of four with bilateral carotid artery ligations survived without complications. Slightly over half of their patients had preoperative irradiation. Of the group undergoing elective ligation, 32 per cent had infection, 22 per cent had a salivary fistula and all of them had necrosis of the vessel wall.

The axion here is that every effort should be made to preserve the integrity of this vessel, and, if its rupture is deemed inevitable, elective ligation is preferable to ligation after exsanguinating hemorrhage.

## Remedial Action

The threat associated with carotid artery ligation could be reduced if there were a preligation test that would determine who could tolerate carotid artery ligation without a complication and who could not. A correlation has been found between the retinal vessels and the carotid artery pressures. Tindall, Dukes and Cupp (1963)[22] reported on this relationship and its applicability to carotid artery surgery. Martinez and his associates (1975)[15] described the development of ophthalmodynamometry. This test evaluates, in a general sense, the competence of the cerebral circulation by evaluating the preoperative changes in the retinal artery upon the temporary ligation of the common carotid artery at a low level in the neck. When this is practical, the surgeon will have information that may indicate high relative safety for elective ligation or a situation in which substitution or rehabilitation of the carotid artery system is mandatory.

When carotid artery resection is anticipated, preoperative angiography of the carotid arteries and vertebral arteries is essential. This graphically demonstrates the character and position of these vessels in the neck and may indicate a dominant vessel. More importantly, it evaluates the competence of the collateral circulation in the brain through the circle of Willis and the anterior and posterior cerebral communicating arteries. When these latter two vessels are minimal in size or congenitally absent, cross-circulation is minimized and a serious catastrophe is probable.

An evaluation of the intracarotid arterial pressure distal to a point of temporary ligation will establish data relative to the collateral pressure produced in the distal portion of the artery. Our experience with this technique indicated that if the pressure in the distal segment fell by more than 50 per cent, elective ligation was extremely hazardous. If it fell by only 30 per cent, the chances of the patient's tolerating ligation were more favorable.

One must further evaluate that in a right-handed individual aphasia may develop from ligation of the left common carotid.

In the final analysis, the surgeon must realize that no test will be a guarantee against mortality and morbidity, regardless of how favorable it might appear. This serious decision in the treatment of cancer in the neck must be weighed against the prognosis, and an elective ligation of the artery following wound complications should be weighed against the possibility that spontaneous rupture may not eventuate.

When this vessel has been ligated, it is absolutely essential that blood volume, blood pressure, aeration, gas exchange and a patent airway be maintained at the optimal functional capacity at all times in the postoperative course. Although a variety of possibilities may present themselves for the reconstitution of the vessel, few are applicable. Partial resections of the artery may be patched with a section of vein. If the upper portion of the vessel contains a significant kink, additional length of 2 or 3 cm. may be attained by straightening the kink, and this may present the possibility for direct anastomosis. The internal carotid artery may be anastomosed with the external carotid artery when the resection is at the level of the bulb or lower. A dacron prosthesis may be considered for total rehabilitation of the vessel. An internal bypass adds security during the interval of repair.

There are certainly times when any attempt at reconstruction of the carotid artery system would be meddlesome and fraught with greater danger than straight ligation.[2, 3, 4] Rehabilitation of the vessel should not be attempted in wounds that are grossly infected. Further relative deterrents are the wounds that have been heavily irradiated and extend into the oral or pharyngeal cavities. These handicaps lead to thrombosis of the graft or prosthesis, secondary hemorrhage, persistent wound infections and rejection.

## Bibliography


### Scope of Operation

1. Boyan, P., and Howland, W.: Blood transfusion: A critical factor in massive transfusion. Anesthesiology, *22*:559, 1961.
2. Frazell, E. L., and Moore, O. S.: Bilateral radical neck dissection performed in stages. Am. J. Surg., *102*:809, 1961.
3. Martin, H., Del Valle, B., Ehrlich, H., and Cohan, W. G.: Neck dissection. Cancer, *4*:441, 1951.
4. Martin, H., and Sugabaker, E. L.: The treatment of cancer of the floor of the mouth. Surg. Gynecol. Obstet., *71*:347, 1940.
5. Moore, O. S., and Frazell, E. L.: Simultaneous bilateral neck dissection. Experience with 151 patients. Am. J. Surg., *107*:565, 1964.
6. Moore, O. S., and Smith, R.: A case of one stage bilateral neck dissection with recovery. Cancer, *4*:1337, 1951.
7. Morfit, H. M.: Simultaneous bilateral radical neck dissection: Total ablation of both internal and external jugular venous systems at one sitting. Surgery, *31*:216, 1952.
8. Perzik, S. L.: Simultaneous bilateral radical neck dissection with recovery: Report of 2 cases. Surgery, *31*:297, 1952.
9. Stell, P. K.: Catastrophic hemorrhage after major neck surgery. Br. J. Surg., *56*:525, 1969.

### Irradiation

1. Bresson, K., Rasmussen, H., and Rasmussen, P. A.: Pharyngo-cutaneous fistulae in totally laryngectomized patients. J. Laryngol. Otol., *88*:835, 1974.
2. Briant, T. D.: Spontaneous pharyngeal fistula and wound infection following laryngectomy. Laryngoscope, *85*:829, 1975.
3. Curutchet, H. P., Terz, J. J., and Lawrence, W., Jr.: The value of the autogenous dermal graft for carotid artery protection. Surgery, *71*:876, 1972.
4. Dibbell, D. G., Gowen, G. F., and Shedd, D. P.: Observations on postoperative carotid hemorrhage. Am. J. Surg., *109*:765, 1965.
5. Gall, A. M., Sessions, D. G., and Ogura, J. H.: Complications following surgery for cancer of the larynx and hypopharynx. Cancer, *39*:624, 1977.
6. Joseph, D. L., and Shumrick, D. L.: Risks of head and neck surgery in previously irradiated patients. Arch. Otolaryngol., *97*:381, 1973.
7. Ketcham, A. S., and Hoye, R. C.: Spontaneous carotid artery hemorrhage after head and neck surgery. Am. J. Surg., *110*:649, 1965.
8. Krause, C. J., Smith, R. G., and McCabe, B. F.: Complications associated with combined therapy of oral and pharyngeal neoplasms. Ann. Otol. Rhinol. Laryngol., *81*:496, 1972.
9. MacComb, W. S.: Mortality from radical neck dissection. Am. J. Surg., *115*:352, 1968.
10. Marchetta, F. A., Sako, K., and Maxwell, W.: Complications after radical head and neck surgery performed through previously irradiated tissues. Am. J. Surg., *114*:835, 1967.
11. Robins, R. E., Budden, M. K., and MacDougall, J. A.: Analysis of mortality and morbidity in 100 composite resections for oral carcinoma. Am. J. Surg., *130*:178–181, 1975.
12. Sellars, S. L., and Jarvis, J. F.: The mortality and morbidity of laryngectomy. S. Afr. Med. J., *50*:428, 1976.
13. Tucker, H. M., Rabuzzi, D. D., Sagerman, R. H., et al.: Prevention of complications of composite resection after high-dose preoperative radiotherapy. Laryngoscope, *84*:933, 1974.
14. Yarington, C. T., Jr., Yonkers, A. J., and Beddoe, G. M.: Radical neck dissection. Mortality and morbidity. Arch. Otolaryngol., *97*:306, 1973.

### Incisions

1. Attie, J. N.: Radical neck dissection via a single transverse incision. Surgery, *41*:498, 1957.
2. Bocca, E., and Pignataro, O.: Radical neck dissection techniques. Ann. Otol. Rhinol. Laryngol., *76*:975, 1967.
3. Conley, J.: Concepts in Head and Neck Surgery. Stuttgart, Georg Thieme Verlag, 1970.
4. Crile, G.: Surgical excision of cancer of the head and neck: 132 cases. J.A.M.A., *47*:1780, 1906.
5. MacFee, W. F.: Neck dissection by transverse incision. Ann. Surg., *151*:279, 1960.
6. Martin, H.: Radical head and neck surgery for cancer. Surg. Clin. North Am., *33*:329, 1953.
7. Moore, O. S.: Bilateral neck dissection. *In* Conley, J. (ed.): Cancer of the Head and Neck. New York, Appleton-Century-Crofts, Inc., 1967, pp. 176–182.

### Dermal Grafts

1. Corso, P. F., and Gerold, F. P.: Use of autogenous dermis for protection of the carotid artery and pharyngeal suture lines in radical head and neck surgery. Surg. Forum, *12*:483, 1961.
2. Loewe, O.: Ueber Haut implantation an Stelle der freien Faszich Plastik. Munch. Med. Wochenschr., *24*:2320, 1913.
3. Peer, L. A., and Paddock, R.: Histologic studies on the fate of deeply implanted dermis grafts. Arch. Surg., *34*:268, 1937.
4. Reed, G. F., Zafra, E., and Ghyselen, A. L.: Self-epithelialization of dermal grafts. Arch. Otolaryngol., *87*:518, 1968.
5. Reed, G. F., and Halsey, W. S.: Protection of the

carotid artery in radical neck dissection. Laryngoscope, *85*:1353, 1975.

6. Reed, G. F., and Harrington, P. C.: Dermal grafts: Clinical experience in head and neck surgery. N.Y. State J. Med., *69*:2563, 1969.
7. Smithdeal, C. D., Corso, P. F., and Strong, E. W.: Dermis grafts for carotid artery protection: Yes or no? A ten-year experience. Am. J. Surg., *128*:373, 1974.
8. Thompson, N.: The subcutaneous dermis graft: A clinical and histological study in man. Plast. Reconstr. Surg., *26*:1, 1960.

**Regional Flaps**

1. Berger, P.: Bull. et. mem. Soc. de chirurgiens Paris, *15*:684, 1889. From Plastic Surgery, John Staige Davis, 1919, P. Blakiston's Son & Company.
2. Conley, J.: Carotid artery protection. Arch. Otolaryngol., *75*:530, 1962.
3. Conley, J.: The use of regional flaps in head and neck surgery. Ann. Otol., *69*:1223, 1960.
4. Corso, P. F., Gerold, F. P., and Frazell, E. L.: The rapid closure of large salivary fistulas by an accelerated shoulder-flap technique. Am. J. Surg., *106*:691, 1963.
5. Foote, P. A., and Chandler, J. R.: Protection of the carotid artery by fascia lata in head and neck surgery. South. Med. J., *65*:1225, 1972.
6. Goldsmith, H. S., and Beattie, E. J., Jr.: Carotid artery protection by pedicled omental wrapping. Surg. Gynecol. Obstr., *130*:57, 1970.
7. Jaques, D. A.: Carotid artery protection by means of a trapezius muscle flap. Am. J. Surg., *122*:744, 1971.
8. Mutter, T. D.: Case of deformity from burns relieved by operation. Am. J. Med. Sci., *4*:66, 1842.
9. Schuler, F. A., III, and Horton, C. E.: A dermal flap for carotid artery protection. Plast. Reconstr. Surg., *58*:694, 1976.
10. Schweitzer, R. J.: Use of muscle flaps for protection of carotid artery after radical neck dissection. Ann. Surg., *156*:811, 1962.
11. Staley, C. J.: A muscle cover for the carotid artery after radical neck dissection. Am. J. Surg., *102*:815, 1961.
12. Zovickian, A.: Pharyngeal fistulas: Repair and prevention. Plast. Reconstr. Surg., *19*:355, 1957.

**Carotid Artery Ligation**

1. Catlin, D.: Carcinoma of the larynx surviving bilateral carotid artery ligation. Ann. Surg., *152*:809, 1960.
2. Conley, J., and Pack, G. T.: Surgical procedure for lessening the hazard of carotid bulb excision. Surgery, *31*:845, 1952.
3. Conley, J.: Carotid artery anastomosis in radical surgery of the head and neck. Trans. Am. Acad. Ophthalmol. Otolaryngol., *56*:910, 1952.
4. Conley, J., and Pack, G. T.: Prevention of cerebral damage after compulsory common or internal carotid artery ligation or excision by ipsilateral anastomosis of external and internal carotid arteries. Surg. Forum, pp. 293–300, 1952.
5. Conley, J., and Pack, G. T.: Prevention of cerebral damage after compulsory common or internal carotid artery ligation or excision by ipsilateral anastomosis of external and internal carotid arteries. *In* Year Book of General Surgery, Philadelphia, W. B. Saunders Co. 1952, pp. 293–300.
6. Conley, J.: Free autogenous vein graft to the internal and common carotid arteries in the treatment of tumors of the neck. Ann. Surg., *137*:205, 1953.
7. Conley, J.: Carotid artery surgery in the treatment of tumors of the neck. Arch. Otolaryngol., *65*:437, 1957.
8. Conley, J., and Pack, G. T.: Procedures for lessening the hazard of carotid bulb excision and carotid artery ligation. *In* Pack, G. T., and Ariel, I. M. (eds.): Treatment of Cancer and Allied Diseases. Vol. 3. 2nd ed. New York, Harper and Row, Publishers (Hoeber), 1959, pp. 608–616.
9. Conley, J.: Carotid artery protection. Arch. Otolaryngol., *75*:530, 1962.
10. Conley, J., Chusid, J. G., and Scheckter, M. M.: Angiography in head and neck surgery. Arch. Surg., *98*:609, 1964.
11. Dibbel, D. G., Gowan, G. F., and Shedd, D. P.: Postoperative carotid artery hemorrhage. Am. J. Surg., *109*:765, 1965.
12. Gandhi, K., and Oppenheimer, P.: Emergency carotid ligation. Arch. Otolaryngol., *75*:541, 1962.
13. Keirle, A. M., and Altemeier, W. A.: Resection of the carotid arteries for neoplastic invasion with maintenance of circulation. Am. Surg., *26*:588, 1960.
14. Ketcham, A. S., and Hoye, R. C.: Spontaneous carotid artery hemorrhage after head and neck surgery. Am. J. Surg., *110*:659, 1965.
15. Martinez, S. A., Oller, D. W., Gee, W., et al.: Elective carotid artery resection. Arch. Otolaryngol., *101*:744, 1975.
16. McCoy, G., and Barsocchini, L. M.: Experience in carotid artery occlusion. Laryngoscope, *78*:1195, 1968.
17. Moore, O. S., and Baker, H. W.: Carotid artery ligation in surgery of the head and neck. Cancer, *8*:712, 1955.
18. Moore, O. S., Karlan, M., and Sigler, L.: Factors influencing the safety of carotid ligation. Am. J. Surg., *118*:363, 1969.
19. Schweitzer, R. J.: Use of muscle flaps for protection of carotid artery after radical neck dissection. Ann. Surg., *156*:811, 1962.
20. Shumrick, D. A.: Carotid artery rupture. Laryngoscope, *83*:1051, 1973.
21. Swain, R. E., Biller, H. F., Ogura, J. H.: An experimental analysis of causative factors and protective methods in carotid artery rupture. Arch. Otolaryngol., *99*:235, 1974.
22. Tindall, G. T., Dukes, H. T., and Cupp, H. B.: Retinal and carotid artery pressures: Simultaneous determinations. Neurology, *10*:623, 1963.
23. Watson, W.L., and Silverstone, S. M.: Ligature of the common carotid artery in cancer of the head and neck. Ann. Surg., *109*:1–27, 1939.

# OROPHARYNGOCUTANEOUS FISTULA

7

*John J. Conley*

The appearance of an unexpected fistula in a composite resection is a serious complication that may infect the entire neck wound, involve the carotid arteries and extend the morbidity. There are multiple technical, biological and physiological factors that contribute to the formation of a fistula. The incidence of fistula varies from approximately 10 to 30 per cent, depending upon the combination of etiological factors present, the management concept and the risk evaluation. From a working point of view, the surgeon should calculate that 10 to 15 per cent of his composite resections will form a fistula. If they are high-risk cases, this figure can be doubled. In the nonirradiated cases with fistula, 5 to 10 per cent may spontaneously rupture the carotid artery, and in the irradiated cases this figure may escalate to as high as 30 per cent. All fistulas will ultimately diminish in size, and approximately 60 per cent will close spontaneously. The presence of a fistula automatically extends the morbidity period, which varies from one to six months. These data, therefore, highlight the necessity of reducing fistula formation to a minimum and direct the course of management.

Robins, Budden and MacDougall (1975)[6] reported a 6 per cent incidence of salivary fistula in 100 composite resections. This was associated with a 28 per cent incidence of wound infection and a 13 per cent incidence of postoperative hemorrhage. Eighty-three per cent of the patients who had fistulas had received preoperative irradiation. One of those patients had a secondary rupture of the carotid artery but did not have any sequelae from emergency ligation. All of the fistulas in this series eventually healed spontaneously.

Shumrick (1973)[8] reviewed 333 major head and neck procedures. Thirteen of these (3.8 per cent) had carotid artery rupture. Twenty-three per cent of those who ruptured had an active fistula, and 46 per cent of those who ruptured had an active fistula in the presence of irradiated tissue. This would indicate that 69 per cent of his cases of carotid artery rupture had an active fistula as a contributory cause.

Mladick and his colleagues (1972)[5] reported a plan of management on the catastrophic postoperative fistula formation. They propose an aggressive diagnostic approach when the diagnosis of fistula is apparent. They inspect and evaluate the size of the intraoral breakdown, and, if it is small, they continue with conservative management. If the breakdown of the mucosal repair is extensive, associated with separation, infection and flap necrosis, they advocate opening of the wound, debridement of the necrotic tissue and diversion of the flow of saliva. They found fusiform bacilli, spirochetes and anaerobic cocci from the oral cavity were common offenders and caused a necrotizing type of infection in the neck tissues. Open saline dressings, aggressive debridement and the use of skin grafts and muscle flaps to protect the artery when the wound is clean enough for their application are emphasized as fundamental points in wound care and prophylaxis against carotid artery rupture.

Bresson, Rasmussen and Rasmussen (1974)[1] stated that in a review of the literature they found the incidence of fistulas to range from 20 to 70 per cent. The physiological status of the patient, size of the ablation and irradiation were all considered to be etiological factors. In their own series

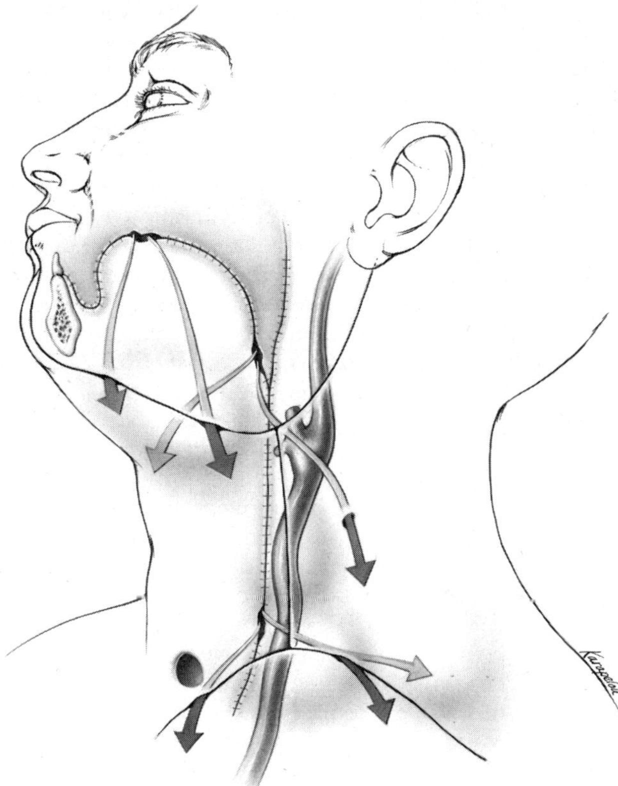

**Figure 7–1** Areas of potential mucosal dehiscence with fistula formation, neck infection and external drainage.

of 148 cases, 65 per cent developed a fistula postoperatively. They found the incidence of fistulas to be doubled when conventional irradiation was used and quadrupled when high-voltage irradiation was used in cancerocidal doses. They advocated reevaluation of the amount of irradiation given preoperatively.

Briant (1975)[2] stated that the most common complication in the early postoperative period following laryngectomy was spontaneous pharyngocutaneous fistula. He reviewed six different series on pharyngeal fistula following laryngectomy and found the incidence varied from 22 to 50 per cent. He reviewed a variety of possible contributory factors, such as early feeding, types of incisions, suture material used; hematoma formation and type of drainage, irradiation, the extent of the operation and the presence of infection. He outlined the rational steps to reduce the incidence of fistula and the methods of definitive management.

Joseph and Shumrick (1973)[4] compared postoperative complications in 105 patients who underwent major surgical procedures in the head and neck. A comparison was set up between those who had preoperative unplanned irradiation (irradiation as the primary method of treatment for cure), those who were in a planned combined program of irradiation followed by surgery and the nonirradiated group. In those who had irradiation for cure and who were subsequently operated on, there was a 73 per cent incidence of fistula, a 77 per cent incidence of dehiscence and a 50 per cent incidence of carotid artery necrosis. In the planned group, the incidence fell to 23 per cent for fistulas, 35 per cent for dehiscence and 2.8 per cent for carotid artery necrosis. In the nonirradiated group, there was 8 per cent incidence of fistulas, 15 per cent incidence of dehiscence and no incidence of carotid artery necrosis.

Gall, Sessions and Ogura (1977)[3] carried out a retrospective study on complications in supraglottic, glottic, superior hypopharyngeal and inferior hypopharyngeal cancers and found no significant difference in the complication rates on the basis of age, sex, race, the site or stage of the primary tumor, preoperative low-dose irradiation, the number of positive cervical nodes, or the size or grading of the tumor. There was an increase in complications when the margins of the tumor were declared abnormal. The most common complications included wound infection, wound necrosis, salivary fistula, hemorrhage and carotid artery catastrophe. The overall incidence of salivary fistulas was 3.9 per cent. The incidence rose to 9.8 per cent in composite resection of cancers of the hypopharynx (pyriform) in combination with lateral neck dissection. Only those patients who received their primary treatment at Washington University Medical Center, under their auspices, were considered in the analysis. This eliminated the group of high-risk patients who had been treated surgically by other doctors or who had had previous irradiation for cure and then developed recurrent cancer.

Sellars and Jarvis (1976)[7] reported an incidence of 15 per cent fistula formation in 147 total laryngectomies. They did not feel that the amount of preoperative irradiation and the extent of the surgery contributed to fistula formation. They had one fatal case of carotid artery rupture, however, and that individual had a wound breakdown and a cutaneous fistula. All the remaining fistulas closed spontaneously and did not require any additional surgical intervention.

## ETIOLOGICAL FACTORS

All of the physiological factors mentioned in Chapter 6 are applicable in the development of fistulas. Nutritional status, metabolic disorders, chronic pulmonary disease, arteriosclerosis and localized infection add a small increment of increased risk.

It is a known fact that individuals who have had cancerocidal doses of irradiation are high-risk patients, prone to wound complications. If the dose has been over 5000 rads and the interval since the termination of treatment has been over six months or a year, the deleterious effect on the wound will be markedly increased. Essentially, this category is made up of irradiation failures and is one of the most dangerous to operate upon. A much more favorable situation exists when irradiation is given in a planned preoperative program and when the dose does not exceed 4000 rads. It is axiomatic that the larger the size of the irradiation port and the higher the dose and longer the interval, the higher the complications associated with surgical intervention. The use of radium needles and seeds circumvented this to a certain degree, in that the effects of irradiation were concentrated directly in the tumor mass, with a minimum of injury to surrounding tissue. These techniques, however, have been largely replaced by the use of supervoltage. The inflammatory reactions associated with the initial application of irradiation change from severe hyperemia with superficial ulceration to the death of a large volume of tissue, associated with endarteritis and severe fibrosis as the years go by. One certainly should not expect this tissue to heal normally following a major resection, and these wounds must be favored in every respect with carefully planned incisions, minimal undermining, creation of oropharyngostomes and pharyngostomes at the termination of the procedure and generous use of regional flaps.

Fistulas are almost exclusively associated with composite resections involving the oral cavity, pharynx and larynx. The incidence of fistula formation in massive resections to critical levels is reduced by the creation of a stoma in the majority of these cases. Extensive removal of the internal lining or external covering, mucosa and skin places additional technical handicaps on the immediate rehabilitation of these wounds and thus, again, predisposes to fistula formation. In these circumstances, the creation of an elective stoma or the use of regional flaps will reduce the incidence of unexpected fistula.

### Technical Factors

The compulsive compliance with the highest concepts of surgical craftsmanship will reduce the incidence of fistula. The accomplishment of a spit-tight closure without tension is a *sine qua non.* Three-O chromic catgut in the uncomplicated cases and #4-0 Vicryl or Dexon suture material in the high-risk cases should be used to close the mucosa. Every effort should be made to avoid kinking, tension and undue stretching or

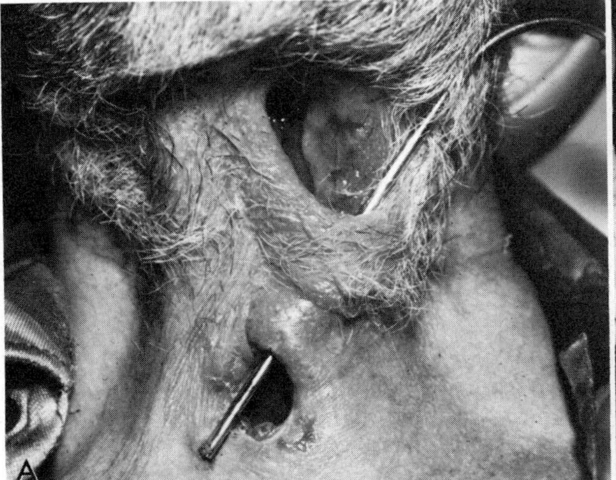

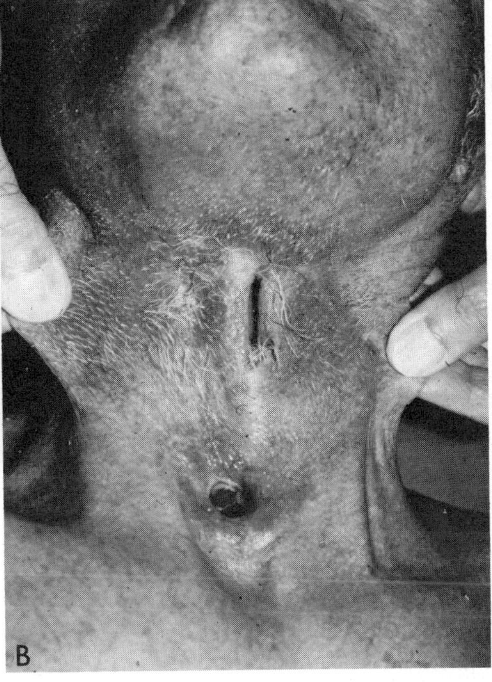

**Figure 7–2** *A,* Large pharyngocutaneous fistula communicating with the tracheostome. The original attempt at closure of the pharynx was carried out with a minimum of mucous membrane closed under tension. This wound contracted and stabilized and was closed with regional tissue in three months. *B,* Same wound after two months' healing and contraction. Closure now requires opening edges and direct approximation.

pressure. When a double layer closure is feasible, it should be used. The draping of mucous membrane about a cut edge of mandible requires careful approximation without tension. An open tooth socket communicating with the wound should be plugged with bone wax or Surgicel (absorbable cellulose gauze). The skin flaps are inspected carefully for bleeding and color. A simple test for viability is to compress the flap with the finger; if the blanched area returns to normal color within four seconds, the flap is, most likely, viable. The skin flaps are closed in layers without tension. If there is unusual tension in any part of the wound, the wound should be adjusted either with the use of regional flaps or by the creation of a stoma. Hemovac drainage is used in the majority of the major wounds, using from two to four suction tubes of small size placed and fixed in critical positions of the wound with a single #3-0 chromic suture. The hemovac should not be placed over the carotid artery. It is important, however, that it be in the position of advantage for drainage, proximal to the mucous membrane repair, should a fistula develop. The area is immobilized with a supportive dressing, and the patient's nutrition is maintained with a nasogastric feeding tube. When healing has progressed normally in the nonirradiated case, and the hemovacs have been removed and the skin flaps appear in a normal state of repair, the patient may be given liquids by mouth on the 7th to 10th day. In all high-risk cases, and particularly in those who have had heavy irradiation or major reconstruction in the pharynx and gullet, feeding is not begun until after an interval of two or three weeks, depending upon the healing process.

## APPEARANCE OF THE FISTULA

### Time Interval

Any fistula that appears within several days of the operation is usually the result of inept mucous membrane closure, a failure to attain a spit-tight closure or stitch dehiscence. It may be difficult to make this early diagnosis because of the mucus and spit being mixed with blood. Once the wound drainage has turned to serum, however, the presence of mucus in the hemovac tubes will be discernible. About 80 per cent of the fistulas are obvious within three weeks of the operation. If the fistula is adjacent to a hemovac tube it may not cause a serious wound disruption. On the other hand, if the contaminated secretions from the oral or pharyngeal cavity flood throughout the cervical wound, the entire operative area will become inflamed and infected, with a thickening and redness of the flap and a copious discharge of both mucus and pus. About 10 per cent of the fistulas will appear after an interval of three weeks. This is almost always associated with postirradiated wounds and has as a precursor an unrecognized mucous membrane dehiscence with the potential for infecting the wound and thus preparing the way for a delayed fistula.

### Position of Fistula

An attempt should be made to evaluate the position and course of the fistula. The location of the break in the mucous membrane pattern by indirect or direct examination will assist in the management program. The position of drainage in the neck supplies information as to the length of the tract and its relationship to the primary repair and the carotid artery. Anterior fistulas that are in a high position in the neck rarely involve the artery, whereas fistulas that drain laterally at the mid or lower level frequently must cross the artery.

The size and position of the fistula may be determined by gentle probing with a soft catheter. Ingestion of methylene blue or 1 per cent neomycin solution will give some estimation of the volume of the leak. It is important to evaluate the condition of the tissues in the lateral neck about the fistula, thus establishing whether it is a single tract that is well localized and contained or whether it is disrupting the major portion of the neck. Suction drainage has been of great advantage in reducing the size of the fistula and in limiting the harmful effects on the operative wound. In many instances, a small leak in the mucous membrane repair can be controlled well by the drainage of a suction tube in that area, thus permitting the major portion of the neck wound to heal per primam. It is important that this critical suction tube not be removed until the cervical wound is well stabilized and has healed over an interval of approximately two to three weeks.

## MANAGEMENT PROGRAM

### Conservative (closed) Method

The majority of small fistulas in uncomplicated cases will heal spontaneously. This group consists of the patients in optimal physiological condition who have a small anterior or lateral positioned fistula, in whom the major portion of the neck wound has healed and there is a minimal reaction of the skin about the fistulous tract. Wound care, under these circumstances, consists of ample drainage, minimal debridement (if, indeed, that is even necessary), elimination of tenting or dead space by pressure dressing or release of the cervical flap. Culture and sensitivity is done to establish the appropriate antibiotic. Feedings are continued with a nasogastric tube, the patient is given sips of 1 per cent neomycin solution throughout the day by mouth in order to irrigate the wound and the wound is packed gently with an antiseptic gauze packing material. These fistulas are usually closed spontaneously within a period of a month.

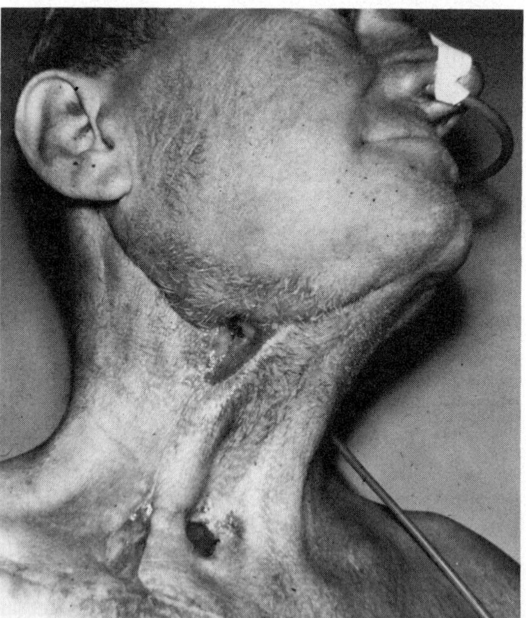

**Figure 7–3** Localized wound infection with fistulization with 90 per cent healing at the neck flaps. The healing process of neck flaps is unquestionably enhanced by the proper use of the hemovac system. This frequently permits the neck to heal and localizes the fistulous tract. This wound healed by secondary intention within an interval of two weeks.

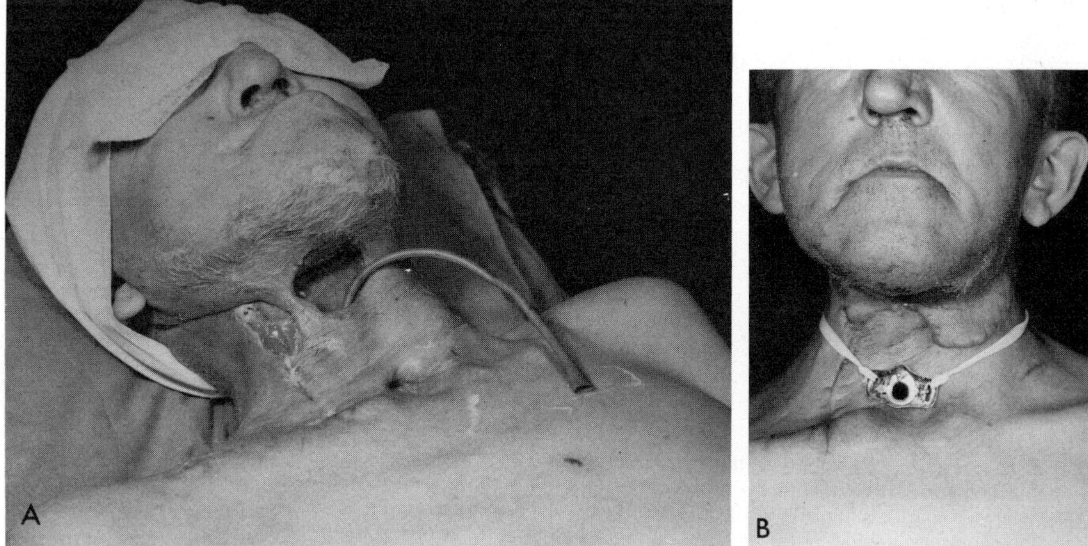


**Figure 7–4** *A,* Secondary wound infection, fistulization and loss of skin following radical resection of lateral neck and larynx. *B,* Repaired after six weeks by use of regional tissue (1951).

## Open Method

This method is applied to the high-risk patients who have some type of physiological or biological deficiency, who are in a postirradiation status or who have a large fistula, drainage over the carotid artery system or a grossly infected fistulous tract with necrosis of the wound in a postoperative condition that is deteriorating rather than improving. These individuals are placed on carotid artery precautions. Cuture and sensitivity studies determine the appropriate antibiotic. There is usually a mixture of *Staphylococcus aureus* and gram-negative bacilli. The wound is opened liberally in the operating room and completely inspected. Particular attention is paid to the status of the carotid artery.

Debridement of necrotic tissue is carried out, and the area is liberally irrigated with saline. If it is technically possible, the wound edges are externalized by suturing mucosa to skin, and thus creating a large stoma. The oral secretions are diverted by local packing or constant oral suction or by covering the wound with rubber or silicone film. If there is inadequate mucous membrane to create a stoma, then consideration must be given to skin grafting over the carotid artery, if the wound contains healthy granulation tissue, or to the use of regional flaps. The regional flap has the advantage of security and viability, solving the resurfacing problem after an interval of two or three days. If healthy granulation tissue is appearing, the behavior of the wound is favorable and it may be

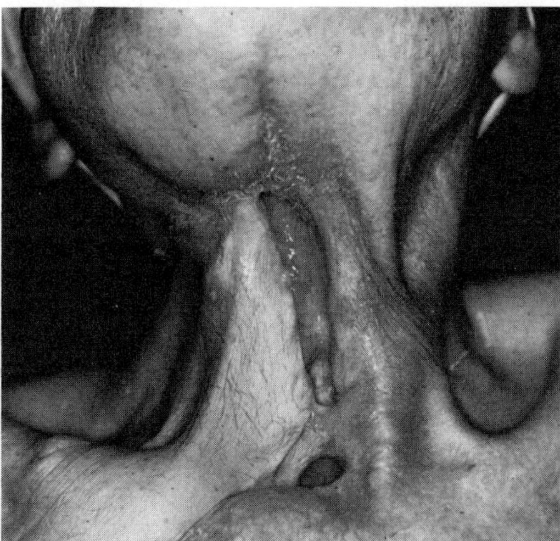

**Figure 7–5** Maximum precautions have been taken in this heavily irradiated radical ablation of the lateral neck, thyroid, larynx and associated skin by creating a large controlled pharyngostome and resurfacing the lateral neck with a thoracoacromial flap. This wound healed per primam. All features of this type of conservative and precautionary management give the best opportunity for healing. The stoma was closed in an interval of six weeks by undermining and direct approximation.

dressed with either a split skin graft or a regional flap. If the wound continues to necrotize, with an extension of the slough toward the carotid artery, one then has the best information concerning the decision for elective ligation.

It is generally recognized that, in the high-risk patient who has a large fistula treated by the open method, with debridement, regional flaps are necessary in the primary resurfacing and also in the secondary closure of the stoma.

## Bibliography

1. Bresson, K., Rasmussen, H., and Rasmussen, P. A.: Pharyngocutaneous fistulae in totally laryngectomized patients. J. Laryngol. Otol., *88*:835, 1974.
2. Briant, T. D. R.: Spontaneous pharyngeal fistula and wound infection following laryngectomy. Laryngoscope, *85*:829, 1975.
3. Gall, A. M., Sessions, D. G., and Ogura, J. H.: Complications following surgery for cancer of the larynx and hypopharynx. Cancer, *39*:624, 1977.
4. Joseph, D. L., and Shumrick, D. L.; Risks of head and neck surgery in previously irradiated patients. Arch. Otolaryngol., *97*:381, 1973.
5. Mladick, R. A., Horton, C. E., Adamson, J. E., et al.: Management of catastrophic postoperative breakdown after massive oropharyngeal cancer surgery. Survival in a perilous situation. Plast. Reconstr. Surg., *49*:316, 1972.
6. Robins, R. E., Budden, M. K., and MacDougall, J. A.: Analysis of mortality and morbidity in 100 composite resections for oral carcinoma. Am. J. Surg., *130*:178, 1975.
7. Sellars, S. L.: The mortality and morbidity of laryngectomy. S. Afr. Med. J., *50*:428, 1976.
8. Shumrick, D. A.: Carotid artery rupture. Laryngoscope, *83*:1051, 1973.

# 8 INFECTION

*Thomas J. Krizek*
*Stephan Ariyan*

. . . among the consequences of toothache are . . . disfigurement of the face and certain death. . . . Very soon after the gums were lanced he suffered from insomnia, delirium and died.

Tulpius, 1694[70]

Throughout life, man harbors on and within his body a most varied and concentrated population of microorganisms, each potentially pathogenic. In the variety of species, number of organisms and potential for virulence, the microbial flora* of the human mouth exceed that of any other area of the body. Health represents not an absence of such microorganisms but rather an exquisite balance between the microorganisms and the local and systemic host defense mechanisms. What is surprising is not that infection is a common complication of treatment but that it is not inevitable.

Surgery in the head and neck region involves surgical wounds that, by bacteriologic standards, should be classified as "dirty" and that are, at best, considered "highly contaminated." The overall incidence of infection in such wounds in other areas of the body would be anticipated to be in excess of 16 per cent.[1] Among the adverse circumstances encountered are the highly virulent nature of the oral microbial flora, their quantitative level of growth, the presence of malignancy and the frequently associated factors of alcoholism, malnutrition, therapeutic radiation and, occasionally, chemotherapeutic agents. Since so many different bacterial and host defense mechanisms are influenced by the disease and its treatment, it seems reasonable to review these factors individually and to determine their potential influence on infection as a complication of treatment.

*Flora — the goddess of flowers. In contrast to *fauna,* which denotes animal life, *flora* refers to vegetative life. Bacteria are now classified into their own kingdom between flora and fauna, but convention dicates that, in the absence of a more suitable word, we continue to refer to the "microflora."

## BIOLOGY OF SURGICAL INFECTION

### Balance

Infection in the patient having head and neck surgery rarely represents a bacterial visitation from without but is rather the end result of a disturbed balance between the patient and a microbial flora for which the patient is himself the reservoir. Although there is a quantitatively spectacular number of microorganisms present in the human oropharynx, they are really "outside" the body, in the sense that they are not established in the depths of the tissues themselves. It is only when they gain such lodgment that there can be proliferation to produce the clinical picture that we accept as "infection." Such an accumulation of bacteria can be relatively innocuous to overall health when it appears in the form of dental "plaque," with the subsequent development of either caries or periodontal disease. On the other hand, the same bacteria gaining access into and proliferating in tissue recently traumatized by surgery can lead to abscess, hemorrhage, fistulas, skin breakdown and carotid rupture.

### Mechanisms of Disturbance

W. D. Miller (1890), the father of oral microbiology, identified six circumstances in which the pathogenic bacteria of the mouth could gain such establishment. Most of these circumstances are applicable today:[50]

1. Infections caused by a breach in the continuity of the mucous membrane, brought about by mechanical injuries (wound, extractions, etc.). . . .
2. Infections through the medium of gangrenous tooth-pulps. These usually lead to abscess at the point of infection *(abscessus apicalis)*, but also sometimes to secondary septicemia and pyaemia with fatal termination.
3. Disturbances conditioned by the resorption of poisonous waste products formed by bacteria.*
4. Pulmonary diseases caused by the inspiration of particles of slime, small pieces of tartar, etc. containing bacteria.**
5. Excessive fermentative processes, and other complaints of the digestive tract, caused by the continual swallowing of microbes and their poisonous products.
6. Infections of the intact soft tissue of the oral and pharyngeal cavities, whose power of resistance has been impaired by debilitating disease, mechanical irritation, etc.†

The entrance portal descriptions of Miller may perhaps be simplistic, but they do show insight into what actually does occur. Although any surgical procedure in the oral cavity should be considered "contaminated," whether it becomes an actual infection depends on the microbial flora that gain access to and proliferate within tissue beyond the critical level, resulting in signs and symptoms of infection. Here, as elsewhere, routine qualitative bacteriologic study often provides inadequate information, for a heavily "contaminated" wound becomes "infected" only when the tissue content exceeds levels of $10^5$ bacteria per gm. of tissue.[64] It is irrelevant biologically that the wounds in composite resections are bathed with oral secretions containing millions (more than $10^{10}$ bacteria/ml.) of microorganisms during surgery or that such levels can be identified in wound washings at the completion of surgery. If the microorganisms fail to become established in tissue or if they do invade but fail to multiply to levels exceeding $10^5$ bacteria per gm. of tissue, there will be no infection.

The therapeutic imperative is to prevent lodgment and growth to such critical levels under circumstances that are favorable to the microorganisms. In order to effect a favorable outcome, it is necessary to have an understanding of not only the microbial flora with which one is dealing but also the local and host defense mechanisms and how they are altered by disease and its treatment.

*Clostridial or gram-negative bacterial endotoxins?
**Contamination of tracheostoma.
†Radiation therapy?

## NORMAL MICROBIAL FLORA OF THE OROPHARYNX

The normal oropharynx is an ideal incubator for microorganisms. It has a temperature of 37°C. (98.6°F.) (1–2 degrees lower in the anterior labial sulcus), which is favorable for most bacteria and for *Candida albicans* but fortunately unfavorable for other types of fungi. There is an abundance of moisture and nutrients and an oxygen tension of such variability as to allow obligate aerobic microorganisms to live side-by-side with obligate anaerobic microorganisms and the facultative and microaerophilic species. The "normal" flora is highly variable and changes not only with age and state of dentition but also at various times of the day. The mouth is sterile at birth, and, although contamination is occasionally seen, the normal flora does not become established until the second or third day of life. During the first months of life, the flora is made up entirely of aerobic organisms, of which 98 per cent are *Streptococcus salivarius* ($\alpha$-hemolytic *viridans* variety). At the end of a year, it consists of 70 per cent *S. salivarius* and also includes *Staphylococcus, Veillonella* and *Neisseria*.[55, 14] There are few anaerobic organisms before the onset of dentition, which provides the sites needed for anaerobic growth. The anaerobic flora then persist throughout life, although predictably declining precipitously after full-mouth extractions. With the appearance of the an-

**TABLE 8–1** BACTERIAL FLORA OF NORMAL ADULT MOUTH MEASURING VIABLE ORGANISMS*

| | Gingiva | Saliva |
|---|---|---|
| *Viable aerobic organisms* | $1.5 \times 10^{10}$ bacteria/gm. | $4 \times 10^7$ bacteria/ml. (range $1 \times 10^7$–$1 \times 10^8$/ml.) |
| *Viable anaerobic organisms* | $3.6 \times 10^{10}$ bacteria/gm. | $1.1 \times 10^8$ bacteria/ml. (range $1 \times 10^7$–$3 \times 10^8$/ml.) |

*Microscopic counts of bacteria show a tenfold increase in number over count of viable bacteria. (Data from Nolte, W. A.: Oral Microbiology. St. Louis, The C. V. Mosby Co., 1968.)

aerobes, the final "normal" microflora becomes established and remains throughout life with approximately equal numbers of aerobic and anaerobic organisms.

## Resident and Transient Flora

The resident flora can best be defined as the quantitatively determined microflora present in a person on repeated examination and can be considered part of that person's "normal" flora. Transient flora are those bacteria present only intermittently, such as after eating, that seem unable to survive any length of time unless the microbial ecology has been disturbed by such therapeutic maneuvers as administration of antibiotics or radiation. Alterations of this flora may also be produced by disease states, such as diabetes; for example, 80 per cent of diabetics are carriers of *Candida albicans*, in comparison with only 56 per cent of normal adults.[14] There is considerable variation among normal persons' flora. Only 47 per cent of healthy dental students carry coagulase-positive *Staphylococcus aureus*, whereas almost 100 per cent of hospital workers carry this organism.[55] Within the oropharynx, the tongue, the gingiva and gingival crevices and the saliva are the three sites that harbor the resident and transient flora.

### TONGUE

The bacterial effluvium of the tongue seems to be the major source of salivary bacteria. Although difficult to quantitate, these bacteria increase in number from the anterior to the posterior of the mouth. They are predominantly facultative, which means that they are either anaerobic with some aerotolerance or aerobic with the ability to grow feebly in anaerobic environments. Some 38.3 per cent are *Veillonella* (gram-negative anaerobic cocci), and 13 per cent are facultative diphtheroids.[55]

### GINGIVA

Bacteria can be identified within gingival tissue and in material extracted from the gingival crevice. These bacteria are almost equally divided between aerobic and anaerobic organisms and their incidence is approximately 100 times that found in saliva (Table 8–1). Studies of material from the gingival crevice show even greater numbers of bacteria, approximately 70 per cent of which are anaerobic. The distribution of these bacteria is seen in Table 8–2.

The gingival crevice is probably not the source of most of the salivary bacteria. Although *Streptococcus salivarius* makes up 47 per cent of the facultative streptococci in saliva, it represents 10 to 55 per cent of such organisms on the tongue and less than 1 per cent of the facultative streptococci found in dental plaque and the gingival crevice.[55] This suggests that the major source of the salivary bacteria is the tongue rather than the gingival crevice.

### SALIVA

Salivary bacteria are the most movable and therefore, the most likely to be inoculated into an operative wound. The flora is almost equally divided into aerobic and anaerobic species, of which *Streptococcus, Veillonella* and *Fusobacterium* are present in the largest quantities (Tables 8–1 and 8–2).[55, 62] Saliva also has a highly variable transient flora that includes *Staphylococcus, Escherichia coli, Pseudomonas aeruginosa* and other coliforms. The bacterial level of saliva is subject to extrinsic factors and has a diurnal variation. The highest levels are found

**TABLE 8–2** IDENTITY AND DISTRIBUTION OF BACTERIAL FLORA IN ORAL CAVITY

| | Gingiva* | Saliva** | Tongue* |
|---|---|---|---|
| *Number of Common Microorganisms* | | | |
| Total *Streptococcus* | $1.4 \times 10^{10}$/gm. | $1.8 \times 10^{7}$/ml. | – |
| Facultative *Streptococcus* | $4 \times 10^{9}$/gm. | $1 \times 10^{7}$/ml. | – |
| *Veillonella* | – | $1.7 \times 10^{7}$/ml. | – |
| *Fusobacterium* | $1.2 \times 10^{7}$/gm. | $5 \times 10^{4}$/ml. | – |
| *Percentage of Microorganisms in Microflora* | | | |
| Gram-positive facultative rods | 29.7% | | 13.0% |
| Gram-positive facultative cocci | 21.9% | | 38.3% |
| Gram-negative anaerobic rods | 16.3% | | 5.3% |
| Gram-positive anaerobic cocci | 16.3% | | 4.2% |
| Gram-negative anaerobic cocci | 8.8% | | 14.5% |

*(Data from Nolte, W. A.: Oral Microbiology. St. Louis, The C. V. Mosby Co., 1968.)
**(Data from Richardson, R. L., and Jones, M.: Bacterial census of human saliva. J. Dent. Res., *37*:697, 1958.)

in the early morning, after a period of fasting ($9 \times 10^7$ bacteria/ml.).[55] A simple saline mouth rinse will reduce this count ten-fold ($1 \times 10^7$ bacteria/ml.). By noon, the count increases to $5 \times 10^7$ bacteria per ml. The noon and evening meals, even without specific oral hygienic measures, reduce the counts five-fold; in fact, they are at their lowest level in the evening. The overnight fast then allows the counts to again reach the early morning peak. It is clear that salivary flow has much to do with the bacterial levels. Although salivary flow is often quoted as being 1 to 1.5 liters per day, it is probably closer to 500 to 600 ml. per day.[24] Of this amount, half is resting and half is stimulated flow. In the unstimulated periods of the day (14–16 hours), the flow is about 200 to 300 ml., of which 70 per cent comes from the submandibular glands and 20 per cent from the parotid gland. With acid stimulation, the parotid and submandibular glands each secrete about 45 per cent, and with mechanical stimulation, the parotid secretes about 50 per cent of the flow. During sleep, the major glands secrete only about 10 ml. of saliva, accounting for the rise in bacteria count during this period.

## DEFENSE MECHANISMS OF THE OROPHARYNX

The oral cavity is a marvelous culture system, and the healthy person is able to maintain an acceptable balance of this variety and concentration of bacteria only as a result of a series of exquisitely sensitive defense mechanisms. The importance of these defense mechanisms can be seen by the tenfold increase in the bacterial flora encountered in persons with dental caries, malocclusion, periodontal disease or any open wound.[55] There are basically two lines of defense employed by the body to protect against bacterial invasion.

### The First Line of Defense

#### MUCOUS MEMBRANE

The most obvious and important defense mechanism against bacterial invasion is the mechanical integrity of the mucous membrane. The human mouth is lined by stratified squamous epithelium that may be keratinized and can become hyperplastic in response to stress. It rarely becomes directly inflamed or ulcerated by bacterial invasion. The teeth, which in good occlusion further protect against stagnation and accumulation of foreign material, may cause an interruption in the mucosal continuity. The gingival crevices, however, are lined by nonkeratinized epithelium and are a ready portal for bacterial invasion in the face of poor oral hygiene or malocclusion.

The bacteria of the mouth become readily attached to surface epithelial cells. The contant shedding of these superficial epithelial cells (saliva contains between $6 \times 10^3$ and $6 \times 10^5$ buccal squamous cells per ml.) washes away much of the flora and helps to maintain the balance. It is well known that small breaks in the mucous membrane allow bacterial invasion. The incidence of bacteremia after dental extractions is reported to be between 16 and 73 per cent depending on the degree of periapical disease.[55] Using *Serratia marcescens* as a marker (not part of the normal oral flora, since the mouth lacks the necessary carbohydrate substrate), bacteremia occurs in 24 per cent of persons with periodontal disease merely from brushing the teeth and in 17 per cent from eating hard candy. Dental manipulation results in bacteremia in 40 per cent of such persons.[55] In addition to tracer *Serratia,* the organisms identified during this bacteremia include bacteroides, *Gaffkya, Actinomyces* and *Fusobacterium.* One may speculate whether such bacteremias are of clinical significance in the healthy person. In persons with foci of decreased host resistance, such as an open wound or deformed heart valve, however, these bacteremias may lead to wound infection[38] or bacterial endocarditis.[55]

It is clear that a more major surgical manipulation or an open wound can break down the single most important defense mechanism and allow bacterial invasion of the soft tissue and blood.

## SALIVA

Another important first line of defense is saliva. Saliva serves both by its mechanical function of flow and by the antibacterial substances it contains.

**Mechanical Function.** Saliva contains mucus, which forms a protective coating over the teeth and the mucous membrane of the oral cavity. Microorganisms are held in this mucus. As saliva flows and is swallowed, the flora are being constantly washed back into the pharynx and ultimately into the stomach, where the bacteria are destroyed by the acidity of gastric juice (except *S. viridans,* which is acid-resistant and thereby also part of the resident flora of the stomach). Tracers (carbon particles) are noted to be completely washed out of the oral cavity within 30 minutes, and nonindigenous bacteria are removed in a similar way within a few minutes to several hours. Clearly, radiation therapy, with its effect of diminishing salivary volume and flow, may interfere with a major defense mechanism and lead to increased bacterial growth.

**Physiologic Function.** In addition to the mechanical action of rinsing, saliva serves important physiologic functions.

MUCIN. The lubricating property of saliva is due to mucins, which are glycoproteins. The mucins entrap bacteria but may also coat and protect them from phagocytosis. Although they make bacteria easier to wash away, the mucins may at the same time protect them.

SALIVARY pH. With a normal pH range of 5.6 to 7.0 (average is 6.7), the hydrogen ion concentration of the oral cavity greatly influences the microflora. A low pH favors aciduric bacteria, whereas a higher pH favors proteolytic bacteria. *Candida albicans* can be found in the saliva of 90 per cent of young adults whose pH is acid (5.0 to 5.5), compared to less than 60 per cent of those whose pH is greater than 6.5

**Antibacterial Substances.** Saliva has been demonstrated to kill many microorganisms. Some antibacterial substances are related to the bacteria themselves. For example, the killing of diphtheroid bacilli by saliva is due to the presence of hydrogen peroxide produced by strains of oral $\alpha$-hemolytic streptococci.[55] More specific substances in saliva that destroy bacteria are lysozymes — mucopolysaccharide enzymes that break the 1–4 link between N-acetyl muramic acid and N-acetyl glucosamine, the two most important mucopeptides of the bacterial cell wall.[44] The exact role of lysozymes in the host defense mechanism is unclear. They are found throughout many tissues of the body, their concentration is high in saliva and they are present in increased amounts in inflamed oral and gingival tissues. Other nonspecific factors identified in saliva include a substance specifically inhibitory to $\beta$-hemolytic streptococci, a factor particularly effective against *Lactobacillus* and factors inhibitory to the growth of *Clostridium tetani.*[44, 55]

An interesting substance is lactoferrin, which is an iron-binding protein present in milk, polymorphonuclear leukocytes and saliva. Since iron is necessary for bacterial proliferation, this substance apparently acts to protect an intact mucous membrane by preventing bacteria from taking up host iron.

It has been shown to inhibit the growth of *Staphylococcus epidermidis, Staphylococcus aureus, Pseudomonas aeruginosa,* and *Bacillus subtilis.*[44]

All of these factors act in conjunction with an intact mucous membrane barrier to protect against bacterial invasion. Once this mechanical barrier is broken the oral cavity has an important and effective second line of defense.

## The Second Line of Defense

### INFLAMMATION

The cellular and humoral defense mechanisms against infection are no different qualitatively in the oral cavity from elsewhere in the body. Certain features of the inflammatory response are present in oral tissues as part of the maintenance of health, however.

The polymorphonuclear leukocytes (PMN), with a life span of some 18 hours in the bloodstream, are present in substantial quantities in oral mucous membrane and gingiva. There is a constant process of phagocytosis of the oral microflora by the PMN, which gradually pass to the surface and are washed away with saliva.[44] Although the PMN count in saliva varies from person to person and even has a diurnal variation, the average count in a normal person ranges from $2 \times 10^3$ to $6 \times 10^5$ PMN per ml.[24] Monocytes have a life span of two to three days in the bloodstream and then migrate to the oral tissues, where they may remain for months as tissue macrophages. Their value to the defense mechanism is sporadic and occurs mostly in response to injury or the presence of a foreign body. It is clear that the cellular response is important to the normal state of health. This normal defense mechanism is altered by chemotherapeutic agents that cause neutropenia, from which oral ulcerations may appear. Furthermore, the inflammatory response itself may be destructive, since the lysosomal hydrolases released by disintegrating PMN's and tissue macrophages may injure the periodontium.[44]

### IMMUNOLOGIC RESPONSE

Although the main immunologic mechanisms operate in a similar way throughout the body, there are specific activities occurring within the oral cavity that may be particularly important in the patient with oropharyngeal cancer. The two main mechanisms reflect the functions of T-lymphocytes and B-lymphocytes.

**T-lymphocytes.** These are derived from precursors in the bone marrow and are thymus-dependent in their proliferation and maturation. T-lymphocytes circulating in the blood are considered long-lived (compared to B-lymphocytes). Both T- and B-lymphocytes migrate to the lymph nodes, the spleen and the interstitial tissues, and both can act alone or with antigen to stimulate the immune response. Stimulated T-lymphocytes release lymphokines, which have the effect of promoting chemotaxis, accumulating activated macrophages and increasing vascular permeability. They also tend to fix macrophages at sites of inflammation. The entire response is known as the "cellular phase" of the immune response.[44]

**B-lymphocytes.** These are responsible for the "humoral phase" of the immune response. So-called because they were first described in the bursa of Fabricius in the gut of chickens, B-cells are not dependent on the thymus, most likely proliferate and mature in the bone marrow and have a shorter life span than T-cells. During the immune response, B-cells differentiate into larger blast cells and into plasma cells that secrete immunoglobulins. Five different classes of immunoglobulins have been described to date (Table 8–3). The two symbols used to represent immunoglobulins are the Greek letter "gamma" ($\gamma$) and Ig, followed by the letters G, M, A, D and E, in their order of discovery. By agreement, the use of the symbol $\gamma$ has been discontinued in favor of the Ig classification system.[69]

IMMUNOGLOBULINS. Antibodies against a given antigen may be found in any one or a combination of the five classes of immunoglobulins in the serum.[2] IgG is the most plentiful immunoglobulin and may be the most important in humans, representing the antibodies to most bacteria and viruses. IgG is transported across the placenta to the fetus and plays a major role in the defense of the infant against infection, for the neonate does not produce IgG for some time after birth. IgM does not cross the placenta but is the first to appear after birth and the first to appear after antigenic stimulation.

**TABLE 8–3** COMPONENTS OF IMMUNE RESPONSE

| Response | Effector | Manifestation |
|---|---|---|
| Cellular | T-lymphocytes (thymus-dependent) | Direct cytotoxic effect on tumor cells; release of factors to stimulate macrophage |
| | B-lymphocytes (gut-dependent; "bursa of Fabricius") | Responsible for production of antibodies<br>Transport information to plasma cells for production of antibodies(?) |
| | Macrophages | Lyse target cells |
| Humoral | IgG (7S) | Antibodies to most bacteria and viruses<br>Transported across placenta and plays major role in newborn defense<br>Formed by plasma cells in lymph nodes and spleen |
| | IgM (19S) | First to appear after antigen stimulus<br>Synthesis diminishes as IgG increases<br>Formed by plasma cells in lymph nodes and spleen |
| | IgA (7S) | Produced by submucosal plasma cells of respiratory tract and intestine and nearly all excretory glands |

IgM is not produced for long periods, however, and generally its production diminishes at a time when IgG is seen to increase. Antibodies to gram-negative bacteria are predominantly of the IgM class, which is probably the reason immunity to these bacteria is usually short-lived. IgD is found only in very small quantities in the serum, and its biologic activity is not certain; IgE has only recently been discovered and not all of its characteristics have been ascertained.

In contrast to IgG and IgM, which are produced by the plasma cells in lymph nodes and spleen, IgA is produced by plasma cells in the submucosal regions of the respiratory and intestinal tracts, as well as in most excretory glands producing saliva. As such, it serves as a defense against invasive bacteria in the oral cavity, in the respiratory and intestinal tracts and in ducts of glands. It is resistant to enzymatic breakdown and may be absorbed from the intestine into the circulation.

### INTACT MUCOUS MEMBRANE (IgA)

Mixed saliva contains large amounts of secretory IgA and small amounts of IgG and IgM. Secretory glycoprotein is conjugated with IgA in cells of salivary glands, making the IgA chemically stable in the oral environment. The IgA is, therefore, present in the mucin coating the oral cavity, and its agglutinating capacity contributes to the "trapping" of bacteria in the mucin and subsequent washing away. Oral bacteria coated with IgA are also more easily phagocytized by leukocytes.

### INJURED MUCOUS MEMBRANE (IgG and IgM)

When the intact membrane barrier is broken, bacterial invasion stimulates transudation of immunoglobulins from serum and local formation of such globulins from B-lymphocytes in tissue. These are primarily IgG with small amounts of IgA and pass through tissue into saliva. IgG functions to neutralize toxins and viruses, and, in the presence of complement, leads to chemotaxis, opsonization and bacteriolysis. These immunologic responses are reflections of cell-mediated immunity, antibody production and other reactions occurring in the body as a whole.[41] In contrast to the broad antibacterial activity of lysozymes, the effects of the immune response are narrow and specific. As a result of salivary secretions, the immune response is active not only on tissues in response to injury but also in the general milieu of the oral cavity to protect the intact mucous membrane barrier.

## ALTERATIONS IN DEFENSE MECHANISMS

The patient with head and neck cancer presents potential problems in altered defense mechanisms that may be either general in nature and not specific to the tumor or local and specific to head and neck cancer. Many of these factors will be present in the same patient, making the problem of infection difficult to predict or prevent.

### General Alterations

There are certain alterations in systemic host defense mechanisms that may render the head and neck cancer patient particularly prone to local or systemic infection problems.

#### MALNUTRITION

Patients with head and neck cancer are often poorly nourished because of pain or difficulty in swallowing together with a lifestyle of alcoholism or poor eating habits. In a large cooperative study of wound infections and ultraviolet light, an incidence of wound infection of 22.4 per cent was observed in patients with malnutrition, compared to an incidence of less than 7.3 per cent in patients with adequate nutritional states.[1] Although short periods (days) of nutritional deprivation may lead to no alteration in the defense mechanisms, chronic wasting, protein deprivation and true hypoproteinemia clearly result in decreased antibody formation and an altered defense mechanism.[2] Dudrick and others have shown the importance of nutrition in the body's ability to withstand surgical stress. In a preliminary report of patients with head and neck cancer, patients on hyperalimentation clearly seemed to tolerate surgery, radiation therapy and chemotherapy better than control patients.[20] A normal person with normal activity requires 2000 to 3000 calories a day to maintain nutritional balance; this increases to 3000 to 3500 calories a day in the early postoperative period and finally reaches more than 5000 calories a day if a complication occurs, such as wound infection. It is reasonable to assume that most patients with head and neck cancer are at a marginal nutritional state at the beginning of treatment, a situation making them more susceptible to infection.

#### DIABETES

The increased incidence of diabetes in the sixth and seventh decades of life would tend to make diabetes a potential factor in the resistance to infection. Galloway showed an increased incidence of infection among diabetics undergoing surgery, and further studies have tended to confirm this.[1, 26] It has also been shown that the elevated blood sugar of the diabetic tends to support the proliferation of gram-positive organisms and fungi.[64] Finally, there is a documented increase of *Candida albicans* in the flora of the diabetic's mouth. Nevertheless, the exact role of diabetes in infection cannot be determined.

#### CHEMOTHERAPY

Virtually all chemotherapeutic agents will have their primary effect on cell populations undergoing the most rapid proliferation. Attempts to alter the cell population of a malignant growth are, therefore, often attended by alterations in the blood cells that are responsible for the host defense mechanisms (leukocytes and lymphocytes). It is clear that altered resistance to infection is the major hazard of chemotherapy and can result in systemic infection, often through local ulcerations in the oral cavity. Because the oral cavity is protected in health by low-grade inflammation, the manifestations of neutropenia and lymphopenia will often be seen initially as ulcerations and infections in the oral cavity.

#### ANTIBIOTICS

Antibiotics are clearly the most important factor introduced into the balance between the oral microflora and the local and systemic host defense mechanisms in the last 30 years. Antibiotics, as discussed in chapters 6 and 7, as part of prophylaxis and therapy also represent a major factor in reducing host defenses against some microorganisms. Each antibiotic has its spectrum of activity, either narrow or broad, but none will produce a germ-free oral environment. Alterations in the bacterial ecology will result from the use of any antibiotic. Administration of penicillin will decrease the population of gram-positive organisms but also will lead to a commensurate rise in the levels of gram-negative organisms. The use of broad-spectrum antibiotics will decrease the levels of both gram-positive and gram-negative organisms, at the expense of a rise in the level of fungi.[14] Ehrenkranz has demonstrated that tetracycline administration will result in a quantitative increase in resistant *Staphylococcus* in the nasopharynx.[21] Patients hospitalized for periods of more than a few days preoperatively acquire the hospital flora, which is often antibiotic-resistant, and there is a linear increase in the chance of infection for any given operation as the hospital stay increases prior to surgery.[1] Therefore, antibiotics, our most potent therapeutic tool against infection, may also represent a hazard and predispose the patient to infection.

#### OTHER FACTORS

There are other systemic host factors that have a variable influence on the systemic resistance to infection but have only occasional and coincidental influence on the patient with head and neck cancer. Included among these are anemia, shock, adrenocorticoid drugs and the rare immunologic disease states. Each may reduce defenses against infection.

### Immunologic Alterations

#### AGED

The increase in incidence of malignancy beyond middle life may be associated with a concomitant decrease in the capability to elicit immunologic defenses against alterations in the biologic milieu. Immunocompetence has been evaluated in man by delayed cutaneous hypersensitivity to a variety of bacterial, viral and fungal agents. The induction of response to a simple chemical such as dinitrochlorobenzene (DNCB), however, avoids the uncertainty of the host's ability to recall previously exposed antigens.

In a study of cutaneous hypersensitivity to DNCB, Gross found a drop in response to 62 per cent in a group of aged patients, in comparison to 97 per cent in the control group of younger patients.[28] There was a further drop to 14 per cent in the group of aged patients with advanced cancer. In a further study of immunocompetence in the aged, Waldorf and his associates noted that, although the number of patients responding to DNCB was significantly decreased with the aged, there was no fall off with age in the response to tuberculin[72] (Table 8–4). This distinction between the response to tuberculin and DNCB supports the contention that the aged may retain the ability to respond to an antigen to which they had been previously exposed, although they may fail to respond to a new antigenic challenge. In addition, Baumgartner has shown a decreased antibody production in older patients.[9] Thus, a decrease in the immunologic response of the host may lead to a higher incidence of malignancy or infection in the aged.

#### IMMUNOSUPPRESSION AND TUMOR IMMUNITY

Immunosuppressive therapy has been in use for many years and has been the mainstay of the spectacular organ transplantation successes in the past decade. The success of the transplant is based on the suppression of the immune mechanism in order to allow the foreign cells to be supported and to survive in the new host. Immunosuppressive therapy has also been used in autoimmune disease as well as in certain other diseases having unknown etiologic factors (e.g., psoriasis). Since the early days of immunosuppression, there has been speculation concerning the potential for increased malignancy developing as a result of the inhibition of the immunologic surveillance mechanism.

The concern for such a consequence of the alteration of the immunologic defenses was well founded, for cases did appear. The first case was reported by McPhaul and McIntosh. It concerned a young woman who developed metastatic squamous cell

**TABLE 8–4** DELAYED CUTANEOUS HYPERSENSITIVITY IN AGED*

| | | | | |
|---|---|---|---|---|
| Gross: | | | | |
| DNCB-positive | *Controls (13–17 years)* 97% | *No Malignancy (60–95 years)* 62% | *Malignancy (60–95 years)* 14% | |
| Waldorf et al.: | *under 70* | *70–79* | *80–89* | *90–99* |
| DNCB-positive | 94% | 69% | 68% | 50% |
| Tuberculin-positive | 60% | 63% | 46% | 50% |

*(Modified from Gross, L.: Immunological defect in aged population and its relationship to cancer. Cancer, *18*:201, 1965; and from Waldorf, D. S., Wilkens, R. F., and Decker, J. L.: Impaired delayed hypersensitivity in an aging population. J.A.M.A., *203*:831, 1968.)

carcinoma following the transplant of a kidney from a patient who died of squamous cell carcinoma of the pyriform sinus.[48] At the time of the transplant there was no gross evidence of kidney metastases in the donor. Cessation of the immunosuppression in this recipient was to no avail, and she rapidly succumbed to the malignancy. Wilson and his associates reported a case of metastatic squamous cell carcinoma of the lung in the operative site and draining nodes of a recipient of a kidney from a patient who had died of bronchogenic carcinoma.[7] In this case, however, the residual cancer disappeared after the cessation of immunosuppression and the removal of the rejected kidney. It is believed that, as a result of the immunosuppression, the transplanted malignant cells flourished and spread, and the cessation of immunosuppressive therapy resulted in the return of immunologic competence in the patient, leading to the search for and destruction of the foreign malignant cells.

Soon thereafter, Starzl reported three *de novo* malignant tumors in the transplant recipients treated in Denver as well as two additional cases reported to him from other investigators.[68] The evidence supporting the contention that these malignancies were a result of immunosuppression increased. Deodhar and his associates reported the development of reticulum cell sarcoma at the site of injection of antilymphocyte globulin (ALG) in their patient.[18] Based on these reports, Penn and Starzl reviewed their Transplant Registry and found 16 malignant tumors in 286 transplant recipients, for an incidence of 5.6 per cent.[58] The most common malignancy was of epithelial origin, and excepting skin malignancy, squamous cell carcinoma of the lip was the most frequently seen. This startling incidence was verified by a prospective study of all transplant recipients in the Scandia Transplant Programme of Denmark,[11] which maintained an exact registration of all necessary information. This study noted a 3 per cent incidence of *de vovo* malignancy developing in a one to four year follow-up period.

A careful review of the transplant recipients demonstrates that, although the incidence of a malignancy developing in an otherwise "healthy" patient was low, there was a 36 per cent incidence of malignancy after transplants from donors with cancer and a 41 per cent incidence of recurrence or me-

**TABLE 8–5** MANIFESTATION OF MALIGNANCY IN TRANSPLANT RECIPIENTS*

| | Number of Patients | Number of Malignant Tumors | Incidence |
|---|---|---|---|
| Pre-existing cancer in donor | 47 | 17 | 36.2% |
| *De novo* cancer | 432 | 24 | 5.6% |
| Pre-existing cancer in recipient | 76 | 31 | 40.8% |
| (*De novo* malignancy) | 76 | 4 | 5.3% |

*(Modified from Penn, I.: Chemical immunosuppression and human cancer. Cancer, *34*:1474, 1974.)

tastasis in recipients who had a pre-existing tumor[57] (Table 8–5). The appearance and progression of malignancy in these patients is a manifestation of immunosuppression. Of particular interest is the 5 per cent incidence of a new malignancy noted in the group with pre-existing tumors, which is the same as the *de novo* group. This study also noted 48 additional cases of malignant tumors developing in nontransplant patients who had been treated by a variety of immunosuppressive agents for other diseases. It is difficult to evaluate the true incidence in this group, however, because the total population at risk is not readily known.

It can be generally stated from the information presently known concerning patients receiving immunosuppressive therapy that their risk of developing a lymphoma is 35 times that expected in normal persons, the risk of skin and lip cancer is 4 times that expected and the risk for other types of cancers is 2.5 times normal.[30] These tumors occur in a younger age group, invariably under age 40, and have occurred as early as age 8.[57] There appears to be no relationship between the development of these tumors and any particular agent used, but there seems to be the effect of general immunosuppression.

## TUMOR IMMUNITY AND IMMUNOGLOBULINS

The immunologic response to tumor in humans is a highly complex multistaged process. It is a manifestation of a cellular response and a humoral antibody response (Fig. 8–1). This antibody response, in turn, may work either antagonistically or synergistically with the cellular antitumor response.[5] In brief, it is believed that T-cells (thymus-dependent lymphocytes) exposed to tumor antigen release migration inhibitory factor (MIF) to attract and immobilize macrophages at the site and macrophage activating factor (MAF), which increases the killing potential of the macrophages (by increasing the activities of lysosomal enzymes). The lysis of tumor cells requires the adherence of macrophages, but phagocytosis is not the mechanism of killing. It is believed that the lysis of the target cells is effected by the release of certain toxic contents by the activated macrophage (Fig. 8–2). This mechanism requires a specific stimulus to activate the macrophage, but the manifestation is not specific, for these immune cells may now respond to a variety of antigens. It is this type of nonspecific activation of macrophages that is believed to be the mechanism of immunologic stimulation by bacille Calmette Guérin (BCG).[6]

The role delegated to the B-cell lymphocytes is the production of antibodies by transforming into mast cells for the production of these antibodies. The role of antibodies against tumors can be either synergistic or antagonistic to the cellular immune response. Although there is evidence through *in vitro* studies that certain antibodies may lyse tumor cells in the presence of complement, such a response has not yet been conclusively described *in vivo*.[3] There is evidence, however, that circulating serum-blocking factors are antigen-antibody complexes that interfere with the binding sites of the cellular immune response.[66]

Although patients with cancer may demonstrate a decreased response in delayed cutaneous hypersensitivity and lymphocyte function, the production of antibodies (immunoglobulins) to bacterial, viral or cancer cell lines in these patients is the same as in normal patients.[67] As a matter of fact, Hughes noted a significant increase in serum levels of IgA in patients with cancer of the oral cavity, larynx and gut.[31] In a further review of salivary IgA production, Mandel noted a significant increase in smokers, in patients with bronchogenic and oropharyngeal cancers and in patients with inflammatory disease of the oropharynx when compared to nonsmoking control patients[45] (Table 8–6).

Since IgA is the predominant immunoglobulin secreted in saliva, the elevated titers in nonsmokers who had tonsillitis or pharyngitis is probably a result of the normal response of the salivary glands to invasion of the oral mucosa by bacteria and viruses. The greater elevation of those who drank as well as smoked may be a result of poor oral and dental hygiene, leading to the same type of response. Since local rather than systemic stimulation leads to IgA production, and since this immunoglobulin has been shown to be elevated in patients with

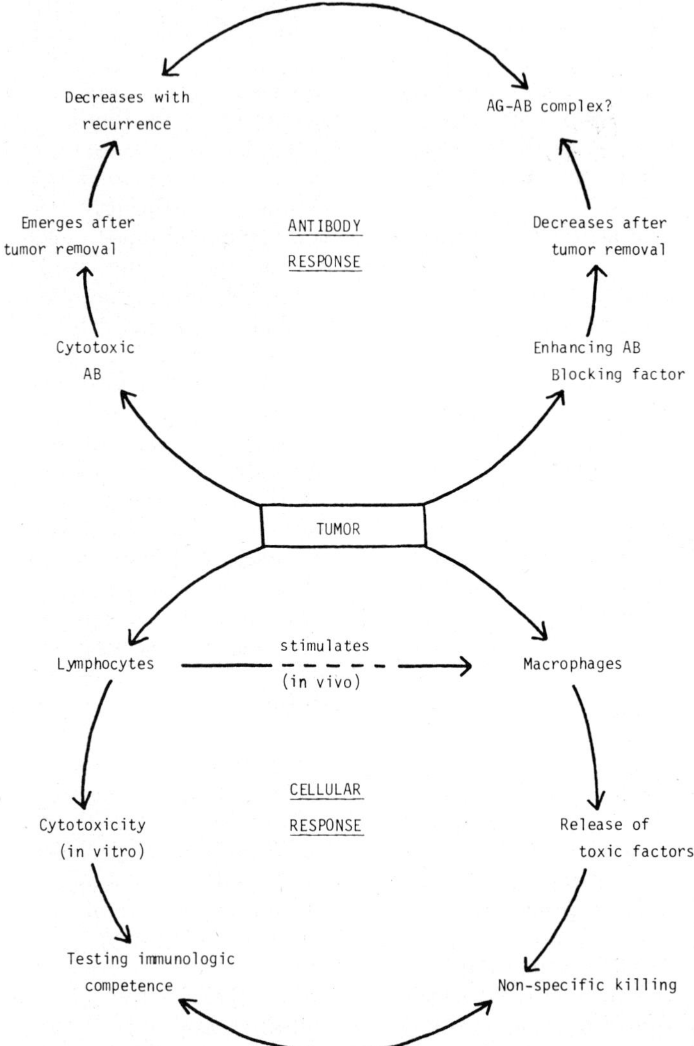


**Figure 8–1** Division of the immune response into antibody and cellular responses. (From Ariyan, S.: Progress of immunotherapy in the treatment of malignant melanoma. Yale J. Biol. Med., *48*:423, 1975.)

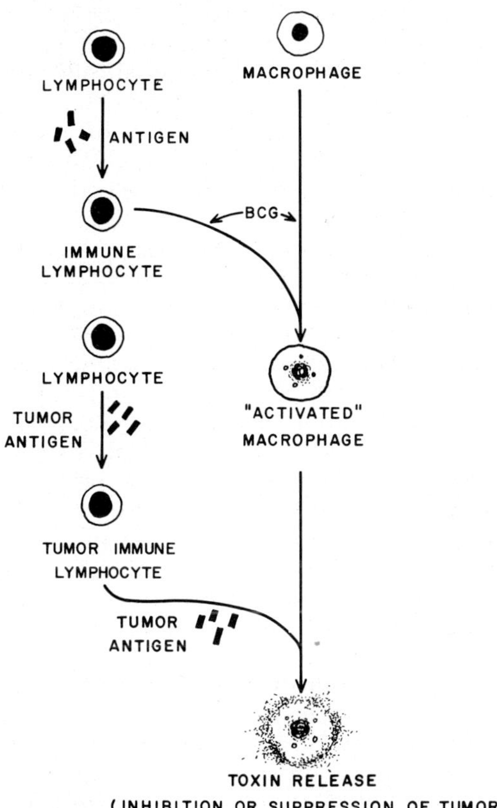


**Figure 8–2** Activation of macrophages. Macrophages may become nonspecifically activated by the injection of BCG in the animal to increase the enzymatic activity, so that the presence of tumor-immune lymphocytes may then cause the macrophages to burst and release their toxic contents, which in turn suppress the tumor. (From Ariyan, S., and Gershan, R. K.: The role of BCG vaccination in producing tumor immunity. Plast. Reconstr. Surg., *56*:430, 1975.)

cancers more directly exposed to local infection, it may be postulated that this increase is a response to secondary bacterial invasion through the neoplastic epithelium. The low levels of IgA in patients with recurrent carcinoma of the oropharyngeal area may be due to radiation atrophy of the salivary glands, since all patients in the group had reportedly received 5000 to 7000 rads to this area preoperatively.

At this time, there is no evidence that immunoglobulins play a significant role in the immune response against solid tumors. They play a significant secondary role in the response to local bacterial and viral invasion of the cancer in the mucosa of the head and neck area, however.

### IMMUNOSUPPRESSION AND INFECTION

Since the advent of penicillinase-resistant penicillins and broad-spectrum antibiotics, the gram-positive organisms have been largely replaced by gram-negative organisms that would otherwise be considered "nonpathogenic."[19] These organisms *(Pseudomonas, Serratia, Klebsiella, Enterobacter, Proteus* and *Escherichia coli)* invade the oral mucosa at sites of local trauma and may precipitate extensive cellulitis and bacteremia. In patients receiving chemotherapeutic agents that result in significant myelosuppression and immunosuppression, these infections may result in septicemia and death.

Renal transplant patients on extensive and prolonged immunosuppression are sus-

**TABLE 8–6** SALIVARY IgA TITERS IN OROPHARYNGEAL IRRITATION AND MALIGNANCY*

| Group | Number of Patients | mg. IgA/15 min. | Standard Deviation | Notes |
|---|---|---|---|---|
| Normal nonsmokers | 30 | 0.58 | ± 0.18 | All nonsmokers |
| Smokers | 35 | 1.35 | ± 0.46 | |
| Smokers and drinkers | 35 | 2.11 | ± 0.46 | |
| Oropharyngeal cancer | 35 | 2.15 | ± 0.65 | One nonsmoker |
| Bronchogenic cancer | 35 | 2.11 | ± 0.48 | One nonsmoker |
| Genitourinary cancer | 25 | 0.71 | ± 0.25 | All nonsmokers |
| Pharyngitis and/or tonsillitis | 25 | 1.47 | ± 0.46 | All nonsmokers |
| Recurrent disease | 10 | 0.70 | ± 0.40 | |

*(Modified from Mandel, M. A., Dvorak, K., and DeCosse, J. J.: Salivary immunoglobulins in patients with oropharyngeal and bronchopulmonary carcinoma. Cancer, *31*:1408, 1973.)

ceptible to malignant disorders and opportunistic infections.[54] Steroids suppress the inflammatory response and the chemotactic response of polymorphonuclear leukocytes and interfere with the intracellular killing of organisms in leukocytes by stabilizing the lysosomal membranes. The commonly used purine analogues, such as azathioprine (Imuran), inhibit the lymphoblast, and antilymphocyte globulin (ALG) inhibits the T-lymphocytes but spares the B-lymphocytes.[56] This suppression of T-cell production accounts for the higher incidence of *de novo* malignancy in this group, but the sparing of the B-cells maintains the humoral antibody responses against infection. Extensive and prolonged immunosuppression in a rejection crisis, however, may result in infections due to the opportunistic organisms noted previously as well as a variety of fungi and viruses.[8, 61]

In a similar fashion, with the general debility associated with the spread of tumor in the terminal stages of cancer, the defense mechanisms are further compromised by the immunosuppressive effects of the chemotherapeutic agents utilized. Therefore, infections are common terminal events in far-advanced cases of cancer.

#### IMMUNOTHERAPY

Stimulation of the immune system with BCG or other agents is part of current investigative work in controlling malignant disorders, particularly melanoma. It is unlikely that such treatment adversely effects the systemic defense mechanism against infection. Our experience with the use of MER-BCG (methanol-extractable residue of BCG) instilled into the wounds at the time of radical neck and groin dissection has demonstrated an occasional intense inflammatory response beginning three to four days postoperatively, lasting for several weeks and subsiding only very slowly. It has not, however, been accompanied by infection.

### Local Alterations in Defense Mechanisms

#### MALIGNANCY

Oropharyngeal cancer has been associated with multiple extrinsic factors, each of an irritative nature, stimulating a local inflammatory response and leading to the repeated reparative efforts characteristically seen in "traumatic" cancers such as Marjolin's ulcers.[7] Among these factors are chronic exposure to cigarette smoking and alcohol and the less common, but more distinctly associated, relationship between the use of chutta (a cigar held with the lighted end against the hard palate for better drainage of the smoke) and the use of khaini (a cud of slaked lime and tobacco held between the lower lip and adjacent alveolar arch).[36] Each is associated with chronic irritation, repair, pseudoepitheliomatous hyperplasia, leukoplakia and, finally, squamous cell carcinoma, often at the exact site of irritation. These and other extrinsic agents result in trauma and discontinuity of the protective mucous membrane barrier and an increase in the tissue levels of bacteria.

The appearance of carcinoma is almost inevitably associated with a break in the continuity of the mucous membrane. The oral microflora becomes established in the tumor tissue itself, erodes and proliferates at the tumor margins and results in the quantitative bacterial documentation of infection. Therefore, therapy in ulcerated oropharyngeal carcinoma is conducted in an environment with more than mere contamination by bacteria; it is in the actual presence of established infection. Palpable regional nodes are often difficult to interpret, since they may represent the inflammatory response to infection in addition to metastases from the tumor. Furthermore, our studies on laboratory animals with tumors have demonstrated that there is decreased resistance to infection in clean operative wounds even where there is no ulceration.[12]

#### SURGERY

Any surgical procedure in the oral or pharyngeal cavity, be it biopsy, dental restoration, extraction or definitive resection, reduces the local defense mechanisms by disrupting the intact mucous membrane barriers. Such procedures do not inevitably result in infection, but they do give a very large inoculum of bacteria access to open tissue. All such procedures must therefore be categorized as "contaminated."

**RADIATION**

Therapeutic radiation lowers the local defense mechanisms to infection as part of its normal biologic alterations. Such alterations are a result of the effects of radiation on salivary flow, as well as being the direct effects of radiation on the tissue itself.

**Saliva.** Therapeutic levels of radiation markedly decrease the volume of salivary flow, resulting in a secretion with a high viscosity and a low pH. Such alterations and their effects on the oral microflora predispose these patients to the formation of dental plaque and subsequent caries. There are increased numbers of lactobacilli and streptococci and decreased numbers of the more harmless *Corynebacterium* and *Neisseria* species. Furthermore, *Streptococcus salivarius,* a normal facultative gram-positive coccus, is replaced by an overgrowth of *Streptococcus mitis.*[44] Since saliva and its washing effect are most important in maintaining the normal balance of the host and the oral microflora, these effects on saliva are profound in reducing some of the defense mechanisms.

**Tissue Effects.** In most centers, there are two methods for applying radiation to tumors that are being considered for surgical procedures. The first is "planned preoperative" radiation. Approximately 4000 rads of external beam radiation is administered, usually in divided doses over a four-week period; after the edema subsides (approximately four weeks), ablative surgery is performed. The rationale in this plan is to "sterilize" the field of microscopic tumor seedings in the tissues, lymphatics and nodes that are not removed by the surgical procedure. The second method of treatment is "curative" radiation doses, in which 6000 rads or more of external beam radiation is administered in divided doses, either alone or in combination with radioactive implants. Those receiving this type of treatment are considered for surgery only if, after a period of time following the radiation, there is demonstration of a recurrence or persistence of the tumor and radiation therapy is deemed to have failed to control the tumor.

With these two methods in mind, two separate studies investigating the major surgical complication rates noted a twofold increase in those treated with the "planned preoperative" radiation doses of 3500 to 4500 rads and a fourfold increase in those patients treated with 6000 rads "for cure."[32, 74] Infection played a major role in the complications noted. Ketcham reported 23 minor and 13 major complications among 60 patients (60 per cent) having surgery after a single dose of 1000 rads that was given 24 hours preoperatively; this is in comparison with 5 minor complications in the 19 nonirradiated control patients (26 per cent).[34] On the other hand, Lawrence reported no difference between the complication rates following composite resection after split doses of radiation (700 rads 24 hours and 48 hours before surgery) and those from a group not receiving radiation (24 per cent vs. 20 per cent).[42] It is not clear from these reports whether there were factors other than radiation that might have influenced the outcome, such as different patient populations, antibiotics or states of nutrition. On theoretical grounds at least, one would anticipate an altered tissue resistance to infection after radiation.

Laboratory investigation of wound complications has been aimed at wound healing from the structural point of view. Retardation of the rate of contraction of wounds was studied by Grillo and Potsaid,[27] as well as by Van den Brenk and his associates.[71] The latter group also studied the biosynthesis of collagen in irradiated tissue. Powers, Ogura and Palmer reported a decrease in the recovery of tensile strength of flaps treated with increasing doses of radiation.[60] The investigation of infection of irradiated wounds and its influence on the final healing of the irradiated tissue has been, for the most part, neglected.

It has been clinically apparent that wound infection is the greatest contributor to wound breakdown, fistula formation, dehiscence, carotid blow out and death. These complications, as well as infection *per se,* are decreased in comparable operations performed on those not receiving radiation. A most important question concerns the effect of radiation on the local tissue resistance to infection. We studied the antibacterial resistance of wounds in irradiated tissues in rats. The radiobiologic equivalent (RBE) of the radiation doses in humans can be estimated in rats based on skin changes and radiation isoeffect curves.[52, 53] From these, the RBE's of 4000 rads ("planned preoperative") and 6000 rads ("curative") in humans were estimated as single-dose equivalents to be 1050 rads and 1800 rads respectively. Standard wounds were inflicted into the skin of the animals at intervals after the radiation was administered, and quantitative bacterial cultures were performed on homogenates of the excised surgical wound four days later.[46]

Infection, defined as the quantitative count of $10^5$, or greater, bacteria per gm. of tissue,[64] was not encountered in the control sham-irradiated animals.[46] In this group, only 3 to 43 animals had bacteria in the wound ($10^2$–$10^3$). There were significantly increased bacterial counts ($10^2$–$10^5$) in the wounds that had been radiated, however. There was a linear increase in the incidence of positive cultures and in the level of bacterial growth as the interval between radiation and wounding was lengthened, the greatest being at four to six weeks in the 1800-rad groups.

Fractionated dosage schemes, usually employed for therapeutic radiation in the head and neck (200 rads per day, 5 days a week, for x number of weeks), result initially in an intense inflammatory response in the mucous membrane and skin. Altered salivary flow and an altered microbial ecology contribute to increased tissue levels of bacteria. There are local adverse alterations in local immune defenses and inflammatory cells. After a few weeks, a new balance becomes established, and some months after radiation the vasculitis and inflammation end in scarring and obliterative vascular changes with local tissue ischemia. A decreased resistance to infection is present both acutely and in the most chronic phases after therapeutic radiation.

Although the mechanisms of this decreased resistance to contaminating bacteria are not yet clear, our data appear to indicate that radiated tissue has a significantly impaired ability to clear the bacterial challenge in surgical wounds.[46] Furthermore, this impairment becomes more significant as the dose is increased and as the time between radiation and wounding is lengthened.

### Other Problems

Dental Caries. The altered salivary flow and microflora after radiation predispose the patient to dental plaque and radiation caries, with an incidence as high as 68 per cent reported in untreated patients.[17]

Osteoradionecrosis. Radiation to the head and neck region and its subsequent alterations in defense mechanisms may lead to osteoradionecrosis. The complication of osteoradionecrosis must be considered in the category of infection, as it is unlikely to occur in the absence of direct bacterial contamination. In a similar way, a patient whose hands had been exposed to 250,000 rads orthovoltage in an industrial accident developed open wounds with the clinical and radiologic picture of osteoradionecrosis. Once infection was controlled and suitable soft tissue (skin flap) coverage was applied, the picture of osteoradionecrosis disappeared completely, without any specific treatment to the bones.[37] Of all patients receiving radiation for head and neck cancer, only those with poor dentition and periodontal disease or those undergoing extractions or surgical manipulation of the bone seemed to be affected. All have in common the exposure of avascular bone to the oral microflora. Areas of relative avascularity with a paucity of soft tissue coverage seem particularly prone to osteoradionecrosis, particularly tumors in the region of the retromolar trigone. Daly emphasizes the importance of performing needed dental extractions well in advance of the beginning of therapeutic radiation, allowing at least 10 days for commencement of suitable wound healing.[17] Among his 304 patients, he noted 74 cases of osteoradionecrosis in 69 bones. Thirty-nine per cent of these appeared to be "spontaneous," 30 per cent followed extractions before the beginning of radiation, 17 per cent were related to surgery, 7 per cent were due to prostheses and 3 per cent were due to nonextraction trauma. All three patients who underwent extractions after radiation developed osteoradionecrosis.

## DENTAL

It is clear that the functional state of the dentition and the degree of oral health are important factors influencing local defense mechanisms against infections. As was stated earlier, there is a ten-fold increase in the microflora of the mouth in the presence of periodontal and periapical disease. Although altered defense mechanisms produced by disease or radiation have an adverse effect on teeth, the teeth themselves are often the foci of areas of diminished resistance. The presence of caries increases the level of microflora. Poor hygiene, poor occlusion and missing teeth may lead to the loosening of other teeth, rupture of periodontal supporting structures and periodontal inflammation or periapical abscesses. The presence of such foci increases the risks of infection following any surgical procedure.

## PROPHYLACTIC MEASURES AGAINST INFECTION

An understanding of the balance between the oral microflora and the host defense mechanisms is the basis on which prophylactic measures may be initiated for the prevention of infection. It is difficult to tease out individual procedures and attempt to document their unique effectiveness by any statistical means because of the multitude of factors influencing the equilibrium present in health and disturbed in disease. Rather, these measures are based on a rational approach to the biology of the disease state.

### General

It goes without saying that the patient's general condition should be at its most favorable state prior to instituting therapy. Once a diagnosis of "cancer" is made, there often is an inherent urgency felt by both the patient and the doctor to proceed quickly. The population group under discussion is particularly prone to additional health problems, however. These "co-morbid" factors may be important determinants in the choice of treatment and its final outcome. For instance, the patient with unstable angina and a history of two myocardial infarctions in the last three years is more likely to die from his cardiac condition than from his oral malignancy. Accordingly, such an associated disease might clearly influence the type of therapy to be employed.

A substantial incidence of associated diseases should be expected because of the age distribution of these patients. Arteriosclerotic heart disease, diabetes and pulmonary disease are common. More specifically, this group has a history of heavy smoking and a high incidence of emphysema and other forms of chronic pulmonary disease. The alcoholic patient may also be likely to have associated cirrhosis, and perhaps portal hypertension. Poor dietary habits with associated pain and difficulty in eating predispose these patients to marginal or frank malnutrition with its associated hypovitaminosis and anemia.

Any of the associated diseases may have either a direct or indirect influence on the systemic and local defense mechanisms against infection. Improvement in the nutritional status, perhaps with oral or parenteral hyperalimentation, should be undertaken. Vitamin deficiencies are easily corrected, and anemia may require preoperative transfusions. Any focus of infection elsewhere in the body should be corrected, since there is an associated increase in the incidence of wound infection as a result of the distant focus.[64] Particular emphasis should be placed on the respiratory tract, where chronic pulmonary disease and respiratory infection may influence not only the chance of wound infection but also the chances of postoperative pulmonary infection.

### Local Measures

The most effective methods of favorably influencing the defense against the oral microflora are local measures designed to correct dental hygiene. The patient should have a complete dental evaluation prior to any form of therapy. Loose and nonrestorable carious teeth should be extracted, and the wound should be allowed to heal for 10 to 14 days prior to the commencement of radiation therapy or, perhaps, definitive surgery. It is our custom to save all healthy teeth, even in patients undergoing radiation combined with surgical treatment. They are useful during reconstructive surgery, and, with proper prophylaxis, radiation-induced caries can often be prevented. The daily topical application of 1 per cent sodium fluoride gel has reduced the incidence of radiation caries to only 31 per cent, from an incidence of 68 per cent in untreated controls.[17] Foci of infection in the gingival, periodontal and periapical tissues should, nevertheless, be corrected prior to either surgery or radiation.

Oral hygiene can be improved by dental prophylactic care, brushing the teeth and rinsing the mouth with saline or very mild antiseptics. Strong antiseptics run the risk of causing local irritation in already irritated tissues and may have a profound effect by altering the ecology of the oral microflora in favor of more resistant organisms.

## Surgical Measures to Prevent Infection

*Good postoperative care begins before the incision is made.* This is particularly true in the efforts to prevent infection.

### PREOPERATIVE CARE

Immediate preoperative measures designed to prevent infection include maintenance of an adequate state of hydration. Fasting, beginning the night before surgery, and the further "drying" effect of atropine and other preanesthetic drugs accentuate the diurnal variation in the oral microflora and tend to bring the patient to the operating room at a time when his bacterial count is at its highest. Mouth rinses and the use of intraoral povidone-iodine in the "prep" of the patient will reduce these microbial levels. Although no agent will sterilize and infection results from a profound disturbance in the *balance* rather than the presence of bacteria, efforts to quantitatively reduce the bacterial side of the balance do make sense.

Hair is an important consideration in operations about the head and neck. Cruse studied the role of hair in many wounds and noted an infection rate of 2.3 per cent when the operative sites had been shaved, 1.9 per cent when hair was clipped and 0.9 per cent when no attempt was made to remove it.[16] In another study, operative sites shaved 24 hours preoperatively had an infection rate of 20 per cent, compared with 3.1 per cent for those shaved immediately preoperatively.[65] Even in the best of hands, shaving produces irritation and small nicks in the skin. These lead to an increase in the bacterial count of the skin, and every surgeon has experienced distress on finding an operative site, which had been shaved the previous night, presenting with multiple microabscesses. Although it is more aesthetically pleasing to have a hairless operative field, the data indicate that it is much safer to merely clip long hairs, and, if a man's beard is to be shaved, it should be done as late preoperatively as possible.

A detailed discussion of skin antiseptics is beyond the scope of this presentation. A mechanical scrub, however, with a soap-base povidone-iodine preparation followed by the "painting" with a povidone-iodine solution would seem to be as nonirritating and effective as is now available.

### INTRAOPERATIVE CARE

The specific value of general operative measures to control exogenous sources of bacteria in surgery of the head and neck requires no documentation. It may be tacitly assumed that hand scrubs, gowns, masks, sterile drapes and so forth are as important here as in any other area of surgery. The realization that one is operating in a contaminated field should not reduce vigilance against extrinsic contamination. An acceptable balance between the indigenous microflora and the host defense may be destroyed by the introduction, even in relatively small numbers, of a new species of bacteria from outside the body.

**Technique.** *A good surgeon knows when to go slowly; a poor surgeon often does not know when to go fast.*

Major surgery of the head and neck is often time-consuming. It is clear that the establishment of bacteria in tissues occurs early in the operative procedure — most often within the first three to four hours. There is, however, an increased chance of accumulation of bacteria the longer an operative wound is exposed, and there is a direct linear increase in the chance of infection the longer any given operation takes to perform.[1] The longer wounds of the neck are exposed to the oral microflora, the more likely is the chance that bacterial accumulation will occur. Irrigations of the wound wash away loose bacteria but have little effect on bacteria already established in tissue.[29] Nevertheless, frequent irrigations during the course of the procedure make good theoretical sense. They also prevent dehydration of exposed tissue, another factor favoring bacterial growth. The value of expedient surgery cannot be emphasized enough and clearly accounts for differences in infection and other complication rates among different surgeons who are apparently employing similar measures in similar fashion.

**Foreign Bodies.** A major predisposing factor to infection is the presence of foreign bodies. These can take the form of seroma, hematoma, necrotic tissue or sutures. Seroma and hematoma are both associated with an increased incidence of infection. Several series have identified hematoma as a contributing factor in as many as 30 per cent of postoperative wound infections.[15, 47] Experimental data have confirmed that hematomas act as an adjuvant to bacterial growth, particularly for gram-negative organisms.[39] Necrotic tissue, in the form of residue after either ligature or coagulation of bleeders, clearly is a focus for bacterial growth, and good surgical technique will minimize this.

Suture material is a particularly adverse foreign body associated with infection. In the classic introduction of quantitative bacterial techniques into surgery, Elek demonstrated that the presence of a silk suture reduced, by a factor of 10,000 times, the number of staphylococci necessary to cause abscess formation.[22, 23] There are also variations among different suture materials, with catgut being the most predisposing to infection.[43] In addition to its presence as a foreign body, catgut elicits a foreign protein "rejection" phenomenon, since it is prepared from New Zealand sheep. Clearly, monofilament sutures lead to less infection than braided or twisted materials. The ideal suture material is nonreactive, handles easily, ties securely, maintains its tensile strength at least 30 to 40 days and dissolves by a chemical process rather than by destruction through the body's inflammatory reaction — it does not exist at this time.

Leakage of lymph from either the thoracic or right lymphatic duct can dissect the neck flaps from the underlying tissue and promote either seroma or hematoma formation in the postoperative period. Chyle (lymph) is bacteriostatic, however, and, in and of itself does not predispose to infection. Therefore, any measure that is effective in preventing the formation of dead space and hematoma is also useful in minimizing those factors predisposing to infection. The authors' preference is the use of large catheter suction (size 20–22 F., since clots in the neck are as big as elsewhere in the body).

**Intraoral Closure.** Routine radical neck dissections without entry into the oral cavity should be considered "clean" operations and should carry an infection rate of less then 2 per cent. The major problems arise in composite resections and other procedures in which the neck contents are resected in continuity with an intraoral or pharyngeal primary lesion, particularly in patients who received preoperative radiation to the area. The microbial flora of the oropharynx is brought into communication with the neck, resulting in a large and very contaminated wound. Careful attention to technique, prevention of hematoma and dead space and careful irrigation will minimize intraoperative bacterial accumulation, and such wounds may be safely closed. Major problems of infection, neck flap necrosis, development of fistulas and carotid rupture occur when the neck contents are bathed in the oropharyngeal secretions and their microflora following the completion of the operation. This most often occurs because of a breakdown in the intraoral closure. The oropharyngeal microflora, with its combination of aerobic and anaerobic bacteria, in the hypoxic environment of the fresh neck wound, in irradiated tissue, creates the ideal environment for a "Meleney type" of infection.[49] This combination of aerobic, microaerophilic and anaerobic organisms produces an infectious process that results in the familiar skin necrosis (cutaneous synergistic gangrene). In our estimation, the breakdown of skin flaps in the neck is more likely due to this type of infectious process than to ischemia of the skin from the surgery itself. The accompanying fistula and the continous bathing of the carotid artery with oropharyngeal bacteria is what leads to ultimate necrosis and rupture of the artery. It is clear that the single-most important factor in preventing this series of events is an adequate intraoral or intrapharyngeal closure — technical maneuvers to control infection.

Healing is unlikely in the wound that is closed with larger suture materials under tension in a heavily contaminated area, particularly if the wound has been irradiated. Tension must be avoided in the closure. Wound margins should remain as near to their original location as possible to avoid any stretching that could result in ischemia. Often, the defect can be closed, primarily when bone has been resected and the tissues collapse together. In nonradiated patients and in rigid nonmobile sites (maxillary and palatal defects) in radiated patients, skin grafts can be used nicely. In other circumstances, we believe closure with a flap is a major factor in preventing infection. The use of local, regional (nasolabial), or more distant flaps (pectoralis major myocutaneous) or free flaps allows closure without tension and prevents the resultant leakage of secretions into the neck. The deltopectoral flap can be introduced through the neck to form a skin-lined, controlled fistula that allows the oropharyngeal secretions to drain to the outside rather than into the neck. If flaps cannot be used and the closure would result in tension, it is better to leave the wound open. The skin may be sutured to mucous membrane at the periphery of the wound to construct a controlled fistula to the outside. Reconstruction of this area can then be performed at a later date.

### POSTOPERATIVE CARE

There seems little doubt that the determinants of infection are established intraoperatively. Contamination occurs during the operation, and bacterial lodgment becomes established during the operation and in the first several hours postoperatively. Epithelial continuity is normally established across primarily closed wounds within a matter of hours, and the possibility of extrinsic contamination beyond the first few hours postoperatively is unlikely. Early feeding may predispose to the disruption of the suture lines, and several days should be allowed for the establishment of a good epithelial seal and fibrin clot and the early development of a fibrous stroma. Openings of esophagostomy and suction catheters can represent potential portals of entry for bacteria, and careful attention must be paid to catheter care, as with intravenous sites.

## Antibiotics

The potential for disrupting the microbial ecology with antibiotics has been discussed previously. The use of prophylactic antibiotics in head and neck cancer surgery should be approached with a sound rationale and with an understanding of their limitations as well as their potential value. The administration of antibiotics, in adequate dosage and at the proper time, should theoretically prevent infection from susceptible organisms. Furthermore, again, theoretically, the broader the spectrum of antibiotic activity, the broader should be the blanket of protection. That antibiotics have failed to produce the germ-free patient or the infection-free operative procedure is clear from the three decades of experience with such agents. That antibiotics can even reduce the incidence of infection for any given operation is open to question in many surgical circumstances. The use of prophylactic antibiotics in head and neck cancer surgery, however, is based on sound theoretical principles, and there are data to support their value. When employed, they should be given at the proper time.

### USE IN RADICAL NECK DISSECTION

Radical neck dissections may be classified as "clean" procedures and carry a minimal risk of infection. The dangers of idiosyncratic reaction from antibiotics or an alteration of the microbial flora, which allows the emergence of resistant organisms, seem to outweigh any potential value of these agents. There are no data to support their value in this operation.

A different situation prevails in neck dissections performed through radiated tissue, however. Radiated tissue is less resistant to infection than normal tissue, and lesser numbers of bacteria will gain access and multiply to critical levels (greater than $10^5$ bacteria/gm.) than would occur in normal tissue. Therefore, the added protection of antibiotics may be warranted in this situation.

**Method of Administration.** Burke has shown that bacterial infection is established the first several hours of operating and that administration of antibiotics after this period fails to inhibit bacterial growth or prevent infections.[13] Administration too early before or for too long after the operation may produce an alteration in the flora and allow the emergence of resistant strains. Therefore, antibiotics should be administered immediately before, during and for a few hours after surgery. The goal is to achieve an adequate tissue level of antibiotics prior to and during the time bacteria are attempting to gain access to and proliferate in the tissue, and the bloodstream is the most dependable distributing system in these circumstances. The antibiotic chosen should carry a sufficient, but no wider, spectrum of activity to protect against the most likely organisms. Since the patterns of infection vary from hospital to hospital and over certain periods, it seems more appropriate to recommend regular careful review of that particular hospital's current experience and to choose the appropriate antibiotic accordingly. For instance, at the present time in our hospital, the most effective agent against gram-positive organisms is erythromycin.

#### USE IN COMBINED PROCEDURES

All procedures that include the oropharynx are contaminated, and the spectrum of the flora has been discussed previously. Polk has shown the value of the administration of preoperative and postoperative antibiotic in contaminated colon surgery.[59] Ketcham reported an infection rate of 8.8 per cent in a series of cancer patients receiving preoperative and postoperative antibiotics, compared with 17.3 per cent in similar patients receiving a placebo.[35] In a small but definitive series, he also demonstrated their specific efficacy in patients undergoing head and neck surgery.[34] Furthermore, it appears to be customary for surgeons to use them, for a recent survey indicated that 62 per cent of surgeons operating in this area use prophylactic antibacterials in composite resections.[40] There is a sound rationale for their use — the wounds are heavily contaiminated, and the local and systemic defense mechanisms may be altered in many patients.

**Method of Administration.** The goal of prophylactic treatment is to achieve an adequate tissue level of antibiotic prior to the time that bacterial penetration occurs and proliferation begins. In this particular situation, administration of antibiotics too early before the surgery will alter the flora in favor of resistant organisms, the very ones that will then contaminate the wound and cause the infection. In a related study, Gabrielson reviewed the effectiveness of 13 antibiotics in 84 patients with odontogenic infection and found that almost half of the patients had more than one organism, and all but one had at least one of the five most common organisms.[25] *Streptococcus viridans* (salivarius) was encountered in 93 per cent of the patients. Although antibiotic sensitivity studies indicated that chloramphenicol was most effective, other less toxic agents should be prescribed; erythromycin (99 per cent), cephalothin (99 per cent) and clindamycin (94 per cent) were the next most effective. Cephalothin is probably preferable at this time because of its wider spectrum, which includes most of the likely organisms. Again, the intravenous route should be employed in the early course of treatment. It should be emphasized once more that this approach is based on the biologic phenomena that are purportedly occurring, rather than on any overwhelming statistical evidence of success.

Other methods of administration, such as intraoperative or postoperative wound irrigations, cannot be defended. Bacteria are established by the end of the operation, and antibiotic washes simply fail to reach into the depths of the tissues. The bloodstream can deliver the drug far more effectively and dependably.

## THERAPY OF INFECTION

If all efforts at prophylaxis fail and infection develops, the likely cause may be either the local wound or seeding of infection from another site (pneumonitis or thrombophlebitis).

### Wound Infections

Although fever in the early postoperative period is most often due to other than wound sepsis (such as pulmonary atelectasis), some of the oral bacteria, particularly

*Streptococcus,* will manifest their presence in the first 18 to 36 hours with high fever, considerable erythema and edema of the wound *(peau d'orange).* The wound should be inspected to confirm the presence of infection. The offending agent may often be identified by inserting 2 to 3 ml. of saline into the wound and then culturing the aspirate. Appropriate therapeutic agents should be chosen on the basis of the diagnostic tests available with culture and sensitivity and with a high degree of suspicion that this infection is due to gram-positive cocci.

The authors contend that most cases of skin necrosis, fistulas, and exposed carotids have as their underlying cause constant contamination by a mixed oral bacterial flora as a result of a breakdown in the intraoral or pharyngeal repair. Impending or frank skin necrosis in these patients is a surgical and infection emergency. The necrotic edges must be debrided and the wound converted to an open wound draining to the outside and not seeding underneath the flaps, which would only potentiate the infection. The site of breakdown should be identified, if possible. A small (12 to 14 F.) Foley catheter inserted through the fistula, with the bag blown up to 2 to 3 ml. and put on slight traction, may perhaps dam the leak, minimize the flow and provide a controlled pathway for egress of the saliva to the outside.[51] In many cases, the fistula has spontaneously closed around the catheter, obviating the need for a secondary closure. Cultures should be obtained for aerobic and anaerobic (as well as microaerophilic) organisms. A review of 1339 anaerobic infections at the Mayo Clinic indicated that infection will result from a single organism in only 15 per cent of cases; in 85 per cent of cases, there will be at least one other organism (two-thirds of the cases were mixed with aerobic organisms).[4] Systemic antibiotic therapy in these cases should presumably cover anaerobic organisms in its spectrum of efficacy.

The open wounds that may result require treatment with topical antibacterial therapy in addition to systemic antibiotics. Although systemic antibiotics will penetrate the normal tissue around the infection site and perhaps limit its further spread, these antibiotics do not penetrate into open wounds that are more than several hours old.[63] An adequate tissue level of such antibacterials can be achieved by the use of the topical antibacterials. Experience with open wounds in burned patients has demonstrated that topical cream-based antibacterials have advantages in their ease of application and their penetration into tissue. Such agents as silver sulfadiazine 0.1 per cent and mafenide acetate 1 per cent have an antibacterial spectrum that includes most of the oral microflora. Such agents, in conjunction with systemic antibiotics, will control the local microbial flora and lessen the likelihood of carotid rupture. Quantitative bacterial counts confirming that such wounds contain less than $10^5$ bacteria per gram of tissue indicate that invasive wound sepsis is not occurring and that definitive secondary closure can be safely performed.

## Other Infections

The most common infection, other than in the wound, associated with head and neck surgery is in the respiratory system. The underlying chronic pulmonary disease that is often present in these patients predisposes to the postoperative problems of atelectasis and pneumonia. In these patients aspiration is not uncommon because of alterations in their ability to swallow and clear secretions. As Miller (1890) stated, infection is caused by "inspiration of particles of slime . . . containing bacteria."[50] Intensive tracheobronchial toilet is mandatory in these patients, and most of these patients deserve a tracheotomy at the time of surgery. Although the tracheotomy provides a secure airway and access to pulmonary hygiene, it also opens an additional portal for infection. Sources of organisms for postoperative pulmonary infection include the following:

1. Respiratory organisms presenting preoperatively
2. Aspiration of oropharyngeal microflora
3. Contamination during suctioning or insufflation of bacteria from contaminated respiratory-assist devices or humidifiers

The diagnosis is established by fever, positive culture of tracheal aspirates and radiologic evidence of changes. Therapy is again directed at tracheobronchial toilet, and the antibiotic choice is based on culture and sensitivity testing.

The occurrence of other sites of infection — venipuncture sites, thrombophlebitis or urinary tract infection—is qualitatively and quantitatively the same in head and neck patients as in any other surgical patient. The prophylactic and therapeutic measures are also the same.

## SUMMARY

The biologic state of the patient with head and neck cancer predisposes to infection. The environment is intensely contaminated with a mixed aerobic and anaerobic microbial flora. The normal defense mechanisms that would enable the person to live in balance with this environment in health are altered by the disease and its treatment. Measures to prevent or treat infection in these patients cannot be undertaken in a cookbook fashion. The multiplicity of factors makes statistical validation of causes or treatments difficult. A rational approach must therefore be based on an understanding of the dynamics of the host–bacteria equilibrium in health and in disease.

## Bibliography


1. Ad hoc Committee of the Committee on Trauma, Division of Medical Sciences, National Research Council Report: Postoperative wound infections; the influences of ultraviolet irradiation of the operating room and the influence of various other factors, Ann. Surg., *160* (Supplement); 1, 1964.
2. Alexander, J. W., and Good, R. A.: Immunobiology for Surgeons. Philadelphia, W. B. Saunders Co., 1977.
3. Allison, A. C.: Interactions of antibodies and effector cells in immunity against tumors. Am. Inst. Pasteur, *122*:619, 1972.
4. Anderson, C. B.: Anaerobic infections. *In* Ballinger, W. F., and Drapanos T. (eds.): Practice of Surgery — Current Reviews. St. Louis, The C.V. Mosby Co., 1975, p. 396.
5. Ariyan, S.: Progress of immunotherapy in the treatment of malignant melanoma. Yale J. Biol. Med., *48*:423, 1975.
6. Ariyan, S., and Gershan, R. K.: The role of BCG vaccination in producing tumor immunity. Plast. Reconstr. Surg., *56*:430, 1975.
7. Arons, M. S., Rodin, A. E., Lynch, J. B., et al.: Scar tissue carcinoma. II. An experimental study with special reference to burn scar carcinomas. Ann. Surg., *163*:445, 1966.
8. Bach, M. C., Sahyoun, A., Adler, J. L., et al.: Influence of rejection therapy on fungal and nocardial infections in renal transplant recipients. Lancet, *1*:180, 1973.
9. Baumgartner, L.: Age and antibody production. J. Immunol., *27*:407, 1934.
10. Beahrs, O. H.: Complications of surgery for cancer of the head and neck in management of surgical complications. *In* Artz, C. P., and Hardy, J. D. (eds): Management of Surgical Complications. Philadelphia, W. B. Saunders Co., 1975, p. 277.
11. Birkeland, S. A., Kemp, E., and Hauge, M.: Renal transplantation and cancer. The Scandia transplant material. Tissue Antigens, *6*:28, 1975.
12. Brin, E. N., and Krizek, T. J.: Resistance of animals with malignancy to experimental wound infection. Surg. Forum, *25*:526, 1974.
13. Burke, J. F.: The effective period of preventive antibiotic action in experimental incisions and dermal lesions. Surgery, *50*:161, 1961.
14. Burnett, G. W., and Scherp, H. W.: Oral Microbiology and Infectious Disease. Baltimore, Williams and Wilkins, 1968.
15. Conolly, W. B., and Golovsky, D.: Postoperative wound sepsis. Med. J. Aust., *1*:643, 1967.
16. Cruse, P. J. E.: Prospective study of 20,105 surgical wounds with emphasis on use of topical antibiotics and prophylactic antibiotics. Presented at the Fourth Symposium on Control of Surgical Infection, Washington, D.C., November 10, 1972.
17. Daly, T. E., and Drone, D. E.: Dental care for irradiated patients. *In* Neoplasia of Head and Neck. Chicago, Year Book Medical Pubs., 1974, p. 225.
18. Deodar, S. D., Kuklinca, A. G., Vidt, D. G., et al.: Development of reticulum-cell sarcoma at the site of antilymphocyte globulin injection in a patient with renal transplant. N. Engl. J. Med., *280*:1104, 1969.
19. Dreizen, S., Body, G. P., and Brown, L. R.: Opportunistic gram-negative bacillary infections in leukemia. Postgrad. Med., *55*:133, 1974.
20. Dudrick, S. J., and Copeland, E. M.: Nutritional concepts in head and neck cancer. *In* Neoplasia of Head and Neck. Chicago, Year Book Medical Pubs. 1974, p. 325.
21. Ehrenkranz, N. J.: Person-to-person transmission of Staphylococcus aureus. Quantitative characterization of nasal carriers spreading infection. N. Engl. J. Med., *271*:225, 1964.
22. Elek, S. D.: Experimental staphylococcal infections in the skin of man. Ann. N. Y. Acad. Sci., *65*:85, 1956.
23. Elek, S. D., and Conen, P. E.: The virulence of Staphylococcus pyogenes for man. A study of the problems of wounds. Br. J. Exp. Pathol., *38*:573, 1957.
24. Ferguson, D. B.: Salivary glands and saliva. *In* Lavelle, C. L. B. (ed.): Applied Physiology of the Mouth. Bristol, John Wright & Sons, Ltd., 1975, p. 145.

25. Gabrielson, J. L., and Stroh, E.: Antibiotic efficacy in odontogenic infections. J. Oral Surg., *33*:607, 1975.
26. Galloway, J. A., and Shuman, C. R.: Diabetics and surgery. Am. J. Med., *34*:177, 1963.
27. Grillo, H. C., and Potsaid, M. S.: Studies in wound healing. IV. Retardation of contraction by local x-irradiation, and observations relating to the origin of fibroblasts in repair. Ann. Surg., *154*:741, 1961.
28. Gross, L.: Immunological defect in aged population and its relationship to cancer. Cancer, *18*:201, 1965.
29. Hamer, M. L., Robson, M. C., Krizek, T. J., et al.: Quantitative bacterial analysis of comparative wound irrigations. Ann. Surg., *181*:819, 1975.
30. Hoover, R., and Froumeni, J. F.: Risk of cancer in renal transplant recipients. Lancet, *2*:55, 1973.
31. Hughes, N. R.: Serum concentrations of G, A, and M immunoglobulins in patients with carcinoma, melanoma, and sarcoma. J. Natl. Cancer Inst., *46*:1015, 1971.
32. Joseph, D. L., and Shumrick, D. L.: Risks of head and neck surgery in previously irradiated patients. Arch. Otolaryngol., *97*:381, 1973.
33. Kerth, J. D., Sisson, G. A., and Becker, G. D.: Radical neck dissection in carcinoma of the head and neck. Surg. Clin. North Am., *53*:179, 1973.
34. Ketcham, A. S., Hoye, R. C., Chretien, P. B., et al.: Irradiation twenty-four hours preoperatively. Am. J. Surg., *118*:691, 1969.
35. Ketcham, A. S., Lieberman, J. E., and West, J. T.: Antibiotic prophylaxis in cancer surgery and its value in staphylococcal carrier patients. Surg. Gynecol. Obstet., *117*:1, 1963.
36. Khanolkar V. R., and Suryabi, B.: Cancer in relation to usages. Three new types in India. Arch. Pathol., *40*:351, 1945.
37. Krizek, T. J., and Ariyan, S.: Severe acute radiation injuries to the hands. Plast. Reconstr. Surg., *51*:14, 1973.
38. Krizek, T. J., and Davis, J. H.: Endogenous wound infection. J. Trauma, *6*:239, 1966.
39. Krizek, T. J., and Davis, J. H.: Role of the red cell in subcutaneous infection. J. Trauma, *5*:85, 1965.
40. Krizek, T. J., Koss, N., and Robson, M. C.: Current use of prophylactic antibiotics in plastic and reconstructive surgery. Plast. Reconstr. Surg., *55*:21, 1975.
41. Lavelle, C. L. B.: Basic immunology. *In* Lavelle, C. L. B. (ed.): Applied Physiology of the Mouth. Bristol, John Wright & Sons, Ltd., 1975, p. 191.
42. Lawrence, W., Jr., Terz, J. J., Rogers, C., et al.: Preoperative irradiation for head and neck cancer: A prospective study. Cancer, *33*:318, 1974.
43. Localio, S. A., Casale, W., and Hinton, J. W.: Wound healing: Experimental and statistical study. V. Bacteriology and pathology in relation to suture material. Surg. Gynecol. Obstet., *77*:481, 1943.
44. MacFarlane, T. W.: Defense mechanisms of the mouth. *In* Lavelle, C. L. B. (ed.): Applied Physiology of the Mouth. Bristol, John Wright & Sons, Ltd., 1975, p. 180.
45. Mandel, M. A., Dvorak, K., and DeCosse, J. J.: Salivary immunoglobulins in patients with oropharyngeal and bronchopulmonary carcinoma. Cancer, *31*:1408, 1973.
46. Marfuggi, R. A., Harder, G., Ariyan, S., et al.: Effects of irradiation on wound infection. (Unpublished data.)
47. May, J., Chalmers, J. P., Loewenthal, J., et al.: Factors in the patient contributing to surgical sepsis. Surg. Gynecol. Obstet., *122*:28, 1966.
48. McPhaul, J. J., and MacIntosh, D. A.: Tissue transplantation still vexes. N. Engl. J. Med., *272*:105, 1965.
49. Meleney, F. L.: Bacterial synergism in disease processes: With a confirmation of the synergistic bacterial etiology of a certain type of progressive gangrene of the abdominal wall. Ann. Surg., *94*:961, 1931.
50. Miller, W. D.: The Microorganisms of the Human Mouth. Philadelphia, S. S. White Dental Manufacturing Co., 1890, p. 275. Reprinted by S. Karger, Munich, 1973.
51. Monihan, R. M., and Lipshutz, H.: Method for closure of a pharyngocutaneous fistula. Plast. Reconstr. Surg., *47*:384, 1971.
52. Moulder, J. E., and Fischer, J. J.: Determination of an optimal treatment plan for rare rhabdomyosarcoma. Radiology, *107*:439, 1973.
53. Moulder, J. E., Fischer, J. J., and Casey, A.: Dose-time relationships for skin and structural damage in rat feet exposed to 250 KVP x-rays. Manuscript #563, Yale Department of Therapeutic Radiology, 1974.
54. Nelson, D. S.: Immunity to infection, allograft immunity and tumor immunity: Parallels and contrasts. Transplant. Rev., *19*:226, 1974.
55. Nolte, W. A.: Oral Microbiology. St. Louis, The C. V. Mosby Co., 1968.
56. O'Loughlin, J. M.: Infections in the immunosuppressed patient. Med. Clin. North Am., *59*:495, 1975.
57. Penn, I.: Chemical immunosuppression and human cancer. Cancer, *34*:1474, 1974.
58. Penn, I., and Starzl, T. E.: Malignant tumors arising de novo in immunosuppressed organ transplant recipients. Transplantation, *14*:407, 1972.
59. Polk, H. C., and Lopez-Mayor, J. F.: Postoperative wound infection: A prospective study of determinant factors and prevention. Surgery, *66*:97, 1969.
60. Powers, W. E., Ogura, J. J., and Palmer, L. A.: Radiation therapy and wound healing delay. Radiology, *89*:112, 1967.
61. Remington, J. S.: The compromised host. Hosp. Pract., *7*:59–70, 1972.
62. Richardson, R. L., and Jones, M.: Bacterial census of human saliva. J. Dent. Res., *37*:697, 1958.
63. Robson, M. C., Edstrom, L. E., Krizek, T. J., et al.: Efficacy of systemic antibiotics in treatment of granulating wounds. J. Surg. Res., *16*:299, 1974.

64. Robson, M. C., Krizek, T. J., and Heggers, J. P.: Biology of surgical infection. *In* Current Problems in Surgery, Chicago, Year Book Medical Pubs., 1973.
65. Seropian, R., and Reynolds, B. M.: Wound infections after preoperative depilatory versus razor preparation. Am. J. Surg., *121*:251, 1971.
66. Sjögren, H. O., Hellstrom, I., Bansal, S. C., et al.: Suggestive evidence that the blocking antibodies of tumor-bearing individuals may be antigen-antibody complexes. Proc. Natl. Acad. Sci., *68*:1312, 1971.
67. Southam, C. M.: The immunologic status of patients with nonlymphomatous cancer. Cancer Res., *28*:1433, 1968.
68. Starzl, T. E.: In discussion of Murray, J. E., et al.: Five year's experience in renal transplantation with immunosuppressive drugs. Ann Surg. *168*:416, 1968.
69. Subcommittee for Human Immunoglobulins of the IUIS Nomenclature Committee, WHD: Recommendations for the nomenclature of human immunoglobulins. J. Immunol., *108*:1733, 1972.
70. Tulpius, 1674, as quoted by Miller, W. D.: The Microorganisms of the Human Mouth. Philadelphia, S. S. White Dental Manufacturing Co., 1890, p. 275. Reprinted by S. Karger, Munich, 1973.
71. Van den Brenk, H. A. S., Onton, C., Stone, M., et al.: Effects of x-radiation on growth and function of the repair blastoma (granulation tissue). Int. J. Radiat. Biol., *25*:1, 1974.
72. Waldorf, D. S., Wilkens, R. F., and Decker, J. L.: Impaired delayed hypersensitivity in an aging population. J.A.M.A., *203*:831, 1968.
73. Wilson, R. E., Hager, E. B., Hampers, C. L., et al.: Immunologic rejection of human cancer transplanted with a renal allograft. N. Engl. J. Med., *278*:479, 1968.
74. Yarington, C. T., Yonkers, A. J., and Beddoe, G. M.: Radical neck dissection. Mortality and morbidity. Arch. Otolaryngol., *97*:306, 1973.

# DYSPHAGIA

*John J. Conley*

# 9

Difficulty in swallowing is associated with an incompetent oral cavity, pharynx or larynx. This handicap is aggravated by various combinations of factors that cripple these organs and regions. The passage of food through a passageway that is shared by the respiratory system to the level of the larynx is a rhythmic act. Dysphagia results from an imbalance in the acts of swallowing, speaking and breathing. This imbalance results from a loss of transport, a defect in the structural architecture or a paralysis of the nerves and muscles responsible for the rhythmic movement.

Passage of a liquid or semisolid bolus begins with entrance through the lips and continues with the sequence of closing the lips, preparing the bolus in the oral cavity by chewing, squashing and molding and then transporting it to the region of the mesopharynx by propulsion of the tongue against the palate. Interference with any of the oral structures responsible for these physiological functions will downgrade the efficiency of the swallowing system.

The movement of the ingestants in the oral cavity is voluntary. Indeed, the preparation and savoring of food in the oral cavity can be made an art or an epicurean delight. Once the bolus reaches the pharynx, however, it comes under the control of a rhythmic reflex movement that propels it into the cervical esophagus with incredible speed. There is no voluntary control over this reflex mechanism. The laryngeal structures constrict to prevent food from entering the trachea. The pharyngeal muscles create a wave of movement with a split second relaxation against the oncoming wave of contraction that is propelling the bolus of food. There is a specific set of muscle balances that protects the airway and permits the food to pass over it without spillage. This wave is a dynamic muscular thrust toward the esophagus. Serious interference with the pharyngeal or laryngeal mechanism will alter or eliminate the coordinated mechanisms of these organs and regions. This cripples the physiological process of swallowing and imposes great handicaps on the patient. In most instances, the patient can adapt to this new stressful situation. A limited number of prophylactic measures have been devised to ameliorate these situations. In certain circumstances, the swallowing or speaking and breathing systems may have to be eliminated to give priority to only one system. It is axiomatic that if no more than 50 per cent of any region is resected, the patient has an excellent chance of recovering function. The most serious complications arise when the resection incorporates several regions or organs. Hoover (1955)[8], Code (1958)[3], Wilkins (1964)[28] and Blakely and his associates (1968)[1] have reported on the anatomy and physiology of swallowing. The pharyngeal muscles contract in a rhythmic way that forces the food bolus toward the esophagus. As this rhythmic wave advances from the pharynx to the esophagus, the cricopharyngeal muscle relaxes in order to create an unobstructed entrance for the bolus. The coordination of these rhythmic contractions and relaxations is the key to normal swallowing. Dysphagia will result from an alteration in the rhythm and an alteration in the anatomy. Kirchner (1958)[11] studied the cricopharyngeal muscle in detail in respect to swallowing and aspiration and its relationship to the vagus nerve and cervical sympathetic trunks. He found that, normally, it was in a constant state of tonus, relaxing somewhat to receive the passage of the bolus and then contracting to assist in the movement of the bolus. Unilateral stimulation of the vagus at the base of the skull reduced this phase of relaxation slightly. Sections of both vagus nerves at the base of the skull abolished the relaxation phase and produced severe dysphagia. Stimulation of the superior cervical ganglion caused a sharp rise in pressure, whereas stimulation to the cricopharyngeal muscle caused a sharp relaxation of pressure. Doberneck and Antoine (1974)[5] reviewed 15 patients who had extensive resections about the mouth, jaw, larynx and pharynx. They found that the loss of an important structure in the deglutition mechanism was more important than the impairment of mobility of the residual structures. They felt that the tongue was the most critical structure.

## REHABILITATION OF THE ORAL CAVITY

Reconstruction of the lips should always be carried out with local tissues of the face that contain a muscular pattern. Inert pedicles are undesirable. Wounds of the buccal mucosa and floor of the mouth are rehabilitated with skin grafts or a regional flap.

Deficiencies of the palate are preferably rehabilitated with a prosthesis. Regional and distal flaps have a secondary role. The loss of the horizontal or ascending ramus of the mandible does not cause serious disability in swallowing. Resections that include the anterior part of the mandible or the entire mandible cause significant difficulty in swallowing, which can be improved by secondary bone grafting.

The tongue is the largest and most important organ in the oral cavity. The patient adapts quite well to partial resections of this organ and, in some specific instances, can adapt to total glossectomy. Fixing the tongue to a rigid mandibular arch causes severe crippling. A much more serious handicap results from large resections at the

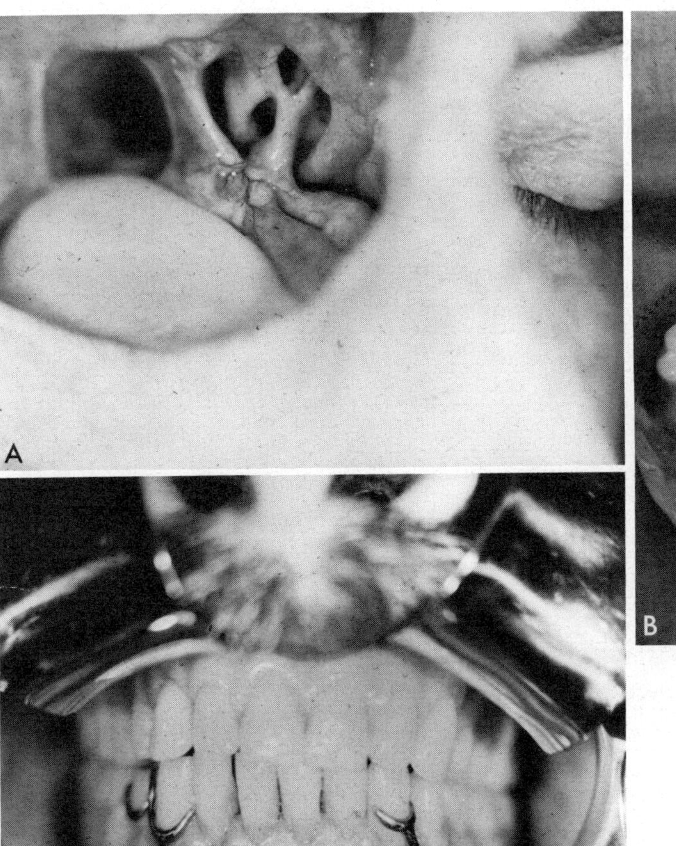


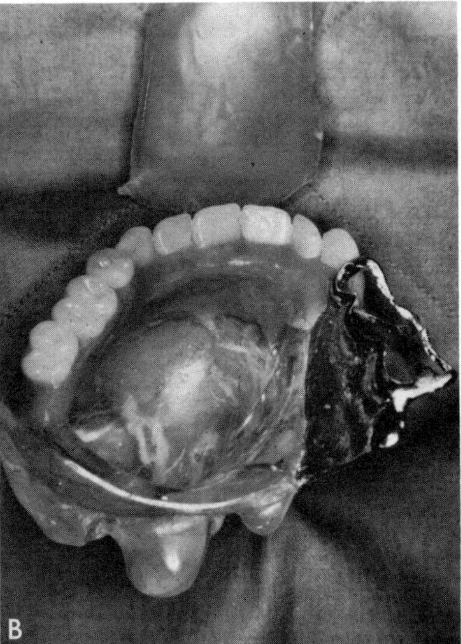


**Figure 9–1** *A,* Palatal-maxillary-orbital deficiency rehabilitated with prosthesis. *B,* Prosthesis. *C,* Prosthesis in place.

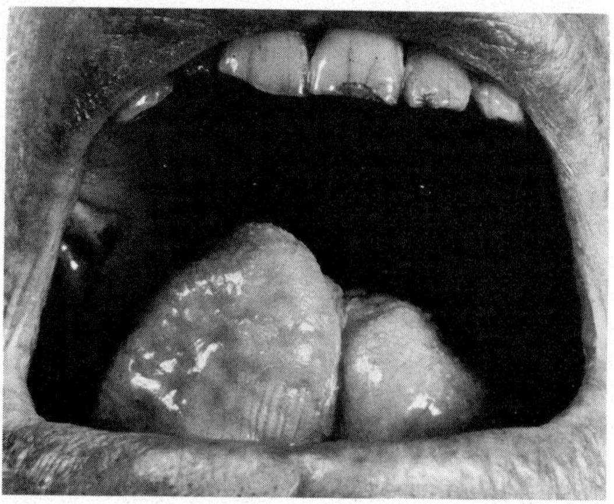

**Figure 9–2** This case represents resection of a large portion of the body of the tongue with limitation of movement, of protrusion and particularly of elevation toward the roof of the mouth. The scars along the floor of the mouth can be excised, and the area skin grafted to liberalize the movement of the tongue but it will not produce bulk or augmentation.

base of the tongue. This is compensated for by hypertrophy of the pharyngeal muscles. The movement of the bolus is facilitated by the formation of a trough. The reduced movement of the tongue can be improved by its marginal release with inlay skin grafts or regional flaps. Total glossectomy with preservation of the larynx places a severe handicap on swallowing, with difficulty in moving the bolus and aspiration. Infirm, poorly motivated individuals with poor pulmonary reserve will not adapt to this type of stress and should have either a feeding esophagostomy, gastrostomy or laryngectomy. The creation of an inert facsimile of the tongue with a tubed flap has no advantage.

The mandibular arch may be stabilized at the time of the primary operation by the use of an indwelling Steinmann pin, Vitallium plates, stainless steel baskets or acrylic prostheses. There is a basic rule operating here

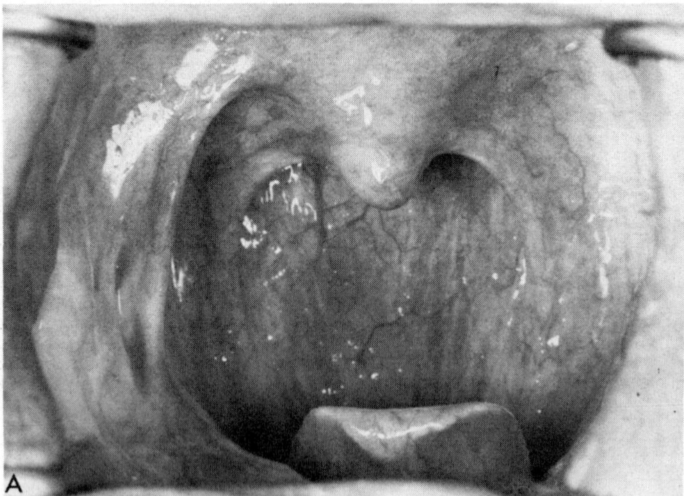


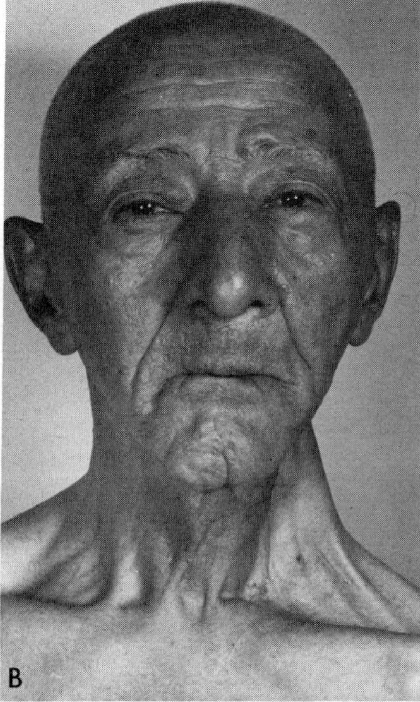


**Figure 9–3** *A,* Postoperative view following total glossectomy and a left radical neck dissection. The sequelae of the operation are associated with severe crippling of the oral cavity in respect to swallowing. Swallowing is actually accomplished with the assistance of gravity and hypertrophy of the inferior constrictor pharyngeal muscles. The presence of an intact larynx, an epiglottis and high motivation will make a satisfactory adaptation to this stress. *B,* This patient survived over 10 years postoperatively, ultimately suffered a stroke but still managed deglutition without gastrostomy or tube feedings.

that controls these principles; namely, the more "hardware" one puts into the wound, the more "hardware" will ultimately have to be removed, and the more elaborate the system of repair, the higher the incidence of failure. The Steinmann pin is perhaps the simplest mechanism to adapt and, also, to remove. The ideal concept of performing an immediate bone graft to reconstitute the mandibular arch is often negated by the fact that there is not enough residual tissue left in the wound to cover the graft securely. The failure of the bone graft technique in extensive reconstructions associated with primary ablation is 40 to 50 per cent. When the bone and soft tissue resection has been minimal, one is justified in going ahead with a primary repair. It is much safer, however, and usually simpler for both the patient and the surgeon, to wait three to six months and then carry out a secondary bone graft through a clean external field.

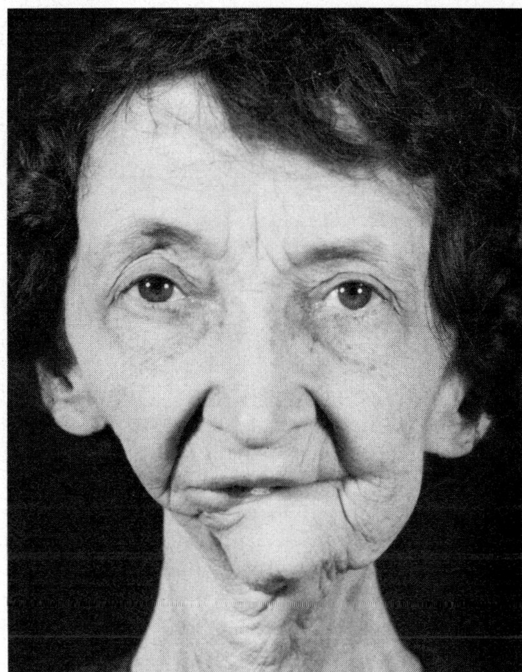

**Figure 9–4** This patient underwent resection of the major portion of the tongue, a little over half the mandible and bilateral neck dissection with primary closure by the use of local tissues (1959). A severe contracture in the region of the right mentum and upper neck is classic for this type of primary closure. This patient carried on with her primary duties as a schoolteacher with a moderately severe impediment in speech, in the functioning of the oral cavity and with the aesthetic appearance. This type of contracture deformity can be eliminated at the time of the primary operation with the use of forehead or chest flaps, or this can be carried out as a secondary technique.

## OPERATIONS AND REHABILITATION OF THE LARYNGOPHARYNGEAL CAVITY

### The Pharynx

Deficiencies in the nasopharynx are corrected by the use of a prosthesis or regional flap. Deficiencies in the mesopharynx and hypopharynx may be repaired by direct approximation or by permitting them to heal by secondary intention if they are minimal in size. When these deficiencies encompass a major portion of the pharynx, they are rehabilitated by free skin grafts and regional flaps. Free skin grafts in this area always contract and may therefore require stenting. The regional flap is preferred. A cricopharyngeal myotomy should be done simultaneously with the repair.

All individuals who have had major resections of the pharynx have dysphagia. The essential portion of the transport mechanism into the esophagus has been removed and an inert nonrhythmical tube is substituted. These patients swallow with the assistance of gravity and by having the base of the tongue milk the bolus into the cervical esophagus. It is important in these instances to have a large entrance into the esophagus and minimal muscular resistance. A cricopharyngeal myotomy at this point will assist in producing this. Dysphagia under these circumstances is often associated with aspiration. If the larynx is completely intact, it will keep aspiration at a minimum. If there has been any crippling of the larynx, such as paralysis of the vocal cord or partial subtotal resection interfering with either the supraglottic protection or the sphincteric action, aspiration may prove to be a serious problem. Minimal laryngeal deficiencies may be improved by injection of Teflon and augmentation with small flaps. If the problem is serious and in an individual who is infirm or not properly motivated, however, a laryngectomy may prove necessary.

Goode (1976)[7] reported on 19 patients who had undergone major resections about the head and neck and who were simultaneously treated with laryngeal suspension and cricopharyngeal myotomy. Half of the 16 patients available for evaluation were able to eat by mouth. Ninety-four per cent of these patients had a normal airway, and 87 per cent had intelligible speech.

## The Laryngopharynx

All operations on the larynx cause varying degrees of dysphagia. This is a direct result of the interference with the synchrony of the rhythmic wave that propels the bolus or of the protective sphincteric closure of the glottis. The slightest alteration in this complex mechanism may cause symptoms. Nature's remarkable adaptive capacities solve the vast majority of these problems. The passage of food into the cervical esophagus has been facilitated in certain paralyses of the pharynx and larynx by cricopharyngeal myotomy. This technique has been applied to a variety of crippling operations about the head and neck relating to the larynx and pharynx, and many authors have reported favorable results. Yet, there are a large number of surgeons who do not use it routinely. Studies on pharyngeal and esophageal motility under normal conditions, in a postsurgical condition and in disease have helped clarify the functions of these structures. There are specific alterations in the automatic rhythm of the swallowing mechanism itself, its nerve and muscle system and all of the structures that support it and participate in it. One of the most conspicuous clinical features is aspiration. This is most directly related to operations on the larynx itself but may also be a manifestation of alterations in the oral cavity, pharynx or esophagus. It is obvious that cricopharyngeal myotomy cannot solve all of the problems, but it can relax the opening into the cervical esophagus to permit an easier passage of food.

The paralysis of one vocal cord may or may not cause hoarseness and rarely causes mild dysphagia. An incompetent larynx results from excision paralysis of one or both cords in conjunction with paralysis, excision or dysfunction of adjacent structures. These conditions are associated with extensions of the supraglottic operation, resection of the superior laryngeal nerves or the vagus nerve high in the neck, partial pharyngectomies, glossectomies or extended partial laryngectomies.

Techniques that can be useful in cases of paralyzed vocal cord are the transposition of a neuromuscular flap to the postarytenoid area, the augmentation of the cord by Teflon injection and the transposition of myothyrocartilaginous flaps for the purposes of augmentation.

Total laryngopharyngectomy is associated with a certain variety of dysphagia but not aspiration. The elimination of the larynx permits the ingested bolus to move only to the esophagus. Reconstruction, therefore, is concerned primarily with the reconstitution of the gullet with skin grafts augmented with stents and regional flaps. Sandburg (1970)[23] studied the functions of the pharynx and esophagus by the measurement of intraluminal pressure in 20 patients who had undergone laryngectomy. The contraction pressures and resting tonus were weaker than preoperatively. Peristalsis in the esophagus was, as a rule, good. None of the patients had spasm of the inferior constructor or cricopharyngeal muscle. They did not feel that any of the alterations in the reduction of muscular power would contribute to dysphagia in any way. Duranceau and his associates (1976)[6] compared the function of the esophagus in 10 laryngectomy cases with that of a control group and found that in individuals who had undergone total laryngectomy, there was considerable derangement in esophageal motility in the upper esophageal sphincteric area and in the middle third of the esophagus. The lower esophageal sphincter remained undisturbed.

## Partial Laryngectomy

There are two operations on the larynx that alter swallowing. The augmented hemilaryngectomy removes significant portions of the larynx involved in the sphincteric action protecting against aspiration. These deficiencies are augmented by regional mucosal or skin flaps and, less frequently, by mucosal or skin grafts. Of primary importance in rehabilitation are the adaptations of the pharynx, the base of the tongue and the residuum of the epiglottis and the return of a simulated sphincteric function of the glottis. Cricopharyngeal myotomy is not essential. Schoenrock and his coworkers (1972)[25] studied 11 patients undergoing hemilaryngectomy with cineradiographic techniques. Seven of these patients aspirated, but only 3 presented with the classic clinical signs and symptoms of aspiration. All 7 patients, however, had significant pulmonary findings associated with aspiration pneumonia. They state that the key to aspiration in these cases is the incompetent glottis and suggest augmentation by Teflon injection, cartilage pedicle flap and muscle grafts. Mladick, Horton and Adamson (1971)[16] reported on 23 cases undergoing immediate cricopharyngeal myotomy to reduce or eliminate the possibility of dysphagia following radical surgery about the area of the head and neck. They state that there is no specific scientific proof that conclusively demonstrates that the myotomy of this muscle helps this type of patient with swallowing. None of their patients had any complications from the technique, and they definitely felt, from the clinical point of view, that there was considerable reduction in dysphagia and aspiration. They urge that it be done immediately at the time of the primary resection, as that is the time when it would be most effective.

## Horizontal Supraglottic Partial Laryngectomy

The horizontal supraglottic partial laryngectomy is always associated with some degree of dysphagia and aspiration. Preservation of the lateral sections of the hyoid bone and suspension of the larynx on the base of the tongue at the time of the primary operation are helpful techniques. Cricopharyngeal myotomy is not indicated in the routine case. If the candidates for these laryngeal operations are carefully selected, the patient will successfully adapt to this stressful situation. In some instances, it may require from one to three months. When aspiration is persistent and troublesome and cannot be eliminated by any locally corrective measure, one can consider permanent or temporary closure of the glottis. This is accomplished by approximating the raw surfaces of the ventricles or vocal cords in a double suture layer. This operation is simpler than total laryngectomy and preserves the structure of the larynx, which may afford the possibility of a reversal of this technique should the situation spontaneously improve. It totally eliminates aspiration and permits the patient to swallow quite normally by mouth. If aspiration and dysphagia are to be corrected by laryngectomy, one should employ the narrow field laryngectomy, thus reducing the scope of the operation and the incidence of possible complications. If the patient is weakened, old or feeble, has poor pulmonary toilet or poor emotional motivation or is an alcoholic, he will probably not be able to adapt, and a partial laryngectomy may have to be converted to a total laryngectomy.

Staple and Ogura (1966)[26] have demonstrated aspiration by cineradiographic studies in 50 per cent of 36 patients undergoing supraglottic laryngectomy. Staple, Ragsdale and Ogura (1967)[27] reported a 4 per cent mortality from chronic aspiration and a 33 per cent incidence of pneumonia in a follow-up study of the supraglottic laryngectomy. Litton and Leonard (1969)[14] presented a 67 per cent incidence of aspiration by cineradiographic studies on 24 patients. There was no doubt that the majority of patients undergoing the horizontal supraglottic laryngectomy had difficulty in swallowing, which was associated with aspiration. They emphasized, from the correlation of their radiographic studies with the clinical course of the patient, that the laryngeal element should be approximated as close as possible to the base of the tongue, that the mobility of the tongue should be assured and that glottic closure was essential. They were not completely convinced that cricopharyngeal myotomy was particularly helpful in overcoming any of these defects. Calcaterra (1971)[2] stated that chronic aspiration had been a problem in more than half of the patients undergoing horizontal supraglottic laryngectomy. He felt that the lack of laryngeal support in these operations was the prime cause for aspiration. He suspended the remaining segment of thyroid cartilage with two heavy chromic or Tevdek sutures through a drillhole in the symphysis of the mandible. He felt that the results on four patients were very gratifying. There was no long-term follow-up to demonstrate the effect or the position of these sutures after protracted pressure on the cartilage and bone. Dayal and Kane (1973)[4] studied the effects of various types of supraglottic laryngectomies in dogs upon swallowing and found no difference in those who had the hyoid bone preserved, those who had a cricopharyngeal myotomy and those who had the standard technique. In addition to the results of these experimental studies, they emphasized the importance of the anatomic integrity of the structures related to swallowing, the coordination of respiration and swallowing and the reflex initiation of swallowing.

Ogura and his associates have been the most active investigators and proponents of the cricopharyngeal myotomy. Their work covers significant investigative studies and clinical trials. They have strongly advocated its use in the subtotal supraglottic laryngectomy. In one of their experimental studies on dogs, Lauerma, Harvey and Ogura (1972)[12] analyzed the sequential events of the hypopharyngeal, thyropharyngeal, thyroarytenoid and cricopharyngeal muscles in normal and subtotal supraglottic laryngectomized animals. They concluded that after subtotal supraglottic laryngectomy associated with cricopharyngeal myotomy these animals showed the same inhibition to the passage of the bolus as that seen in the normal situation. When the myotomy was not performed under these circumstances, there was a spasmodic contraction of the cricopharyngeal muscle concurrently with the thyroarytenoid muscle as the bolus moved downward in the pharynx. These data, combined with favorable experience in a large number of clinical trials, supports their contention that it is a helpful technique to reduce dysphagia and aspiration under these circumstances.

## DYSPHAGIA IN RELATION TO THE THYROHYOID COMPLEX AND TRACHEOSTOMY

Severe dysphagia may result from interference with the elevation of the thyrohyoid complex in the act of deglutition. This type of crippling follows resection in this area of structures that reduce or eliminate the upward movement of the thyroid cartilage. This upward movement positions the larynx somewhat anteriorly and higher as it closes to prevent aspiration of the ingestant. Ardran and Kemp (1951, 1952)[1,2] have described the mechanism of swallowing and the protection of the laryngeal airway during swallowing. This movement is assisted directly by the ribbon muscles in the neck and, secondarily, by the suprahyoid muscles with their attachments to the mandible and base of the temporal bone. Any operation that resects these muscles or their bony attachments will immobilize this upward movement and predispose to aspiration. Single interference with one of these groups of muscles will only cause temporary dysphagia, since the region has the residual capacity to adapt to this function. If, however, the tongue, pharynx or larynx is afflicted in this procedure, the dysphagia is severely exaggerated.

Edgerton and McKee (1959)[5] emphasized the importance of the hyomandibular complex and its association with swallowing. They also pointed out that resections of large neoplasms involving these structures interfered with the elevation of the thyroid cartilage and larynx and downgraded the swallowing act. They pointed out the necessity of keeping the thyroid cartilage suspended. Conley (1960)[4] outlined a large group of swallowing dysfunctions associated with radical surgery in the head and neck. He emphasized the pertinent combinations that created severe dysphagia and suggested methods of ameliorating them. Jabaley and Hoopes (1964)[7] and Rappaport, Swinsky and Chiv (1969)[8] further emphasized the importance of the hyomandibular complex in the suspension of the larynx during the act of swallowing. Many of the techniques of suspension have included wire or suture support that will certainly help initially but will relax with the passage of time.

It is very unusual for dysphagia to complicate tracheostomy. Immediately after the tracheostomy there may be some temporary dysphagia with aspiration, which is most likely due to alterations in intraluminal air pressures. Feldman, Deal and Urquhart (1966)[6] reported 3 patients out of 328 (approximately 1 per cent) undergoing tracheostomy who had postoperative dysphagia. Those patients affected had had an anterior tracheal flap technique performed on the trachea. X-ray studies indicated that there was an incoordination of the swallowing mechanism. There was also subsequent tracheal dilatation, but they felt this was secondary. They stated that once the condition developed, it was very difficult to treat successfully. Bonanno (1971)[3] reported 3 patients out of a group of 43 undergoing tracheostomy who developed severe dysphagia and aspiration. He felt that this was primarily due to a restriction in the elevation of the thyroid cartilage upon the act of swallowing secondary to immobilization caused by the tracheal tube. In tracheostomy wounds that have abundant granulation tissue and a localized inflammatory process, the trachea becomes relatively attached to the strap muscles and the skin of the neck along the tract of cicatrix. This restricts the upward mobility of the larynx and trachea upon the act of swallowing and sets the stage for aspiration.

### Cranial Nerve Involvement

The paralysis of certain cranial nerves with the resultant alterations in function can have a serious effect on swallowing. The most important nerve in this respect is the vagus nerve. Its lysis has a profound effect upon swallowing and speaking. When it is realistic, direct approximation or nerve grafting should be done. Resection of the vagus nerve high in the neck causes an interference with the palate, the entire unilateral pharyngeal musculature and the ipsilateral vocal cord. The patient has severe dysphagia and hoarseness associated with aspiration. This may present a critical handicap that persists for three to six months. Gradually, the patient's adaptive capacities overcome it, and, in most instances, no remedial surgery need be carried out. When the symptoms persist and are troublesome, however, a reduction in the size of the choana in the nasopharynx will cause improvement in nasality, air-leak and food regurgitation. This is accomplished by direct suture or the use of regional flaps in the nasopharynx. The flaccid portion of the paralyzed pharyngeal muscle may be fixed to the prevertebral fascia with nonabsorbable suture material or resected and directly approximated. This causes a moderate improvement in the act of swallowing, as it permits the normally functioning contralateral pharyngeal muscle to become stabilized. Cricopharyngeal myotomy usually causes significant improvement in all of these cases. Teflon injection into the paralyzed cord reduces the tendency to aspirate and improves vocal quality.

Chodosh (1975)[2] reported on the use of cricopharyngeal myotomy for a group of individuals with dysphagia following ablative surgery to the head and neck, dermatomyositis, cerebrovascular accidents and cricopharyngeal achalasia, with significant improvement in most instances. Dayal and Freeman (1976)[3] reported on a case of oculopharyngeal muscular dystrophy with dysphagia that was improved by cricopharyngeal myotomy. Calcaterra, Kadell and Ward (1975)[1] reported on six patients who had neuromuscular dysfunction of the cricopharyngeal muscle with dysphagia. They were improved by cricopharyngeal myotomy. Zehm (1977)[5] described the rehabilitation of the paralyzed pharynx due to resection of the vagus nerve at a high level. This serious impediment to swallowing is overcome by the resection of the denervated pharyngeal muscle on the paralyzed side in the same way one would do a partial pharyngectomy. A new food passage is reconstructed with the residuum of the pharynx, and this permits a balanced sphincteric rhythmic movement for swallowing with considerable improvement. He further proposes the use of two local flaps for any associated velopharyngeal insufficiency. Mills (1973)[4] reported on 13 patients who had paralysis secondary to motor neuron disease who were treated by cricopharyngeal sphincterotomy. There was marked improvement in 10 patients.

The fifth, seventh, ninth and twelfth cranial nerves are frequently involved in radical resections about the head and neck. With the exception of the facial nerve, they do not ordinarily require any specific rehabilitative program.

## BOWEL TRANSPLANTATION

Dysphagia is uncommon in rehabilitation of the pharynx by bowel transplantation. The risks of wound infection and wound slough are certainly more threatening (Brain and Reading, 1966)[1] Both the stomach and the colon have been used to reconstitute the gullet. It has been accomplished with preservation of the larynx, but, in the vast majority of cases, the larynx is resected along with the pharynx, thus eliminating the possibility of aspiration. The extensive use of regional chest and cervical flaps to reconstruct the gullet has greatly reduced the necessity for bowel transposition. The unavailability of regional flap tissue, the resection of the esophagus at a low level and the subtotal resection of cancer locally when immediate reconstruction is unrealistic all proffer the possibility for bowel transplantation. Harrison (1964, 1969)[2, 3] has reported an extensive experience in reconstruction of the gullet by colonic transfer but has not emphasized dysphagia as a complication. Higton and Lord (1970)[5] have reported on seven patients who had postoperative swallowing difficulties after colon grafts. They outlined the possible hazards of this technique, indicating that angulation, stricture, external pressure, muscle inertia, antiperistalsis, kinking and aperistalsis may all lead to some variety of dysphagia. LeQuesne and Ranger (1966)[6] have reported on the immediate reconstruction of the pharynx by transposition of the stomach and anastomosis to the residuum of the pharynx. Although the technique of pharyngeal resection and immediate reconstruction may be carried out by some variety of bowel transplantation in the individuals who qualify for such an extensive technique, it has its limitations. Many of these patients are in the older age group, have had difficulty in swallowing for weeks or months, are malnourished and infirm or are in a postirradiation status failure group. These patients certainly do not qualify for simultaneous surgery in the neck, abdomen and chest. One therefore carries out the primary resection in the neck, closes off the pharynx, transfixes the cut cervical esophagus at a low level and drops it into the mediastinum and then creates a tracheostoma and a gastrostomy. Postoperative irradiation to the low neck and mediastinum may be a part of the program. In these advanced and high-risk problems, one should wait six to 12 months to evaluate the condition. If there is no contraindication, the reconstruction can then be carried out by using the colon or stomach. It is good to bear in mind that all preliminary gastrostomies under these circumstances should be positioned so that the wall of the stomach is still available for tubing and anastomosis with the hypopharynx. The segment of stomach or colon is passed through the chest to the neck. There is a recognized hazard to the great vessels in passing it through scar and postirradiated tissue at the base of the neck. Tip viability is absolutely essential and is established by proper planning of the vascular arcade and by eliminating kinking, torsion and pressure. This complex reconstructive process is carried out by a surgical team with capabilities in the neck and abdomen.

## PROSTHESES

Prosthetic devices play a specific role in dysphagia. Their application relates primarily to the substitution of a mechanical device to reduce an anatomic and physiologic deficiency.[1, 2, 3, 4, 5] They are of little functional value about the lips. They are essential, however, in deficiencies of the hard and soft palate and are the most effective method of rehabilitating this type of crippling in the oral cavity. Their use to stabilize the jawbone in hemimandibulectomy has proved to be less rewarding. The intent of keeping the jaw in alignment with braces, bars and flanges depends upon the presence of stable teeth that must be put under the pressure of the appliance. It is, of course, not applicable in the edentulous patient and is restricted in individuals who have poor teeth or are in a postirradiation status. In skillful hands, however, it can accomplish its purpose, but most patients either cannot or will not wear the device consistently. Prosthetic devices have been made to establish continuity between the mesopharynx and cervical esophagus. These plastic tubes are fitted into this void with a snug fit above and below and act as an internal or external conduit for the passage of food. They always leak to a certain degree but do provide the opportunity for the patient to eat by mouth under limited circumstances. This device is rarely needed because of the availability of a variety of surgical techniques to reconstruct the gullet by the use of regional flaps.

## NASOGASTRIC FEEDING TUBE

The nasogastric feeding tube is an essential element in all major head and neck operations. It is the most satisfactory method of maintaining nourishment after surgery and has eliminated the need for gastrostomy in the vast majority of cases. The tube may be used preoperatively to augment nutrition in the preparation of a debilitated person for an operation and is essential in the postoperative phase during wound healing and until the patient can swallow.

The tube is placed through the nose into the lower esophagus or stomach. Its position should be verified first by auscultation and then by passing 10 cc. of water slowly through it. The tube is secured in position with a silk suture in the melonasal sulcus or by adhesive tape applied to the cheek and nose. Replacement of the tube in certain circumstances may be hazardous and is almost always undesirable for both patient and surgeon.

The tube is attached to the Gumko apparatus postoperatively. When peristalsis begins, the patient may be started slowly on a feeding program through the tube. About 50 cc. of water are given with the patient in an upright position. This is gradually increased, and then a prescribed diet is substituted. The diet is regulated according to the patient's condition and needs and is designed to prevent solute overloads and protein and electrolyte imbalances. Tubes are cleared after each feeding with a wash of water to prevent clogging.

The tubes used in adults are usually a #16 catheter or nasogastric tube and #5 and #8 French feeding tubes. Smaller tubes are more comfortable but have a tendency to block. A short feeding tube of catheter length is indicated when a patient has a reflux with the nasogastric tube. If it has been decided that the patient will have to wear the tube for months, it may be advisable to insert it directly into his esophagus through a controlled esophageal fistula in his low neck. It is important that, when the tube is inserted in the root of the neck, it does not come in direct contact with any of the great blood vessels, since pressure necrosis and hemorrhage could result.

Many individuals master the technique of "swallowing" the tube for each feeding, thus eliminating the discomfort and inconvenience of having it constantly in position. A patient usually "swallows" the tube through his oral cavity as he would swallow a long piece of spaghetti. After a feeding is completed, he removes the tube, washes it and sets it aside for the next feeding. All nasogastric feeding tubes cause a certain amount of discomfort and distress, and all patients are anxious to be rid of them. Although the healing process cannot be speeded, this emotional reaction to the tube can be used as an incentive for the patient to swallow on his own.

Complications from the nasogastric tube are rare. Many wear these tubes for weeks or months. Any complications arise primarily in debilitated patients whose tissues have a lowered tolerance for local pressure, when there is postirradiation or when a tube is too large or distorted. These pressure points cause localized pain and ulceration. Small, soft tubes should be used in these individuals or one should go directly to a gastrostomy. Some patients have reflux with aspiration. The position of the tube and the status of the esophagus, stomach and upper bowel are evaluated. Repositioning the tube or using the short catheter usually solves this problem.

In the uncomplicated case of a composite resection of the oral, pharyngeal or laryngeal areas, it is safe to begin the taking of food by mouth within one or two weeks of the operative date. With individuals who have had extensive resections and preoperative irradiation, it is appropriate to wait from two to three weeks for the healing of the wound. One has a fairly accurate evaluation of the condition of the neck flaps by inspection and palpation. If they are red or thickened, one must assume that the integrity of the wound is threatened by an internal process that is secondary to a salivary leak, by a primary or secondary infection or hematoma or by a collection of serum or chyle. These circumstances would certainly delay the taking of an ingestant by mouth until the condition of the wound was stabilized.

## PRACTICING SWALLOWING

The most primitive swallowing act — devoid of the thinking process and under automatic control — is the "gulping" technique. Many patients are reluctant to attempt this because they fear aspiration. If, however, they have the courage to gulp down a glass of water, they have proved to themselves that the swallowing act is possible and are prepared to go ahead. Fluids are the most difficult to swallow, but they are the only substances that can be gulped. The patient's food, therefore, is prepared in a blender after a trial with water.

In many instances of total glossectomy and supraglottic resection, a small amount of fluid accumulates over the cords. This is cleared automatically at the end of the swallowing act by a small expulsive cough followed by another swallow. Perseverance and practice are the prime ingredients for success.

The purpose behind practicing is to attain automaticity. The thyrohyoid complex must be elevated in order to accomplish swallowing. This maneuver is demonstrated to the patient by his surgeon. The patient then imitates this act and confirms the elevation of the thyrohyoid complex by placing his finger on the thyroid cartilage. He practices this in front of a mirror several hundred times a day. The understanding and organization of this first step will usually lead to successful swallowing within a few days or a few weeks. This act is carried out with the nasogastric tube in position. If the patient still cannot swallow or persists in aspirating, he is taught to swallow the nasogastric tube for each feeding. After many trials he can do this on his own and become quite expert at it. This, hopefully, will actually cause an improvement in the swallowing mechanism as it is practiced and will lead the patient to the point where he is anxious to try a bolus of food. The best indicator as to whether he is ready to swallow food is the absence of mucus and saliva in his tracheal cannula. The patient should never be decannulated until the swallowing act is quite secure.

It is obvious, from this potpourri of circumstances, that the patient can adapt to serious anatomic and physiologic deficiencies as sequelae or complications to surgery in the area of the head and neck. He has an astounding capacity for adaptation in developing a modified swallowing mechanism, adapting to it and, ultimately, accepting it. The pharyngeal muscles and the vagus nerve high in the neck are the most critical structures associated with dysphagia. It is axiomatic that if no more than 50 per cent of any region is resected, the patient has an excellent chance of recovering his function. The most serious complications arise when the resection incorporates several regions simultaneously. Any operation preventing the elevation of the hyoid-laryngeal complex will complicate the act of swallowing and induce aspiration. If such an operation is extended to include a portion or all of the pharynx, the vagus nerve high in the neck and the ipsilateral hypoglossal nerve, adaptation to this severely altered functional system is impossible from a swallowing and aspirational point of view. If this is combined with scar tissue contraction and distortion or incompetence of the glottis in a poorly motivated patient, a chronic alcoholic or older person with poor pulmonary function who cannot tolerate stress, the dysphagia will be so persistent, so crippling and so threatening that it may only be resolved by laryngectomy. Before this is suggested, however, the patient should be given an interval of 6 to 12 months to rehabilitate his swallowing spontaneously and with persistent practice. He should be told that there are alternate methods of nourishing him by the operations of esophagostomy or gastrostomy. All aids and techniques that are rational should be applied. If he fails to retrain or adapt to this stress of dysphagia and aspiration, he should then decide to accept a definitive procedure to assure his nourishment and to protect his pulmonary system.

## Bibliography

1. Blakely, W. R., Garety, E. J., and Smith, D. E.: Section of the cricopharyngeus muscle for dysphagia. Arch. Surg., *96*:745, 1968.
2. Calcaterra, T. C.: Laryngeal suspension after supraglottic laryngectomy. Arch. Otolaryngol. *94*:306, 1971.
3. Code, C. F.: An Atlas of Esophageal Motility in Health and Diseases. Charles C Thomas, Springfield, Illinois, 1958.
4. Dayal, V. S., and Kane, N.: Supraglottic laryngectomy and swallowing — an experimental study. Can. J. Otolaryngol. *3*:581, 1974.

5. Doberneck, R. C., and Antoine, J. E.: Deglutition after resection of oral, laryngeal, and pharyngeal cancers. Surgery, *75*:87, 1974.
6. Duranceau, A., Jamieson, G., Hurwitz, A. L., et al.: Alteration in esophageal motility after laryngectomy. Am. J. Surg., *131*:30, 1976.
7. Goode, R. L.: Laryngeal suspension in head and neck surgery. Laryngoscope, *86*:349, 1976.
8. Hoover, W. B.: Observations on the hypopharynx and cricopharyngeus area. Ann. Otol. Rhinol. Laryngol., *64*:874, 1955.
9. Kawasaki, M., Ogura, J. H., and Takenouchi, S.: Neurophysiologic observations of normal deglutition. I. Its relationship to the respiratory cycle. Laryngoscope, *74*:1747, 1964.
10. Kawasaki, M., and Ogura, J. H.: Interdependance of deglutition with respiration. Ann. Otol. Rhinol. Laryngol., *77*:906, 1968.
11. Kirchner, J. A.: The motor activity of the cricopharyngeus muscle. Laryngoscope, *68*:1119, 1958.
12. Lauerma, K. S. L., Harvey, J. E., and Ogura, J. H.: Cricopharyngeal myotomy in subtotal supraglottic laryngectomy: An experimental study. Laryngoscope, *82*:447, 1972.
13. Levitt, M. N., Dedo, H. H., and Ogura, J. H.: The cricopharyngeus muscle. An electromyographic study in the dog. Laryngoscope, *74*:122, 1965.
14. Litton, W. B., and Leonard, J. R.: Aspiration after partial laryngectomy: Cineradiographic studies. Laryngoscope, *79*:887, 1969.
15. Mills, C. P.: Dysphagia in pharyngeal paralysis treated by cricopharyngeal sphincterotomy. Lancet, *1*:455, 1973.
16. Mladick, R. A., Horton, C. E., and Adamson, J. E.: Immediate cricopharyngeal myotomy: An adjunctive technique for major oral-pharyngeal resections. Plast. Reconstr. Surg., *47*:6, 1971.
17. Ogura, J. H.: Supraglottic subtotal laryngectomy and radical neck dissection for carcinoma of the epiglottis. Laryngoscope, *68*:983, 1958.
18. Ogura, J. H., Saltzstein, S. L., and Sojut, H. J.: Experiences with conservation surgery in laryngeal and pharyngeal carcinoma. Laryngoscope, *71*:258, 1961.
19. Ogura, J. H., Kawasaki, M., and Takenouchi, S.: Neurophysiologic observations on the adaptive mechanism of deglutition. Ann. Otol. Rhinol. Laryngol., *73*:1062, 1964.
20. Ogura, J. H., and Mallen, R. W.: Partial laryngopharyngectomy for supraglottic and pharyngeal carcinoma. Trans. Am. Acad. Ophthal. Otolaryngol., *69*:832, 1965.
21. Ogura, J. H., and Mallen, R. W.: Conservation surgery for cancer of the epiglottis and hypopharynx. Proceedings of the International Workshop on Cancer of Head and Neck, 1967, pp. 407–422.
22. Ogura, J. H., and Biller, H. F.: Conservation surgery in cancer of the head and neck. Otol. Clin. North Am., *2*:641, 1969.
23. Sandberg, N.: Motility of the pharynx and esophagus after laryngectomy. Acta Otolaryngol., *263*:124, 1970.
24. Schobinger, R.: Spasm of the cricopharyngeal muscle as cause of dysphagia after total laryngectomy. Arch. Otolaryngol., *67*:271, 1958.
25. Schoenrock, L. D., King, A. Y., Everts, E. C., et al.: Hemilaryngectomy: Deglutition evaluation and rehabilitation. Trans. Am. Acad. Ophthal. Otolaryngol., *76*:752, 1972.
26. Staple, T. W., and Ogura, J. H.: Cineradiography of the swallowing mechanism following supraglottic, and subtotal laryngectomy. Radiology, *87*:226, 1966.
27. Staple, T. W., Ragsdale, E. F., and Ogura, J. H.: The chest roentgenogram following subtotal supraglottic laryngectomy. Am. J. Roentgenol., *100*:583, 1967.
28. Wilkins, S. A.: Indications for section of the cricopharyngeus muscle. Am. J. Surg., *108*:533, 1964.

#### Dysphagia in Relation to the Thyrohyoid Complex and Tracheostomy

1. Ardran, G. M., and Kemp, F. H.: The mechanism of swallowing. Proc. Roy. Soc. Med., *44*:1038, 1951.
2. Ardran, G. M., and Kemp, F. H.: The protection of the laryngeal airway during swallowing. Br. J. Radiol., *25*:406, 1952.
3. Bonanno, P. C.: Swallowing dysfunction after tracheostomy. Ann. Surg., *174*:29, 1971.
4. Conley, J. J.: Swallowing dysfunctions associated with radical surgery of the head and neck. Arch. Surg., *80*:602, 1960.
5. Edgerton, M. T., and McKee, D. M.: Reconstruction with loss of the hyomandibular complex in excision of large cancers. Arch. Surg., *78*:425, 1959.
6. Feldman, S. A., Deal, C. D., and Urquhart, W.: Disturbance of swallowing after tracheostomy. Lancet, *1*:954, 1966.
7. Jabaley, M. E., and Hoopes, J. E.: A simple technique for laryngeal suspension after partial or complete resection of the hyomandibular complex. Am. J. Surg., *118*:685, 1964.
8. Rappaport, I., Swinsky, A., and Chiv, S. C.: Functional considerations after resection of the hyomandibular complex. Am. J. Surg., *116*:581, 1969.

#### Cranial Nerve Involvement

1. Calcaterra, T., Kadell, B. M., and Ward, P. H.: Dysphagia secondary to cricopharyngeal muscle dysfunction, surgical management. Arch. Otolaryngol., *101*:726, 1975.
2. Chodosh, P. L.: Cricopharyngeal myotomy in the treatment of dysphagia. Laryngoscope, *85*:1862, 1975.
3. Dayal, V. S., and Freeman, J.: Cricopharyngeal myotomy for dysphagia in oculopharyngeal muscular dystrophy. Report of a case. Arch. Otolaryngol., *102*:115, 1976.
4. Mills, C. P.: Dysphagia in pharyngeal paralysis treated by cricopharyngeal sphincterotomy. Lancet, *1*:455, 1973.
5. Zehm, S.: Reconstructive procedures on the denervated gullet. Trans. Am. Acad. Ophthalmol. Otolaryngol., *84*:57, 1977.

**Bowel Transplant**

1. Brain, R. H. F., and Reading, P. V.: Colon transplantation into pharynx and cervical esophagus. Br. J. Surg., *53*:933, 1966.
2. Harrison, D. F. N.: The use of colonic transplants and revascularized jejunal autografts for primary repair after pharyngolaryngoesophagectomy. Proc. Roy. Soc. Med., *57*:1104, 1964.
3. Harrison, D. F. N.: Pharyngoesophageal replacement in postcricoid and esophageal carcinoma. Ann. Otol. Rhinol. Laryngol., *73*:1026, 1964.
4. Harrison, D. F. N.: Surgical management of carcinoma of hypopharynx and cervical esophagus. Br. J. Surg., *56*:95, 1969.
5. Higton, D. I. R., and Lord, I. J.: Dysphagia following colon pedicle grafts. Br. J. Surg., *57*:825, 1970.
6. Le Quesne, L. P., and Ranger, D.: Pharyngolaryngectomy with immediate pharyngogastric anastomosis. Br. J. Surg., *53*:105, 1966.

**Prosthesis**

1. Ackerman, A. J.: The prosthetic management of oral and facial defects following cancer surgery. J. Pros. Dent., *5*:413, 1955.
2. Cantor, R., Curtis, T. A., and Rozen, R. D.: Prosthetic management of terminal cancer patients. J. Pros. Dent., *20*:361, 1968.
3. Cantor, R., and Hildestad, P.: A material for epitheses. Odont. Tidskr., *74*:32, 1966.
4. Scannell, J. B.: Practical considerations in the dental treatment of patients with head and neck cancer. J. Pros. Dent., *15*:764, 1965.
5. Silverman, S., Jr., and Galante, M.: Oral cancer monograph. San Francisco, University of California Medical Center, Printing Division, 1966, p. 1.

# 10 NEURAL SEQUELAE

*John J. Conley*

The entire region of the head and neck is interlaced with a network of sensory, motor and regulatory nerves. It is always necessary to sacrifice some of these nerves in major resections. This results in loss of sensation, motor power, vital function, regulatory response and muscle volume in that region. The severity of this combination of deficiencies will be directly proportional to the number of nerve elements obliterated and their functional capabilities. The loss will allow some function or it may create severe crippling. The most significant losses stem from destruction of the cranial nerves and those nerves supplying special sense organs. Much of this deficit is accepted as a sequela of the surgical experience.[12]

## CRANIAL NERVES

The olfactory nerve (I) is routinely resected in the majority of tumors of the nasal cavity and sometimes in extensive neoplasms about the orbit. It is fortunate that these operations are unilateral, with olfaction remaining on the opposite side. There is no rehabilitation.

The optic nerve (II) and orbital contents are resected in approximately 40 per cent of the cancers of the nasal sinuses and in most high-grade neoplasms occurring in the orbit. This condition is usually unilateral. Surgery always results in a certain amount of mutilation about the orbital structures, thus adding an aesthetic deficiency to the physiological one. The decision whether to resect both sides of the optic system is a challenging biologic and philosophic problem. Sight cannot be restored, but the deformity can be improved.

The oculomotor (III), trochlear (IV) and abducens (VI) nerves supply the muscles in the orbit and are only rarely affected by head and neck surgery. Partial resections inside the orbit and intracranial techniques may interfere with their function. This may be improved by muscle-balancing techniques.

The trigeminal nerve (V) is the dominant nerve in the region of the face, supplying most of the sensation in this area and innervating the muscles of mastication. Portions of it are frequently resected during surgery on the sinuses, oral cavity, mandible and pterygoid areas. The deficiencies are usually unilateral. The patient can accommodate these alterations.

The facial nerve (VII) is both motor and sensory. The striking feature of its resection is the resulting facial paralysis. This affects closing of the eye, movement of the face, chewing, speaking and appearance. This nerve has exceptional capacities for rehabilitation. Microsurgical techniques, including special instrumentation and #10-0 monofilament suture material, have greatly perfected the craft of nerve repair. Free autogenous nerve grafting from the proximal stump, cross-over from the hypoglossal nerve, nerve implantation, grafting from the contralateral side, regional muscle transposition and free blood vessel, nerve–muscle transplantation all have a place in rehabilitation of the paralyzed face. It is reasonable to state that the sequelae of facial paralysis can be improved to some degree in every instance by one or a combination of the above techniques. Improvement extends over several years and may require a series of operations.

The acoustic nerve (VIII) has a cochlear and a vestibular component, responsible for hearing and balance, respectively. Unilateral radical resections in this area obliterate these functions, but there is compensation and adjustment within two to four weeks from a normally functioning system on the

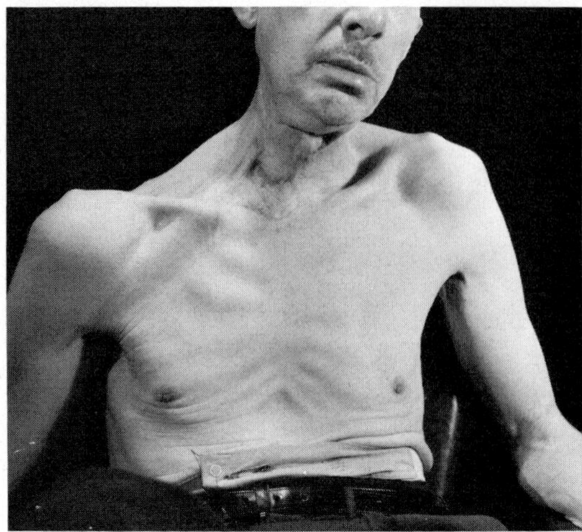

**Figure 10–1** Severe shoulder drop following neck dissection. This situation can be improved by preserving the nerve supply to the levator scapula and also by an exercise program.

opposite side. This adaptation will never be total but will reach levels for adequate functioning.

The glossopharyngeal nerve (IX) contains both sensory and motor fibers. Its primary function is sensory, with branches going into the area of the tonsils, palate, pharynx and posterior tongue. It is routinely resected in radical operations in these areas. Dysphagia is a temporary sequela. There is adequate adaptation from the opposite side within two to four weeks.

The vagus nerve (X) is both motor and sensory, with branches about the pharynx and larynx. It supplies motor power to the pharyngeal muscles and larynx and sensation in the region of the supraglottis. The resected vagus nerve in the mid or low neck causes vocal cord paralysis. It is partially rehabilitated by free nerve grafting. This may require one to two years for incomplete return of function to appear. Cross-over of the fascicle of the recurrent laryngeal nerve from the vagus may assist the paralyzed vocal cord. If this is unrealistic, the vocal cord paralysis can be improved by cord transposition, Teflon injection or neuromuscular implantation. Resections of the vagus and its connections at the base of the skull are much more serious. It causes weakness in the pharyngeal musculature from the palate down to the esophagus, loss of sensation in the supraglottic area and paralysis of the vocal cord. Cricopharyngeal myotomy facilitates swallowing. Suture stabilization or resection of the paralyzed pharynx improves the dysphagia. This serious affliction in swallowing and speaking may require a year for the patient to adapt satisfactorily. A certain amount of crippling is permanent. The majority of patients struggle with these sequelae and adapt. In those who cannot tolerate this type of stress, there is reasonable hope for improvement with the above techniques.

Paralysis of the spinal accessory nerve (XI) causes shoulder drop with some limitation of movement of the arm and shoulder and local discomfort. Most patients adjust to this disability. In some, however, it may cause prolonged pain and interfere with work and sport. This deficit has stimulated surgeons to seek ways of salvaging the spinal accessory nerve. In certain circumstances, this nerve may be preserved, for example, in an elective neck dissection, in minimal metastasis to lower jugular compartments and in a low-grade cancer of the thyroid.

Most undifferentiated cancer and melanomas and all gross metastases of squamous cell and adenocarcinomas in the superior deep jugular and spinal accessory triangle warrant a complete neck dissection. It is a fact that the more tissues one saves in cancer surgery, the more one increases the chance of saving cancer and thus worsening the prognosis.

The spinal accessory nerve may be injured in the simple excision of a lymph node in the spinal accessory chain. Most of these lymph nodes prove to be merely hyperplastic; a much smaller percentage turn out to be lymphosarcoma or metastatic cancer. The lysed nerve should be repaired immediately by direct nerve approximation or a nerve graft.

The trapezius muscle helps stabilize the scapula, and its paralysis will cause a shift in scapular position and movement. This ultimately affects the shoulder joint, the sternoclavicular joint, the vertebrae and associated muscles. The trapezius acts in harmony with, or as an antagonist to, other regional muscles in the upward and downward movement of the scapula and is assisted in these movements by the levator scapulae and the rhomboid muscles. Abduction of the shoulder is limited; when the patient attempts to abduct his arm laterally, he usually compensates by flexing his spine to the opposite side. If the spinal accessory nerve is lysed, the trapezius muscle usually becomes completely atrophic. On rare occasions, however, there may be a functional cross-over with the nerves of the brachial plexus, which allows the patient to move his shoulder quite normally. Nerves to the levator scapulae muscles should be preserved.

Pain in the joint restricts movement and causes additional stiffness and muscle atrophy. Both the shoulder joint and the sternoclavicular joint are strained under torsion. Stress in these joints may cause contraction of the capsule, stiffness and swelling.

The spinal accessory nerve has been rehabilitated with free autogenous nerve grafts consisting of other branches of the sensory cervical plexus or sural nerve. The rehabilitation has been only partially successful; hence, the concept has never become well established.

Considerable improvement can be achieved through a program of active and passive physiotherapy and exercise. Within a week or two after the operation, the patient is told how to elevate his paralyzed shoulder in order to strengthen his levator and rhomboid muscles. He should stretch his serratus anterior muscles by pulling his shoulders backward and then exercising them in this position. His scapulohumeral joint should be kept mobilized with active arm exercises of abduction posteriorly, laterally and anteriorly.

The patient is also trained to touch the top of his head and "climb the wall" with his weakened arm, using those arm and hand muscles that function or elevating his impaired arm with the good one. Swimming, golf, tennis, gardening and regular calisthenics are all helpful. Hydrotherapy and physiotherapy contribute to rehabilitation. Ideally, the program is continued for a year. The alternative to a rehabilitation program such as this is total inaction, with the patient living within the perimeters of his disability, his movements restricted, his joints stiffening and his muscles atrophying. Most patients are anxious to take the route of action and have a positive hand in their own well-being.

Anderson and Flowers (1969)[1] have reported on the use of spinal accessory nerve grafts. Beahrs and Roy (1969)[2] and Roy and Beahrs (1970)[10] have detailed the relationship of the spinal accessory nerve in radical neck dissection. Saunders and Johnson (1975)[11] have reported on the disabilities associated with resection of the spinal accessory nerve and a program of exercise to rehabilitate the affected parts. Bocca (1972, 1976)[3,4] has reported extensively on the salvage of the spinal accessory nerve in the conservative neck dissection.

The hypoglossal nerve (XIII) is the motor nerve to the tongue. The fact that the tongue is the most important organ in the oral cavity gives this special significance. Resecting one hypoglossal nerve causes a moderate impediment that is physiologically adjustable without serious sequelae. When a portion of the tongue is resected along with the hypoglossal nerve, functional disability worsens. Bilateral hypoglossal nerve resection immobilizes the tongue and severely cripples swallowing and speaking. Some patients can adapt to this severe handicap, but it requires persistent practice, alertness, a change in diet and eating habits, discipline and a well-functioning respiratory system. If this is too much stress for the individual, he can solve the nourishment problem with a gastrostomy or the aspiration problems with an elective laryngectomy. Nerve grafting is usually not feasible.

## SENSORY NERVES

In addition to the sensory branches associated with the cranial nerves restricted to the anterior and lateral portions of the face, forehead and anterior scalp, there are sensory branches from the cervical nerves. The C-2, C-3 and C-4 supply the cervical area and upper chest about the clavicle. Branches from C-5, C-6, C-7 and C-8 supply the upper and lower arm and hand. The primary complications of surgery arise from regional anesthesia associated with the trigeminal nerve, which may lead to corneal abrasion and a loss of sensation about the upper and lower lip on one side, the floor of the mouth, palate and buccal area, thus interfering with eating.

A neuroma forming at the end of a cut nerve may cause pain or an abnormal sensation. One in the neck must be differentiated from recurrent cancer. In the lingual or alveolar nerve, a neuroma may produce severe pain. Pain is also produced by irritation of the trigeminal and glossopharyngeal nerves. Sectioning these nerves creates a sensation of numbness and, in some instances, phantom pain. All of the cut deep branches of C-2, C-3 and C-4 have some sensitivity, which is usually subclinical.

## CERVICAL SYMPATHETIC SYSTEM

There are three cervical ganglia located in the neck. They are interconnected and linked to the cervical nerves and certain cranial nerves. The principal effect of interference with the cervical chain is Horner's syndrome, which does not cause any symptomatology.

## INTRACRANIAL COMPLICATIONS

Intracranial complications in surgery of the head and neck are rare, but when they occur they may be profound. They consist of meningitis, brain abscess, herniation of the brain, cerebrospinal fluid leaks, ischemia, infarction and hemorrhage.

## MENINGITIS AND BRAIN ABSCESS

These infections are uncommon because the patient is amply protected by prophylactic antibiotic therapy. The dura and brain are frequently exposed in radical procedures on the sinuses, nasal cavity, orbit and temporal bone. Approximately 1 per cent of these high-risk cases will develop an intracranial complication. *Staphylococcus, Streptococcus* and gram-negative bacilli are the common organisms. Prophylaxis is the best treatment. When this type of operation is planned, the patient is started on large doses of penicillin (6,000,000 per day) preoperatively and continued for at least a week after the wound has healed. Identification of the organism by culture of the spinal fluid usually necessitates the injection of the specific antibiotic into the subthecal space. Brain abscess requires neurosurgical consultation. Bray and Calcaterra (1976)[5] have reported the successful treatment of three patients who underwent major head and neck resections with resultant cerebrospinal fluid leaks and who developed *Pseudomonas aeruginosa* meningitis. The antibiotics used for these patients were gentamicin and carbenicillin systemically and gentamicin intrathecally.

## HERNIATION OF THE BRAIN

This condition is due to a lack of support. It is the result of bone removal, lack of adequate soft tissue and dural covering and constant intracranial pressure. Most of these cavities are dressed with a split skin graft in order to cover the dura and eliminate all raw surfaces. If the skin graft "takes" perfectly, herniation is unlikely. There may be some localized bulging that reestablishes an equilibrium. A skin graft will grow directly on the pia mater.

This technique is satisfactory if the dural deficiency is minimal. It is not satisfactory for large wounds, does not afford protection and may lead to herniation. These large dural deficiences are repaired with a fascia lata graft, which is then resurfaced with a regional scalp or cervical flap. If the patient is scheduled for postoperative radiotherapy or has had radiotherapy preoperatively, repair by use of a flap is essential.

## CEREBROSPINAL FLUID LEAKS

Cerebrospinal fluid leaks are common in radical operations about the cribriform plate and temporal bone. The cribriform plate is perforated by multiple branches of the olfactory nerve passing from the intracranial cavity into the upper portion of the nasal cavity. They are accompanied by a small circular tube of dura. When the plate and nerve filaments are resected, there is an automatic spontaneous leakage of cerebrospinal fluid. In a nonirradiated patient, this is controlled by the application of a split skin graft. In resection of the deep part of the temporal bone, the internal auditory meatus becomes engaged, with a resultant cerebrospinal leak. The cavity in the temporal bone is dressed with a split skin graft directly over the dura and pia. All of these patients who have had intensive radiotherapy or who are scheduled for postoperative radiotherapy should be rehabilitated with a regional flap. The majority have a temporary leak of cerebrospinal fluid for one to three weeks postoperatively. When the graft or flaps heal, the leak is obliterated by sealing and contraction. There may be an accumulation of spinal fluid under the flap that is aspirated and then compressed with a pressure dressing. This fluid may escape into the eustachian tube and provide a channel for infection and meningitis. When it is necessary to reenter the wound because of persistent cerebrospinal fluid leak, one must identify the anatomy of the leak and its channel and then cover it with a supporting structure. Fascia and dermis are readily available for implantation. Septal flaps in the nasal cavity and regional soft tissue flaps are necessary for external covering. The patient should be given ample antibiotic therapy during this interval.

## NEUROGENOUS TUMORS

These tumors are derivatives of neural tissues and their supporting structures. The complications and sequelae of neurogenous tumor resection are associated with the tumor's previous clinical behavior and postoperative nerve deficit. Neurogenous tumors may involve any nerve in the area of the head and neck that has a neural sheath. Neurilemomas may pass through adjacent foramina into the spinal cord or the intracranial cavity, with signs of compression of the central nervous system or the spinal cord. They commonly cause pain and paresthesia. Only rarely is it possible to preserve the integrity of a neural pathway when it is intrinsically involved with a tumor of neurogenous origin. Nerve grafting is helpful in partially rehabilitating an essential motor nerve. Sensory nerves are not grafted. Conley (1955)[6] and Conley and Janecka (1969, 1973, 1974)[7,8,9] have reviewed 92 cases of neurilemoma in the head and neck and 21 neurilemomas of the facial nerve. They detailed the diagnosis, management and prognosis.

## Bibliography

1. Anderson, M. D., and Flowers, R. S.: Spinal accessory nerve grafts. Am. J. Surg., *118*:796, 1969.
2. Beahrs, O. H., and Roy, P. H.: Spinal accessory nerve in the course of radical neck dissection Am. J. Surg., *118*:800, 1969.
3. Bocca, E.: Critical analysis of the techniques and value of neck dissection. Nuovo Arch. Ital. Otol., *4*:151, 1976.
4. Bocca, E.: Chirurgie der Halslymphknoten. *In* Naumann, H. H. (ed.); Kopf und Hals-Chirurgie, Stuttgart, Thieme, 1972, Bd. 1, pp. 153–187.
5. Bray, D. A., and Calcaterra, T. C.: Pseudomonas meningitis complicating head and neck surgery. Laryngoscope, *86*:1386–1390, 1976.
6. Conley, J. J.: Malignant schwannoma of tip of the nose. Arch. Otolaryngol., *62*:638, 1955.
7. Conley, J., and Janecka, I. P.: Neurilemmoma of the facial nerve. Plast. Reconstr. Surg. *52*:55, 1973.
8. Conley, J., and Janecka, I. P.: Schwann cell tumors of the facial nerve. Laryngoscope, *84*:958, 1974.
9. Conley, J., and Janecka, I. P.: Neurilemmoma of the head and neck. Trans. Am. Acad. Ophthalmol. Otolaryngol., *80*:459, 1975.
10. Roy, P.H., and Beahrs, O. H.: Spinal accessory nerve involved in radical neck dissection. Am. J. Surg., *119*:701, 1970.
11. Saunders, W. H., and Johnson, E. W.: Rehabilitation of the shoulder after radical neck dissection. Trans. Am. Laryngol. Assoc., *96*:105, 1975.
12. Swift, T. R.: Peripheral nerves and their involvement in radical neck dissection. Am. J. Surg., *119*:694, 1970.

# COMPLICATIONS IN EAR-SURGERY

11

*Adolf Miehlke*

*Dedicated with respect to George E. Shambaugh, Jr.*

## INTRODUCTION

This is written for those who find themselves confronted, either accidentally or through negligence, by an otosurgical complication and who want to understand clearly how such a misfortune could have occurred and what is the most rational way to help their patient. This means that this chapter is addressed to those who are completely versed in otosurgery.

Operations in *acute inflammatory ear disease* and their complications have become far less common during the last few decades since the introduction of antibiotic treatment. *Operations designed to improve hearing*, however, both in chronic infections of the middle ear and their residues and in otosclerosis have greatly increased in importance.

These operations, designed both to cure and to improve function, must, as a matter of course, be carried out under the operating microscope. They demand special training of the surgeon in specialized microsurgery. Extensive equipment is mandatory for each technique. If one of these two factors — appropriate skills or equipment — is not available and the operation is attempted nevertheless, it may provoke the first complication.

## THE AURICLE

### Postoperative Perichondritis of the Auricle

Operative enlargement of the outer meatus as part of radical mastoidectomy or limited excision of cartilage in the surgery for meatal atresia is part of the planned operation. Infection may start at the exposed edges of cartilage. Occasionally, it will be due to *Pseudomonas aeruginosa (P. pyocyanea)* or *Proteus*. Specific antibiotic treatment will have to be started at once.

The picture of loss of contour of the outlines of the auricle is well known. If fluctuation occurs in small areas, incision and counterincision should be done early. When the auricle is widely infected, the necrotic cartilage should, according to Herrmann, be excised far into intact cartilage from a retroauricular incision; an incision alone will not be sufficient. If large areas of the auricle are involved, all of the cartilage except the helix edge will have to be removed. The edge of helix will have to be fixed temporarily with a few sutures to the scalp. With this technique disfiguring shrinkage of the auricle can be prevented.

### Injuries and Scarred Stenoses of the External Meatus

The lining of the outer meatus may be damaged during faulty extraction of foreign bodies either by abrasions or by loosening skin flaps. By way of the operating microscope, such skin-flaps have to be adapted with great care. They are covered by a specially cut strip of silicone, and the meatal canal is loosely filled by a strip of gauze soaked in cortisone ointment. This strip is changed only on the 12th day.

If a definite stenosis of the meatus has already been formed, it will have to be dilat-

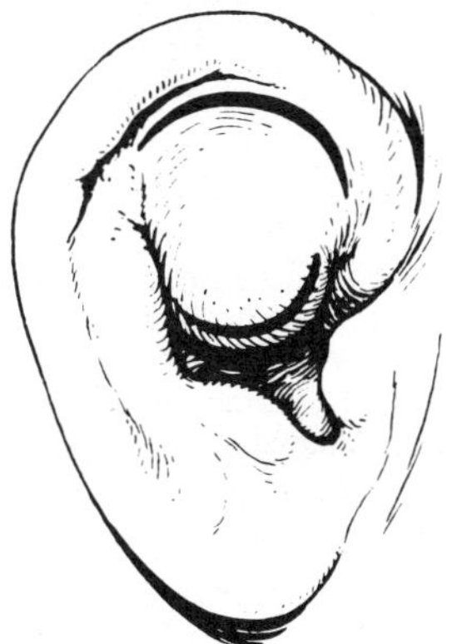

**Figure 11–1** Incision and contraincision of an otohematoma, respectively abscess. (After von Eicken, C., and Schulz van Treeck, A.: Atlas der HNO-Krankheiten. Stuttgart, Thieme, 1951.)

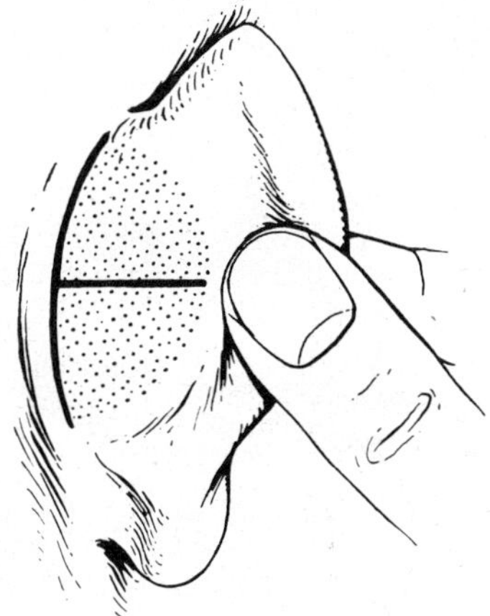

**Figure 11–2** Excision of cartilage in perichondritis of the concha. Dotted area shows extension of cartilaginous parts to be removed. (After von Eicken, C., and Schulz van Treeck, A.: Atlas der HNO-Krankheiten. Stuttgart, Thieme, 1951.)

ed via a retroauricular incision. After elevating the stenotic meatal lining, the bony meatus is enlarged using a rose drill and bur. The scarred stenotic ring is excised and the remainder of the meatal lining replaced on the bony bed; the uncovered areas of bone are covered with split skin grafts. Once again, they are covered with a specially cut strip of silicone. This is followed by the insertion of the cortisone ointment–soaked gauze strip for 12 days.

## Foreign Bodies in the Meatus

The following observation was made by the well-known German otologist Marx: "One can say without exaggeration that — with few exceptions — foreign bodies in the meatus are harmless if left alone. Only faulty attempts at extraction will render them dangerous for the patient."

The following complications of faulty attempts at extraction of foreign bodies are known: injuries to the meatus and eardrum, pushing the foreign body farther beyond the bony meatus and into the tympanum, dislocation and even removal of the ossicles and injury to the facial nerve in its tympanal course. Medicolegal consequences often cannot be avoided. Such regrettable incidents can be prevented if the doctor in charge follows a few rules:

1. One should never forget to ask the patient whether he has ever had otitis media and whether a perforation in the drum was found.
2. If a perforation of the drum is suspected or if the foreign body is of potentially swelling material, aural wash-outs are contraindicated.
3. Except in the incidences just mentioned, one ought to use aural wash-outs in order to remove a foreign body.
4. If a properly performed wash-out does not succeed, then removal of the foreign body with a small blunt hook is indicated.
5. Forceps are not suitable for the removal of foreign bodies from the meatus. Using them would be a gross mistake.
6. Fixed foreign bodies that cannot be washed out are extracted with less risk under a short general anesthetic, particularly in children.
7. When these rules are heeded, only a few cases remain that may require surgical exposure and enlargement of the meatus by removing a corresponding part of the posterior bony meatus with a bur.

## Congenital Auricular Fistula

Surgical removal of an auricular fistula malformation at the line of closure of the first and second branchial arches does not involve real dangers from operative tech-

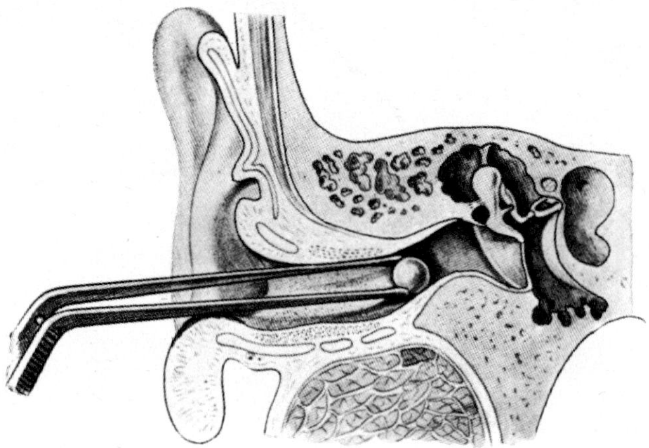

**Figure 11–3** Improper attempt at extraction of a spheric body with simple forceps. The foreign body slips and slides in deeper (After Lüscher, E. L.: Kurze Klinik der Ohren-, Nasen- und Halskrankheiten. Basel, Schwabe, 1948.)

nique. The sinus is generally a cul-de-sac lined with squamous epithelium, mostly opening in front of the ascending crus of the anthelix.

These fistulas should not be excised at a stage of acute infection. There is danger of a spread of infection into surrounding tissue and, possibly, of perichondritis of the tragus and of Santorini's meatal cartilages. It is safer to wait and make do with the incision. Once inflammation has subsided, excision of the whole of the sinus should be carried out. Before this operation, it is advisable to fill the sinus with methylene blue, which will indicate its course. The incision should not be too short or the danger of complications will increase, e.g., the tearing of the "tube" of the sinus. This may happen if one attempts to improve exposure by pulling on the track of the sinus from too narrow an operative field. Once this track is torn, the field of operation will be stained with methylene blue and the stump of the tract will retract into the depth. If one now searches for it without great care, the temporofacial branch of the facial nerve may be damaged. In any case, unless the whole of the sinus is removed intact, recurrence is inevitable. For this reason, a sufficiently long incision is mandatory.

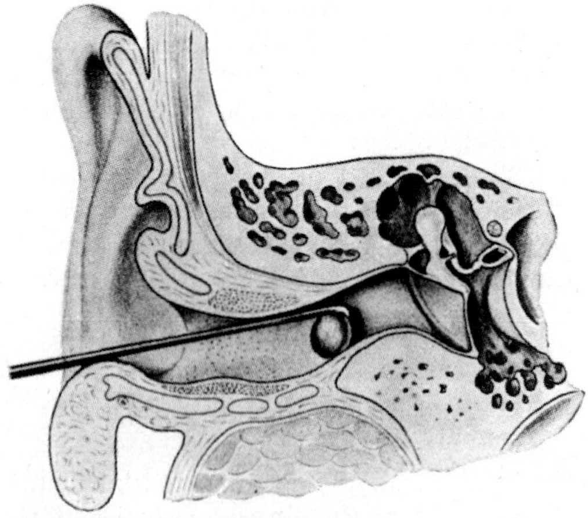

**Figure 11–4** Proper extraction with a hook. (After Lüscher, E. L.: Kurze Klinik der Ohren-, Nasen- und Halskrankheiten. Basel, Schwabe, 1948.)

## Neck and Ear Fistulas

Removal of neck and ear fistulas may, at times, be difficult, since they run more or less closely to the extratemporal course of the facial nerve. Incorrect surgery may damage the nerve and produce facial paralysis.

Rankow and Hanford as well as Ungerecht have pointed out that, owing to the ontogenesis, otocervical fistulas open distally below the angle of the mandible and at about the level of the hyoid bone. Proximally, however, they either end blindly at the junction of bone and cartilage or open into the external meatus. These hyomandibular fistulas are lined with squamous epithelium. Their walls may contain hair, sebaceous glands or cartilage. Their lumina are often filled with detritus. They run anterolaterally to the posterior belly of the digastric muscle and the external carotid artery.

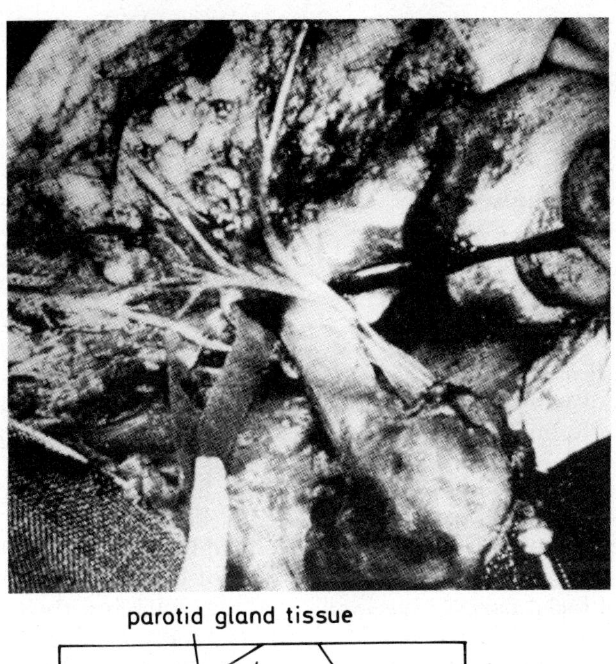

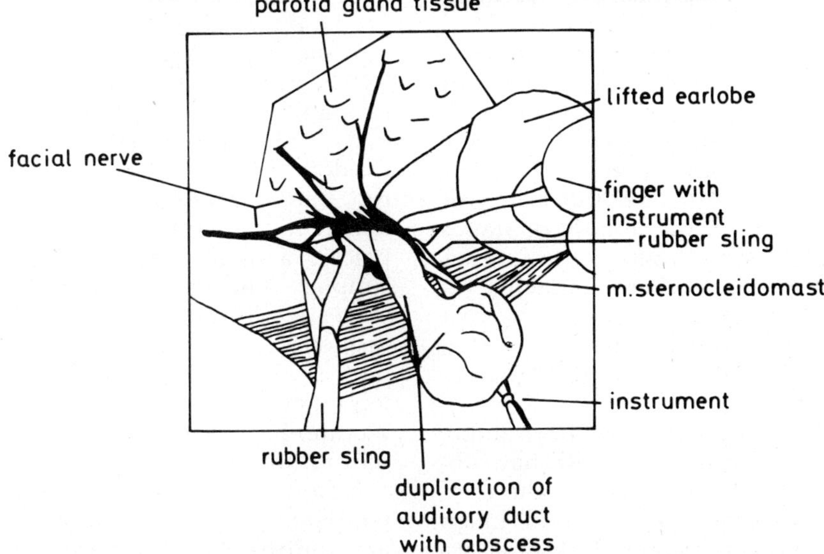


**Figure 11–5** Hyomandibular fistula—reduplicated outer meatus (ear-neck fistula). Note the course of the second meatus through the bifurcation of the facial nerve (embryonically of great interest).

According to Altmann, their topographic relation to the facial nerve may vary. Ungerecht emphasizes that branches of the fistulas remain near the surface and pass the facial nerve laterally when the ectoderm of the first branchial arch persists. If, however, the ectoderm is retained in the deep parts of the branchial arch, then the resulting fistulas will run medially to the facial nerve. One may assume that there might be transitional cases.

Actually, we have had two cases in which the tract of the fistula ran between the cervicofacial and temporofacial main branches of the facial nerve. We agree with Ungerecht that, when excising a deep hyomandibular fistula, one should, as in parotidectomy, first dissect the trunk of the facial nerve at its exit from the stylomastoid foramen in the retromandibular fossa. Its course should then be followed beyond its bifurcation. After this, it is not difficult to expose the hyomandibular fistula from its origin in the meatus to its end in the upper cervical triangle, using the operating microscope. The course of the facial nerve can be clearly seen. The track of the fistula can be removed safely. Any other operative approach carries the danger of an iatrogenic injury to the facial nerve.

## The Middle Ear

There is an indication for *paracentesis* (myringotomy) in all cases of closed otitis media with a strongly bulging drum, high temperature and severe pain. The indication is absolute in the following conditions: cerebral irritation (meningism), labyrinthine irritation or labyrinthitis (reduced hearing down to deafness, vomiting, dizziness and nystagmus) and facial paresis due to inflammation.

If myringotomy is not performed correctly, at the top of the bulge or in its inferior posterior quadrant, there is a danger of injury to the ossicle chain, particularly for the incus and stapes. Dislocation of the joint between them, fractures of the crura of stapes and division of the tendon of stapes are found after such faulty paracenteses. Since the inner ear in these situations remains closed, the general dangers are not too great, but a conduction deafness with a loss of hearing of 50 to 60 decibels will result.

If such types of damage have been done, the tympanic cavity, after the otitis has subsided, will have to be opened and the tympanoplastic measures will have to be taken to restore sound conduction. A possible injury to the facial nerve would have to be repaired according to the rules of the surgery of the facial nerve.

### Dislocation of the Stapes

Dislocation of the stapes due to faulty paracentesis is very dangerous, because it is followed rapidly by labyrinthitis and, possibly, by otogenic meningitis. Intensive antibiotic treatment, starting with a wide-spectrum drug and continued after immediate testing for resistance with the most suitable antibiotic, has to be started at once in order to save whatever possible.

If dislocation of the stapes has occurred, the damage should be repaired immediately. If the vestibulum has been opened, it will have to be closed immediately and temporarily with Gelfoam. The definitive repair will have to follow. Wash-outs are dangerous because bacteria might thus be introduced into the vestibulum. Careful sucking off of blood from the tympanic cavity is less dangerous, but the tip of the sucker should not be placed near the oval window.

If the stapes is dislocated after its tendon has been torn, it tends to tilt toward the promontory. The foot plate, correspondingly, will protrude obliquely from the oval window. Under the operating microscope, the stapes is gently realigned and maintained in the restored normal position by placing a small plug of fat laterally for its support. The joint between the incus and stapes is reduced and covered with a tube fashioned from a vein (Dietzel) that will support it in the corrected position until the joint has healed. Additional fixation with 2-cyano-butyl-acrylate fixative (Histoacryl) has not proved successful.

Following removal of polyps from the tympanic cavity, dislocations of the stapes are unfortunately not rare. Hinsberg reported 25 instances, and Günther reported 10. Removal of granulation polyps endangers the ossicle chain. If the drum is absent

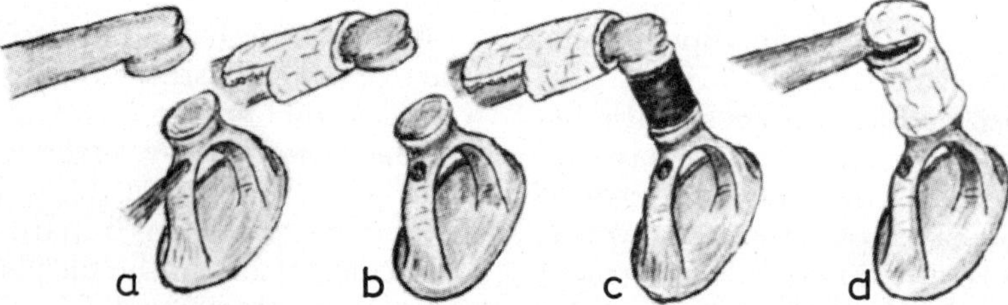


**Figure 11–6** Luxation of the joint between incus and stapes. Correction and support by vein graft according to Dietzel (HNO, *7*:209, 1966.) *A*, Covering the process of the incus with an inverted vein tube; eventual cutting of the stapedius tendon. *B*, Interposition of a cartilage implant between stapes head and processus lenticularis. *C*, Securing the implanted link of the transformation chain by flapping over the inverted vein tube.

and the granulations are located in the upper posterior part of the tympanic cavity, granulations and polyps should be removed only under the operating microscope, after careful anesthesia and with the aid of a sucker. A preoperative audiogram should be taken so as to protect the surgeon against possible unjustified claims.

### Drainage of the Tympanic Cavity

Using an hourglass PVC tubule for draining the tympanic cavity through the drum in cases of effusion or mucotympanon has lately become popular again. The dangers of paracentesis are the same as those mentioned previously. If such a tubule should accidentally slip into the cavity, this is no disaster. Generally, the tubule is shed via the eustachian tube, or it remains in the hypotympanum without harm.

## CURATIVE OTOSURGERY

Curative operative techniques will be dealt with only in so far as they are needed for insight into dangerous stages and possible complications. In principle, one should in all curative operations proceed "as radically as necessary and as conservatively as possible."

As mentioned before, there are now two basic types of operations: curative and corrective (for the improvement of hearing).

### Mastoidectomy

#### INDICATIONS

Destruction in the retrolabyrinthine area in acute or chronic otitis media. Approaches for saccotomy and part of the translabyrinthine approach to the inner meatus.

#### PRINCIPLE

With purulent processes, the retrotympanal cell system attacked by infection is cleared, and a wide access to the tympanic cavity is created, preserving the bony posterior wall of the meatus.

The first dangers present themselves with the incision. If this is done too far upward, the dura may be exposed on the way to the antrum. Particularly when using the older chisel technique, wedging or *perforating bone splinters* may possibly slide between dura and temporal bone without the surgeon being aware of it. Headache confined to the side of operation will suggest this complication to the experienced otologist. Since these bony splinters from the infected mastoid generally are themselves infected, they may produce intracranial complications.

Should it prove difficult to locate the antrum, the dura should be routinely exposed. It is then used as a guide along which one will safely reach the antrum. Whether one accepts this routine procedure or not, it is important to always check whether the dura lies closely along the bone throughout at the end of the operation. If there is even the smallest gap, i.e., an elevation of the dura, then one has to consider the possibility of an interposition of a hidden bone splinter.

Wider exposure of the dura will now be required. Under the operating microscope, removal of the splinter with a small hook will not be difficult. Conditions in the intentional or unintentional exposure of the *sigmoid sinus* are somewhat similar. Here, too, perforation by bone or tearing of the vessel by chisel or drill may occur. When this happens, the often severe bleeding has to be temporarily plugged. Then, the operation intended should be carried out with all care, and the sinus is repaired.

As suggested by Herrmann, sterile rubber flaps fashioned from a surgical glove are put directly on the lesion. On top of this one should put gelatin sponges soaked in penicillin and an additional gauze strip covered with antibiotic ointment. Open postoperative treatment is necessary after this. The first change of dressing should follow on the 12th day.

A further complication due to ill-advised handling of instruments (particularly with the so-called "spoon antrotomy," still used for small children in older techniques) is dislocation of the incus at its short limb in the posterior fossa. The same mishap may occur during unskillful manipulations in the antrum; a little hook is often used to explore the location and size of the antrum. During this stage, dislocation of the incus may be caused by the little hook wrongly being directed anteroinferiorly, instead of correctly toward the posterosuperior parts of the antrum. Dislocation of the incus causes interference with hearing. Such injury will have to be dealt with by tympanoplasty.

Iatrogenic injury to the lateral semicircular canal will be dealt with next; iatrogenic damage to the facial nerve and its correct treatment will be described in a special total survey that applies to all operations on the ear (see p. 157).

## Radical Operation of the Ear (Radical Mastoidectomy)

### INDICATIONS

Chronic otitis media with cholesteatoma that has entered the retrotympanic spaces, particularly with fistulas of the semicircular canals. Possibly benign tumors (e.g., neuromata of the facial nerve in its tympanomastoidal course and others).

### PRINCIPLE

A long-lasting, wide opening between the retrotympanic spaces and the outer meatus is created, sacrificing the bony posterior wall of the meatus and lining the surgical cavity with epidermis. In the past, "radical operation" also implied removal of drum and ossicles except the stapes, with excision of the tympanic mucosa down to the eustachian tube and its closure to shut off the tympanic cavity. Today this does not apply. Instead, we attempt to preserve ossicles and the residual drum (the so-called "conservative radical operation"). At the same or a second stage, sound transformation (Wullstein), i.e., ossicle chain and drum, is reconstructed.

One can proceed in two ways: (1) starting from the mastoid plane opening of the antrum and removing, step-by-step, the bony posterior wall of the meatus (retroauricular approach) or (2) starting from the meatus opening of aditus and antrum and removing the bony posterior wall of the meatus toward lateral and coinciding clearance of the retrotympanal cells as far as demanded by the extent of the pathologic process (enaural approach). There are two inherent dangers of the radical operation of the ear which demand special consideration: *intraoperative facial paralyses* (see p. 157) and *iatrogenic injury to the labyrinth,* i.e., injury to the semicircular canals or to the stapes.

In lesions of the labyrinth, the lateral semicircular canal is most often involved. Incorrect use of chisel or drill near the bulge of the lateral semicircular canal may lead to the top of the canal being directly cut or drilled off because of faulty assessment of the level when trying to find the antrum. Such faults of localization may occur particularly where the mastoid process shows limited pneumatization or is compact.

Another danger to the semicircular canal arises from the effort to shape the entrance to the radical cavity in the mastoid process so that it is as accessible as possible for postoperative treatment. The surgeon will thus try to grind the so-called "facial spur," after dividing the "bridge," as far down to the level of the floor of the meatus as possible.

When faced with so serious a lesion, we must try to save what we can. Following a suggestion of A. Herrmann, we cover the gap in the bone with a split skin graft dusted with bone. At times, it proves possible to save hearing function in this way. Intensive antibiotic treatment is mandatory.

Chronic osteomyelitis of the ear may have spontaneously involved the semicircular canal. *Circumscribed labyrinthitis* may have developed before the surgeon ever got near it. In chronic otitis, granulations or the matrix of a cholesteatoma may cover up a fistula of the semicircular canal. Occasionally, one will be unable to observe the fistula symptom in such erosions of the semicircular canal. When working near such a fistula without due care, granulations of the matrix may be torn out of the hole, and diffuse labyrinthitis would follow.

There are various views as to the appropriate attitude to a spontaneous labyrinthine fistula. Some surgical schools advocate the gentle removal of the matrix of cholesteatoma or granulations covering the fistula; others are against it because of the danger of provoking labyrinthitis.

In order to explain this author's attitude to this problem, a few words on the special morbid anatomy of circumscribed labyrinthitis are needed:

Circumscribed labyrinthitis is a granulating infection. It arises regularly and immediately from an osteomyelitis that has perforated the capsule of the semicircular canal with its granulations. This granulating labyrinthitis is clearly perilymphatic. In time, it expands over major parts of the perilymphatic space, sometimes even the whole vestibular apparatus. The endolymph space at first is not involved. Only later, at the healing stage, will the vascular granulation tissue be changed to connective or bone tissue. Thus the endolymph space may become constricted secondarily, even partially or wholly obstructed from the perilymph space.

If the intrusion into the bony labyrinth capsule lies at the semicircular canal, we generally will find the fistula symptom. In accordance with the creeping progress of the infection, the tests of vestibular function will show no or only minor abnormality, as long as the endolymph space is not, or only mildly, involved. When the endolymph tube is narrowed or shut off, however, it may be seen, especially in calorization, in the reduction or abolition of the sensitivity of the sensory final loci. The result of the rotatory test is more ambiguous, but occasionally one will find the symptom of the so-called "peripheral position nystagmus" (Vogel, Miehlke). As long as the process is confined to the balance apparatus, a further reduction of hearing beyond that already existing does not need to be present.

Ordinary granulating labyrinthitis usually heals spontaneously after its cause in the middle ear is removed. One has to remember, however, that the creeping, purely proliferative, form of labyrinthitis just described is not always as harmless as that. If the osteomyelitis in the middle ear runs a stormy course, then the granulation tissue that attacks the capsule and enters the inner ear is still young and slack and has little resistance. When pus builds up in the middle ear or manipulation near the fistula is inappropriate, infection may use the existing port of entry to invade the whole of the inner ear via the still young granulating focus.

All this should make clear that early and particularly gentle radical operation of the ear will have to be carried out for creeping granulating circumscribed labyrinthitis. The author agrees with many ear surgeons that one should not touch the fistula in the horizontal semicircular canal. It will close spontaneously once the circumscribed intralabyrinthine inflammatory processes have formed new bone and subsided.

This therapeutic concept, however, also means that one abandons the idea of employing an even gentler curative surgical technique, i.e., posterior tympanotomy, meatoepitympanotomy or osteoplastic epitympanotomy.

Accidental *dislocation of the stapes* while clearing granulations and residual matrix of cholesteatoma from the oval window in the course of radical mastoidectomy is a highly dangerous complication, since it is often followed by purulent labyrinthitis or meningitis.

This complication can be prevented by working with the small forceps *only in the longitudinal direction* of the stapes tendon, i.e., parallel to the crura of the stapes. Here one should work very gently, step-by-step, and never use a tight grip or even pull. Any procedure performed near the legs ought to be done extremely gently and be well planned. Should operative instrumental dislocation of the stapes occur, it should be immediately repaired, as mentioned previously. Massive antibiotic treatment is mandatory.

## Posterior Tympanotomy ("Intact Canal-wall Technique")

### INDICATION

Chronic otitis media and decompression of the facial nerve in the tympanum (C. Jansen, J. Sheehy).

### PRINCIPLE

The creation of a cavity should be avoided by preserving the posterior wall of the meatus with a wide opening of the tympanic cavity through the chorda-facial recess. This retroauricular approach is combined with the transmeatal approach.

This approach to the tympanic cavity following transcortical mastoidectomy was originally developed by H. L. Wullstein in 1952. It is used for the so-called lower control of the tympanum, for decompression of the facial nerve in its tympanal course and for the control of the round window. It was later used by Jansen in Germany and Sheehy in the U.S.A. for the clearance of middle ear cholesteatomata and, since then, by many ear surgeons all over the world. Wullstein was unwilling to accept the procedure because, in his opinion, it provided insufficient access. Even experienced surgeons have to count on up to 35 per cent residual and recurrent cholesteatoma (Sheehy). The areas below the pyramidal process and in the pretympanum are especially problematic.

Complication may therefore develop because this approach does not provide full access in individual areas to the cholesteatoma and other pathologic changes in the middle ear. Even if the cholesteatoma is completely eradicated, however, there is the further danger of the development of a pocket of retraction into the surgically created opening at the chorda-facial recess and thus the possibility of the formation of a second retraction cholesteatoma.

In order to prevent this complication, Sheehy inserted a Silastic foil into the recess. He started from the premise that the dangerous retraction pockets in a formerly infected area would form from fibrous adhesions between the drum or drum transplant and the raw surface of the bone in the facial recess. According to Sheehy, it would be possible to prevent such adhesions by inserting Silastic foil.

This author has, on occasion, seen such retraction pockets with cholesteatoma formation, in spite of using this technique via the chorda-facial angle with the purpose of decompressing the facial nerve in Bell's palsy. It appears that retraction is not due to preceding infection. Such retraction and its complications might be explained by the rerouting of the natural aeration pathways of the middle ear following the wide opening of the chorda-facial angle (S. R. Wullstein). This could be prevented by inserting an exactly shaped autologous bone transplant into the surgically created opening at the chorda-facial recess at the end of the "intact canal-wall technique." This technique demands considerable surgical skill, and certain dangers to the facial nerve cannot be ruled out. The use of the "intact canal-wall technique" remains a question of conscience, since leaving behind even the smallest remnant of matrix in one of the many recesses of the tympanic cavity, with the branches of the various cell lines, will inevitably lead to recurrence of the cholesteatoma. Only quite recently, we were forced to reoperate on a cholesteatoma that had been overlooked elsewhere during posterior tympanotomy and that grew via the posterior lower and anterior upper cell lines into the tip of the pyramid. In addition, this cholesteatoma had infiltrated the inner meatus via these cell lines beyond the facial nerve and had caused ever-recurring bouts of meningitis. A possibly deadly complication threatened unless surgery was performed immediately. In such a situation, the inner meatus must be exposed via the translabyrinthine route according to the principles of its surgery, and the cholesteatoma in the inner meatus must be cleared out while preserving the facial nerve.

## Meato-epitympanotomy

### INDICATION

Curative for chronic otitis media with cholesteatoma; reconstructive for transplantation of ossicles, drum and meatal tube; tumor of the middle ear; purposes of surgery of the tympanal course of the facial nerve.

### PRINCIPLE

There is osteoclastic epitympanotomy and temporary removal of posterior and upper bony wall of the meatus.

The temporary meatotomy (H. Gerlach) had its original indication in the exposure of antrum, aditus and retrotympanal spaces for clearance in chronic otitis media.

Dr. Ralf Arold at our department in Göttingen extended this technique by lengthening the anterior incision into bone anteriorly beyond the petrotympanic fissure in order to achieve wide exposure of the area of the anterior cupola, including the supratubal recess (S. R. Wullstein). This *meato-epitympanotomy*, as we call it, facilitates not only clearance in chronic otitis media but also transplant of homologous ossicle chains and drums.

The meato-epitympanotomy is also applicable for various aspects of surgery of the facial nerve in the tympanic area, including the repair of lesions of the facial nerve at the ganglion geniculi.

Postoperative complications may arise when the temporarily removed segment of the meatus cannot be exactly refitted into its original site. This can be prevented by using the "pointed cone diamond drill" designed by H. L. Wullstein so that the bone gaps resulting from the removal of the segment can be kept extraordinarily small, always providing the technique performed is correct. A posterior tilt of the bony segment can be prevented by fixing it at a point with the 2-cyano-butyl-acrylate fixative (Histacryl) Braun, Melsungen).

Like J. Marquet, we do not incise the dermal meatus but detach the meatal tube from its bony support bluntly toward the front or laterally in one piece. The completely preserved meatal tube will later be returned and serve to support the replaced bony segment and revascularization of the homeotransplants.

### Osteoplastic Epitympanotomy

#### INDICATIONS

Chronic otitis media with cholesteatoma and tympanic sclerosis; purposes in surgery of the facial nerve in its tympanal course.

#### PRINCIPLE

The cupolar space is temporarily exposed by cutting out the lateral wall in order to restore physiologic aeration while obtaining optimal views of the pathology of the cupola.

A bony cover is shaped according to S. R. Wullstein along the tegmen close to the dura. The cortex of the dura is used at the same time as a landmark for the upper limit of the cover. The anterior landmark for the cover is the petrotympanic fissure; the posterior limit corresponds to the fossa incudis posterior.

In contrast to the posterior tympanotomy and the meato-epitympanotomy, the chorda-facial recess is left intact in this procedure, according to S. R. Wullstein. This prevents the formation of retraction pockets with their threat of secondary cholesteatomata from the start. Shaping of the bony cover is carried out by excavating with the bur the bony meatal wall in its upper medial aspect. The surgeon must decide the thickness of the cover individually, corresponding to the degree of pneumatization (a relatively large thickness with pneumatization is extensive, and vice versa). Depending on the nature of the disease, the whole of the retrotympanal space can also be exposed and cleared with this technique.

One can imagine the possible complications, for instance, a lesion of the *dura* due to faulty guidance of the bur. A *lesion of the facial nerve* in its pyramidal course could be caused when the fossa incudis posterior has not been unequivocally located as a limiting landmark beforehand. This can be avoided if one preserves a thin bony bridge above the posterior fossa of the incus. The bridge is broken with the elevator for the removal of the bony cover. This intentional fracture should be produced *at right angles* to the course of the facial nerve over the fossa incudis. On the other hand one should not leave a residual bony edge over the fossa incudis so as not to overlook possible remnants of cholesteatoma in the angle. This danger threatens particularly in cases in which a Körner septum is present. It is exceptionally important to check the inner aspect of the bony cover meticulously for possible cholesteatoma buds.

## OPERATIONS TO IMPROVE HEARING

### Complications of Tympanoplasty

Among the *tympanoplastic procedures* proper there are various postoperative complications that follow clearance after chronic otitis media. These are contained in a list compiled by Harry Jakobi:

1. Damage to the ossicle chain
2. Necroses
3. Blocking of drainage
4. Allergies
5. Interference with the drum (blowing the nose, sucking, damage by instruments or faulty inlay dressing)
6. Perichondritis
7. Labyrinthitis

Damage to the ossicle chain may be due to ill-advised actions on the part of the surgeon, e.g., premature politzeration, or on the part of the patient, e.g., unnecessarily rapid head movements. This may lead to a collapse of the columella, which in turn causes a reduction in the size of the tympanic cavity, with the chance of adhesions forming. Damage leading to depression of the

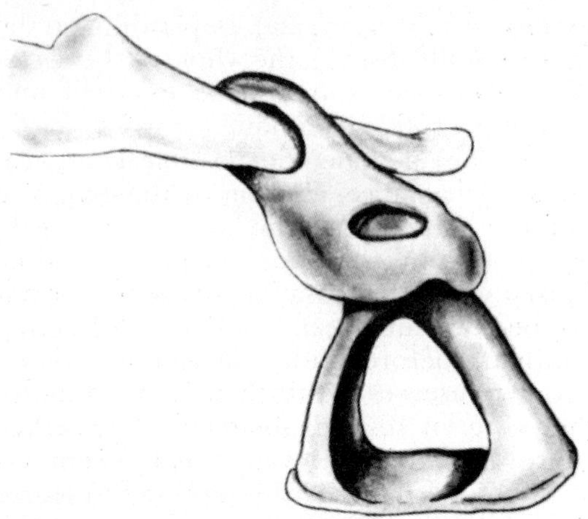

**Figure 11–7** Creating and stabilizing of a new sound transmission between malleus and stapes by incus shaped according to Marquet. (Marquet, J. F.: Homoiotransplantationen von Trommelfell und Gehorknöchelchenkette. HNO, *25*:157–163, 1977.)

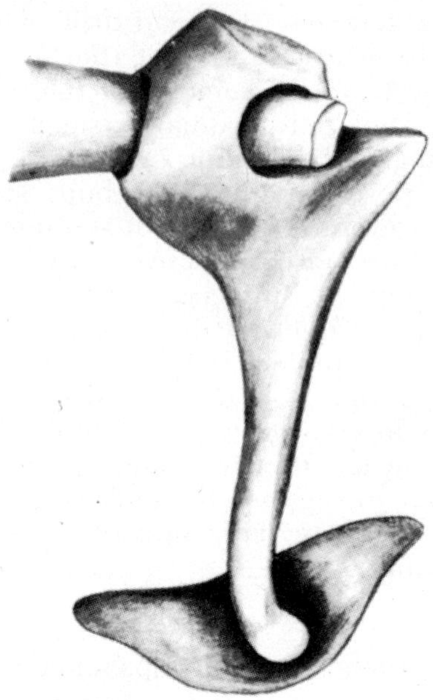

**Figure 11–8** Creating and stabilizing of a new sound transmission between malleus and footplate by incus transposition, according to Marquet. (Marquet, J. F.: Homoiotransplantationen von Trommelfell und Gehorknöchelchenkette. HNO, *25*:157–163, 1977.)

oval window, from which involvement of the inner ear with loss of hearing and threatened labyrinthitis may develop, is rather worse.

One can prevent instability of columellization as a main cause of damage to the chain by using a columella technique used by Marquet. The ossicle transplant to be used as columella is drilled in its upper and lower part. The drill holes are arranged in such a manner that both the handle of the hammer and the head of the stapes will fit into them, and thus safely stabilize the columella. Occasionally, considerable necroses may be seen in the operative field, e.g., if antibiotic protection was wrong or insufficient, clearance was not complete or aeration of tympanic cavity and antrum is deficient. These three dangers have to be taken into account during surgery of the tympanic cavity if they are to be guarded against from the start.

Blocking of drainage with renewed infection that may spread further and the resulting further complications will have to be prevented by adequate drainage at the end of the operation.

Many people, particularly chronically ill patients, have more and more allergies, a fact that must be realized. Detailed history-taking is, therefore, of prime importance. In some patients, exanthemas or enanthemas, with all their usual side effects, occur for *the first time* only after the operation. Immediate countermedication and revision of antibiotic protection is needed, since many patients have become allergic to many antibiotics.

Disturbances of the drum occur when shifts of the drum transplant are caused by nose blowing, sucking, wash-outs, incorrectly applied gauze-strip dressings or pulling with instruments. These prevent proper healing. All such manipulations must be avoided. This complication may be automatically prevented by covering the drum or plastic drum at the end of the operation with crossed strips of silicone foil, placing Gelfoam plugs soaked with nutrient fluid on top of this and, finally, applying a strip soaked in penicillin or oxytetracycline hydrochloride-hydrocortisone (Terra-Cortril) ointment, which should be left untouched within the outer meatus for 12 days.

This dressing of the ear should be removed on the 12th day. At this time it is no longer needed, since the graft as a rule is sufficiently linked to the nutrition. The Gelfoam plug, on the 11th or 12th day, has already undergone such changes that it can easily be sucked out with a sterile sucker. If the dressing remains *in situ* beyond the 12th to 14th day, the formation of granulations is provoked, the plug disintegrates and infection rapidly spreads in the cavity. Removal of the Gelfoam plug in good time favors the process of epithelization. The next goal is far-reaching exclusion of air from the surgical cavity and simultaneous creation of the most sterile conditions possible. After the removal of the Gelfoam plug, using the utmost gentleness, we can achieve this by brushing the cavity with the old, established Castellani solution* and by introducing triamcinolone ointment (Volon A). Castellani solution acts antiphlogistically, antimycotically and antibacterially. Triamcinolone ointment is strongly antibacterial over a wide spectrum and because of its prednisolone content prevents the formation of granulations. Far-reaching exclusion of air from the radical cavity is safeguarded by the introduction of the ointment on a firm strip plug that is best kept *in situ* for one week.

The identical dressing with Castellani solution and firm triamcinolone ointment–plugging is repeated at weekly intervals. It is important to realize that treatment with either the solution or the ointment alone does by no means yield results equally good as with their combination. The uncontrollable, and often forgotten, use of eardrops has been abandoned. As a rule, postoperative treatment ends after two to three weekly changes of this dressing. The ear should be dry. Conventional radical cavities usually require four to six weekly changes. Exceptions to this rule are rare.

The most dangerous complication is postoperative labyrinthitis. Should it occur, massive antibiotic treatment will have to be started at once. We strongly recommend a combination of several antibiotics that pass into the cerebrospinal fluid and act in the inner ear.

## Stapes Transplant

For the *surgical improvement of hearing* in otosclerosis, the stapes transplant with the fat and wire prosthesis (Schuknecht) or the Teflon piston (Shea) has become accepted as a routine technique. It is a major surgical misfortune when the foot plate or one of its parts is dropped into the vestibulum. Experience has taught us that it is wise not to try extraction in any way. Such manipulations are dangerous to the inner ear. Instead, the stapes transplant should be completed with the greatest care.

Fabian reports this surgical complication in 3.4 per cent of all stapes operations and adds that it was followed only once by deafness, in 8 cases by gradual deterioration of the improved hearing and in two instances by return to the preoperative level.

Dropping of the foot plate or one of its parts into the vestibulum is followed by a dizziness that lasts longer than that usually following stapes transplants. Only one of Fabian's cases with this complication led to considerable vestibular irritation similar to that exhibited in the "Dandy syndrome" and was combined with an otherwise good effect on hearing.

If iatrogenic dislocation of the incus occurs during the stapes transplant, malleolabyrinthopexy with fat and wire prosthesis offers a technical way out that must be modified accordingly. The wire sling around the handle of the malleus must lie *below* the drum or the prosthesis will become unhinged. In other words, before fixing the prosthesis at the handle of the malleus, part of the drum will have to be detached. The wire sling may be pulled through this surgical gap and fixed around the handle of the malleus.

Bleeding into the open vestibulum is not of great moment. Even more severe hemorrhage can be controlled by an inlay of Gelfoam sponges and gentle sucking away from the vestibulum.

## Postoperative Perilymph Fistula

*Postoperative perilymph fistula* exhibits symptoms similar to those of endolymphatic hydrops, although permanent loss of perilymph, not excess endolymph, is responsible for reduction of hearing, vertigo, a feeling of fullness and tinnitus.

Correction of this surgical mishap first requires exploration of the tympanic cavity and exact localization of the site of perilymph leakage. The entire membrane must

*Solutio Castellani: 5 g. phenolum liquefactum, 1 g. boric acid, 5 g. acetone, 10 g. resorcinol, solutio fuchsini spirituosa 10 per cent, aqua dest. ad 100 ml.

be removed from the oval window and be replaced by a fat and wire prosthesis or a wire and foam prosthesis. This usually will stop the leakage. As far as hearing is concerned, the treatment of perilymph fistula is unsatisfactory in most cases; but it satisfactorily eliminates vertigo and the risk of meningitis (Shambaugh, Jr.).

### Loss of Hearing Gain Due to Stapes Surgery

*Loss of the original gain in hearing following a stapes operation* may have different causes: ankylosis of incus or malleus; slippage of a prosthesis from the incus or its insufficient fixation; and necrosis of the tip of the long process of the incus.

In addition to these surgical errors, sound conduction deafness, occurring only at a later date, may be due to renewed osseous closure of the oval window by osteosclerotic bone after stapedectomy.

Although the surgical mistakes mentioned previously are easily identified at the reoperation and can be corrected by another stapes transplant, it is advisable to treat recurrent closure of the oval window by osteosclerotic bone with *fenestration of the lateral semicircular canal*. Another attempt to operate on the oval window would only lead to renewed osteogenic activity.

Damage to nerve structures, the chorda tympani and the facial nerve ought not to happen with a stapes operation. Following tearing or removal of the chorda tympani at the access to the oval window, patients will complain during the first postoperative weeks of a metallic taste on the homolateral side of the tongue. This taste disturbance usually subsides in time. The chances of damaging the facial nerve during a stapes operation will be discussed next.

## MALFORMATIONS

In the *surgery of malformations of the ear*, there are no really typical surgical complications. Each case has to be assessed and surgically dealt with differently, because malformations vary a great deal. It would be beyond the scope of this chapter to go into detail. The reader interested in the pathogenesis and varieties of malformations of the ear and their surgical problems is referred to the contributions of Miehlke, Shambaugh, Jr., Altmann, House, Rüedi and others. In this type of surgery, the often atypical course of the facial nerve provides a very special problem. Intraoperative damage to it is not rare. Careful preoperative explanation to the patient and his family is of the very greatest importance. This author agrees with George Shambaugh, Jr., who made it clear how easily the facial nerve or the labyrinth can be damaged in malformation cases during the search for the tympanic cavity. In cases of obvious danger, he recommends stopping any further search in order to save the patient, who already has a disability, additional damage. The surgeon undertaking to treat a malformation of the ear should always be aware that he might bring about an additional tragedy — iatrogenic facial paralysis.

Unfortunately, this author must often deal with reconstruction of intraoperative facial nerve damage in patients with malformations of the middle ear. It is exceptionally difficult to localize the often abnormally situated nerve or nerve remnant in such cases.

The difficulty of reaching the tympanic cavity through a compact mastoid process is acknowledged by all who have experience with operations designed to improve hearing in the malformed middle ear. Vogel and his coworkers and Shambaugh, Jr. have described useful landmarks at the base of the skull.

The dangerous path to the tympanic cavity can be rendered much easier if one follows the recommendation, first made by Denecke, of using *the facial nerve itself as a safe guide to the tympanic cavity*. In order to prevent possible surgical complications, Denecke recommends the following:

> The facial nerve is exposed at its exit from the stylomastoid foramen.... This is even easier than with normal ears, since in microtia and anotia there is a shallow "valley" over the stylomastoid foramen. Below this the facial nerve is easily reached. Now one proceeds from distally proximally, using the operating microscope and, step by step, various burrs, down to the diamond drill. The last slender bony wall of the Fallopian canal is preserved. Through it the nerve can be seen. If, in the mastoid segment of the course of the facial nerve, one keeps anterior, the tympanic cavity will be reached without endangering the

semicircular canal. The origin of the chorda tympani is a landmark indicating that advancing proximally one will soon reach the tympanum. Before this is entered, one sees a small, rounded, gradually enlarging dark structure. Once the cavity has been entered, the opening is enlarged with small osteotomes or drills.

## OPERATIONS ON THE INTERNAL MEATUS

### Indications

Menière's disease resistant to conservative treatment, small- or medium-sized acoustic neurinoma and fractures of the petrous bone with facial nerve involvement.

### Principle

Translabyrinthine or middle cranial fossa approach to the internal auditory meatus is achieved.

### Transtemporal Approach

For the transtemporal approach via the middle cranial fossa, one may either employ the 60° - technique, according to Fisch, for

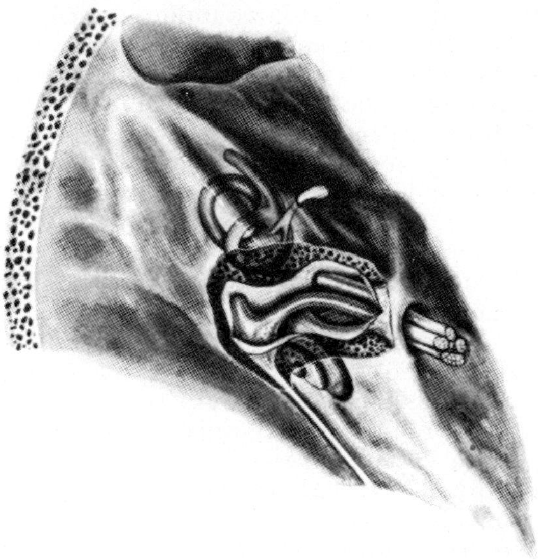

**Figure 11–10** Inner ear shown from above. To facilitate understanding of the relative position of the facial nerve, the cochlea and vestibular organ are drawn as if transparent. (After Miehlke, A., and Bushe, K. A.: Chir. Plast. Reconstr., *3*:37, 1967.)

the safe exposure of the internal meatus or the approach, originally recommended by W. House, via the major superficial petrosal nerve, the ganglion geniculi and the facial nerve. Problems in opening the inner meatus may arise from the fact that the dis-

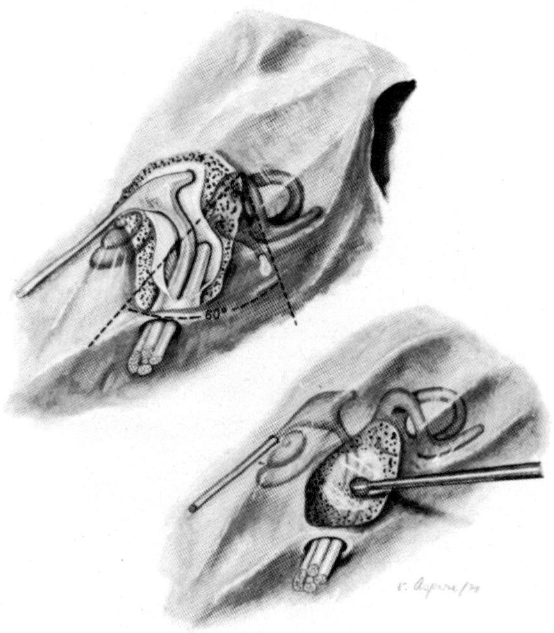


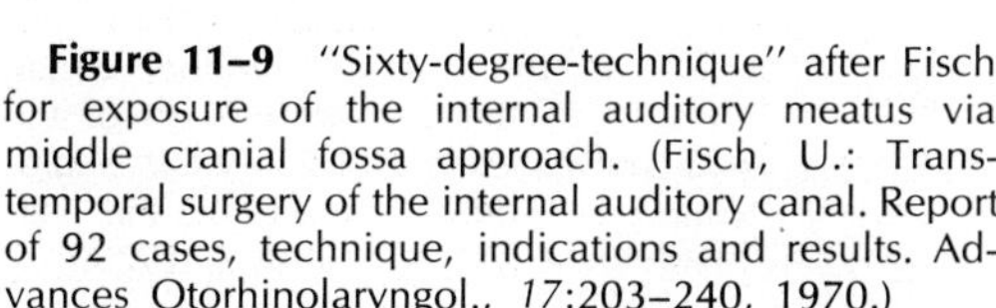

**Figure 11–9** "Sixty-degree-technique" after Fisch for exposure of the internal auditory meatus via middle cranial fossa approach. (Fisch, U.: Transtemporal surgery of the internal auditory canal. Report of 92 cases, technique, indications and results. Advances Otorhinolaryngol., *17*:203–240, 1970.)

tances between the surrounding structures vary. The anatomic structures that limit access are shown in (Figure 11–10.) Because of these variations, it may happen, in spite of exact surgery with the diamond bur (size 3–6), that vestibulum or cochlea is opened inadvertently. For operations of Menière's disease, the author prefers the 60°-technique of Fisch, since the purpose of the operation is the direct localization of the inner meatus.

For surgery of the facial nerve, however, we use the original approach of W. House, lifting off the temporal dura from the petrosal pyramid and exposing the major superficial petrosal nerve. Starting from this important landmark, the hiatus of the fallopian canal is opened with a diamond drill and the ganglion geniculi is exposed by retracing along the major superficial petrosal nerve.

This procedure demands the greatest care, since in 5 per cent of all people the ganglion geniculi has no, or only a paper-thin, cover against the middle cranial fossa. If dissection is careless, the ganglion may be damaged. If one proceeds from the ganglion with the diamond drill quite closely along the course of the facial nerve, one will drill, as in a deep furrow, between the cochlea in front and the vestibulum behind without touching, let alone damaging, either. The reader will realize that this type of surgery is not without risks for various structures, i.e., the cochlea, the vestibulum and the facial nerve.

Although damage to the cochlea and vestibulum will produce irreversible loss of function, surgical damage to the facial nerve should be repaired at once. According to the well-tried techniques of facial nerve surgery, the stumps of the damaged nerve have to be directly apposed. For only superficial loss of nerve substance, up to one third of the total diameter of the nerve, an "inlay graft" may be considered; more extensive damage in the labyrinthine course or near the ganglion should be treated by "rerouting" the facial nerve. In such instances, the fallopian canal can be shortened by drilling toward the semicircular canal, and end-to-end suture of the labyrinthine and tympanic facial nerve stumps can be accomplished.

### Retroauricular Translabyrinthine Approach

What has been said about the chances of injury during the transtemporal approach to the inner meatus applies in a similar manner to the *retroauricular translabyrinthine approach to the inner meatus*. Here, one first clears all of the labyrinth and then, starting from the vestibulum, searches for the superior ampullary nerve, a very important landmark. Retracing its course, "Bill's barr" is exposed.

It is essential that the surgeon exposes these two landmarks clearly before entering the inner meatus proper because only in this way can he make sure of the course of the facial nerve within the inner meatus.

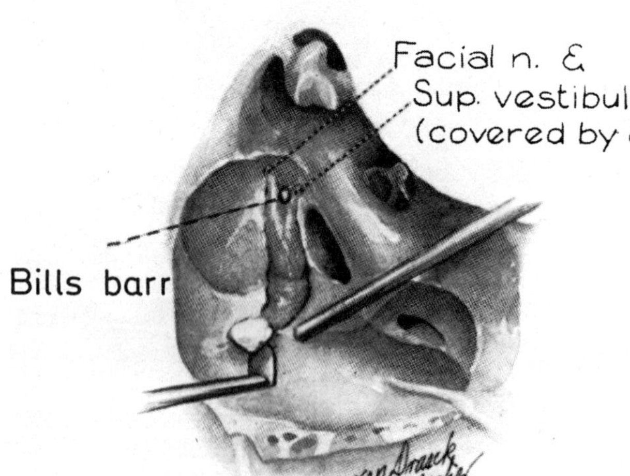


**Figure 11–11** Translabyrinthine approach to the internal auditory canal. Exposure of the petrous portion of the facial nerve. (After House, W.: *In* Shambaugh, G. (ed.): Surgery of the Ear. Philadelphia, W. B. Saunders, 1973.)

If, in spite of all precautions, the facial nerve is damaged in its labyrinthine or meatal segments or near the ganglion, the modern techniques of surgery of the facial nerve will once more have to be applied in order to repair the damage. Here, too, rerouting, as described before, is available. The results of such repairs of the facial nerve in the inner meatus and in its tympanal course are extraordinarily favorable. The rule that such repair has to be done immediately following the iatrogenic lesion applies here also.

## IATROGENIC FACIAL NERVE PALSY

What has just been said leads straight to the center of the discussion concerning the complication most feared by every otologist and most visible to everyone after ear surgery — the *iatrogenic facial nerve palsy*.

Technical progress in otosurgery has reduced to a minimum the danger of iatrogenic damage to the facial nerve. Nevertheless, this complication still occurs.

It comes as a severe shock to both patient and surgeon when an operation that was meant to be curative results in the catastrophe of facial paralysis.

Statistics on the frequency of intraoperative facial paresis vary a great deal. They lie between 0.6 per cent (Pöllmann) and 3.6 per cent (Körner). In reoperations, their incidence may even be 4.6 per cent to 11 per cent. In the experience of this author, those departments in which many assistants receive their specialist training have to expect a larger number of intraoperative facial palsy than those in which all operations are done solely by an experienced otologist. There is no doubt that routine use of the operating microscope and improvements in surgical techniques have contributed to a further decrease in the incidence of iatrogenic facial nerve lesions. In Germany, at present, less than 1 per cent iatrogenic nerve damage occurs among all operations on the ear.

Recognition of a facial nerve paralysis is, of course, easy. It is, however, a curious fact that those palsies that are caused by the hands of the otosurgeon, i.e., the iatrogenic lesions, are not recognized because one does not want to.

### Simple Mastoidectomy

When, during a *simple mastoidectomy,* a surgeon loses his way to the antrum (and this happens most frequently to beginners and inexperienced surgeons), he may place his bur too low, i.e., too far toward the mastoid tip, probably because he fears damage to the dura.

In working his way into the depth, he endangers the facial nerve in its mastoid portion, near the level at which the chorda tympani branches off. We call this the "lesion of the beginners."

### Radical Mastoidectomy

During the course of a *radical mastoidectomy*, the facial nerve is in danger near the second bend when the facial "spur" is taken down, which is one of the goals of the well-trained ear surgeon. We call this, therefore, the "lesion of the experienced surgeon." The following is a concrete example:

*Case report*

Mastoidectomy was to be performed on a young woman with mastoiditis. The operation was carried out by a resident in a West German ENT department. During the course of the operation, the facial nerve was injured at a typical site — the branching off point of the chorda tympani ("lesion of the beginner"). The chief of the department was called in immediately and set out to transform the prepared cavity into a radical mastoid cavity. In doing so, he injured the facial nerve in front of the facial spur, a site typical for radical mastoidectomies ("lesion of the experienced surgeon"). At reoperation at the

*Text continued on page 163*

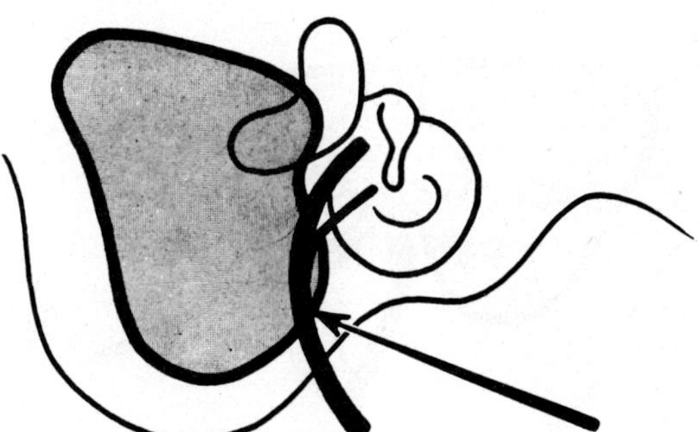

**Figure 11–12** Typical site of intratemporal facial nerve lesion during mastoidectomy. (After Jongkees.)

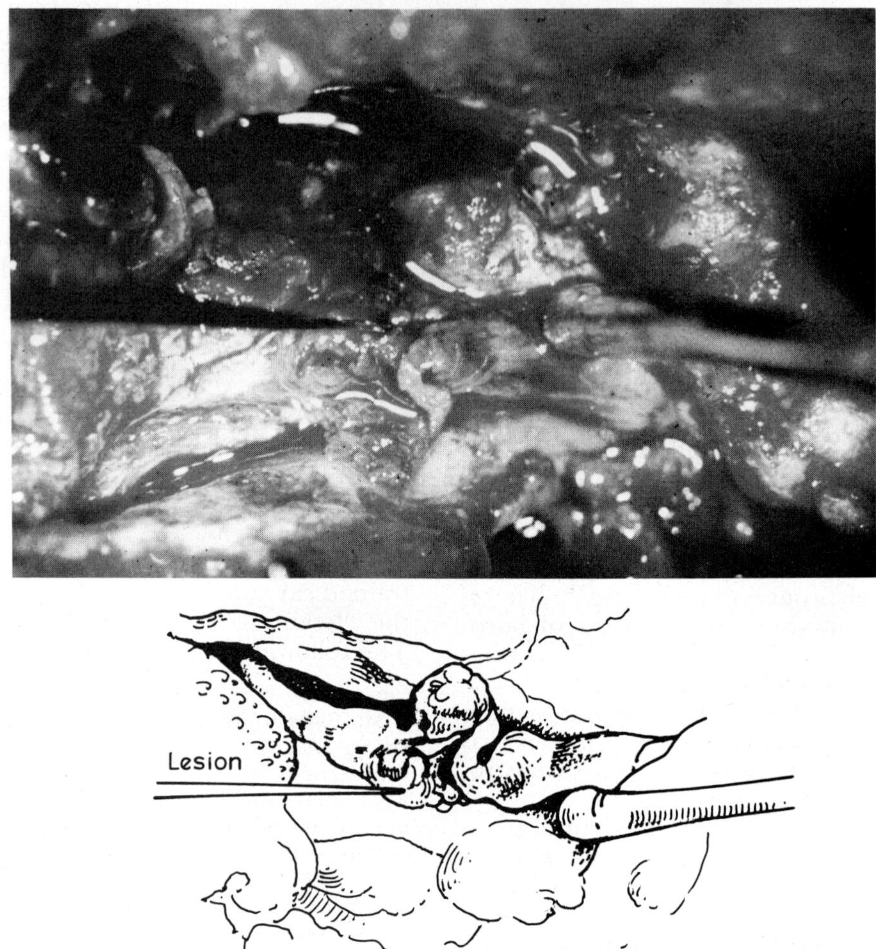


**Figure 11–13** Severe iatrogenic damage to the mastoid segment of the facial nerve during mastoidectomy; typical site.

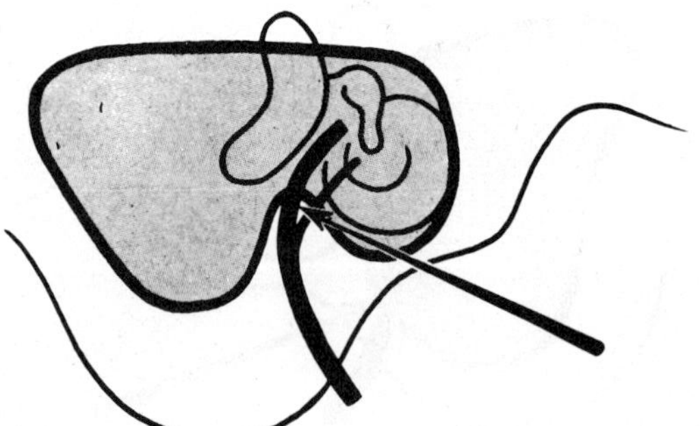

**Figure 11–14** Typical site of intratemporal facial nerve lesion during radical mastoidectomy. (After Jongkees.)

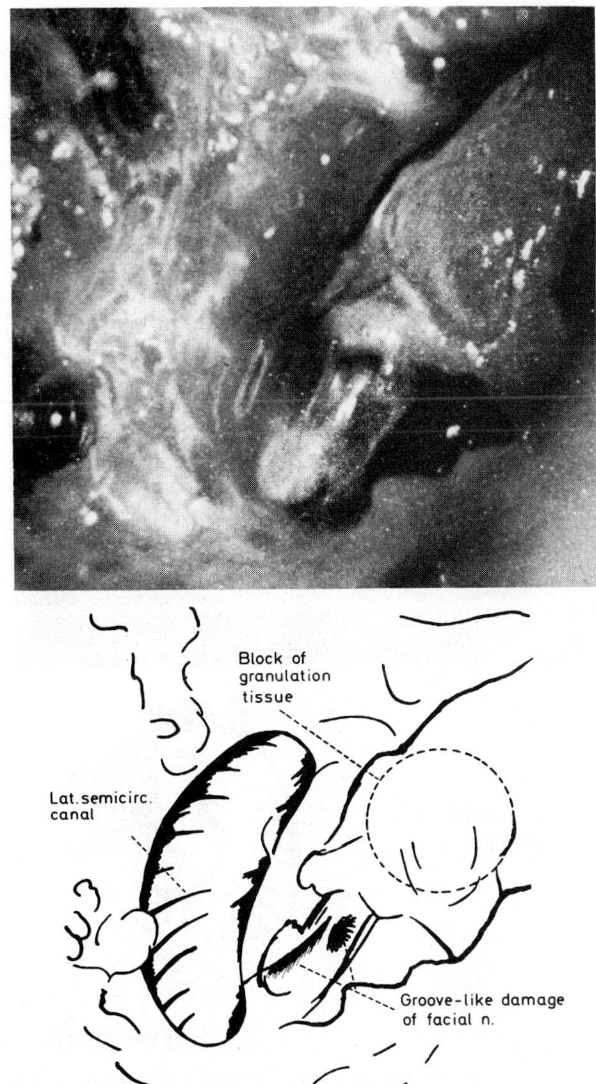


**Figure 11–15** Severe damage to the facial nerve at its pyramidal segment. Finding eight weeks after radical mastoidectomy. About half of the diameter of the Vth nerve is destroyed. Distally ample inflammatory granulations.

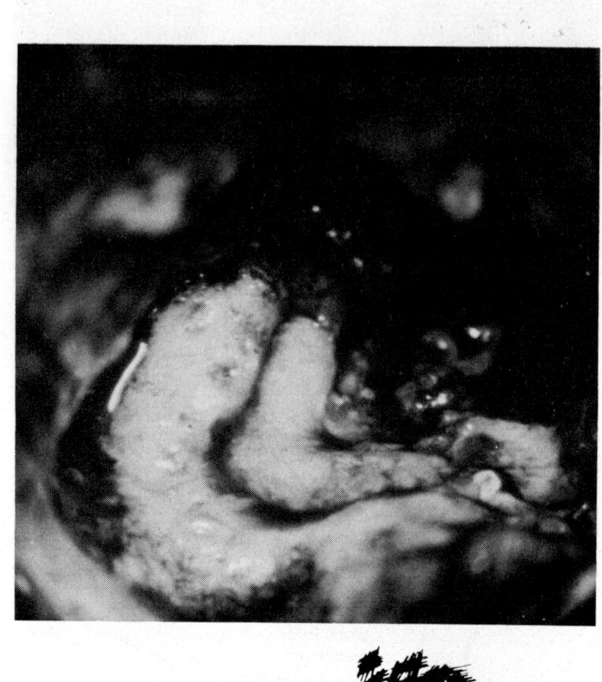

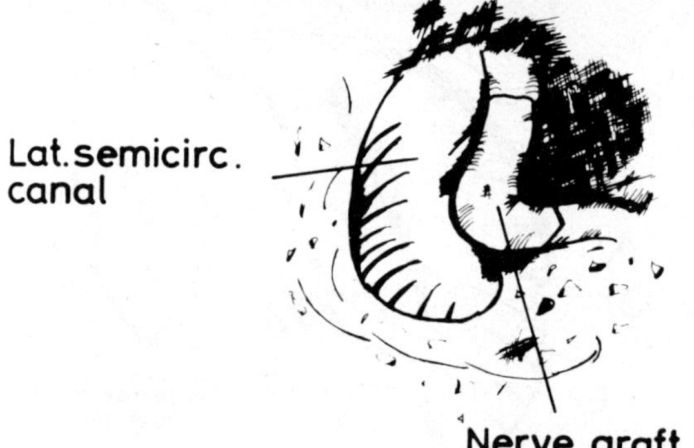


**Figure 11–16** Reconstruction of the facial nerve by autogenous nerve transplantation after resection of the destroyed part of that nerve.

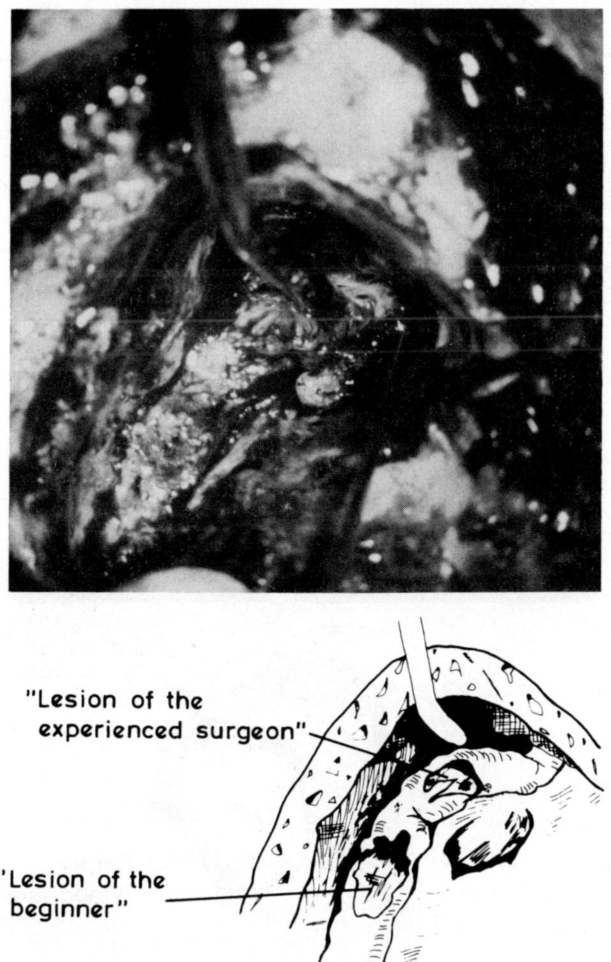


**Figure 11–17** Severe iatrogenic damage to the pyramidal *and* tympanic segments of the facial nerve; a double lesion.

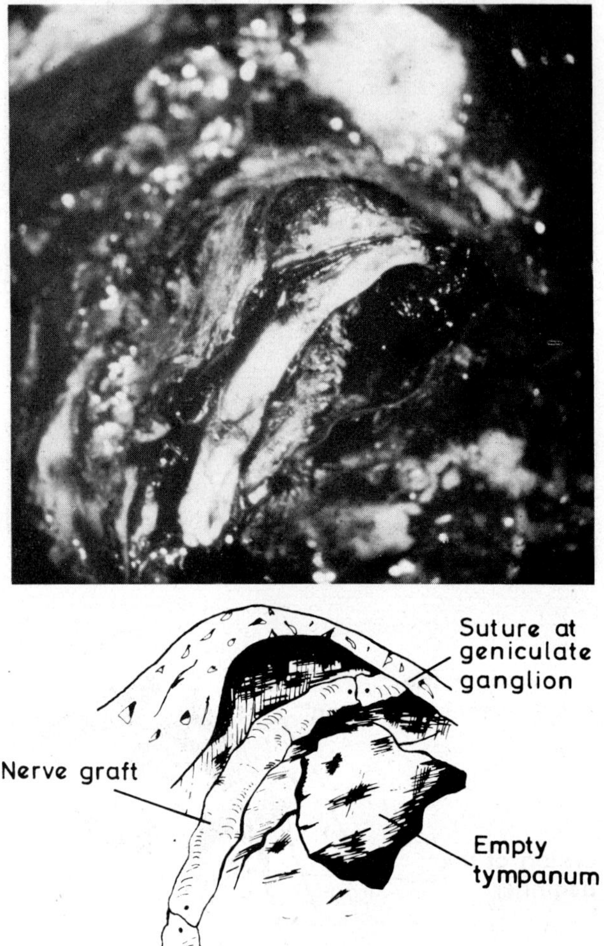


**Figure 11–18** After resection of the destroyed segment of the facial nerve, bridging of the defect by free autogenous nerve graft following suture at the geniculate ganglion.

ENT department of Göttingen University the author cut the facial nerve transversely both proximally and distally to the lesions and then inserted an autogenous nerve graft to bridge the defect. Facial nerve function was restored after one year.

### Fenestration

In general, fenestration of the lateral semicircular canal has been abandoned in favor of stapedectomy as the method of choice in the surgical management of otosclerosis. Nevertheless, fenestration still remains the superior method, especially with malformations of the ear and, occasionally, with tympanosclerosis. In Germany, which only a few years ago witnessed the thalidomide tragedy, there are now many children growing up who, in the future, will become definite candidates for fenestration. During the course of this operation, the surgeon may suddenly lose control of his drill, especially at the semicircular canal, causing a lesion of the facial nerve in the posterior third of its horizontal portion. These lesions may be facilitated by an anatomic variant. In this area, the nerve is protected by nothing but a paper-thin bony wall. To make matters worse, the nerve often lies exposed owing to dehiscences of varying sizes in the fallopian canal.

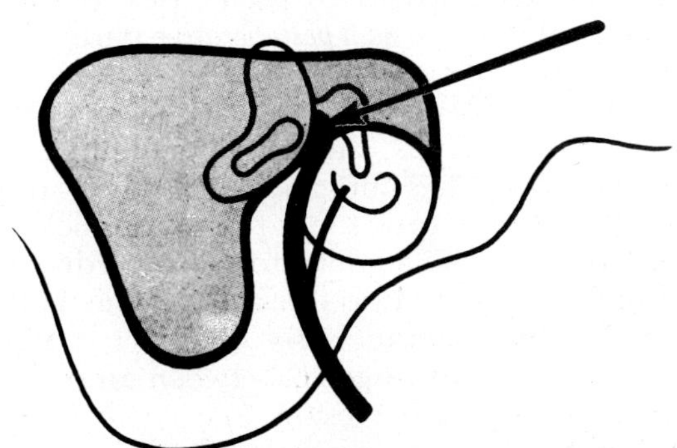

**Figure 11–19** Typical site of intratemporal facial nerve lesion during fenestration operation. (After Jongkees.)

### Tympanoplasty

Tympanoplasties of various kinds now occupy a major place in the daily schedule of the otosurgeon. I need not dwell on the difficulties encountered in the attempt to determine the anatomic outline of the tympanic cavity in cases of chronic otitis media. It is this difficulty in orientation that in such cases may be directly responsible for surgical lesions of the facial nerve within its tympanic portion. Such lack of orientation may occasionally lead to very serious damage of the nerve in the region of the geniculate ganglion.

For the surgeon who later has to reoperate on such cases, this type of lesion presents one of the most unpleasant experiences. Often seemingly never-ending efforts are required in order to find the stumps of the severed nerve. The only logical management of the restoration of function of the facial nerve is its anatomic reconstruction. In most cases, this is done by means of autogenic nerve grafts.

The tympanic opening of the eustachian tube is frequently the first and only landmark for locating the nerve stump at the site where it emerges from its translabyrinthine course. In this case, one will have to feel one's way from the eustachian tube to the last portion of the geniculate ganglion or what has remained of it.

### Stapedectomy

The last of the typical surgical lesions of the facial nerve within the tympanic cavity are those that occur during *stapedectomy*. One would think that a procedure of such clear-cut anatomic definition, which usually permits a complete survey of the entire situation within the tympanic cavity, could hardly lead to facial nerve injuries. The fact is, however, that they do happen occasionally. One such lesion was quite remarkable. It came about in the following way. After a well-executed stapedectomy, a Schuknecht wire prosthesis was inserted and the wire left after cutting was too long. The upper end of the wire, which could not be seen during the procedure, twisted sideways, entered the fallopian canal through a dehiscence and penetrated the nerve from below.

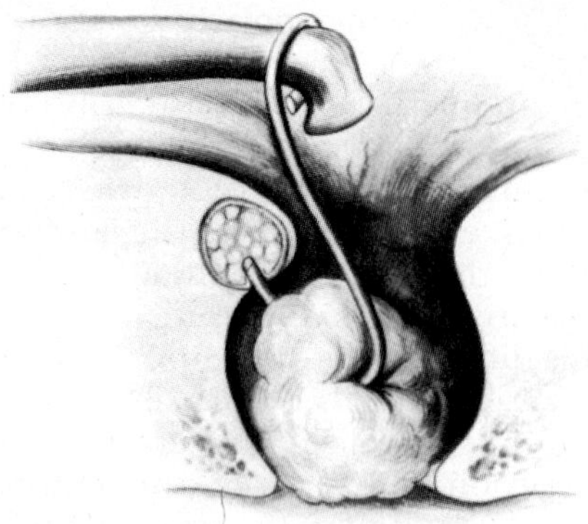

**Figure 11–20** Injury to the facial nerve by an erroneously placed wire fat prosthesis with an excessively long wire tilted up and fitted through a dehiscence into the facial nerve.

Facial paralysis ensued.

If the nerve does not take a normal course, there will, occasionally, also be lesions during stapedectomy.

This author recently had to give a medical opinion on a case of facial nerve damage, because its course was a kind of anatomic rarity. The nerve passed between the two "feet" of the stapes, which itself was somewhat plump. Its "feet" were almost merged into one, and the stapes looked rather like a pyramid. During its excision, the facial nerve was divided.

Other injuries may occur if the facial nerve runs through the tympanic cavity, a very rare curiosity described by Plester. Here, too, the surgeon might damage it, feeling quite certain that it could not possibly be the facial nerve.

Iatrogenic lesions of the facial nerve may, medicolegally, be of two different kinds. They will have to be precisely defined and differentiated between the surgeon's "causing" nerve damage and "being guilty" of causing it. Paralysis of the facial nerve may be *caused* when it is deliberately produced by the surgeon, e.g., during resection of a parotid tumor or of an acoustic neurinoma. A surgeon will be *guilty* of damaging the facial nerve, however, when this could have been avoided by a more careful technique. Moreover, this usually happens at typical sites.

This brings me to the final point of my discussion: the occasional misjudgment of iatrogenic lesions of the facial nerve at typical sites. The consensus of opinion of those with experience in this field is that surgical lesions of the facial nerve have a very poor prognosis if left alone.

Fortunately, this prognosis can be reversed by reconstructive surgery, because these lesions at typical sites are easily accessible by virtue of the preceding operation that caused them.

Despite the fact that the surgeon has at his disposal a wide variety of alternative decisions on what may be the appropriate indication in any particular case, e.g., in facial palsy due to herpetic infection or the much-discussed Bell's palsy, this is not so in iatrogenic lesions.

This author agrees with Jongkees' belief that the many relevant aspects of the individual patient exert the most decisive influence on our attitude toward an indication for reconstructive operation. An elderly man who may feel no need to be too concerned about his facial appearance will present a problem entirely different from that of a beautiful woman.

The catastrophic consequences of an iatrogenic lesion, however, provide a challenge to the surgeon of quite a different kind.

As Jongkees so rightly emphasizes, "the sun must not be allowed to set before reoperation is undertaken." Surgery will have to be carried out immediately. The chance of converting a poor prognosis into a good one must always be impressed in the surgeon's mind. The necessary prerequisites are, of course, the recognition of the mishap and a critical assessment of what might actually have happened. At times, this is not as easy as it sounds.

As we all know, there are cases in which paralysis develops only after a certain time-interval has elapsed. In such cases, the lesion is referred to as a *postoperative* paralysis, as opposed to the *intraoperative* types of lesion we have been discussing so far. In postoperative paralysis, the nerve has not been severed and has not been handled too roughly. Nerve function is probably blocked temporarily by a hematoma or edema. Usually, but not always, lesions of this kind will recover spontaneously. At times it may be difficult to distinguish between an intra- and a postoperative lesion.

Two kinds of error may confuse the issue: First, a surgeon is only human. Subconsciously he may tend to refuse to realize that he has made a mistake and has injured the facial nerve. This is understandable, but this self-deception often leads to the assumption that, before paralysis actually manifested itself, there was a "free interval." This, of course, would suggest a "postoperative paralysis," with its more favorable prognosis. Second, even in the case of a complete intraoperative paralysis, the upper eyelid will always be closed to some degree during sleep and especially during anesthesia. This, however, is due to relaxation of the superior levator palpebrae muscle, which is innervated by the oculomotor, not the facial, nerve. Therefore, the statement of the nurse in the recovery room — that the eyelid was closed normally immediately after the operation — should always be taken with a grain of salt.

Function tests of the facial nerve, conducted immediately after surgery or after the patient has regained consciousness, are therefore of great value. When in doubt, it is always better to assume the worst, i.e., to act as if there is a serious surgically produced paralysis. Immediate surgical exploration cannot do any additional harm, but it can certainly help to clear up any doubts. There is nothing worse than a "wait-and-see attitude" while "hoping for the best." In reality, this can only make matters worse.

We know that early reoperation is often followed by restoration of function and complete success. If the chance of immediate reoperation is missed, one should at the very least decide to carry out the surgical reconstruction within the first two to three weeks after the first operation in order not to rob the patient of the great advantages of *early* reoperation. This, no doubt exceptionally difficult, situation requires that the otosurgeon should carefully weigh every aspect with special care. His decision to reoperate at once or at least very early will make all the difference between his having "caused" the nerve injury and being "guilty" of overlooking, misinterpreting or neglecting it.

Legal liability will only apply if, having "caused" the nerve injury, he exposes himself to the charge of being "guilty" of not recognizing and immediately repairing it.

The otosurgeon might be guilty of damaging the facial nerve on the ground of ignorance or of incompetence. Ignorance hardly applies, since his professional training has taught him that in operating on certain parts of the ear he will have to work close to the facial nerve. Incompetence may be a matter of lack of technical skill. Even the most skillful otologist may, on occasion, cause a lesion to the facial nerve. A professional blunder would have as little to do with this as, for instance, it would with postoperative paralysis of the recurrent laryngeal nerve following a thyroid operation. The most experienced goiter surgeon may "cause" this misfortune.

In this context, a decision of the German Supreme Court (1912) is important and may have a bearing on future decisions in the courts in the U.S.A. "We can assume that even the most skillful physician does not act with the certainty of a machine. In spite of all his qualifications and care, a 'grip,' an incision or a prick might not 'come off' which never before has failed this same surgeon." In such cases, nobody would be entitled to talk of incompetence.

We have to remember the occasional existence of anomalies, that reoperations have to be carried out in conditions that are difficult to predict or survey and that following fractures of the skull the topography of the tympanic cavity does not correspond to the normal state. All this does not mean that real negligence would be condoned.

Therefore, in coming to the end, the author wants to point out once more the criteria that in his opinion characterize a conduct as extremely careless and inexcusable:

If matters are hushed up;

If one lets things slide;

If the only chance of restoration is disregarded: exploration and rehabilitation at the proper time.

It is indeed true, as John Conley once so aptly put it: "Your surgeon can be your fate."

## Bibliography

Altmann, F.: Missbildungen des Ohres. *In* Handbuch der HNO-Heilkunde III/1, Stuttgart, Thieme, 1965.

Denecke, H. J.: On the surgery of ear abnormalities with reference to the facial nerve. Z. Laryngol. Rhinol. Otol., *39*:425–428, 1960.

Dietzel, K.: Arch. Ohr.-Nas.-Kehlk. Heilk., *185*:845, 1965.

Dietzel, K.: HNO, 7:209, 1966.

von Eicken, C., and Schulz van Treeck, A.: Atlas der Hals-Nasen-Ohren-Krankheiten. Stuttgart, Thieme, 1951.

Fabian, G.: Stapesoperationen. *In* Oeken, F. W., and Kessler, L. (eds.): Fehler und Gefahren bei Routineeingriffen im HNO-Fachgebiet. Leipzig, Thieme, 1978.

Fisch, U.: Transtemporal surgery of the internal auditory canal. Report of 92 cases, technique, indications and results. Advances Otorhinolaryngol., *17*:203–240, 1970.

Gerlach, H.: Die hintere Gehörgangswand bei der Tympanoplastik. Z. Laryngol. Rhinol. Otol., *48*:214–218, 1969.

Günther: quoted from Marx, H.

Herrmann, A.: Gefahren bei Operationen an Hals, Ohr und Gesicht und die Korrekturen fehlerhafter Eingriffe. Heidelberg, Springer, 1968.

Hinsberg, G.: Zentralblatt Ohrenheilkunde, *4*:488, 1966.

House, H. P.: Management of congenital ear atresia. Laryngoscope, *63*:916–946, 1953.

House W.: Surgical exposure of the internal auditory canal and its contents through the middle, cranial fossa. Laryngoscope, *71*:1363–1385, 1961.

House, W.: Middle cranial fossa approach to the petrous pyramid. Report of 50 cases. Arch. Otolaryngol. (Chicago), *78*:460–469, 1963.

Jakobi, H.: Tympanoplastische Eingriffe als Behandlung chronischer Mittelohreiterungen. *In* Oeken, F. W., and Kessler, L. (eds.): Fehler und Gefahren bei Routineeingriffen im HNO-Fachgebiet. Liepzig, Thieme, 1978.

Jansen, C.: HNO, *11*:90, 1963.

Jongkees, L. B.: Les opérations plastiques du nerf facial dans le cas de traumatisme endotemporal, Acta Oto-rhino-laryng. Belg., *10*:36–44, 1956.

Jongkees, L. B. W.: Deutsche Med. Wochenschr., *83*:865, 1958.

Jongkees, L. B.: On intratemporal facial paralyses and their surgical treatment. Z. Laryngol. Rhinol. Otol., *40*:319–336, 1961.

Körner, O.: Z. Ohrenheilk., *22*:182, 1892.

Lüscher, E.: Kurze Klinik der Ohren-Nasen- und Halskrank-heiten. Basel, Schwabe, 1948.

Marquet, J. F.: Homoiotransplantationen von Trommelfell und Gehorknöchelchenkette. HNO, *25*: 157–163, 1977.

Marx, H.: Kurzes Handbuch der Ohrenheilkunde. Jena, Fischer, 1947.

Miehlke, A.: Tierexperimentelle Untersuchungen über die Ursache und den Ort der Auslösung des peripheren Lagenystagmus. Arch. Ohren- Nasen- u. Kehlkopfh., *166*:327–349, 1955.

Miehlke, A.: Surgery of the facial nerve, 2nd ed. München, Urban and Schwarzenberg; Philadelphia, W. B. Saunders, 1973.

Miehlke, A.: Etiology and varieties of congenital malformations involving the ear. *In* Shambaugh, G. E., Jr., and Shea, J. J. (eds.): Proceedings of the Shambaugh Vth International Workshop on Middle Ear Surgery and Fluctuant Hearing Loss. Chicago, Northwestern University Medical School, 1976.

Miehlke, A., and Bushe, K. A.: Chir. Plast. Reconstr., *3*:37, 1967.

Plester, D.: personal communication.

Pöllmann, L.: Monatsschr. Ohrenheilk., *71*:1068, 1937.

Rankow, R. M., and Hanford, J. M.: Congenital anomalies of first branchial cleft. Surg. Gynecol. Obstet., *96*:102–106, 1953.

Ruedi, L.: Surgical treatment of atresia auris congenita; clinical and histological report. Laryngoscope, *64*:666–684, 1954.

Schuknecht, H. F.: Gelfoam as an implant in oval window following stapedectomy. Ann. Otol. Rhinol. Laryngol., *80*:415–418, 1971.

Shambaugh, G. E., Jr., and Derlacki, E. L.: Primary skin grafting of fenestra and fenestration cavity; early and late results. A.M.A. Arch. Otolaryngol., *64*:46–49, 1956.

Shambaugh, G. E., Jr.: Surgery of the Ear. Philadelphia, W. B. Saunders, 1967.

Shea, J. J., Jr.: The management of repeat stapes operations. Laryngoscope, *78*:808–812, 1968.

Shea, J. J., Jr.: Arch. Otolaryng., *89*:431, 1969.

Sheehy, J. L.: Radikaloperation mit Tympanoplastik (die Technik mit Erhaltung des ausseren Gehorganges). HNO, *19*:97–111, 1971.

Sheehy, J. L., and Crabtree, J. A.: Tympanoplasty: staging the operation. Laryngoscope, *83*:1594–1621, 1973.

Ungerecht, K.: HNO, *10*:14, 1962.

Vogel, K.: HNO-Wegweiser, *2*:309, 1950–1951.

Vogel, K.: Arch. Ohr.-Nas.-Kehlk. Heilk. u. Z. HNO-Heilk., *157*:89, 1951.

Wullstein, H. L.: Die Eingriffe zur Gehörverbesserung. *In* Uffenorde, W. (ed.): Anzeige und Ausführung der Eingriffe an Ohr, Nase und Hals. Stuttgart, Thieme, 1952.

Wullstein, H. L.: Die Tympanoplastik als gehörverbessernde Operation bei Otitis media chronica und ihre Resultate. *In* Proceedings of the Vth International Congress on Oto-Rhino-Laryngology, Amsterdam, 1953.

Wullstein, H. L.: Operationen zur Verbesserung des Gehörs. Stuttgart, Thieme, 1968.

Wullstein, S. R.: Die osteoplastische Epitympanotomie und die Pathologie des Mittelohres. I. Das operative Vogehen. Z. Laryngol. Rhinol. Otol., *52*:34–44, 1973.

Wullstein, S. R.: Osteoplastic epitympanotomy. Ann. Otol. Rhinol. Laryngol., *83*:663–669, 1974.

Wullstein, S. R.: Z. Laryng. Rhinol., *54*:32, 1975.

# 12 COMPLICATIONS OF SURGERY OF THE NASAL CAVITY, SINUSES AND PHARYNX

*Joseph L. Goldman*
*Stanley M. Blaugrund*

Complications involving surgery of the nasal cavity, sinuses and pharynx are inevitable. A large segment of complications are avoidable, however, and one should be particularly concerned with these complications. Many factors, operating alone or together, may lead to complications. It is especially true in this field, where small errors may lead to serious complications because of the confined area of manipulation. Errors in complete knowledge of the anatomy or in full comprehension of physiopathology or inadequate instrumentation or light, alone or in conjunction, may be the origin of complications. As will be indicated, however, the method of performing a procedure may also contribute to complications. It should be appreciated that many complications involving surgery of the nasal cavity, sinuses and pharynx are avoidable with technical precision, and the effort to accomplish surgical precision should be ever-present.

## EPISTAXIS

Epistaxis can be a simple or troublesome problem. Usually this depends on whether the source of bleeding is situated anteriorly or posteriorly. Here is an instance in which the knowledge of the source of blood supply is helpful to the management of severe bleeding.

Terminal branches of both the internal and external carotid arteries contribute to the blood supply of the nose. The anterior and posterior ethmoidal arteries are terminal branches of the internal carotid artery by way of the ophthalmic artery that transverses the orbit. *The anterior ethmoidal artery* is usually the larger of the two and is distributed to the anterior third of both the lateral and mesial area of the nasal cavity. *The posterior ethmoidal artery* supplies a confined area in the region of the superior concha and a corresponding portion of the adjacent nasal septum.

The *sphenopalatine artery* passes into the nose via the sphenopalatine foramen, which is a branch of the internal maxillary artery. The various branches of the sphenopalatine artery supply a major portion of the posterior nasal cavity. A limited portion of the lower posterior area of the nasal cavity is supplied by terminal branches of the descending palatine artery, also a branch of the sphenopalatine.

Major vessels supplying the nasal septum include (1) the superior labial branch of the external maxillary, (2) the greater palatine artery, (3) the nasopalatine branch of the sphenopalatine artery and (4) the anterior ethmoidal artery. These vessels are situated within the mucosa and form abundant anastomoses in the caudal septum known as Kiesselbach's or Little's area.

It is usually the nasopalatine artery, a branch of the sphenopalatine artery, that is responsible for severe posterior epistaxis. It should be remembered that the sphenopalatine artery from each side has a communicating branch, sometimes a fairly large one. In attacking the problem of severe epistaxis, it may be necessary to deal with one or more arteries, depending on the success, while always remembering the interrelationships.

The most common source of bleeding is in the well-known Kiesselbach's area, and these vessels may come from several sources, as mentioned previously. After application of topical anesthesia, 4 percent xylocaine or 10 percent cocaine hydrochloride, cauterization with 50 per cent trichloracetic acid or silver nitrate stick will usually control the bleeding. It is advisable to follow with an application of alcohol to counteract the continued and undesirable effect of trichloracetic acid or silver nitrate. Occasionally, the bleeding is profuse, owing to a large vessel or a small hemangioma. In such instances, electrocoagulation is required after a local injection of 1 per cent xylocaine. Care must be taken not to injure the perichondrium or cartilage.

Repeated cauterization with trichloracetic acid or other chemicals or by electrocoagulation can result in septal perforation. Such perforations as a rule can be closed by using a posterior flap of mucoperichondrium and mucoperiosteum. The senior author prefers to bring the flap, properly measured, through the perforation and attach it to the mucoperichondrium of the other side. The most peripheral layer of mucous membrane should be removed. This can be accomplished with an instrument to denude the mucous membrane. The same approach is directed superiorly and inferiorly to the perforation. A large flap can be brought forward on the same side but must be long enough, and the perforation small enough, to permit torsion of the flap posteriorly. The procedures can be carried out with topical and local anesthesia. Again, we prefer 1 or 2 per cent lidocaine (Xylocaine), depending on the amount, and topical 10 per cent cocaine hydrochloride. An intraoral labial pedicle flap may be brought up into the nose by way of a partial lateral rhinotomy incision and used for this purpose.

Severe posterior epistaxis may be a source of anxiety for the patient and may require considerable ingenuity on the part of the surgeon. The senior author, after years of experience in controlling many instances of severe epistaxis, may be overcritical in making the statement that our younger surgeons are resorting to the ligation of the internal maxillary artery by way of the pterygopalatine approach too quickly.

The care of severe posterior epistaxis should not be continued under casual conditions if the bleeding cannot be controlled. Such a patient should be taken to an operating room and be thoroughly anesthetized topically; a Good light should be used under the same operating room conditions used for intranasal surgery. Under such a controlled situation, the bleeding area usually can be seen, cauterized or packed with a nasopharyngeal plug tightly secured high in the nasopharynx.

The presence of anterior and posterior nasal packing sufficient to arrest a massive hemorrhage can and often does produce secondary problems that could be termed complications in themselves. These include totally obstructed nasal breathing resulting in varying degrees of respiratory insufficiency. Dryness and encrustation of the mouth, headache, epiphora, disturbed eustachian tube function with occasional otitis media and sinusitis may also develop. After packing sequelae occasionally include nasal synechiae and pressure ulcerations of the nasal vestibule and upper lip. These complications can be minimized by the manner in which the packing is secured in the nose. The hazards of repeated blood transfusions when packing fails to stop the bleeding are obvious. We are aware of the reported fatalities using this method but have never seen one, and one inevitably questions the techniques used if fatalities do occur.

The patient should be managed in the semisitting position for a minimum of 36 hours and in an intensive care facility for this period of time if one is available. Vital signs as well as blood gas determinations are closely monitored while feet and legs are encased in elastic bandages or stockings. Pain medications are administered judiciously to avoid respiratory depression. Ice packs are helpful in reducing pain and swelling of the nose and face. The patient is maintained on a soft diet, and laxatives are given to prevent constipation. Antibiotics are administered routinely, and blood is replenished if necessary. Complete medical survey is performed to rule out underlying bleeding diathesis. These patients should be closely watched.

In our opinion, ligation of the internal maxillary artery should be a rare procedure but should be done when judgment warrants such surgery. Competence, experience and specialized instrumentation are essential for this procedure, however. A torn internal maxillary artery can be the source of still more serious hemorrhage. One should not forget that the external carotid artery is a vessel easily available and that on unusual occasions both internal maxillary and external carotid arteries need to be ligated because of the communication between both sphenopalatine arteries. On occasion, the ethmoidal arteries must be ligated as well. Attention should be given to these vessels before considering the ligation of the external or even the internal carotid arteries.

## SEPTAL SURGERY COMPLICATIONS

Submucous resection and septoplasty are attended by the possibility of several complications: (1) septal abscess; (2) perforation of septum; and (3) collapse of dorsum of nose. Septal abscess will be discussed later.

Meticulous care during submucous resection and septoplasty should always be used. Approximating tears of the mucoperichondrium, or mucoperiosteum, usually will result in a perforation. If such a situation is recognized at surgery, attempts to repair the tear or tears should be made by suturing. If possible, creating an immediate flap on one side to cover the tear on the other side might be attempted.

Nasal collapse (saddle nose, eventually) results from removal of too much cartilage and bone superiorly, causing lack of adequate dorsal support. This must be gauged with precision and accuracy, leaving at least one-quarter inch of cartilage and bone superiorly. Correction of a saddle nose requires corrective, reconstructive surgery.

## SEPTAL ABSCESS

Septal abscess can follow (1) traumas, which usually involves a laceration of the mucoperichondrium or mucoperiosteum and septal fracture, (2) submucous resection and (3) rhinoplasty. An unexpected high fever, a swollen, red, tender nose and sometimes a septic patient should make the surgeon suspicious of this condition. Examination of the nose will show bulging or a reddish mucoperiochondrium and mucoperiosteum on each side. If any doubt exists about the complication, an aspirating needle will solve the problem. The offending microorganism is usually *Staphylococcus aureus,* although any upper respiratory pathogen can be isolated. A posterior vertical incision should be made after using topical anesthesia and the pus evacuated. A drain never remains in place; instead, the incision should be opened daily until no further pus is obtained. Gentle suction can be helpful. Culture of the pus and appropriate antibiotic therapy are obvious details.

In the days before antibiotics, septal abscesses were responsible for cavernous sinus thrombosis and meningitis. One should remember in this instance, as well as other siutations to be discussed in this text, that old-fashioned complictions can and still do occur in spite of antibiotics.

## SINUS IRRIGATIONS

A good deal of the technical aspects of rhinology is becoming a lost art. This is unfortunate and could be a factor contributing to complications. At this point, we wish to stress the expertise required to irrigate the paranasal sinuses. All the sinuses, with exception of the ethmoidal labyrinth, have natural orifices, and, in our opinion, the ideal approach is irrigation through the natural orifices. The sinus that becomes particularly involved in this consideration is the maxillary sinus. It is fair to say that this sinus is irrigated more frequently by puncture through the nasoantral wall in the inferior meatus, and more recently through the anterior wall of the maxillary sinus.

It is essential that cannulas enter the cavity of the sinuses and not be placed under the mucosa. Freedom of movement of a cannula is a tactile sensation in the fingers that comes from experience. It is assumed that a warm saline solution is used for irrigation. Great care should be taken to remove all air from the irrigating system. Under no circumstances is air used at any time during or after the irrigation. As an aside, it should be understood that irrigation of a sinus may be a diagnostic lavage or a therapeutic irrigation.

From our experience, the maxillary sinus can be entered through the natural orifice in about 90 per cent of attempts, the sphenoid sinus in 75 per cent and the frontal sinus in 50 per cent. Thus, our main concern with complications from this procedure involves the maxillary and sphenoid sinuses in particular.

Obviously, the most serious complication is death, which is completely avoidable under the circumstances to be mentioned. The teaching of years ago, and possibly in some places even now, recommended that the warm saline, which is injected into the maxillary sinus, should be expelled by the injection of air. It is now known that death has followed such a procedure, and air embolism has been found at autopsy. At our institution, the injection of air is forbidden, and it really isn't necessary. Retained saline drains from the sinus after irrigation.

Bleeding rarely is a problem but can on occasion be profuse, particularly following the method of perforating the nasoantral wall in the inferior meatus. The application of adrenalin usually controls the bleeding; rarely is packing required.

One of the hazards in attempting to irrigate the maxillary sinus through the natural orifice lies in the possibility of perforating the lateral wall either too high or too far anteriorly. This results in the solution entering the orbit. This is why the eye should be observed closely during the injection of fluid. If recognized immediately, no serious harm is done. The patient will have proptosis for several days and the saline will be absorbed. A prophylactic antibiotic is recommended. Rarely will intraorbital hemorrhage take place. If it is not too large, the hematoma will also be absorbed without harm to the patient.

If too much saline enters the orbit or too much blood collects and proptosis and lack of movement of the eye are severe enough to damage sight, however, then the aid of an ophthalmologist should be sought to relieve pressure. This can become an urgent procedure when hemorrhage occurs.

Orbital cellulitis resulting from fracture of the lamina papyracea is a very rare complication following irrigation of the maxillary sinus, but this will be discussed in more detail in relation to ethmoidal surgery later.

The thrusting of cannulas into the sinus can produce dangerous consequences. This is one of the main reasons why entering through the natural orifice offers a greater degree of safety. In irrigating the maxillary sinus with a trocar, there have been instances in which the instrument was pushed through the floor of the orbit, through the posterior wall of the maxillary sinus into the pterygopalatine space and even through the lateral wall. Knowledge of the anatomy of these areas suggests all the possible complications that can ensue.

In irrigating the sphenoid and frontal sinuses, care obviously must be exercised. Pushing a cannula through the lateral or posterior wall of the sphenoid sinus can produce a number of serious complications, such as injury to the cavernous sinus, the maxillary and mandibular nerves, the motor nerves to the orbit and, remotely, the optic nerve and the internal carotid artery. Posteriorly, of course, is the hypophysis, and, in some instances, the wall between the sphenoid sinus and hypophysis is comparatively thin.

The frontal sinus orifice can be capricious and does not always open into the infundibulum. Infraction of the middle turbinate at times helps to gain access to the frontal duct. The attempt to force entry medial to the frontal sinus orifice may cause injury to the cribriform plate. The need for care here is emphasized by the fact that such an injury can lead to meningitis. In other words, forcible thrusting or pushing should be avoided. There are times when impossible situations arise with regards to irrigation, and a surgical procedure in the operating room avoids the undesirable complications.

## SINUS SURGERY

The term "sinus surgery" encompasses a wide variety of procedures. This alone implies that sinus surgery can be responsible for a number of complications, some simple, others serious. To understand this fully, one only needs to appreciate the closeness of the sinuses to numerous vital structures. The difficulty of performing desirable surgery in a confined area requires excellent illumination and precision in technique with essential, fine instrumentation.

The operations that can be included under sinus surgery are:

1. Antrostomy
2. Sphenoethmoidectomy and antrostomy
   a. Intranasal approach
   b. External approach
   c. Transantral approach
3. Anterior ethmoidectomy to open nasofrontal duct
4. Frontal sinus surgery
5. Exposure of hypophysis for biopsy (Hypophysectomy will not be considered in this chapter.)
6. Caldwell-Luc operation
7. Pterygopalatine fossa surgery
   a. Ligation of internal maxillary artery
   b. Vidian neurectomy

Accurate and intimate knowledge of the anatomy associated with these operations, as stated before, is essential to avoid or minimize complications. The operator is *always* close to such structures as branches of the internal and external carotid arteries, branches of the V nerve and parasympathetic nerves, the cavernous sinus, the dura, the optic nerve, neural branches of the V nerve to the orbit and the orbit.

### *Antrostomy*

This operation should be confined at most to the anterior two thirds of the nasoantral wall of the inferior meatus. The posterior third contains fairly large branches of the sphenopalatine and descending palatine arteries. If injured, an attempt to control the bleeding should be made by crushing the vessel or by electrocoagulation; packing should be a last resort. In bringing the antrostomy opening forward to the nasal process of the maxilla, one should be on guard not to approach the opening of the nasolacrimal duct superiorly. This is truly an unnecessary complication. The antrostomy should be brought down to the floor of the nose. This will usually avoid the complication of atresia. If the nasoantral wall is brought down to the level of the floor of the nose, atresia occurs very rarely.

### *Sphenoethmoidectomy*

It should be stated at the outset of our discussion that we always accompany this operation with an antrostomy. As already indicated, there are various approaches to accomplish a sphenoethmoidectomy. In all procedures, the landmarks for safety are the same, and violation of these landmarks can lead to serious complications. It seems to us in considering complications in relation to this operation, one should emphasize the avoidance of such complications. This can be accomplished by adhering to the following landmarks, beyond which the operator should not go:

1. The level of the roof of the sphenoid and adjoining large ethmoid cell
2. The lateral wall of the sphenoid, which is continuous with the lateral walls of the ethmoid cells
3. The posterior border of the nasal process of the maxilla
4. The frontal duct, which exists at the point of junction of the posterior border of the nasal process and the roof and lateral wall of the nasal cavity
5. The insertion of the middle turbinate (The operator should never work medial to the insertion of the middle turbinate to avoid injury to the cribriform plate.)
6. The middle meatus

If these boundaries are violated, the complications that follow may occur.

#### ORBITAL CELLULITIS

Cracking the lamina papyracea and exposing orbital fat may lead to orbital cellulitis. Once fat is recognized, it is prudent not to proceed further in this area. Orbital cellulitis is a mild complication and will clear with the passing of time. Antibiotics are advisable.

#### HEMORRHAGE

Severe hemorrhage can originate from three sources: injury to the anterior ethmoidal artery, the posterior ethmoidal artery and the nasopalatine branch of the sphenopalatine artery. For the first two arteries and involved areas, local pressure is advised, or possibly very superficial and localized electrocoagulation. If bleeding into the orbit becomes a problem, then electrocoagulation of these vessels or ligation, if preferred, through an external ethmoidal incision should be undertaken. We wish to emphasize that electrocoagulation in this area should be performed as judiciously as possible in order to avoid optic nerve damage. The nasoplatine artery is located in the mucoperiosteum of the basisphenoid, just below the floor of the sphenoid sinus. The mucoperiosteum should be elevated and reflected away from the basisphenoid. The vessel should then be crushed or electrocoagulated laterally. Occasionally it becomes necessary to resort to packing.

#### MENINGITIS

This is a dreaded complication but need never occur if admonitions previously specified are followed. The cribriform plate should not be injured, which means that the surgeon should not work medial to the insertion of the middle turbinate. Curettes should be avoided, particularly in enlarging the nasofrontal duct. This should be accomplished by punch forceps, usually 45° angle punch forceps. (We always use punch forceps on a universal handle.) Exposure of the dura, especially anteriorly, can eventuate in meningitis. By not going above the level of the roof of the sphenoid and posterior ethmoid cell, such an injury should be avoided. Inept exposure of the anterior face of the hypophysis can result in meningitis.

It should be appreciated that meningitis may eventuate in a brain abscess. The treatment of meningitis in such instances involves opening the traumatized intranasal area widely and treating the meningitis in the classic way, in consultation with a neurologist. It should be borne in mind that there may be an associated bacteremia.

#### OPTIC NERVE INJURY AND BLINDNESS

This can occur if the operator violates the boundaries in the posterior ethmoidal region or lateral wall of the sphenoid. Such damage is usually irreparable.

#### HEMORRHAGE FROM THE CAVERNOUS SINUS

An attempt should be made to pack with one-half inch iodoform packing. Packing should be left in place for from 10 to 14 days. Cavernous sinus thrombosis today is treatable with antibiotics, which cares for the associated bacteremia usually present.

It is very difficult to injure the maxillary and mandibular divisions and the internal carotid artery through the lateral wall of the sphenoid. It can happen with very gross and inexpert manipulations, but we have not heard of these complications.

### *Anterior Ethmoidectomy to Open the Nasofrontal Duct*

This operation should be performed early in acute progressive suppurative frontal sinusitis. Once the duct is opened, pus gushes forth and the problem is under control. Irrigations are instituted later. The need to take a culture and the administration of antibiotics are mentioned in passing.

In our opinion, this type of surgery has more rationale than the trephine procedure. Either technique is acceptable in overcoming the acute process. Early control of the suppuration prevents the complications that were common years ago, namely, osteomyelitis of the frontal bone, meningitis, brain abscess and even cavernous sinus thrombosis.

### *Frontal Sinus Surgery*

This type of surgery still needs to be a part of our armamentarium in sinus surgery. There are instances of uncontrolled infections, osteomas, mucoceles and tumors. Although at times we still approach the sinus by way of the floor of the sinus, we are leaning, more and more, toward the osteoplastic flap. We would like to emphasize the fact that a sphenoethmoidectomy should also be performed in every case of chronic suppurative frontal sinusitis, perhaps as a later procedure.

Again, the complications to be concerned about are osteomyelitis of the frontal bone, meningitis, brain abscess and possible cavernous sinus thrombosis. Antibiotics have changed the entire approach to the occurrence and treatment of these complications. They have become practically nonexistent. Nonetheless, one must be on guard to recognize and treat rare cases.

We might mention that in osteomyelitis of the frontal bone the progression of infection is by way of the venous system. Should this complication occur and become evident on a roentgenogram, all diseased bone should be removed after a reasonable trial with antibiotics.

### *Exposure of the Hypophysis for Biopsy*

Removal of the hypophysis by the nasosphenoidal approach will not be considered in this chapter. This is very specialized surgery and really not in the category of sinus surgery. It is our belief, however, that needle biopsy of tumors of the hypophysis can be executed by the experienced sinus surgeon.

Any approach to the sphenoid sinus can be used. We prefer the intranasal method. A sphenoethmoidectomy is performed on one side and a portion of the nasal septum is removed posteriorly. Then, the intersphenoidal septum is removed. The enlarged tumorous hypophysis can be seen bulging forward. The bone over the enlarged hypophysis is usually very thin and can be removed easily. A biopsy needle can then be easily inserted into the tumor and a specimen obtained.

The patient has the potential for developing the usual complications associated with sphenoethmoidectomy. Bleeding from the hypophysis can usually be controlled by mild pressure or the application of a small adrenalin sponge.

### *Caldwell-Luc Operation*

We reserve this operation for biopsy of tumors and removal of persistent polyps and thickened polypoid membrane after an antrostomy has failed. Otherwise, we rely on the intranasal antrostomy operation, which, incidentally, should be performed in conjunction with the Caldwell-Luc operation. The reason that this operation should not be regarded lightly is that paresthesias of varying degrees can follow the Caldwell-Luc operation. In some patients, this symptom can be very troublesome and is difficult to treat. As a last resort, in some instances, it may be necessary to subject the patient to permanent anesthesia of the maxillary division.

### *Pterygopalatine Fossa Surgery*

The two main procedures that presently are performed in this area after removal of the posterior wall of the maxillary sinus are (1) ligation of the internal maxillary artery for severe epistaxis and (2) vidian neurectomy.

As has been indicated, expertise in working in this area through the operating microscope is essential. The internal maxillary artery is tortuous, and injury to this vessel can produce severe hemorrhage.

Vidian neurectomy also requires considerable competence. A variety of neural complications can ensue that can affect the movement and sight of the eyeball. Any improvement must be spontaneous. The use of cortisone may be helpful.

### *Lateral Rhinotomy*

This is a very useful nasal and sinus operation, usually employed for the removal of tumors both benign and with limited malignancy. The incision begins as a frontoethmoidal incision and extends down in the fold between the nose and cheek and around the lobule of nose. The incision should be carefully made so that ultimate approximation will leave a hairline scar with no distortion. A poor approximation should be considered a complication.

The technique of lateral rhinotomy is not in the province of this discussion, but it should be mentioned that the patient is usually left with a complete sphenoethmoidectomy, a Caldwell-Luc procedure and a complete removal of the nasoantral wall.

All the potential complications mentioned before relating to sphenoidethmoidectomy, antral surgery and septal surgery pertain to this operation. In addition, there may be a need for reconstruction of the nasofrontal duct, should it be removed, by inserting a plastic tube and leaving it in place for eight weeks. This requires firm anchorage. Failure to restore a nasofrontal duct can lead to frontal sinus problems and the need for future obliteration of the frontal sinus. This is an undesirable complication.

### *Maxillectomy*

This operation is performed for malignant disease of the maxillary sinus, which usually extends into the ethmoid cells but can spread in any direction, and is carried out as a planned procedure to encompass all the areas of involvement. When there is evidence of spread beyond the confines of the maxillary antrum, then ablative surgery is carried out with preoperative radiation therapy. If it is reasonably certain that the lesion is well confined to the antrum, surgery may then be the initial modality of therapy followed by irradiation to those areas where further spread is encountered at the time of operation. It is the opinion of the senior author that all cases of squamous cell carcinoma of the maxillary sinus should have preoperative irradiation.

Complications of maxillectomy include (1) infection and necrosis of the flap with development of a cutaneous fistula, (2) sagging of the globe, (3) lower lid edema and ectropion, (4) contracture of the skin of the cheek, (5) loss of visual acuity (when the eye is saved) and (6) cerebrospinal fluid leak.

Necrosis with cutaneous fistulization usually develops at the inner canthus of the eye. It is not frequently encountered, however, and develops most often following preoperative radiation therapy. Under these circumstances, when not limited by tumor encroachment, the flap from this area should be made as thick in subcutaneous tissue as possible and placement of closing sutures should be meticulous.

The development of edema and of ectropion are minimized by inclusion of the orbicularis oculi muscle on the facial flap when possible and by the performance of temporary mesial and lateral tarsorrhaphy prior to making the incision.

Contracture of the skin of the cheek, cerebrospinal fluid leak and sagging of the globe are minimized by completely lining the cavity and cribriform plate areas with split thickness skin.

When attempt is made to save the eye, great care should be taken to avoid damage to the globe through excessive pressure by retractors and other instruments and through attention to appropriate landmarks to avoid damage to the optic nerve. The bony cut, which is made along the frontoethmoidal suture, should not extend beyond the posterior ethmoidal foramen, and the posterior dissection in the pterygomaxillary space should be performed with great care.

## CEREBROSPINAL FLUID LEAK

Cerebrospinal fluid leak may result from trauma associated with an accident or from surgical injury or it may be idiopathic, without causative explanation.

A variety of accidents affecting the head may cause fractures of the floor of the anterior fossa of the brain, including fracture of the cribriform plate with tear of the dura, creating the serious and difficult problem of cerebrospinal fluid leak. The complication may also be a consequence of faulty sinus surgery in the area of the cribriform plate, and reference to this has already been made. Spontaneous cerebrospinal fluid leak may happen without any explainable traumatic experience. We label such a leak as idiopathic, but most likely an underlying structural defect has existed. The dynamics of the spinal fluid, we hypothesize, cause a breakthrough of the unprotected dura.

The detection of cerebrospinal fluid, unless it is profuse and obvious, can be difficult. The fluid, if possible, should be collected in a test tube so that tests for sugar content, specific gravity and protein content can be performed. The presence of sugar is not necessarily diagnostic, since lacrimal secretions also contain glucose. Protein content of cerebrospinal fluid is much less than in nasal discharge. Another important differential point is that nasal secretion will develop sediment while cerebrospinal fluid remains clear.

A more precise method of ascertaining the site of leakage is by the intrathecal injection of either fluorescein or indigo carmine dye. The nose is first decongested. Separate plegets of cotton are then inserted into the sphenoethmoidal recess, the olfactory slit and the anterior superior nasal cavity. With the patient in the sitting position, fluorescein (1 cc. of 5 per cent solution) is injected intrathecally. The cotton plegets in the nasal cavity are then inspected at regular intervals using an ultraviolet light source. This may be repeated after 10 minutes in the recumbent position if no dye is seen initially.

The treatment of these leaks can be carried out by the neurosurgeon, using the intracranial route. Fascia is usually used to close a demonstrated rent of dura.

As rhinologists, we are interested in the new intranasal technique being used to cover the leaking area. This is accomplished by removing the endothelium of the surrounding area and covering the leak site and surrounding area with a pedicle flap obtained from mucous membrane in the nose. Flaps are best procured from the septum high in the region of the olfactory groove. On occasion, it may be necessary to perform this technique by an external approach in order to gain adequate exposure. The septomucosal flap is rotated into the area of leakage and a layer of Gelfoam saturated in antibiotic solution is carefully packed over the graft. A pedicle flap from the lateral nasal wall can also be used. These flaps should be buttressed with antibiotic-impregnated iodoform gauze, which should remain in place for a minimum of one week. These methods have been successful in a growing number of cases. The advantage of this technique over the intracranial approach is obvious.

## TREATMENT OF HYPERPLASTIC VASOMOTOR INFERIOR TURBINATES

The enlarged, hyperplastic, swollen, vasomotor inferior turbinates are responsible for nasal obstruction in a multitude of patients. If these patients cannot be helped by allergenic therapy, we treat them by submucosal electrocoagulation. At the same time, a posterior mulberry tip is removed, if one exists, with a snare, under topical anesthesia. The results are most gratifying. Occasional bleeding can be a complication. If this cannot be controlled by an adrenalin pack, then packing with iodoform gauze for 24 to 48 hours should be instituted. Very rarely, sequestration of bone from the inferior turbinate may form and this can be easily removed *after* it has become detached.

## TONSILLECTOMY AND ADENOIDECTOMY

No operations have been so frequently and strongly criticized, both rightly and wrongly, as have tonsillectomy and adenoidectomy. The fact that tonsillectomy and adenoidectomy are performed more often than any other surgical procedure contributes to both the favorable and abusive attitudes toward the operations. The fact that tonsillectomy and adenoidectomy are performed in many instances by other than well-trained otolaryngologists also contributes to contradictory and unreasonable issues. It is difficult to establish a common, universally acceptable base line for indications for surgery and for treatment of complications.

In our view, which is shared by almost all well-trained otolaryngologists, the issues are clear. We consider tonsillectomy and adenoidectomy as separate entities with regard to the indications for treatment of the diseased processes of these separate lymphoid organs and to the complications of these operations themselves.

Beginning with very young children, adenoiditis of varying degrees and kinds of inflammations may produce acute otitis media or serous (or secretory) otitis media with the usual concomitant conductive hearing impairment. Acute otitis media can be treated by antibiotics alone or myringotomy with antibiotics, according to the otologic judgment. Serous otitis media may be treated by aspiration or myringotomy followed by appropriate nonantibiotic medication and allergenic therapy. Cultures and sensitivity tests are always indicated. Repeated attacks of acute adenoiditis causing repeated episodes of acute otitis media (how many attacks? — enough to warrant helping a sick child become well) are a valid indication for adenoidectomy. In children under the age of two, possibly three, with no evidence of tonsillar disease, the operation is definitely limited to an adenoidectomy.

In children of the same age group with repeated serous otitis media associated with conductive deafness, adenoidectomy with myringotomy and insertion of a plastic tube for middle ear ventilation is indicated. Untreated serous otitis media can lead to retraction of the tympanic membrane in the attic area with possible ultimate formation of cholesteatoma. Adhesive processes may ensue with permanent conductive hearing impariment.

Repeated attacks of tonsillitis with high fever usually associated with adenoiditis raise the question of the need for tonsillectomy. How many attacks? Possibly more than four or five. More important is an evaluation of the health of the child. It still should be remembered that 50 per cent of attacks of acute tonsillitis are caused by $\beta$-hemolytic streptococcus, and it is believed that this microorganism under certain immunologic conditions is responsible for rheumatic fever or rheumatic heart disease.

In our opinion, the adenoids should always be removed with a tonsillectomy. Tonsillectomy and adenoidectomy in patients with cleft palates require special consideration.

The indication for tonsillectomy in adults is the same as is stated for children. In adults, if there is no adenoidal condition, the operation can be performed under local anesthesia, which removes the problem of general anesthesia.

This preliminary discussion has been developed because we appreciate that tonsillectomy and adenoidectomy are far from simple operations. In fact, thorough procedures should be considered difficult operations that require considerable care and precision in technique to avoid especially troublesome complications. It should also be mentioned that the art of medicine, with its associated judgments, should play a role in these diagnostic and therapeutic decisions.

We remove tonsils by the dissection and snare method. The capsule is dissected away from the surrounding tissue, preserving the anterior and posterior pillars. Every effort should be made to avoid tearing the pharyngeal fascia and muscles. In preserving the pillars, the palate is thereby protected, and, of course, the uvula should always be inspected during and after closure of the snare. Removal of the uvula should be avoided.

The adenoids are removed by sharp currettes and punch forceps. The punch forceps are used under direct vision with bright illumination, such as provided by a Good light, with the palate elevated. This technique is used because all the adenoidal tissue can be removed and minimal trauma afflicted on the nasopharyngeal fascia and muscles.

Bleeding or hemorrhage is the most common complication of tonsillectomy and adenoidectomy. Technique plays an important part in avoiding bleeding at the operation or postoperatively. As in all surgery, less trauma to the tissues will cause minimal and controllable bleeding. Clamping of the vessels, ligatures and electrocoagulation efficiently applied should result in a completely dry field. As has already been indicated, all adenoid tissue must be removed, for a piece of remaining adenoid tissues can be a source of continuous bleeding.

In elevating the palate, care must be used for gentle retraction. Strenuous retraction or pulling of the palate or the palatopharyngeal muscles can result in temporary nasality, which usually clears in a month.

It is assumed that all tonsillectomies and adenoidectomies in children are currently performed by intubation general anesthesia. This limits aspiration, which can be controlled by suction through the intratracheal tube by the anesthesiologist. With intubation, respiration can be monitored and also controlled. All children should have continuous intravenous fluid during the procedure plus continuous cardiac monitoring. This kind of care avoids catastrophic situations. Postoperative bleeding can usually be cared for much more effectively in an operating room, where excellent illumination, exposure and suction are available. An obvious bleeding vessel should be clamped, ligated or electrocoagulated. Pressure with pack may be all that is necessary to control the bleeding. The use of adrenalin has been a subject of much discussion because of the possible adverse effects. Packs containing diluted adrenalin with excess adrenalin squeezed out, used cautiously with close observation, can be very effective in controlling bleeding areas, particularly in the nasopharynx.

Dysphagia and pain can be troublesome symptoms postoperatively. Appropriate analgesics and soft foods and fluids will make most children comfortable. Swallowing should be encouraged because activity of the pharyngeal muscles lessens the amount of pain more quickly.

Postoperative injection of suspensions containing corticosteroids should be used with caution because of possible visual disturbances.

Severe injury of the muscles of the nasopharynx and palate can result in atresia of the nasopharynx, a most serious complication. The senior author has had two occasions to repair such postadenotonsillectomy atresia by plastic procedures and the insertion of a plastic nasopharyngeal stent for a matter of six months. Yet, there is no need for such complications. That is why we stress the need for precise adherence to sound principles of surgical technique and competence in the performances of the tonsillectomies and adenoidectomies. These admonitions are not directed toward well-trained otolaryngologists.

### *Complications of Acute Tonsillitis*

Fifty per cent of acute tonsillitis is infected with $\beta$-hemolytic streptococcus. A severe acute tonsillitis can lead to suppurative adenitis, peritonsillar abscess and jugular phlebitis. These complications can occur in spite of the use of antibiotics, the primary method of therapy.

Suppurative adenitis and peritonsillar abscess require incision and drainage. The presence of pus is sometimes misleading owing to the findings, however. When there is question concerning the existence of a collection of pus, an aspirating needle will quickly settle the issue and should be used readily.

Jugular phlebitis presents a more involved problem. In a septic patient, the diagnosis can only be established by proving the existence of a bacteremia. We have seen several cases of jugular phlebitis (including lateral sinus thrombosis) cured by antibiotics. If a bacteremia and septic course persist, however, ligation of the jugular vein must be considered.

## NASOPHARYNGEAL ABSCESS (THORNWALDT'S ABSCESS)

Thornwaldt's disease is most commonly seen in adults. It has been attributed to inflammation of a pharyngeal bursa representing a diverticulum in the midposterior wall of the nasopharynx. The apex of the pouch extends superiorly toward the tubercle of the occipital bone.

Various theories have been advanced concerning the etiological factors, several claiming aberration in embryonic development, since bursae have been found in contact with notochord remnants of embryos. Others postulate an adult type, resulting from proliferation of pharyngeal epithelium.

Since the disease is found more often in adults, the most accepted theory is that Thornwaldt's disease results from retention cysts that develop in the medial cleft of the adenoid. These are very often infected.

The disturbing symptoms are frequently not recognized because the nasopharynx has not been adequately examined. This may require anesthesia of the pharynx (4 per cent lidocaine [Xylocaine] or 10 per cent cocaine). Unexplained fever, adenitis, ear problems and headache may have their origin in a Thornwaldt abscess.

Treatment of Thornwaldt abscess involves not only incision and drainage but also removal of the anterior wall by punch forceps. This can be accomplished under topical anesthesia. Working through the Yankauer nasopharyngeal boot can be very helpful. Cultures should be made from the evacuated secretions and the appropriate antibiotic should be administered. It is interesting how certain ear problems that seem to have the eustachian tube as a factor will clear after the removal of a Thornwaldt abscess. Uncontrollable bleeding is rarely a complication.

## RETROPHARYNGEAL ABSCESS

Retropharyngeal abscesses as a result of suppuration of a retropharyngeal adenitis are rare these days. Antibiotics are most likely responsible for this. The condition can occur and complications can be serious if not disastrous, however. Careful observation must be used to avoid the possibility of spontaneous rupture. This can lead to aspiration and suffocation. Even incision and drainage, or recognition of the entity, must be carefully carried out to avoid these complications. This means that the procedure should be performed without general anesthesia and strong suction should be in readiness to aspirate the evacuated pus.

One must also be on guard against supraglottic edema in cases of descending retropharyngeal abscess.

## ORAL-ANTRAL FISTULA

Oral-antral fistula is a complication that results from extraction of teeth whose roots extend into the maxillary sinus. When these roots are infected, a foul smelling infection of the maxillary sinus develops, usually caused by the *α-Streptococcus viridans.* The foul odor is not due to an anaerobe.

The fistula obviously communicates with the maxillary sinus and the temptation is to irrigate this sinus through the fistula. This should not be done. On occasion, irrigation through the intranasal natural orifice may bring about closure of the fistula. At least the infection will be cleared with the additional use of antibiotics.

If the fistula persists, plastic surgical closure by way of the mouth is required. If the fistula is small, mucoperiosteal flaps on each side of the alveolus are fashioned and these flaps are brought together in a two layer closure. If the fistula is large, closure can be accomplished by rotation of a palatal flap and brought under the buccal mucous membrane. The uncovered and bare palatal bone of the donor site will heal spontaneously in a matter of weeks.

## Bibliography


1. Angell, James, J.: Transethmoidal hypophysectomy. Arch. Otolaryngol., *86*:256, 1967.
2. Bacher, J. A.: Fatal air embolism after puncture of the maxillary antrum. Calif. State J. Med., *21*:443, 1923.
3. Ballenger, J. J.: Disease of the Nose, Throat and Ear. 11th ed. Philadelphia. Lea and Febiger, 1969.
4. Bateman, G. H.: Transsphenoidal hypophysectomy. A review of 70 cases treated in the past two years. Trans. Am. Acad. Ophthalmol. Otolaryngol., *66*:103, 1962.
5. Berkstein, A.: Safeguards in anchoring a posterior nasal packing. Can. J. Otolaryngol., *23*:390–392, 1973.
6. Bernstein, L.: The Caldwell-Luc operation. Otolaryngol. Clin. North Am., *4*:69–77, 1971.
7. Bordley, J. E., and Cherry, J.: The use of the rhinotomy operation in nasal surgery. Case reports. Laryngoscope, *70*:258–270, 1960.
8. Briant, T. D. R.: Transsphenoidal hypophysectomy. Proc. Can. Otolaryngol. Soc., *18*:159, 1964.
9. Chandler, J. R., and Serrins, A. J.: Transantral ligation of the internal maxillary artery for epistaxis. Laryngoscope, *75*:1151–1159, 1965.
10. Conley, J.: Concepts in head and neck surgery. New York, Grune & Stratton, Inc., 1970.
11. Cook, T. A.: Analysis of the alterations of blood gases produced by nasal packing. Laryngoscope, *83*:1802–1809, 1973.
12. Golding-Wood, P. H.: Pathology and surgery of chronic vasomotor rhinitis. J. Laryngol. Otol., *76*:969–977, 1962.
13. Goldman, J. L., and Morgenstein, K. M.: Boundaries and principals of intranasal surgery. Sinus Surgery Course, Page and Wm. Black Post Graduate School of Medicine, Mount Sinai School of Medicine, C.U.N.Y.
14. Hallberg, O. E.: Severe nosebleed and its treatment. J.A.M.A., *148*:355, 1952.
15. Hara, H. J.: Severe epistaxis. Arch. Otolaryngol., *75*:258, 1962.
16. Harpman, J. A.: Management of epistaxis other than from Little's Area. Arch. Otolaryngol., *75*:254, 1962.
17. Hirsch, C.: Ligation of internal maxillary artery in patients with nasal hemorrhage. Arch. Otolaryngol., *24*:589–593, 1936.
18. Jackson, C., and Jackson, C. L.: Diseases of the Nose, Thoat and Ear, 2nd ed. Philadelphia, W. B. Saunders Co., 1959.
19. Juselius, H.: Epistaxis. A clinical study of 1,724 patients. J. Laryngol. Otol., *88*:317–327, 1974.
20. Kirshner, J. A., Yanigasawa, E., and Crelin, F. S., Jr.: Surgical anatomy of the ethmoidal arteries. A laboratory study of 150 orbits. Arch. Otolaryngol., *74*:382—386, 1961.
21. Kuhn, A. J., and Halberg, O. E.: Complications of postnasal packing for epistaxis. Ann. Otol., *62*:62, 1955.
22. Levitt, G. W.: Cervical fascia and deep neck infections. Laryngoscope, *80*:409–433, 1970.
23. Macbeth, R.: Caldwell-Luc operation, 1952–1966. Arch. Otolaryngol., *87*:630–636, 1968.
24. Malcomson, K. G.: The surgical management of massive epistaxis. J. Laryngol., *77*:299–314, 1963.
25. Montgomery, W. W.: Surgery for cerebrospinal fluid rhinorrhea and otorrhea. Arch. Otolaryngol., *84*:538–550, 1966.
26. Montgomery, W. W., Katz, R., and Gamble, J. F.: Anatomy and surgery of the pterygomaxillary fossa. Ann. Otol. Rhinol. Laryngol., *79*:606–618, 1970.

27. Montgomery, W. W.: Surgery of the upper respiratory tract. Philadelphia. Lea and Febiger, 1971, pp. 269–291.
28. Mosher, H. P.: Submaxillary fossa approach to deep pus in the neck. Trans. Am. Acad. Ophthalmol. Otolaryngol., *34*:19–26, 1929.
29. McCoy, G.: Cerebrospinal fluid rhinorrhea: A comprehensive review and definition of the responsibility of the rhinologist in diagnosis and treatment. Laryngoscope, *73*:1125–1157, 1963.
30. McKinney, R.: Traumatic pneumoencephalon. Ann. Otol., *41*:597–600, 1932.
31. Ogura, J. H., Nelson, J. R., and Dammoehler, R., et al.: Experimental observations of the relationships between upper airway obstruction and pulmonary function. Trans. Am. Laryngol. Asso., *85*:40–64, 1964.
32. Ogura, J. H.: Nasal surgery. Physiological considerations of nasal obstruction. Arch. Otolaryngol. (Chicago), *88*:288–295, 1968.
33. Pang, L. Q.: Air embolism during lavage of the maxillary sinuses. A report of two cases. Laryngoscope, *62*:1205–1224, 1952.
34. Pearson, B. W., MacKenzie, R. G., and Goodman, W. S.: The anatomical basis of transantral ligation of the maxillary artery in severe epistaxis. Laryngoscope, *79*:969–984, 1969.
35. Ritter, Frank N.: The paranasal sinuses anatomy and surgical technique. St. Louis, The C. V. Mosby Co., 1973.
36. Ritter, Frank N.: A clinical and anatomic study of the various techniques of irrigation of the maxillary sinus. Laryngoscope, *87*:215–223, 1977.
37. Shaheen, O. H.: Arterial epistaxis J. Laryngol. Otol., *89*:17–34, 1975.
38. Slatin, H. P.: On the late clinical condition after septum hematomas and septum abscesses. Mschr. Ohrenheilk., *102*:641–644, 1968.
39. Tardy, M. E., Jr.: "Practical suggestions on facial plastic surgery — How I do it." Sublabial mucosal flap. Repair of septal perforations. Laryngoscope, *87*:275–278, 1977.
40. Van Alyea, O. E.: Nasal polpys and sinusitis. Ann. Otol., *75*:881–887, 1966.
41. Yankauer, S.: Nasopharyngeal Abscess. A Report of 155 Cases. Trans. Am. Acad. Ophthalmol. Otolaryngol., 1929, p. 364.
42. Yankauer, S.: The complete spheno-ethmoid operation. Transactions of the 27th Annual Meeting of the American Laryngology, Rhinology and Otology Society, 1921, p. 115.

# COMPLICATIONS OF CLEFT LIP AND CLEFT PALATE SURGERY

13

*Leslie Bernstein*

In general, complications arising from cleft lip and cleft palate surgery are not very common. As with any form of surgery, some of these complications may occur during the operative period or shortly therafter. Of far greater importance, however, are the long-term complications that result from improper planning or timing of the various operative procedures that may be employed for the complete rehabilitation of these patients. Because these cleft deformities affect the appearance of the patient as well as certain of his social functions, long-term surgical complications may be categorized as both aesthetic and functional.

## EARLY COMPLICATIONS OF CLEFT LIP SURGERY

### *Unilateral Clefts*

The only possible functional complication following repair of a unilateral cleft lip is breakdown of the suture line. This happens very rarely, indeed, and is usually associated with some postoperative trauma, such as may result from sucking on a finger or a nipple, from an impact with a solid object or when the infant may have been allowed to lie prone. Of course, it is conceivable that wound dehiscence may occur as a result of systemic causes; however, this is quite a remote possibility in view of the widely accepted tenet that this elective procedure be done when the child is at least 10 weeks of age, weighs at least 10 pounds, has over 10 gm. of hemoglobin and is in apparent good health.

Should dehiscence of the repair line occur, it is prudent to allow the wound to heal by secondary intention. After ascertaining the cause of the complication and taking the necessary steps to preclude its recurrence, the revision of the procedure should not be undertaken for at least three months. If a reasonably broad band of residual scar tissue survives to hold the lip segments together, albeit in an unsightly fashion, it may be prudent to leave the lip for a longer period and do a well-planned revision at an older age. The overall results of such an approach are far more satisfactory, since in the interim the orbicularis oris muscle sling will have been functioning and the larger size of the tissues in the older child permits easier reconstruction.

Cosmetic complications of unilateral cleft lip operations depend on the choice of the particular surgical procedure, the skill and artistry of the surgeon and the postoperative care rendered. An additional basic consideration is the extent of the cleft and whether or not it is associated with an underlying cleft of the alveolar process. The accepted principle is that, all other things being equal, the more extensive the cleft, the more difficult it is to achieve a good cosmetic result.

Specifically, cosmetic complications of the lip may consist of a readily apparent scar, a vertically foreshortened lip, absence of a symmetric Cupid's bow, improperly aligned segments, a notch in the vermilion (the so-called whistling deformity) and unequal substance to the vermilion on each side of the repair line.

To a certain extent, these deformities may be precluded. To avoid tension along the

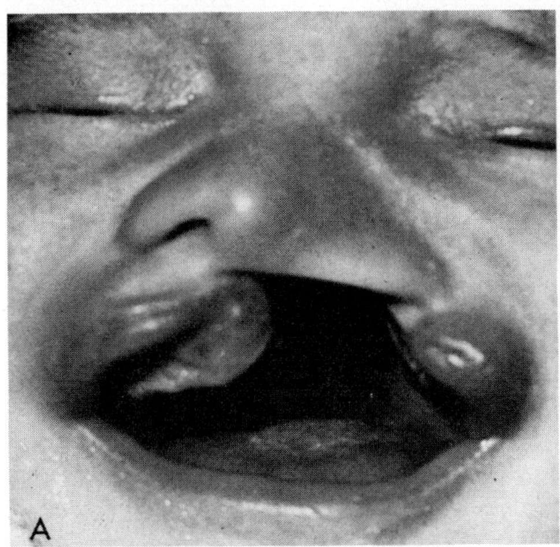


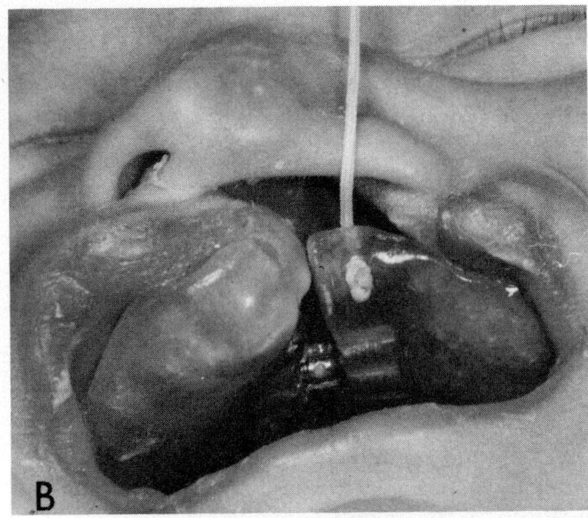


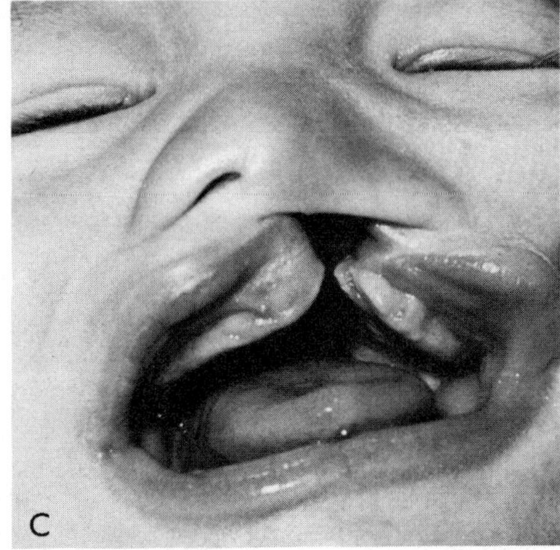


**Figure 13–1** Maxillary orthopedics. *A*, pretreatment condition; *B*, appliance in place — string is for securing to cheek; *C*, condition two weeks later.

suture line in widely divergent lip segments with an underlying complete cleft of the palate, preoperative maxillary orthopedics may be instituted by means of a removable dental appliance in order to narrow the palatal cleft and, concurrently, bring the lip segments closer together (Fig. 13–1). Additional lip length may be gained by choosing a suitable surgical procedure for this purpose, such as one of those described by Millard,[5] Randall,[6] Skogg[8] or Bernstein.[3] These procedures are also designed to obtain a symmetric Cupid's bow.

### *Bilateral Clefts*

Postoperative wound dehiscence is more likely to occur in complete bilateral clefts of the lip when repair is attempted with a tight surgical closure in the presence of a protrusive premaxilla. To preclude this from happening, it is mandatory to institute preoperative maxillary orthopedics in order to line up the palatal segments into a more favorable position and to bring the lip segments closer together or to repair the clefts in two operations, or both.

An uncommon complication of the Schultz[7] operation is the postoperative downward displacement of the premaxillary segment (Fig. 13–2). This tends to occur when the protruding premaxilla is tilted somewhat upward. The inclination causes the repaired lip to slide into the angle formed between the nose and the premaxilla. In response to the vector of the muscle pull, the premaxillary segment becomes

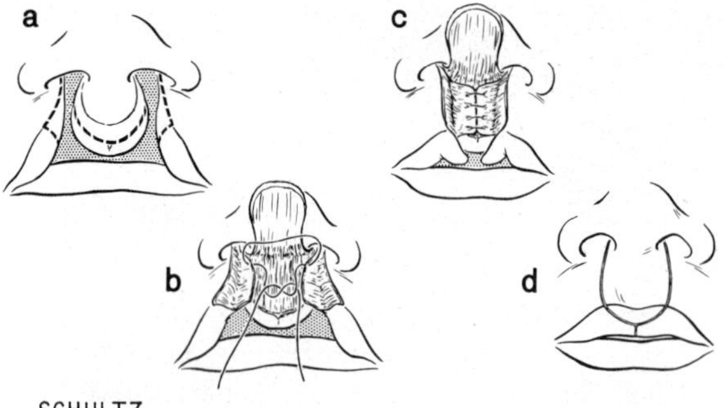


**Figure 13–2** The Schultz operation.

gradually displaced downward and backward. Eventually, it will require surgical reduction (Fig. 13–3).

The correct management of the protrusive premaxilla, which has become trapped in its forward location after the cleft palate has been repaired, may pose a considerable problem. In certain instances, correction may be amenable to orthodontic treatment, possibly with subsequent bone grafting to stabilize the segments. In other cases, the offending premaxilla may require surgical recession or resection. A word of caution is in order, however, against performing this

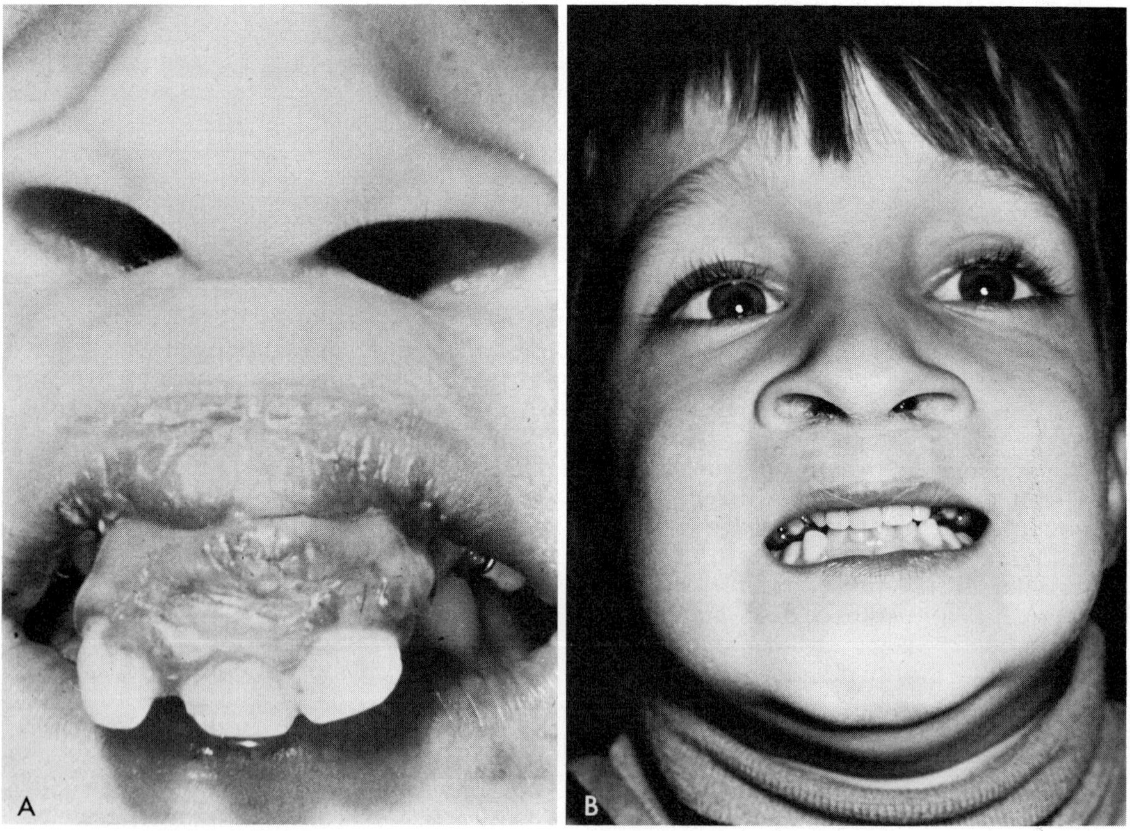

**Figure 13–3** *A,* Downward displaced protrusive premaxilla resulting from Schultz procedure. *B,* After resection and fitting with appliance.

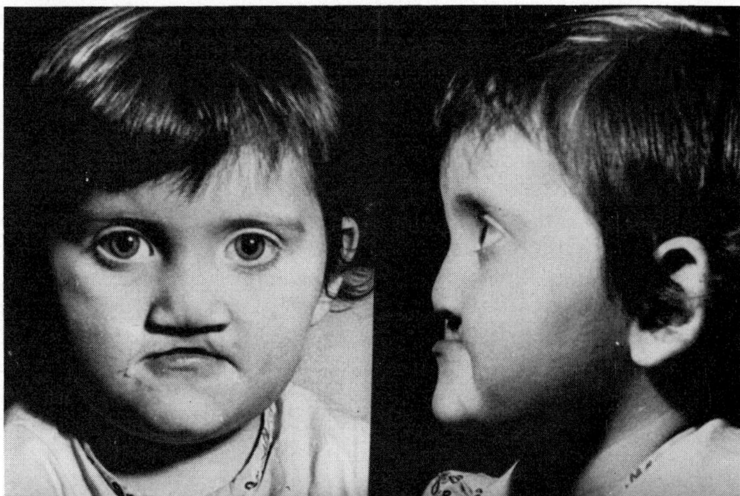

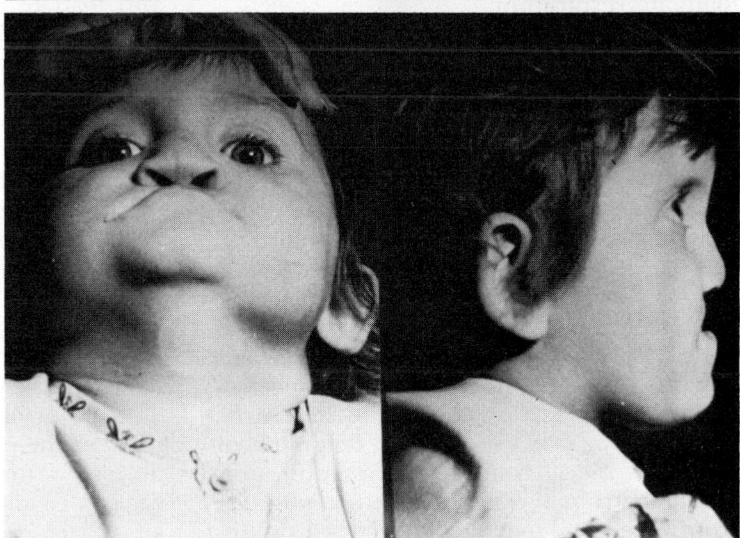

**Figure 13–4** Effect of resecting the premaxilla in infancy. Note underdevelopment of middle third of face at age of three. Condition progressed with age.

surgery before the age of four years to avoid traumatizing the area lest it interfere with subsequent growth of the face (Fig. 13–4).

The overall cosmetic complications of bilateral cleft lip surgery are similar to those of a unilateral defect. Ironically, however, because the defect of the bilateral cleft lip is usually fairly symmetric, the deformities are not as readily noticed by the lay public.

## EARLY COMPLICATIONS OF CLEFT PALATE SURGERY

Certain patients with a cleft of the secondary palate, especially those with Down's syndrome or even with the so-called Pierre Robin syndrome, may sustain airway difficulties immediately after the palatal repair. The reason for this is that, in spite of their proportionately big tongue, these patients have been enjoying relatively easy respiration by augmenting their breathing through the cleft. Moreover, in many of these clefts, the palatal processses are inclined at a rather steep vertical angle, affording more accommodation for the tongue. Immediately after the repair, the mucoperiosteal flaps are located at a lower level in the midline, so that there is less room for the tongue. If one adds edema to the tongue that may have resulted from a tightly fitting gag, the result may be quite alarming — especially in the immediate postoperative recovery period.

Prophylaxis of this complication is not feasible, except to delay the age of the operation, especially in those with Down's syndrome. If the airway is compromised during recovery from the anesthetic, administration of cortisone may improve matters by reducing any edema. Otherwise, it is prudent to keep the mouth wide open by separating the teeth until the child recovers. The tongue may have to be kept forward by a suture through its tip. An oropharyngeal airway is contraindicated, lest it tear the flaps apart; however, bilaterally placed nasopharyngeal tubes may help ease the problem. Once full consciousness has been reached, the patient quickly learns to keep the tongue away from the palate in order to maintain respiration.

More commonly, the sequelae of repair of palatal clefts may include immediate postoperative hemorrhage. Later, breakdown of the suture line or necrosis of tissue may follow, leading to fistula formation or to reconstitution of at least some part of the cleft.

Hemorrhage is a rather rare complication in cleft palate surgery and is seldom of serious consequence. Worrisome intraoperative bleeding may occur from a severed greater palatine artery. If the vessel retracts into its palatine canal, it may be electrocoagulated or the canal may be stoppered with bone wax or with a small fragment of bone or wood from a cotton applicator. Bleeding from the lateral wound edges or from bare bone may at times be a little disturbing; however, this is usually easily controlled with electrocautery, by inserting Gelfoam into the lateral relief incisions and by holding down the flaps against the bone for several minutes with a moist gauze pack.

Palatal or nasal hemorrhage around the 5th to 10th postoperative day may herald wound breakdown. Since this is usually associated with infection, it may at times be of help, at this late stage, to give the child an appropriate antibiotic.

Breakdown of the repair line in palatoplasty may also be precluded by giving the patient a liquid diet for three to four weeks after surgery in order to avoid undue strain on the suture line. Feedings should be given by cup only. The child's arms should be restrained for the same period to prevent him from inserting harmful objects into his mouth.

Necrosis following palatoplasty is most likely due to traumatic handling of the tissues during the operation. Anyone performing this surgery should know that the mucoperiosteum on the oral surface of the palate is fairly brittle and tends to tear if manipulated too roughly. Therefore, the elevation must be done very carefully and patiently, and it must proceed under the innermost layer of the mucoperiosteum. The rough surface of the underlying bone of the palate may make this chore somewhat difficult.

It should be remembered that the palatal mucoperiosteum is thinnest in its posterior part, along the medial edge. Consequently, tight sutures will tend to cut into this tissue and lead to tears. Therefore, especially in wide clefts, forceful manipulation must be avoided, and the flaps should be approximated with a minimal amount of tension. If the flaps do not come together readily, the cause of the restraint should be determined and corrected. Common restraints may be located at one or both greater palatine neurovascular bundles, at the attachment of the velum to the bony palate or along the relief incision lateral to the soft palate.

Another etiologic factor that may lead to eventual necrosis is poor design of the flaps in a complete bilateral cleft of the palate. The major blood supply to the mucoperiosteum of the palatine process of the maxilla is derived from the greater palatine artery. Exiting from the greater palatine canal, this vessel runs forward toward the cleavage between the palatine process of the maxilla and the premaxilla, where it anastomoses with terminal capillaries of the lateral nasal branch of the sphenopalatine artery and of the infraorbital artery. Capillaries from the greater palatine artery also anastomose at the gingivae with capillaries of the buccal surface of the maxilla. This anastomosis is always severed when making the lateral relief incisions.

Accordingly, both the anterior and the posterior flaps of a four-flap palatoplasty may be at risk. When the posteriorly based flaps are made too long, especially if the neurovascular bundles have been cut, there is risk of postoperative necrosis of the tip of the flaps. In a wide bilateral cleft, if the anteriorly based flaps are cut too short, they cannot be rotated sufficiently medially to cover the defect. Consequently, the anterior part of the cleft may remain unrepaired. On the other hand, if these two flaps are forced together, the risk of necrosis is increased.

In order to preclude these complications, it is suggested that (1) maxillary orthopedics be instituted early in order to approximate the divergent segments; (2) the lateral relief incisions be placed at the necks of the teeth so that the flaps may be as wide as possible; (3) the neurovascular bundle be preserved whenever possible; (4) each bipedicled mucoperiosteal flap be divided along a line from the cuspid tooth to the medial point at the back of the hard palate, which gives each flap satisfactory length; and (5) the mucoperiosteum be dissected very carefully from its bony attachment, that it be handled with the least amount of trauma and that tight suturing be avoided.

Another site of tissue breakdown is at the junction of the mucoperiosteum with the velum in the midline. This point lies more or less midway between the insertion of the neurovascular bundles into the mucoperiosteum. Hence, it is at risk of tight suturing when the neurovascular bundles restrain medial approximation of the flaps. Occasionally, the fault may be an insufficient relief incision lateral to the soft palate.

A tight closure in this area may be overcome by freeing up the neurovascular bundle and by making certain that the lateral relief incisions have served their purpose. Infraction of the hamular process of the medial pterygoid plate may provide additional relief. Further strain may be taken off the repair line by supporting it with one or two vertical mattress sutures placed 5 to 10 mm. lateral to the midline.

## LONG-TERM SEQUELAE OF CLEFT LIP AND CLEFT PALATE SURGERY

The long-term complications of cleft lip and cleft palate operations also may be divided into functional and cosmetic entities.

### Functional Sequelae

The functional problems are primarily connected with speech or, more specifically, with nasal escape during speech. This is associated either with velopharyngeal incompetence or with fistulas that communicate the oral with the nasal cavities. Of lesser consequence is the crossbite malocclusion that may result from collapsed palatal segments.

A not uncommon cosmetic complication may be related to actual or latent velopharyngeal incompetence. This is manifested by facial grimacing during speech, especially about the base of the nose. It is actually an unconscious effort to reduce nasal escape.

#### *Velopharyngeal Incompetence*

Velopharyngeal incompetence following palatoplasty has been variously reported in 20 per cent to 40 per cent of cases.[2] Naturally, the degree of incompetence varies from almost acceptable speech at one extreme to marked rhinolalia aperta at the other. The incidence of velopharyngeal incompetence is somewhat lessened when a pushback technique is employed in the original repair.

Borderline cases may be helped by speech training in many instances, or they may benefit from the injection of Teflon paste into the posterior pharyngeal wall. Some may be treated successfully by a pushback procedure. Severe cases can only be helped by a pharyngeal flap and, under certain rare circumstances, by a pharyngeal obturator.

It should be mentioned that the pharyngeal flap operation also carries a certain operative risk. One immediate complication is bleeding, either from the donor site in the pharyngeal wall or from the raw surface of the flap or even the recipient pocket in the palate. A delayed complication may be stenosis of the lateral airway portals. This not only interferes with nasal respiration but also may give a denasal quality to the subject's speech. At the other extreme is the infrequent possibility that the flap had been poorly constructed or that there was postoperative breakdown, resulting in inadequate correction of the rhinolalia aperta.

An oronasal fistula may allow for nasal escape of speech as well as for nasal ingress of ingested food. Figure 13–5 shows a method of closing such a fistula that utilizes two flaps so as to line both the oral and the nasal surfaces. These fistulas may be closed at any time recommended by the speech therapist.

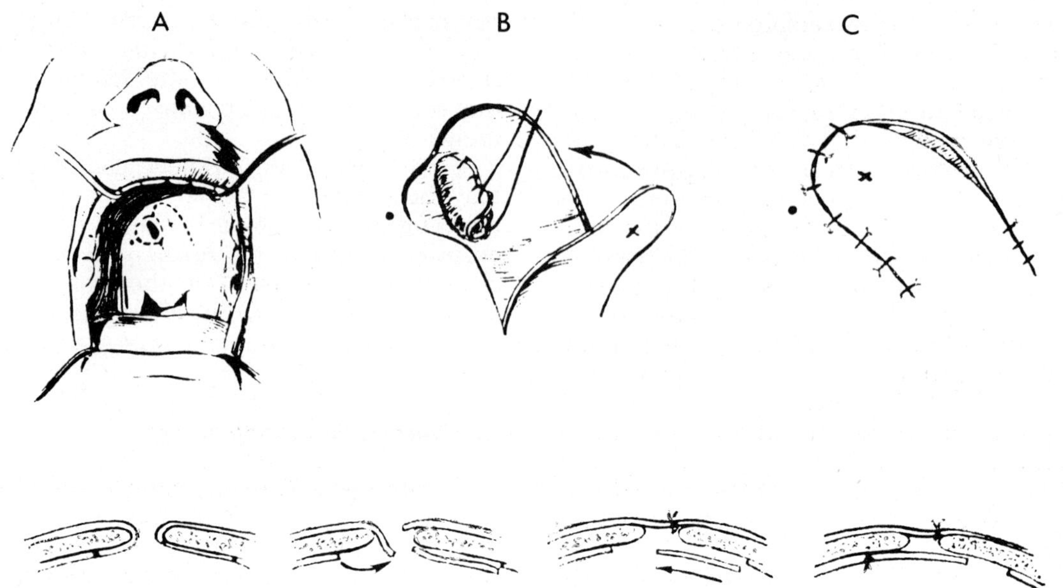


**Figure 13–5** Closing an oronasal fistula with the two-flap technique. *A*, Operative planning; *B*, suturing minor flap to line nasal floor; *C*, transposed larger flap to provide oral coverage. Bottom shows details in coronal section.

A useful preoperative evaluation of the success of the closure with regard to speech may be obtained by blocking the fistula with soft dental wax.

Nasolabial fistulas may also be responsible for poor speech and regurgitation of food into the nose. A technique for repairing such a defect is shown in Figure 13–6. This operation should be delayed until after the permanent incisors have fully erupted. In many instances, the nasolabial fistula may be continuous with a nasoalveolar cleft that extends onto the palatal surface. This fistula should be closed in the same procedure if it is deemed to be symptomatic.

## Long-Term Cosmetic Complications

Cosmetic complications may relate to unsightly labial scars, malformations of the lip and nose and mandibulomaxillary disproportions.

### *Lip Scars*

In instances of a conspicuous scar on the lip, revision of the scar should be undertaken at an age when the patient becomes aware of the deformity and is mature enough to cooperate during the healing phase.

When a markedly depressed, or broad, scar is present, it may well be prudent to excise the entire width of scar tissue and reconstitute the lip as in a primary repair. In such cases, the basic advancement-rotation procedure of Millard is recommended, particularly because its resultant scar assumes the shape and position of a philtral ridge.[5]

If the problem is that of asymmetric height of the lip, the scar having contracted to effect a "whistling" deformity, the operative revision should incorporate an elongation procedure. This is best performed by staggering the repair line to preclude recurrent contracture of the new scar. Bearing in mind that the upper half of the lip is invariably in shadow, care should be taken to plan the lower half of the scar so that it assumes symmetry with the contralateral ridge of the philtrum — this, for a more acceptable cosmetic result (Fig. 13–7).

### *Absent Cupid's Bow*

Whether unilaterally or bilaterally absent, it is best to create a Cupid's bow by incising

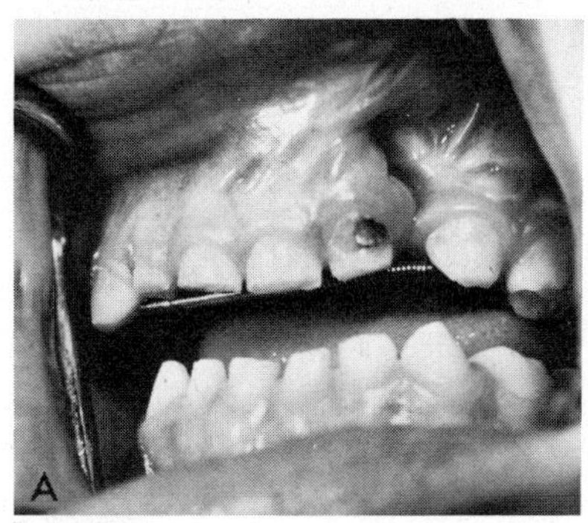


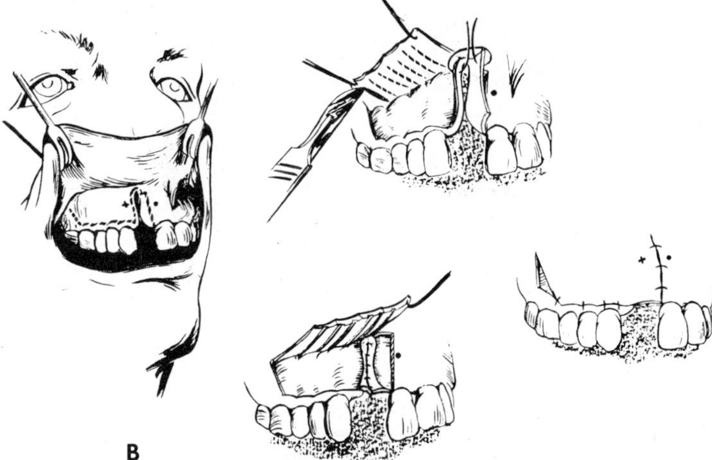


**Figure 13–6** *A,* nasolabial fistula on left side. *B,* Method of closing fistula using two flaps.

across the entire lip. The reason for this is that the symmetric scar will be less conspicuous than a scar placed over only part of the lip.

The generally available method of creating a Cupid's bow is that described by Gillies and Millard,[4] and this author recommends a minor technical modification, which is shown in Figure 13–8.[1] This produces a more acceptable vermilion-cutaneous margin with a fairly prominent scar that resembles the normal linea alba often found at this junction.

In those lips in which the Cupid's bow is entirely absent and when the vermilion-cutaneous border is reasonably symmetric, the bow may be created in a rather simple fashion. An ovoid area is excised in the mid-

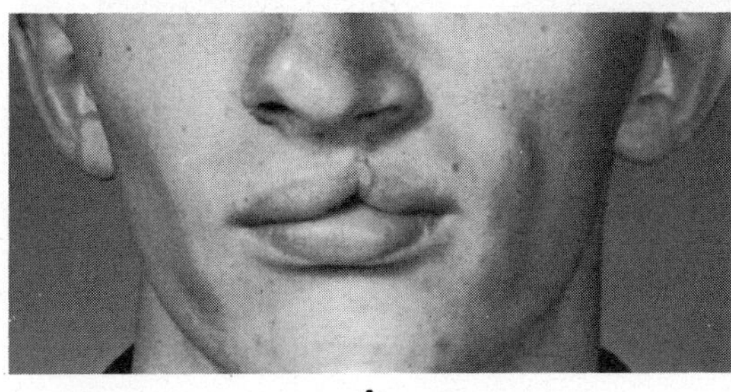
A

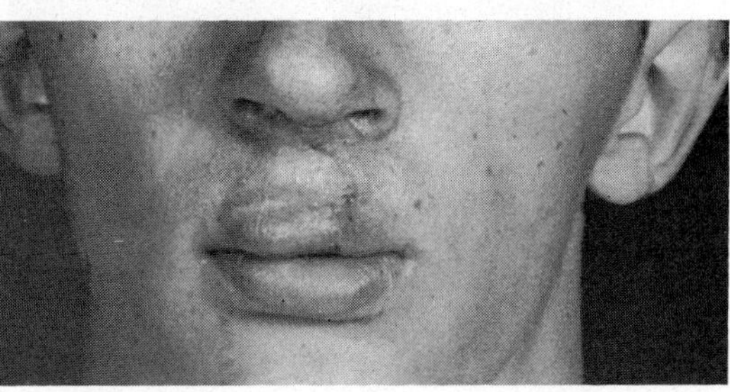
B

**Figure 13–7** *A,* Cleft lip and nose revision using the rotation-advancement technique. *B,* Postoperative view obtained after three weeks.

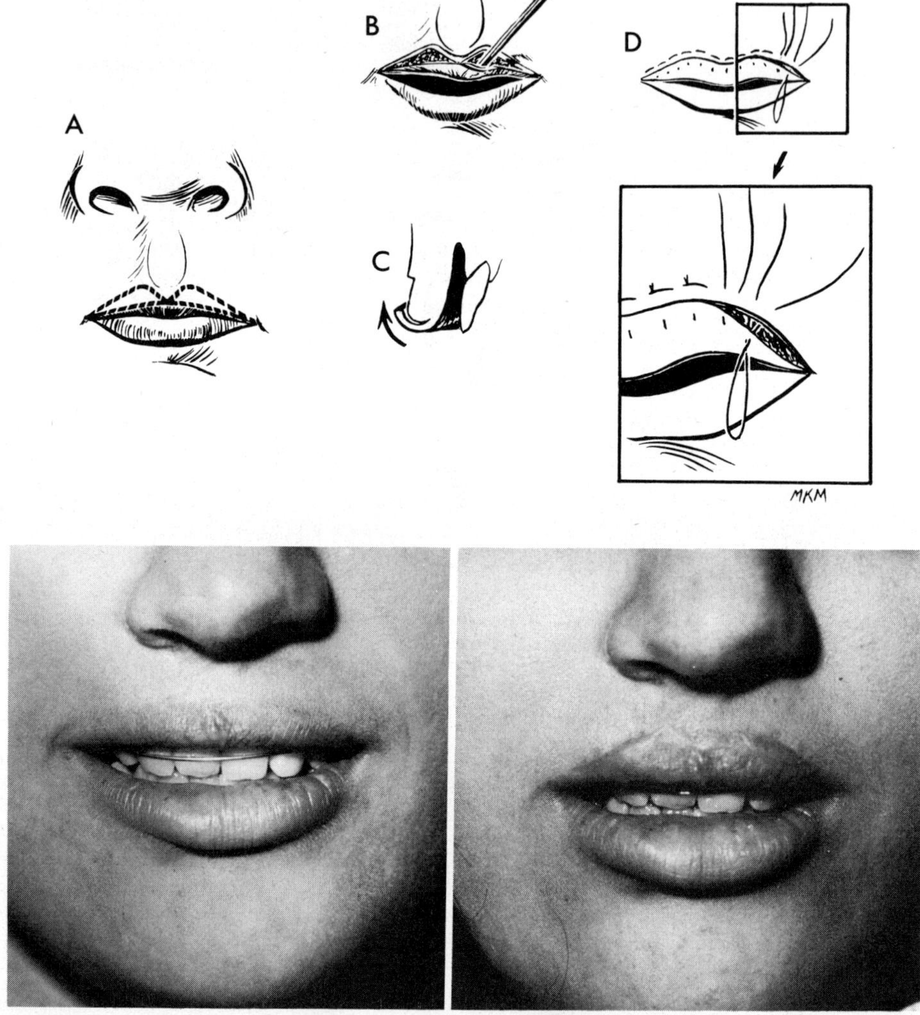


**Figure 13–8** Vermilion advancement technique for creating a Cupid's bow. The suture is triangular in shape, having a horizontal mattress component on the skin and a vertical component on the vermilion. The wound gapes slightly to produce a broad scar. The photograph on the right was obtained one year postoperatively.

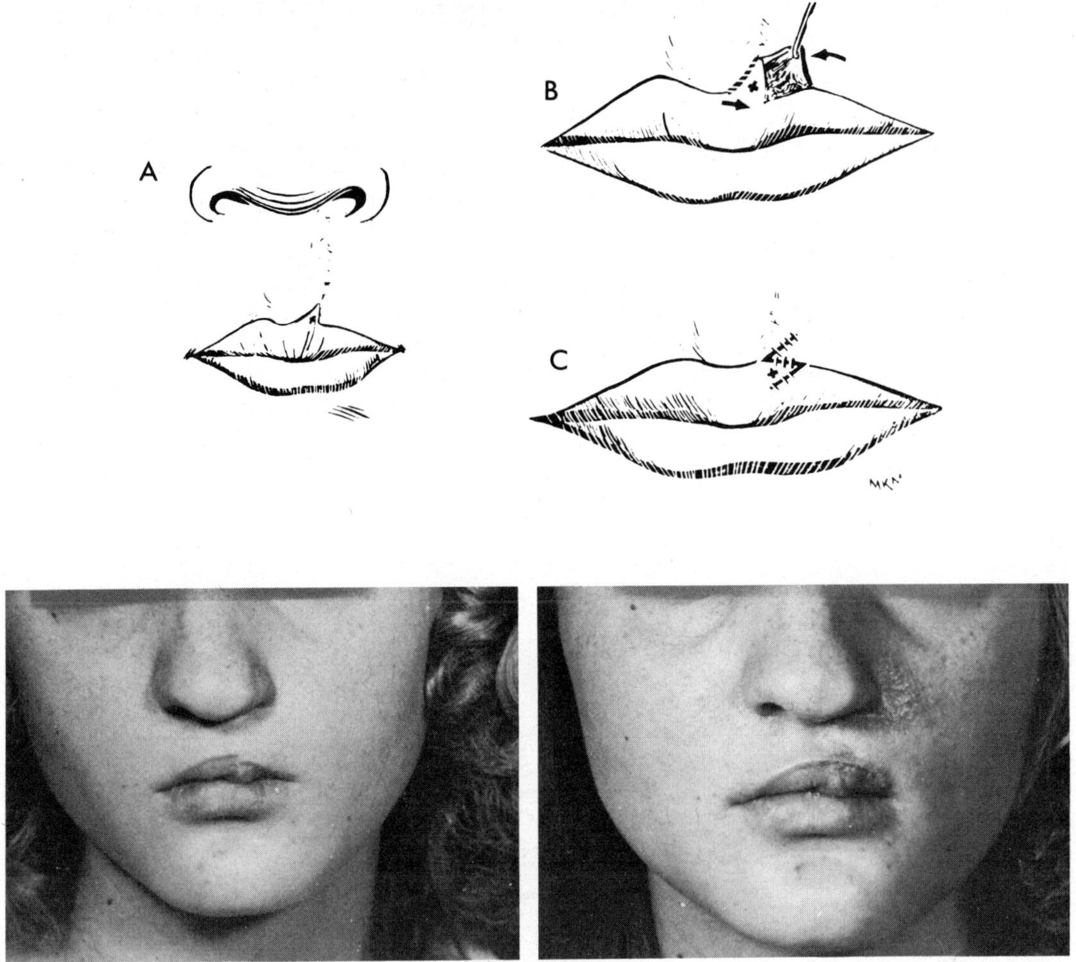


**Figure 13–9** Z-plasty technique for correcting unequal vermilion edges. Photographs show pre- and postoperative views. Note redundant vermilion substance that was resected later.

line at the vermilion-cutaneous junction and the skin of the philtral area is undermined and advanced into the defect (Fig. 13–8).

### *Poorly Aligned Lip Segments*

If the vermilion-cutaneous junction of each lip segment was not meticulously apposed in the original lip repair, the discrepancy usually becomes more obvious with the growth of the child. At times, there may also be a tendency for the epithelium of the vermilion to grow into the lower part of the lip scar. This, no doubt, happens if there is some wound separation at this site. The end result is a vermilion-like triangle at the bottom of the lip scar.

Both of these defects are readily corrected, either by revising the operative line or by means of a Z-plasty (Fig. 13–9).

### *Problems of the Vermilion Substances*

The vermilion substance may have unequal thickness on each side of the cleft, and it is always somewhat meager in the prolabial segment of the bilateral cleft. Moreover, the surgical design or procedure may lead to additional asymmetry, so that the ultimate problem is usually a deficiency, as compared with the contralateral side or with the lower lip. Very occasionally, there may be localized redundancy.

### REDUNDANT VERMILION SUBSTANCE

Only seldom is one presented with a redundancy of the vermilion substance that needs to be reduced (Fig. 13–9). The removal should be planned so that the suture line will be out of sight. The incision is, therefore, placed at the lower vermilion margin, where it meets the lower lip in the closed position. Thus, the suture line should be out of direct sight.

### INSUFFICIENT VERMILION SUBSTANCE

The only way vermilion can be augmented in cleft lip deformities is at the expense of the inner portion of the lip. This may be done by rolling out a flap made up of inner mucosa and half the thickness of the lip musculature. The residual defect on the inner aspect of the lip is closed by the V-Y method. This technique is especially suitable for broad deficits (Fig. 13–10).

Narrow defects may be corrected quite easily by fashioning two opposing, horizontally oriented, Y-V's. By bringing the apices of the V's toward each other, or even by overlapping them somewhat in some cases,

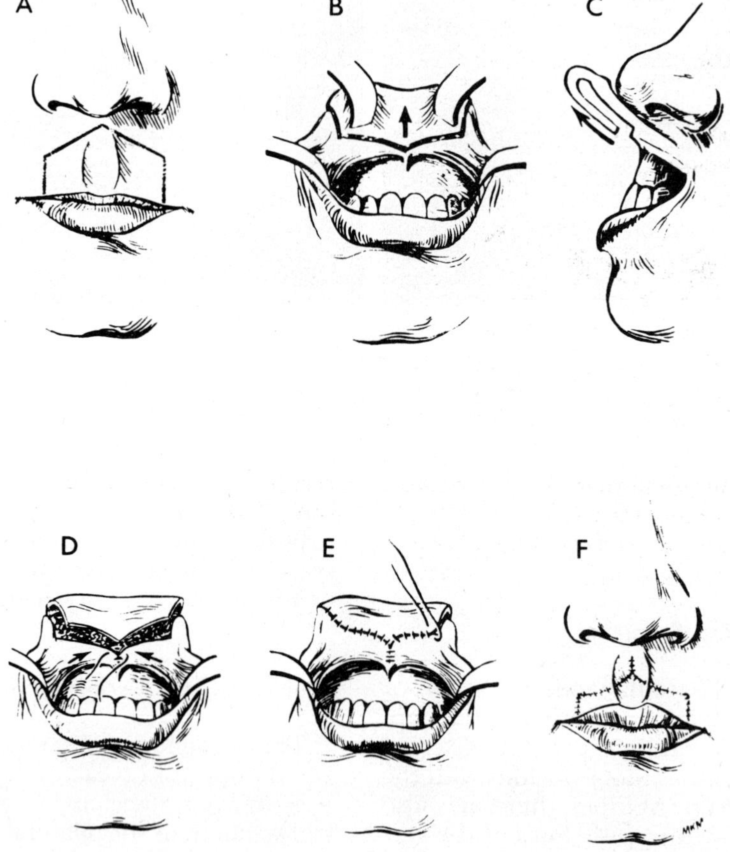


**Figure 13–10** Two examples of vermilion augmentation by means of an advancement flap of the inner half of the lip, using the V-Y technique for closure of the resultant defect. *A–F,* Midline augmentation; *G* and *H,* unilateral procedure. Photographs show pre- and postoperative examples of each.

*Figure 13–10 continued on opposite page.*

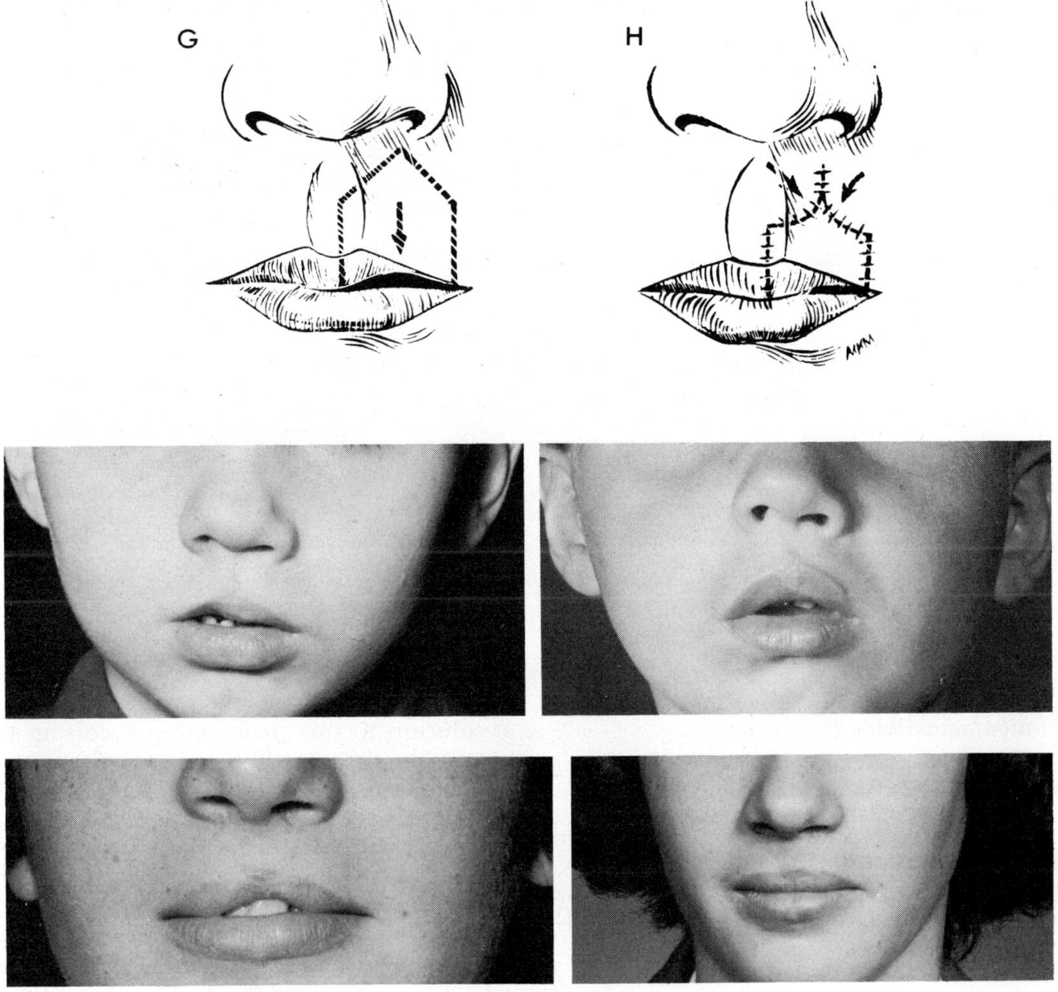


the intervening triangular flap of vermilion that is based superiorly is advanced in a cephalad direction. Consequently, this flap is forced to bow out, thus augmenting the vermilion (Fig. 13–11).

### *Discrepant Sizes of the Lips*

As a consequence of certain primary operations for bilateral cleft lip, there may be marked discrepancy between the upper and lower lips. Very occasionally, this may be encountered with unilateral clefts as well. The discrepancy is more obvious in profile and is characterized by a tight upper lip and a protruding lower, usually with an excessive pout to it. Cupid's bow is invariably absent.

This cosmetic complication lends itself quite naturally to correction with the Abbe transposition flap from the lower lip. In those cases in which this procedure is well planned and executed, each of the defects enumerated above may be corrected (Fig. 13–12).

When the upper lip is considered to be of adequate shape and size and does not need augmentation, the protruding lower lip may be reduced by a midline wedge excision. Prior to undertaking this, however, consideration should be given to whether there may be a need to augment an existing microgenia, since such an augmentation often tends to correct the lip protrusion to some degree.

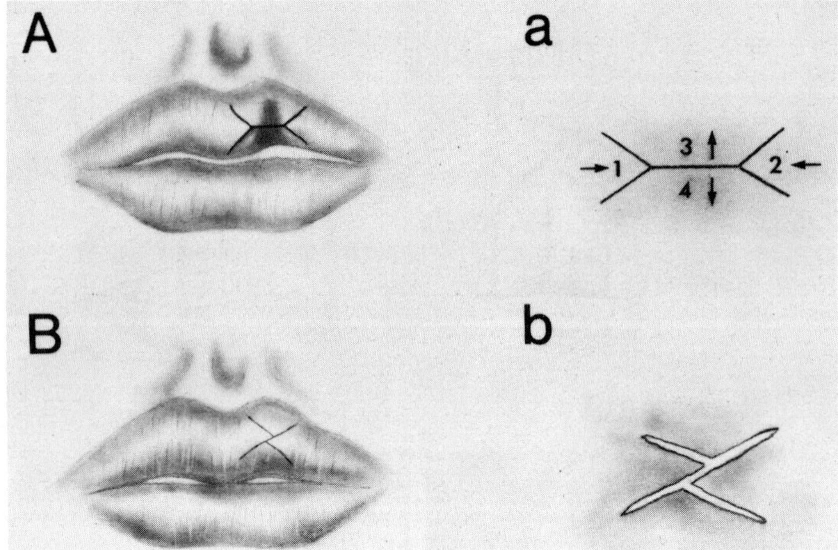


**Figure 13–11** Illustrations of double Y-V technique for correcting localized defect of vermilion substance.

### *Mandibulomaxillary Discrepancies*

#### PROTRUSIVE PREMAXILLA

A protrusive premaxilla may be a complication of poor planning of the case from the start. Failure to align the fragments prior to repairing the lip may have locked the maxillary palatine processes behind the premaxilla, and this relationship may have been ignored at the time of the palatoplasty. Under these circumstances, the best approach is to institute orthodontic treatment, and, if this fails to correct the problem, recession of the premaxilla should be undertaken. In any event, the operation should be delayed until after the incisor teeth have erupted so as to interfere as little as possible with midfacial growth (Fig. 13–4). It is prudent to correlate the operation with orthodontic expansion of the dental arches. The overall result should be more satisfactory.

#### PROGNATHISM

Aggressive surgery on the bony palatal structures may lead to underdevelopment of the middle third of the face, so that the mandible may appear to be relatively prognathic. Since it is much easier to attain a resolution to this problem by recessing the mandible, this should be done in those cases in which the appearance of the middle third of the face is in an acceptable relationship to the rest of the upper facial features. Otherwide, the maxillary segment may have to be moved forward. It is strongly recommended that these cases be evaluated preoperatively in close consultation with an orthodontist who is experienced in the management of such cases. Not only should the work-up include preoperative cephalometric radiographs and dental casts but there also may be a need for presurgical orthodontic treatment.

## NASAL PROBLEMS

Practically every cleft lip patient is born with a coexisting nasal deformity. Some of these deformities may be further complicated by the surgery, especially when there is a concomitant cleft present in the underlying alveolar process. To best understand the residual postoperative sequelae that may complicate the original nasal malformation, the reader should be familiar with the nasal deformities that accompany unilateral and bilateral clefts of the lip.

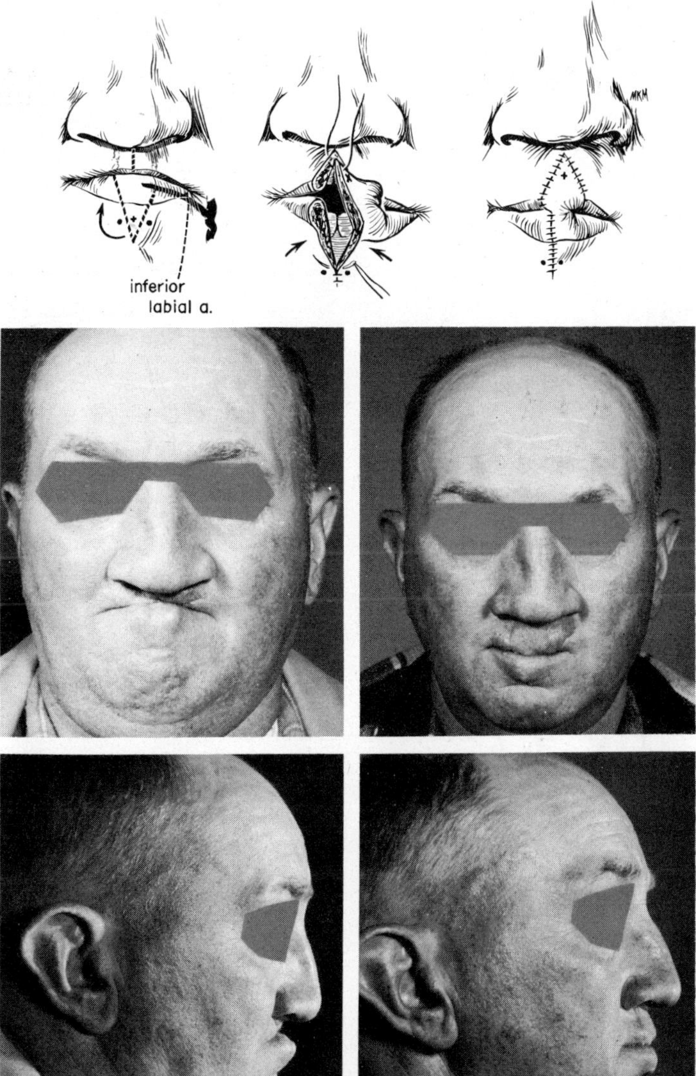


**Figure 13–12** Correction of lip discrepancies with Abbe flap. Note spontaneous improvement of nose and chin a year later.

### *Unilateral Cleft Lip Nasal Deformity*

Whether the lip is entirely cleft or not, the floor of the nasal vestibule is wide. The columella is inclined toward the cleft, and its vertical height on the cleft side is shorter than that on the uncleft side. The dome of the lower lateral (tip) cartilage on the cleft side is wider than that of its counterpart, and it is displaced backward and caudally. Consequently, the rim of the naris is flattened, sometimes with a distinct depression about its midpoint. The natural apex of the naris is flattened, giving the impression of a web at this site. Often, the ala on the affected side is smaller and lower set on the face than the ala on the other side. Its base is usually posteriorly displaced, in accordance with the underlying maxillary segment.

It is to be noted that the previous description applies more in those cases with extensive clefts. It should also be stated that in all unilateral clefts of the palate, the nasal septum is attached to the uncleft portion of the

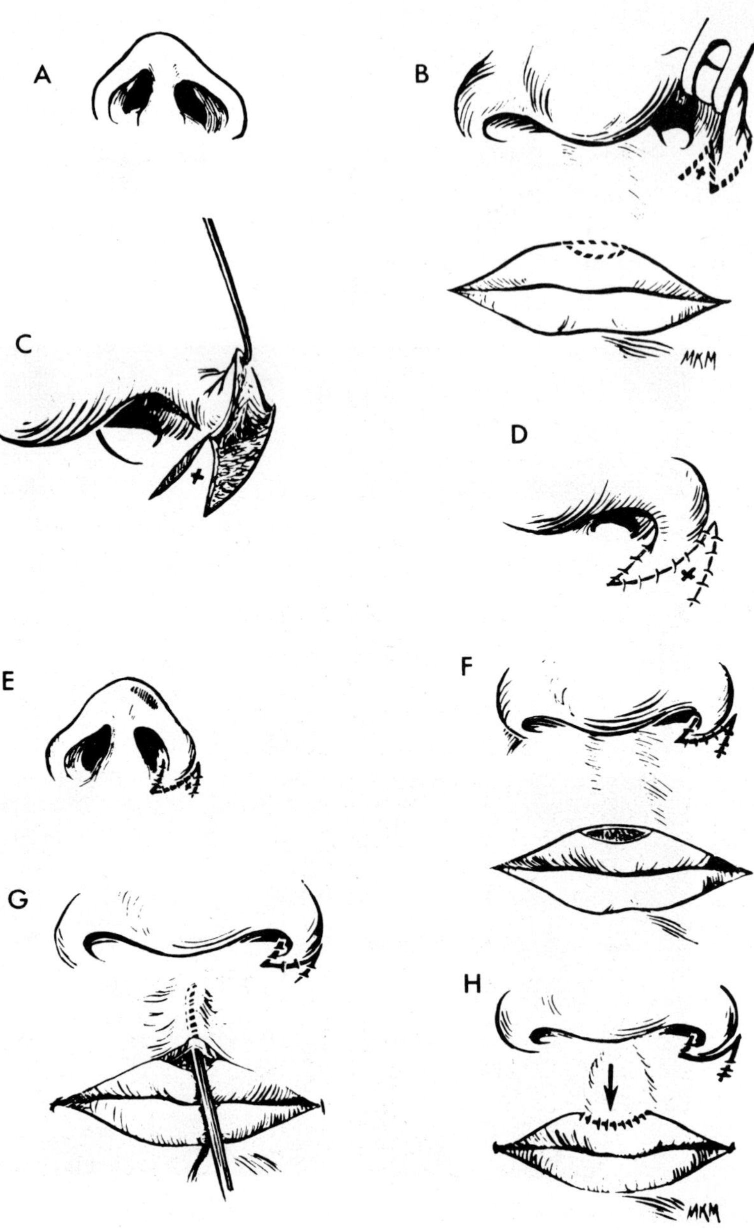


**Figure 13–13** Technique of correcting nasal defect in unilateral cleft lip by narrowing the wide vestibule with a Z-plasty and augmenting the depressed dome with a cartilage graft. A method of creating Cupid's bow is also shown.

palate and is inclined, or deviated, toward the cleft.

Modern cleft lip repair invariably includes some correction of the nasal deformity. Accordingly, the postoperative stigmata will usually bear evidence of the original deformities as well as those that may have been inflicted by the surgeon, both at the primary operation and subsequently.

The main technical objective to be achieved in these cases is the attainment of symmetry. Invariably, this requires a bilateral approach. Various operative procedures are available to achieve this end. One such technique is illustrated in Figure 13–7 and another in Figure 13–13.

### *Bilateral Cleft Lip Nasal Deformity*

The most striking feature of the nose in a bilateral cleft of the lip is the short columella. In extreme cases, it may be barely discernible. Consequently, the cartilaginous vault is flat, a fact that is made worse when there are underlying bilateral clefts of the alveolar process. The nares then appear very flared, with horizontal orientation of their long axes. The alae may be rather small and set backward. When the premaxilla is protrusive, the entire deformity may appear much worse.

The nose in a bilateral cleft may well appear less deformed after lip repair than it would in an equivalent unilateral deformity. This is because the residual nasal deformity is symmetric and, consequently, not as readily perceptible by the average lay observer (Fig. 13–3). The main technical objectives to be achieved in these cases are elongation of the short columella and reconstruction of the cartilaginous framework of the lobule. Several techniques are available for this purpose.

## CONCLUSION

Surgery for cleft lip and cleft palate, like any other elective procedure, carries a minimum of surgical risk. Most of the immediate complications are readily correctible with basic surgical or medical techniques or a combination of the two.

Of far greater importance are the long-term functional and cosmetic complications. In clefts of the lip and palate, such complications are invariably due to badly planned management and poor surgical technique. Most of the complications are avoidable and have dropped in incidence in recent years because of the following factors: (1) institution of preoperative maxillary orthopedics; (2) proper timing of the various operations; (3) improved surgical techniques; and (4) overall planning and management of the patient's problems by a multidisciplinary team.

## Bibliography

1. Bernstein, L.: Secondary reconstructive procedures for cleft lip and nose. Trans. Am. Acad. Ophthalmol. Otolaryngol., *71*:71–80, 1967.
2. Bernstein, L.: Treatment of velopharyngeal incompetence. Arch. Otolaryngol., *85*:67, 1967.
3. Bernstein, L.: Modified operation for wide unilateral cleft lips. Arch. Otolaryngol., *91*:11–18, 1970.
4. Gillies, H. D., and Millard, D. R.: The Principles and Art of Plastic Surgery. Boston, Little, Brown, & Co., 1957.
5. Millard, D. R.: A primary camouflage in the unilateral hare lip. *In* Skoog, T. (ed): Transactions of the First International Congress of Plastic Surgeons. Baltimore, Williams & Wilkins Co., 1957, p. 160.
6. Randall, P.: A trianglular flap operation for the primary repair of unilateral clefts of the lip. Plast. Reconstr. Surg., *23*:331, 1959.
7. Schultz, L. W.: Bilateral cleft lips. Plast. Reconstr. Surg., *1*:338, 1946.
8. Skoog, T.: A design for the repair of unilateral cleft lips. Am. J. Surg., *95*:223, 1958.

# COMPLICATIONS OF SURGERY OF THE SALIVARY GLANDS

14

*Robin M. Rankow*
*Irving M. Polayes*

It is axiomatic that a surgeon operating in the head and neck, and particularly on the major and minor salivary glands, be highly knowledgeable concerning the anatomic details of these regions. Moreover, the surgeon must be fully acquainted with the clinicopathologic entities that may be encountered during the course of the surgical procedures. The adequacy and appropriateness of the excision may require sacrificing structures that, of themselves, can produce intraoperative and postoperative complications.

In an effort to clarify and organize the discussion of complications of surgery of the salivary glands, the authors plan to discuss first those complications resulting from diagnostic procedures, second those complications following the intraoperative exposure and excisions and third those complications appearing early or later in the postoperative period. The management of these potential and actual complications will be described in clinical and technical detail at the appropriate instances.

## SURGICAL ANATOMY

In brief, there are three major bilateral salivary glands — the parotid, submandibular and sublingual — and a multitude of minor accessory salivary glands widely distributed in the mucous membranes of the oropharynx, including the lips, palate, retromolar area, floor of the mouth, tongue, buccal tissues, paranasal sinuses and larynx (Fig. 14–1).

## DIAGNOSTIC PROCEDURES

Numerous diagnostic techniques have been developed to facilitate identification of the congenital, traumatic, inflammatory, neoplastic and non-neoplastic disorders affecting the salivary gland. The treatment of both benign and malignant tumors represents the bulk of surgical interventions. Despite the advances in roentgenographic studies and siabiology, the diagnostic solution to the tumors of the salivary glands most often rests upon a tissue diagnosis. It is well established that the specimen for this tissue diagnosis of the major salivary glands should be obtained as a lateral or medial partial parotidectomy with preservation of the facial nerve or as a total excision of the submandibular and sublingual salivary glands. This approach is often rewarding both as a diagnostic and therapeutic maneuver with minimal seeding of the surgical wounds. In the instance of the widely dispersed minor salivary glands, however, it is prudent to first obtain an incisional biopsy. Then, based upon the clinicopathologic diagnosis, a three-dimensional block excision can be contemplated to encompass the mass, with due concern for the anatomic structures of bordering sound tissue, the margins of which must be included in an appropriate excision.

## DUCTAL INJURY AND OBSTRUCTION

Sialography is a pertinent diagnostic procedure for the evaluation of salivary ducts

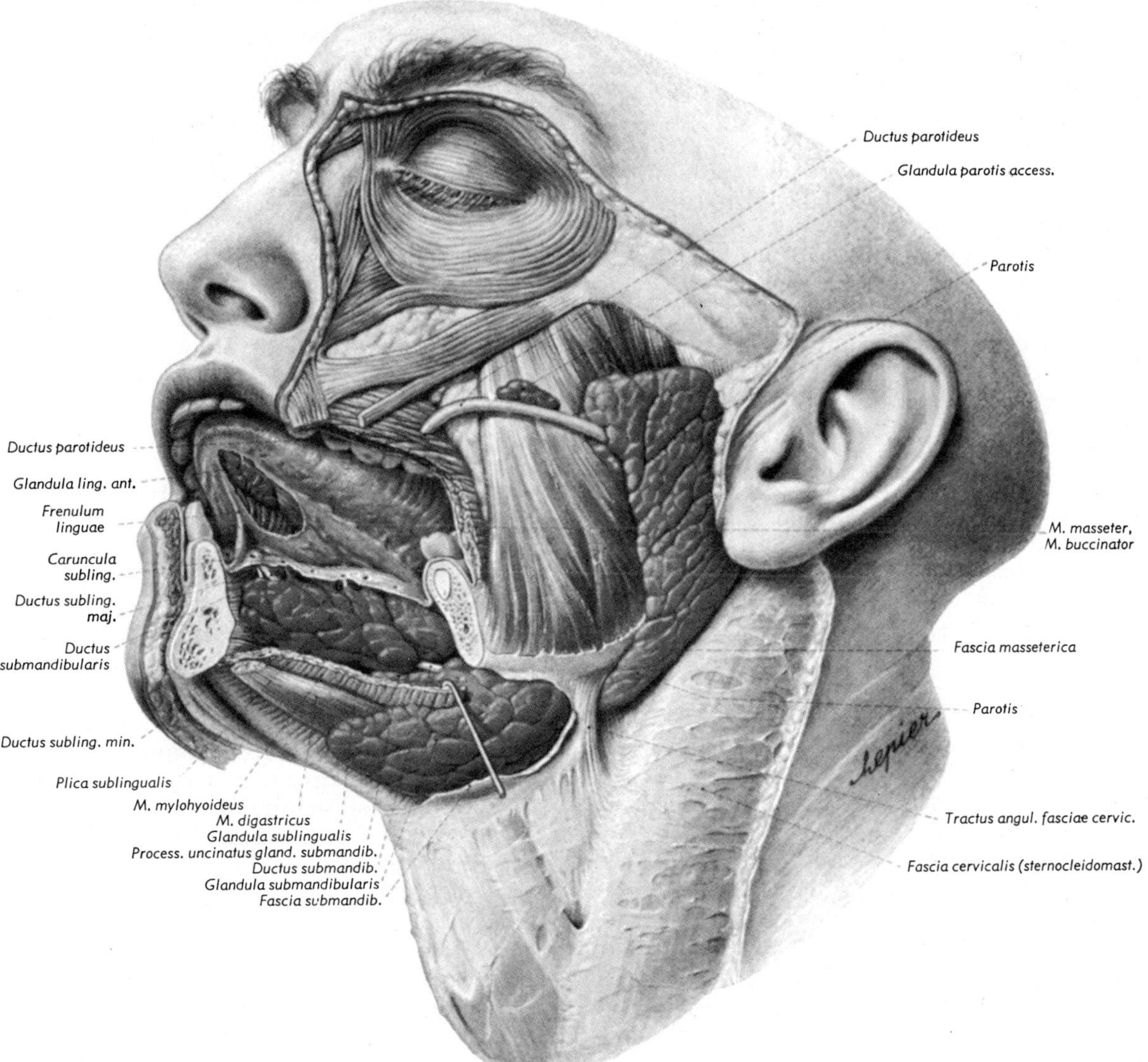


**Figure 14–1** The major salivary glands and their ducts. The body of the mandible has been removed. (From Pernkopf, E.: Atlas of Topographical and Applied Human Anatomy. Vol. 1, Head and Neck. Philadelphia, W. B. Saunders Company, 1963.)

by the introduction of an opaque medium into the ductal system of the major salivary glands. It is usually limited to the parotid and submandibular glands. It is useful in differentiating the benign lymphoepithelial lesion of Sjögren from local inflammatory changes that may accompany stenosis, calculi and, at times, tumors.[21] Patients with history of sensitivity or of anaphylaxis to iodine compounds should not be subjected to sialography.

The use of sialographic techniques and instrumentation during acute inflammation is hazardous and may cause disruption of ductal epithelium. The passage of the contrast medium into the parenchyma of the gland may result in a severe, painful foreign body reaction, especially when oily contrast media are used. The removal of this material is hazardous to the preservation of critical structures in the involved region and best not attempted. The use of water-soluble iodinated organic media is preferable in that foreign body reactions to these media are extremely rare. The retention of iodinated contrast material may interfere with subsequent thyroid function tests, and these studies, if indicated, should be performed prior to the sialography. In addition, the amount of contrast material injected into the gland should be governed by the production of pain and not be a preconceived volume.[34]

Knowing the site of a ductal perforation either by external trauma or by sialography is helpful in deciding whether to repair or permit fistulization of the perforated duct. In general, distal perforations of the duct require no correction. Oral fistulization is preferred and flow of saliva should not be a problem. If the perforation is in the proximal duct or within the gland, then saliva will collect and a cystic diverticulum or extravasation will persist until the duct is repaired. External fistulas and associated symptoms of painful obstruction and infection or ultimate stenosis may follow.

Acute bacterial infections (Fig. 14–2) can produce parenchymal destruction by suppuration and necrosis. Antibiotics and careful cannulation and dilation of the obstructed duct may permit release of mucous or purulent exudates. If this is not successful, then external applications of moist warm compresses will help outline the sites of involvement and the need for external drainage. The incisions for drainage must be so placed as to preserve the branches of the facial nerve (Fig. 14–3). If normal salivary function fails to return to the submandibular or sublingual glands or repetitive episodes of inflammatory obstruction occur, then it is best to totally excise these glands. The parotid gland is more likely to recover adequate function after external incision and drainage of an isolated abscess because of the greater number of functioning alveoloductal segments. If extensive fibrosis and repetitive episodes of parotitis occur, segmental resection of the involved portion of the gland with preservation of the facial nerve will help resolve the disease process (Fig. 14–4).

## POSTSURGICAL SIALOLITHIASIS

Generally, calculi in the parotid gland or duct are infrequent. Seventy-five to 80 per cent of calculi occur in the submandibular gland or duct, about 19 to 20 per cent in the parotid gland or duct and but 1 per cent in the sublingual gland or ducts.[20]

Postsurgical calculi are usually a manifestation of alveoloductal obstruction with persistent or chronic infection, stasis and ductal stenosis. The submandibular duct may be probed with a fine lacrimal dilator to locate an intraductal calculus. If this is the patient's initial obstruction by a solitary calculus, oral removal of the calculus should be attempted. A temporary ligature of #4-0 silk or nylon is passed around the duct proximal and distal to the calculus. The duct is

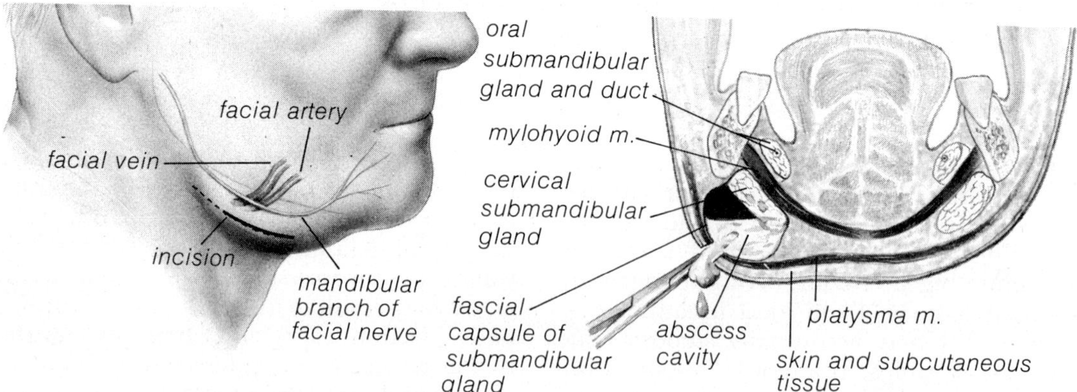


**Figure 14–2** Incision and drainage of submandibular abscess. (From Rankow, R. M., and Polayes, I. M.: Diseases of the Salivary Glands. Philadelphia, W. B. Saunders Company, 1976.)

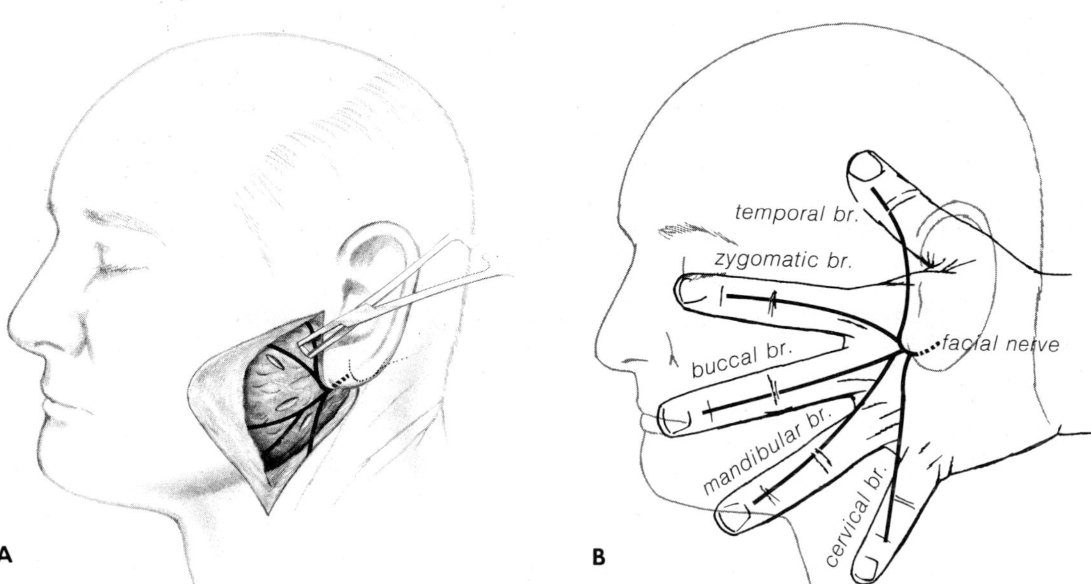


**Figure 14–3** *A,* Blunt expansion of parotid incisions made parallel to general direction of facial nerve branches. *B,* Facial nerve branches fan over the face in the direction simulated by spreading the fingers of the hand. (From Rankow, R. M., and Polayes, I. M.: Diseases of the Salivary Glands. Philadelphia, W. B. Saunders Company, 1976.)

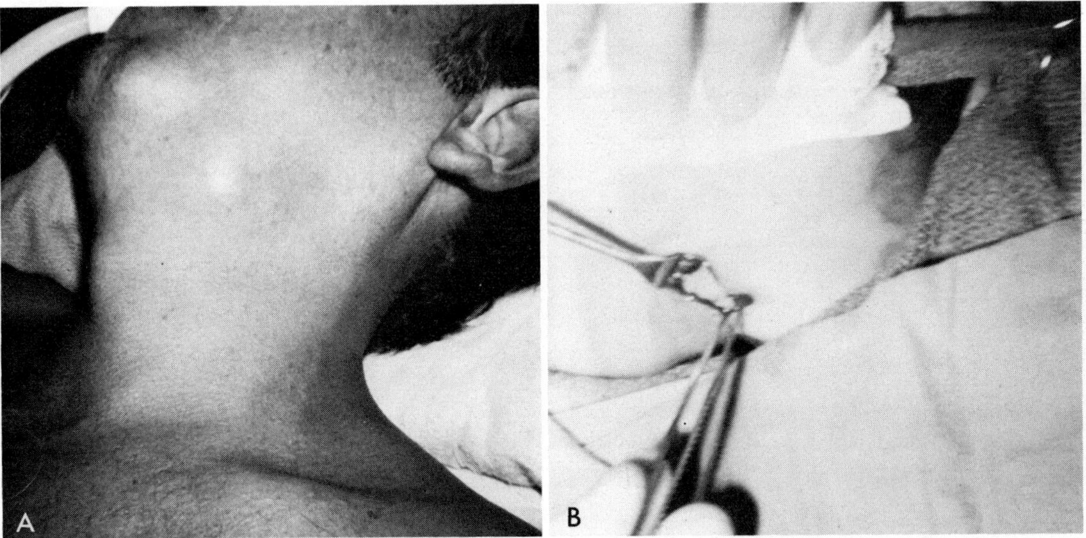


**Figure 14–4** Incision and drainage of acute suppurative submandibular gland abscess.

opened longitudinally between these two sutures and the calculus is removed. If recurrent obstruction appears, it is treated by total excision of the submandibular gland and duct. If the sublingual gland is involved by obstructive calculi or cysts, the gland should be totally removed.[31]

The solitary calculus in the distal portion of the major salivary duct of the parotid gland can be treated by distal and proximal isolation of the calculus with circumferential temporary duct ligatures in a fashion similar to that described previously for the submandibular duct. A Silastic tubular stent may be used as a guide for immediate closure of the duct. Simple removal of the calculi is often followed by recurrent sialadenitis and sialithiasis.

Chronic obstruction of the parotid gland following removal of calculi is often associated with retention cysts due to partial or total obstruction of accessory ducts and stasis of involved acini. The treatment of choice is partial or total parotidectomy of the involved portion of the gland with meticulous identification and preservation of the facial nerve and its branches in a hazardous field.[9, 10] Antibiotics are useful for the inevitable secondary infection associated with chronic inflammation.

## INTRAOPERATIVE PROCEDURES — PAROTID GLAND

The most frequent operations on salivary glands are for the excision of benign or malignant tumors. Inadequate wedge excision and enucleations of salivary gland tumors with surgical margins transecting tumor or biopsies that implant tumor cells lead to a high incidence of recurrences. The majority of parotid tumors (80 per cent) occur in the superficial portion of the gland lateral to the facial nerve. In all these instances, the operative specimen should consist of the entire superficial portion with preservation of the nerve and frozen tissue section diagnosis of the contained tumor. If the tumor mass lies in the deep portion of the gland, the superficial parotidectomy must be completed and the preserved facial nerve elevated carefully from the deep portion, which is then removed. Accordingly, the most frequent and most distressing complication to the patient is that of a temporary, partial or complete paralysis of the facial nerve and its branches (Fig. 14–5). All things being equal, the incidence of this complication, excluding intentional resection of portions of the nerve involved by malignancy, is a direct measure of the anatomic knowledge and meticulous

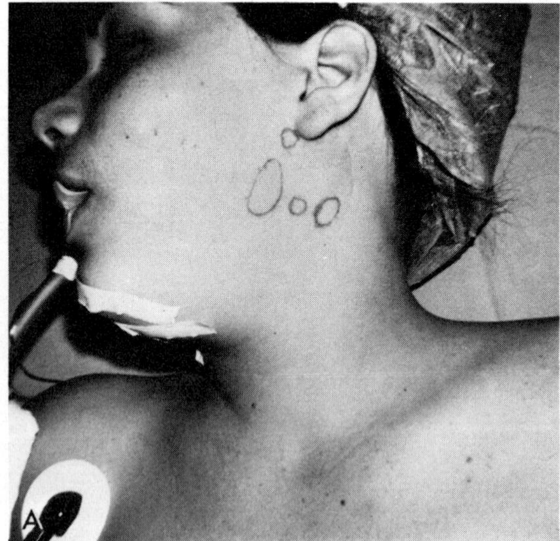


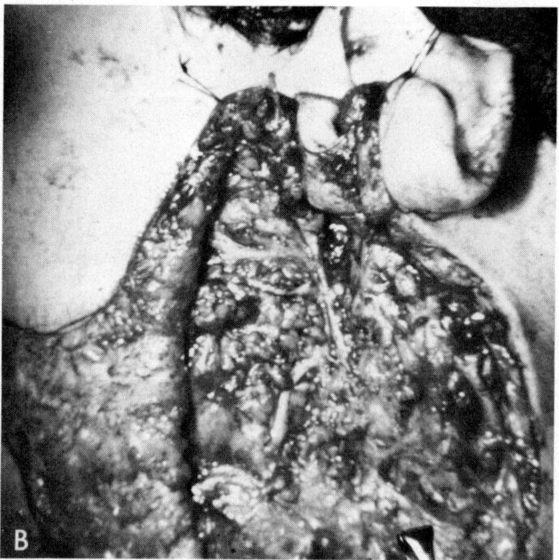


**Figure 14–5** *A*, Recurrent mixed tumor of the parotid gland two years after inadequate excision of tumor margin. *B*, Operative view of recurrent tumor nodules. Note deep parotid segment below facial nerve.

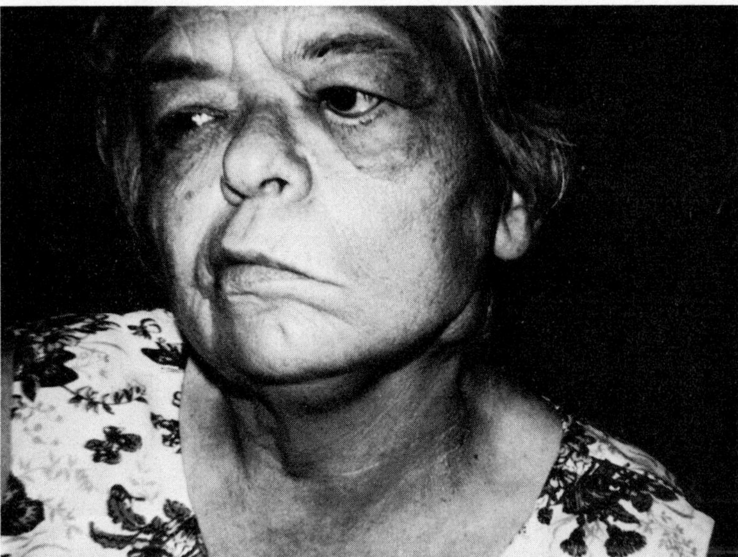

**Figure 14–6** Complete paresis of the facial nerve following parotidectomy, with recurrent cancer in upper neck two years post surgery.

skill of the operating surgeon. It is good practice to habitually observe the function of the facial muscles shortly after the patient's recovery from anesthesia. Good muscle function at that time assures the integrity of the nerve. Devascularization or edema from handling the nerve may still result in a facial weakness, but initial recovery is usually evident within six to eight weeks. Because of this danger, galvanic stimulation of the nerve during operation should be minimal (Fig. 14–6)

Soft rubber drains and, in selected instances, suction catheters are placed at the superior and inferior portions of the surgical wound. These drains should not rest upon the exposed main trunk or branches of the facial nerve. The wound is closed in layers, with #4-0 chromic catgut (or any other absorbable suture material) for the subcutaneous tissues and fine silk or dermalon for the skin. A pressure dressing is applied to protect the operative site and restrain the head and neck. The superior suction tubing or drain is removed in 24 to 48 hours, at the first dressing. The inferior drain or suction is discontinued after three to four days, and by the sixth to seventh postoperative day sutures are removed. A salivary fistula may persist through the drain site for seven to 10 days but usually seals spontaneously. Persistent accumulation of retained salivary secretions within the parotidectomy site that does not respond to simple aspiration beyond a three week postoperative period may require surgical drainage procedures. Maintaining the patient on a citrus-free, bland diet postoperatively is advisable; however, the use of antisialagogues is of no benefit.

Numbness of the preauricular tissues and lower auricle and lobule of the ear may persist for four to six months until the severed, sensory, great auricular nerve regenerates. At times, a painful neuroma may occur at the cut end of the great auricular nerve.[18] Although sharp excision of the neuroma has been practiced, treatment is usually ineffective. Sweating of the face anterior to the auricle may appear during eating owing to the disturbance of reflex pathways from both the great auricular and the auriculotemporal nerves to the skin (Frey's syndrome)[13, 16] (Fig. 14–7). This requires the reassurance of and an explanation to the patient, since the syndrome may persist for several years. Excessive annoying gustatory sweating persisting beyond one to two years may be relieved by simple re-elevation and closure of the entire surgical skin flap without drainage. Tympanic neurectomy has also been suggested as a method of treating the excessive and uncontrolled sweating by interrupting Jacobson's nerve, which contains the secretomotor preganglionic parasympathetic fibers.[14] To date, no definite

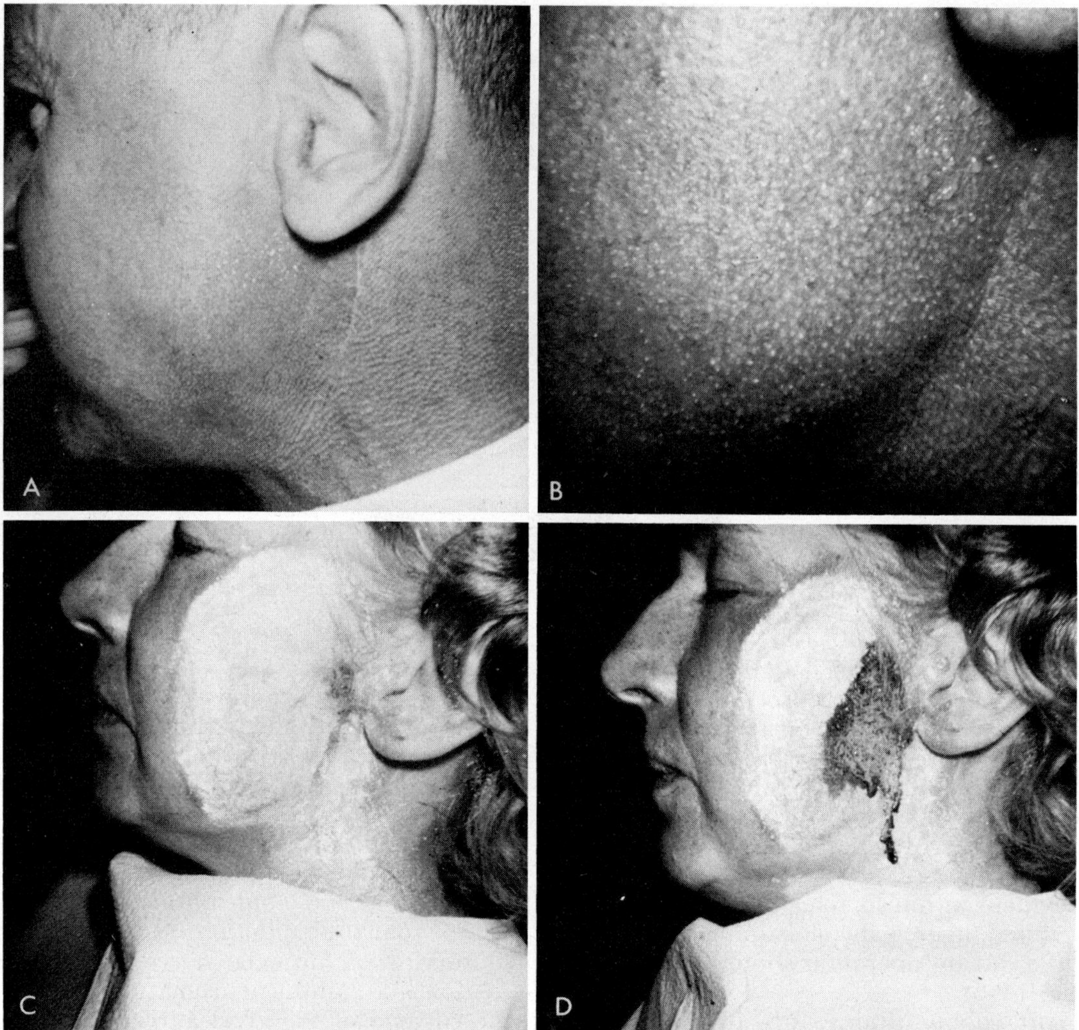


**Figure 14–7** *A,* Postparotidectomy patient chewing celery stalk. *B,* Beads of sweat evident on skin overlying site of parotidectomy. *C,* Tincture of iodine applied over skin at site of parotidectomy and covered with starch paste. *D,* Stained area of sweating after gustatory stimulus. (From Rankow, R. M., and Polayes, I. M.: Diseases of the Salivary Glands. Philadelphia, W. B. Saunders Company, 1976.)

cure for Frey's syndrome has been found, and its incidence remains in 20 to 50 per cent of the patients six months following parotidectomy.

Except for the slight depression of the lateral facial tissues, the overall physiologic and cosmetic results following parotidectomy are satisfactory. De-epithelialized composite rotation of skin or myocutaneous flaps can help fill out the soft tissue defect, if indicated in the late postoperative period.

Intraoperative complications may follow inappropriately designed incisions for exposure of the parotid gland. A useful design consists of a preauricular limb of an incision joined to a postauricular limb behind the lobule of the ear that is then joined vertically by a gently curving transverse incision passing anteromedially from the junction of the preauricular and postauricular limbs along an upper crease of the neck approximately one to two finger breadths below the inferior border of the mandible. The curved incision should be posterolateral to the gland, especially if a distorting mass is present, in order to avoid entry into the tumor.

In general, the most favorable depth of the incision is just beneath or through the subcutaneous fat of the skin flap. This exposes the parotid fascia and gives a protective guide and cover for the parotidectomy.

There are several acceptable approaches to the facial nerve, but the authors prefer early identification of the facial nerve by exposure and palpation of anatomic bony landmarks encircling the main trunk of the nerve at its exit from the stylomastoid foramen. This gives a secure guide for elevation and adequate removal of the lateral portion of the gland while preserving the underlying facial nerve divisions and branches under direct vision. If the tumor mass rests within the portion of the gland deep to the facial nerve, the preserved nerve should be gently elevated and freed from the underlying gland, which can then be anatomically removed.

The mandible may be dislocated and displaced anteriorly to assist in the excision of the less accessible medial expansion of the deep (retromandibular) parotid portion. Care should be taken not to damage the condyloid process and ligaments of the temporomandibular joint and to restore the joint to its normal position in the glenoid fossa in order to prevent troublesome joint complications characterized by pain and limitations in mandibular function.

The pterygoid venous plexus may be the source of troublesome bleeding that can be controlled by compression with tampons or suture ligatures. The external carotid artery and its maxillary and superficial temporal branches and the retromandibular vein (posterior facial) and its tributaries should each be identified, divided and carefully ligated if the deep portion of the parotid gland is being removed. Hypotensive anesthesia is useful when acceptable for the patient, but the blood pressure should be restored to normal well before closing the wound to minimize postoperative hemorrhage and hematomas. All bleeders are best grasped by fine mosquito clamps to visualize adjacent nerve fibers, using care to protect them from being crushed by the instrument. Preferably, all ligatures should be fine chromic catgut or silk tied meticulously at the points of the beaks of the clamps to avoid ligation and damage to the exposed nerve fibers. It is best to promptly ligate these vessels and remove the clamps in the course of the dissection. This will prevent accidental injuries to the nerve branches by mechanical traction on the vessels.

The cartilaginous portion of the external auditory canal is bared during the reflection of the superficial portion of the gland and may be damaged by tumor or surgery. Although the external canal is presumably sterilized during the preparation of the surgical field, perforation may cause late infection. If penetrated, the canal should be reapproximated and repaired with a fine suture joining the perichondrium but not entering the canal, if possible. In general, preoperative, intraoperative and short postoperative courses of appropriate antibiotics are optional but more likely are useful, since the parotid duct does pass to a contaminated oral cavity, and there is questioned sterility of the external ear canal in the surgical field.

## INTRAOPERATIVE PROCEDURES — SUBMANDIBULAR GLAND

Several important nerves are present in the submandibular compartment and should be identified and protected by the surgeon. The gland is innervated by the lingual nerve, the sympathetic plexus upon the facial artery and the submandibular ganglion (parasympathetic secretory fibers from the chorda tympani). The mandibular branch of the facial nerve passes on the undersurface of the platysma and superficial to the facial vessels at the mandibular notch and is particularly vulnerable to submandibular incisions along the surface of the gland. Injury to this nerve results in distortion of the corner of the mouth in motion because of partial paralysis of the orbicularis oris muscle of the lip. The hypoglossal nerve, the motor nerve to the tongue, passes beneath the posterior belly of the digastric muscle along the surface of the hypoglossus muscle. It runs close to the lingual veins and may be injured if obscured by venous bleeding during surgery. Paralysis of the ipsilateral tongue follows injury to the nerve. The lingual nerve is located at the uppermost surface of the gland beneath the mandible and is also subject to injury during surgery.

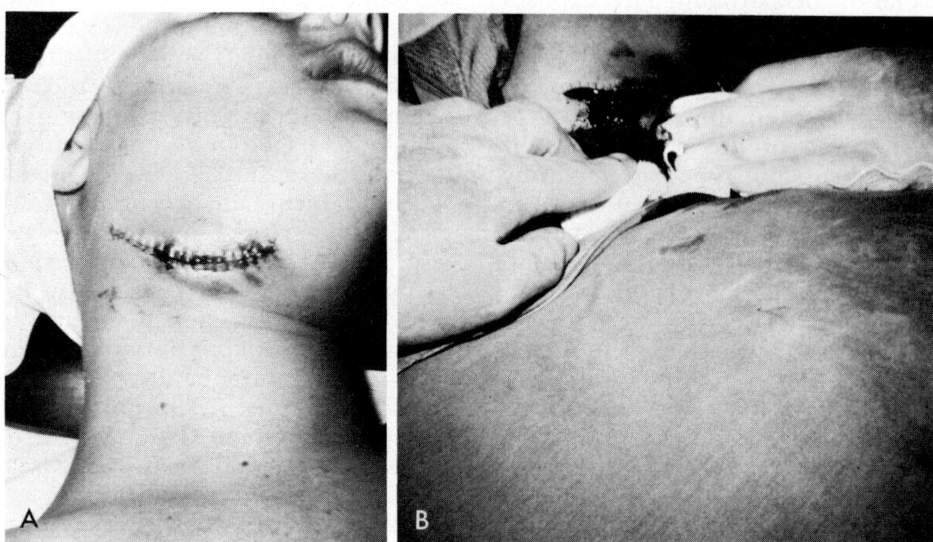


**Figure 14–8** Clinical. *A,* Hematoma appearing five days after submandibular and sublingual gland excision. *B,* Patient was returned to operating room for evacuation of clots and control of bleeding vessels.

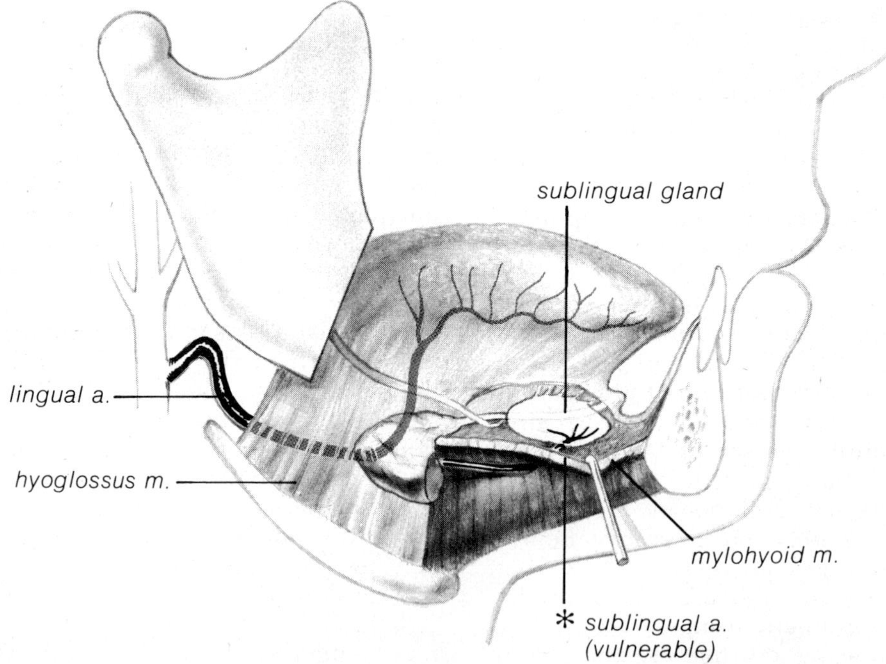


**Figure 14–9** The sublingual branch is the chief arterial supply of the sublingual gland. It is vulnerable to surgical injury as it passes along the floor of the mouth to the gland. (From Rankow, R. M., and Polayes, I. M.: Diseases of the Salivary Glands. Philadelphia, W. B. Saunders Company, 1976.)

Such injury results in anesthesia of the anterior two thirds of the tongue.

The facial artery courses through the submandibular gland to reach the mandibular notch. It is important to carefully ligate this vessel beneath the posterior belly of the digastric muscle where it leaves the external carotid artery as well as at the mandibular notch. Vigorous bleeding can follow loss of control of the facial artery. Persistent ooze from numerous branches of the facial vein also may result in hematoma formation (Fig. 14–8).

The submandibular and sublingual glands are both managed best by a total excision in chronic obstructive situations other than obvious acute abscesses. This prevents postoperative recurrent sialadenitis and sialolithiasis. In the presence of a suspicious primary tumor mass in these two glands, it is particularly important to achieve a total removal. The incidence of a malignant mass in the submandibular glands is about 60 per cent and in the sublingual glands it is well over 80 per cent.[11, 17, 30] When partial excisions or biopsies are attempted, there may be seeding of tumors with reduced survival rates and creation of recurrent fistulas and infections.

## INTRAOPERATIVE PROCEDURES — SUBLINGUAL GLAND

The sublingual artery is the chief vessel to the sublingual gland and is particularly vulnerable to injury during excisional surgery of the gland. It is a branch of the lingual artery passing through the mylohyoid muscle onto the floor of the mouth, upon which the gland rests (Fig. 14–9). If this artery is ignored or not ligated securely, brisk bleeding and dissecting hematomas elevate the tongue and floor of the mouth and may compromise the oral airway. In such instances, the surgical field should be re-explored promptly under endotracheal general anesthesia in order to suture ligate the bleeding vessel and remove all blood clots and drain the wound.

The sublingual gland enfolds the submandibular duct, and excisional surgery of the gland requires prior ductal cannulation with fine lacrimal probes for protection of the duct. A total block excision of the sublingual gland requires that the distal segment of the submandibular duct and the multiple sublingual ducts opening into the floor of the mouth should be excised with the specimen. The proximal stump of the submandibular duct is then transposed to adjacent sound mucosa to maintain salivary flow and prevent pain and swelling of obstructive recurrent sialadenitis. Fibrosis that follows recurrent sialadenitis in the remaining submandibular gland may mimic metastatic disease and complicate judgment in the management of such patients.

The lingual nerve passes inferior to the submandibular duct and medial to the sublingual gland to supply sensory fibers to the tongue. The nerve should be identified and preserved to avoid damage during excisional surgery of the gland that may result in paresthesias of the tongue and floor of the mouth. If the nerve is divided and the cut ends are readily available, end to end anastomosis is feasible. In general, no repair is necessary, since the probability of recovery of the sensory nerve is high.

## RADICAL SURGERY FOR CANCER

### *Parotid Gland*

Total parotidectomy and partial mandibulectomy often includes resection of the condyle, portions of the ascending ramus and the underlying external carotid artery to the take off of the superficial temporal arteries, as indicated by the clinicopathologic diagnosis. The entire retromandibular (posterior facial) vein and its tributaries down to its junction with the external jugular vein are included in the specimen. The regional lymph nodes should be excised as encountered during the course of the dissection along the jugulodigastric level. Depending upon the pathologic diagnosis of these nodes as reported by frozen section tissue, a clinical decision can be made as to the need for radical neck dissection incontinuity with the primary excision.

The complications of radical neck dissections are discussed in Chapters 4 to 9. The special complications of specific salivary gland excisions will be highlighted in this discussion.

### *Submandibular and Sublingual Gland*

There is a high incidence of occult neck metastases in submandibular and sublingual gland cancers (40 per cent)[28] and incontinuity radical neck dissection is usually advisable except for low-grade mucoepidermoid cancer of the glands. The decision to combine excision of the floor of the mouth, partial mandibulectomy and both submandibular and sublingual glands with an incontinuity radical neck dissection is supported by positive frozen tissue section of any compartmental glandular nodes evident in the surgical field or in the regional jugular lymph nodes. The hypoglossal nerve should not be spared if radical neck dissection is elected, nor is there any need to reconstruct the excised nerve since margins of adjacent sound tongue, mylohyoid muscle and floor of mouth are added to the primary resection. The patient will have atrophy of the homolateral tongue and anesthesia of the floor of the mouth due to lingual nerve inclusion with the primary resection, but these complications are well tolerated by the patient and rarely require reconstructive or reparative surgery.

Drainage of the neck is accomplished best with catheters attached to suction that extend into the site of the glandular defect. It is prudent to fix the catheters to the soft tissue bed with plain catgut sutures and avoid suction damage to critical vessels and nerves. Care should be taken to have the nursing attendants check the effectiveness of the suction apparatus at regular, frequent intervals during the first 24 to 48 hours to assure proper drainage of serum or blood collections. If hematomas form, they may require irrigations and forced suction or opening of portions of the incision for control of bleeding sites and evacuation of the hematomas.

Anesthesia of the lingual and alveolar tissues of the floor of the mouth and mandible is expected following radical sublingual and submandibular glandular resections. The patient should also be advised of the possibility of similar anesthesia if the mandibular ($V_3$) nerve is excised with the deep pyterygoid portion of the parotid gland or if division of the ascending ramus is required in a radical parotidectomy.

Facial and hypoglossal nerve division may be repaired immediately in the interoperative phase by anastomosis or autografts from the anterior cervical plexus. If the nerves of the plexus are adherent to metastatic cervical nodes, then the contralateral neck or sural nerve from the leg may be the preferred choice for obtaining the nerve graft.

It is best not to attempt immediate mandibular bone grafting simultaneously with major glandular resections; however, a simple rigid wire may be used to retain the uncontrolled fragments in a more normal and functional position, and an autogenous bone graft may be inserted at a later date. This order of management will minimize orocutaneous fistulas and reduce the incidence of wound infection that may extend into the soft tissues of the neck dissection and threaten the integrity of the common carotid artery.

Complications of local three-dimensional resections of malignant minor salivary glands generally result from persistent tumor due to the anatomic restraints in achieving sound tissue margins. Persistent wound infections and cellulitis are complications that follow inadequate cover of exposed bone and soft tissues in the surgical wound. Immediate split-thickness skin grafts, rotation of adjacent pedicle flaps or regional flaps are useful at this intraoperative phase to avoid these complications. Free grafts with arterial and venous microsurgical revascularization as well as microneural anastomoses are being used more frequently in recent years and may provide a sound method for immediate reconstruction.

## LOSS OF FACIAL NERVE FUNCTION

Reconstructive efforts following complications of salivary gland surgery are most often concerned with the sequelae produced by loss of facial nerve function, the cosmetic soft tissue deficits resulting from the ablative salivary gland procedure and those complications resulting from hematoma, infection and loss of skin flaps.

Surgery of the parotid, submandibular and sublingual glands may involve injury to

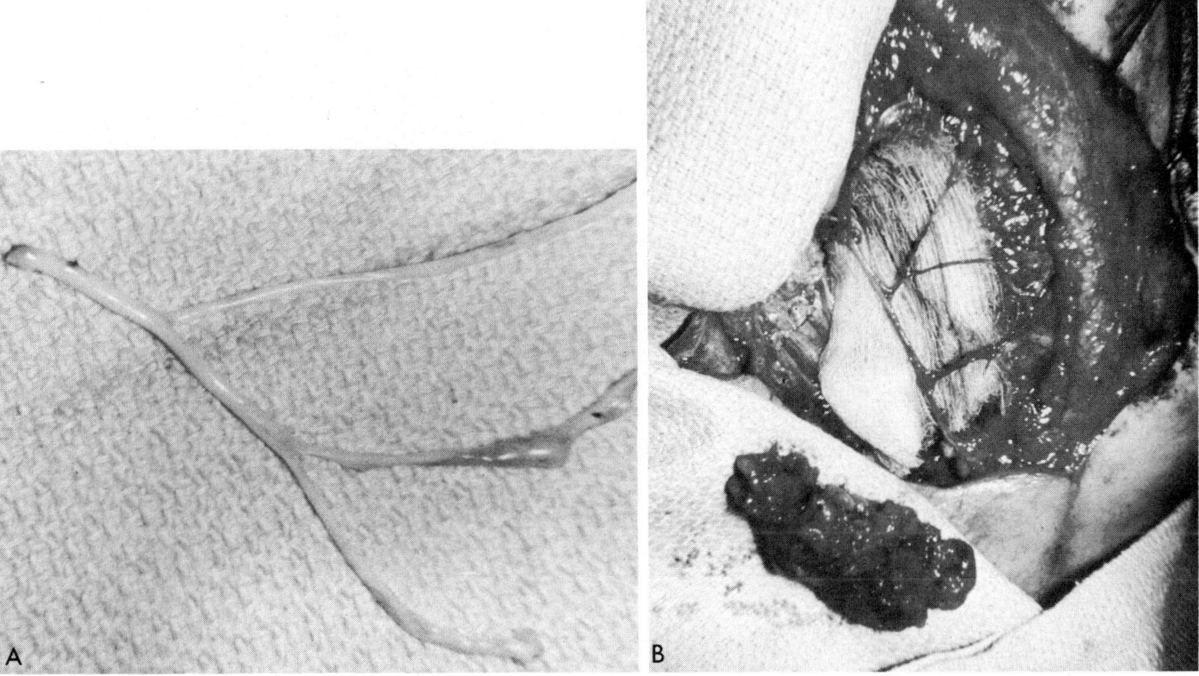

**Figure 14–10** *A,* Branched graft of same diameter as the facial nerve obtained from the anterior cervical plexus. *B,* Interpositional autograft following resection of facial nerve for parotid malignancy. Excised specimen at bottom of field. (From Rankow, R. M., and Polayes, I. M.: Diseases of the Salivary Glands. Philadelphia, W. B. Saunders Company, 1976.)

the mandibular ramus of the facial nerve. Most often such injury is due to careless retraction, handling, or prolonged electrostimulation of the nerve and is usually followed by recovery of nerve function within four to six months. In many instances in which fibers of the facial nerve are severed anterior to a vertical line drawn from the lateral canthus down through the mental foramen, nerve repair is unnecessary, since these terminal fibers are one of many connecting branches supplying the same area.[7] Facial nerve trunks severed posterior to this line (Fig. 14–10), however, usually require microreanastomosis for return of function.

## TARSORRHAPHY

Surgery of the parotid area when complicated by facial nerve injury to the main trunk distal to the stylomastoid foramen will result in loss of function in all areas innervated by its severed branches. Immediate nerve reconstruction or anastomosis is indicated. Even if primary reanastomosis is performed or nerve grafts are inserted to reconstitute the lost segments of the trunk, however, paresis will exist for 6 to 12 months, which can be both functionally and cosmetically disabling. Immediate temporary measures must be taken to protect vital structures and augment weakened muscle action while awaiting recovery of nerve function. A temporary tarsorrhaphy is indicated when the patient is unable to adequately close the eyelids for protection of the cornea on the affected side.[6, 32] When the Bell's phenomenon is not demonstrable, a tarsorrhaphy is mandatory until the protective closure of the eyelids has returned or has been restored by reconstructive procedures. Two types of tarsorrhaphies are illustrated in Figure 14–11. The temporary nonfusion tarsorrhaphy can be held in place for only four to six weeks, but the temporary fusion variety can be maintained as long as necessary. Either procedure will not deform or distort the eyelids to any significant degree when they are separated. The fusion

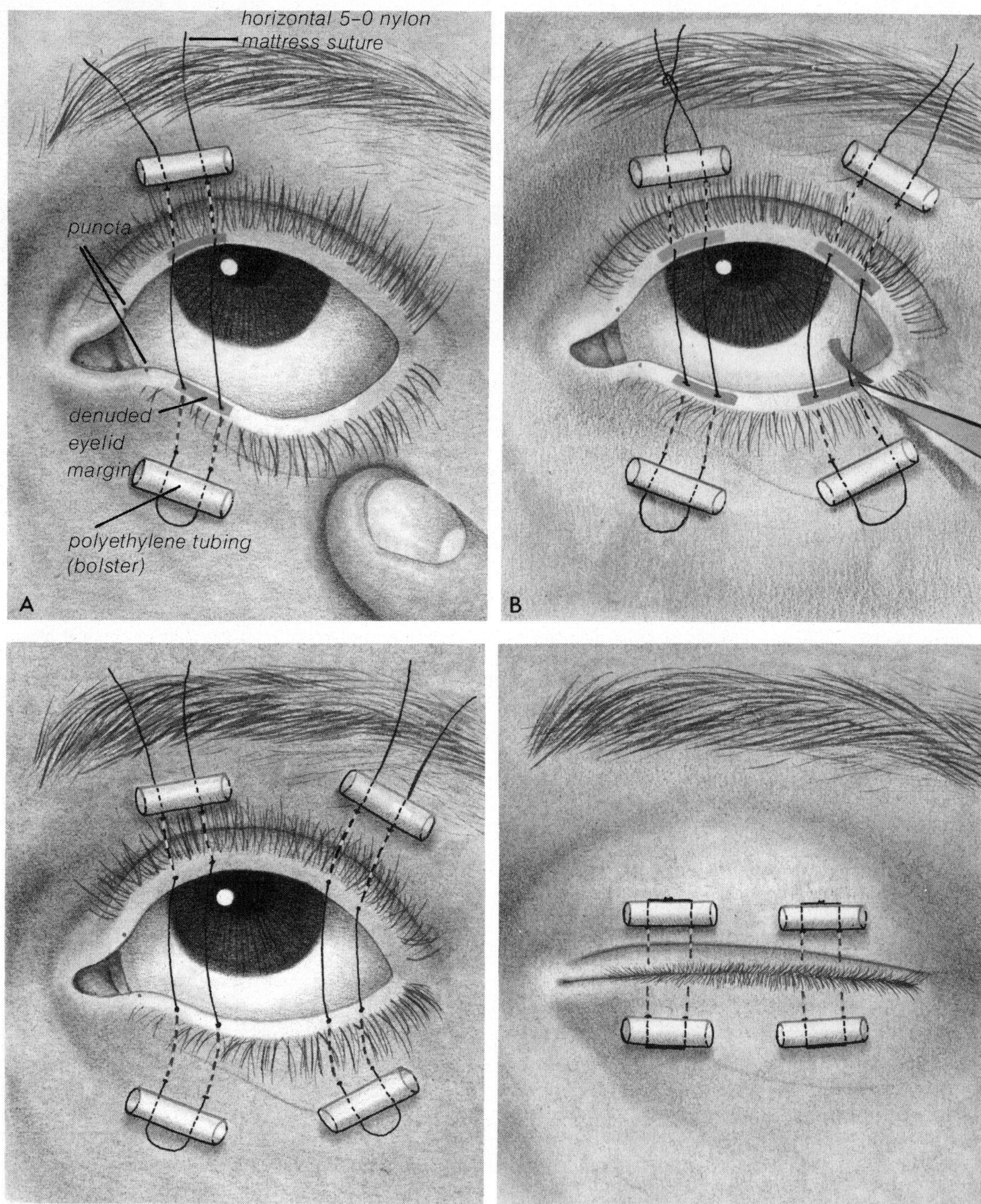


**Figure 14–11** Temporary fusion tarsorrhaphy. *A,* A rectangular 5 mm. length of eyelid margin is denuded, using a #11 knife blade, from the lateral and medial thirds of the upper and lower eyelids. The upper and lower lids fuse at the areas of denuded epithelium. *B,* A #5–0 nylon simple horizontal mattress suture is placed through 1.0 cm. lengths of polyethylene or Silastic tubing and then through the tarsal area of the eyelids, exiting in the denuded areas of eyelid margins. Suture is placed so that the knot remains on the upper eyelid bolster. Bolster and sutures are removed in three weeks. Fused upper and lower eyelids can be actively opened in the central area for vision. *C* and *D,* Temporary nonfusion tarsorrhaphy. Using #5–0 nylon sutures passed through bolsters of 1 cm. polyethylene or Silastic tubing, the eyelids may be closed by a simple horizontal mattress suture through the eyelid margins. This method protects the cornea while allowing a central opening of the eyelids for vision. The epithelium of the lid margin is left intact. (From Rankow, R. M., and Polayes, I. M.: Diseases of the Salivary Glands. Philadelphia, W. B. Saunders Company, 1976.)

type of tarsorrhaphy should be used when long-term recovery of the facial nerve is anticipated, or it can remain as a permanent fusion if indicated.

## STATIC FASCIAL SLINGS

Weakness at the corner of the mouth and after injury to the mandibular and buccal branches of the facial nerve with its attendant dropping and incompetent oral sphincter action on the affected side presents both disabling functional and cosmetic difficulties for the patient. Drooling is a constant problem while eating and drinking, and control of the normal accumulation of saliva is also a difficult task. When nerve repair has been performed by either primary anastomosis or nerve graft, the prolonged period of recovery before adequate functional return can be made more comfortable for the patient by the use of a supportive, static, fascia lata sling.[2, 12] This sling utilizes a strip of fascia lata taken as an autograft from the patient's thigh and split longitudinally as a "V" at one end. The split end is sutured to the orbicularis oris muscle of the upper and lower lips as well as at the oral commissure. The remainder of the fascia lata is passed upwards beneath and around the malar arch to be brought back down toward the oral commissure. By placing tension on the end of the fascia lata passed around the malar arch, correct elevation and positioning of the affected oral commissure can be determined when compared with the resting and active positions of the normal side. The correct tension is then secured by suturing the fascia lata to itself as well as to the periosteum of the malar arch to maintain the position of the oral commissure. Access to these areas is gained through incisions in the nasolabial fold, at the malar arch and in the upper and lower lips on the affected side. These incisions are kept small and in normal skin lines or folds so that scarring can be minimal.[33]

A static sling may also be used to correct a lagophthalmus in the affected lower lid resulting from facial nerve injury. Such a sling is used when a temporary fusion tarsorrhaphy cannot be performed or when full return of facial nerve function has not been realized. This procedure again utilizes autogenous fascia lata that is tunneled through the lower lid and fixed to the medial canthal ligament as well as to the temporal fascia. The fascia lata is fixed in position by #4-0 or #5-0 white silk sutures or clear proline suture material in both of the static slings described previously.

## ACTIVE MYOFASCIAL SLINGS

If facial nerve function has been lost permanently, the static fascia lata slings can be augmented by active muscle transfers to the fascia lata segments. The masseter muscle transfer has proved useful in adding an active component to an already existing static support.[1, 8, 33] The anterior third of the masseter muscle is split longitudinally to the level of its neurovascular supply, being careful to preserve nerve and vessels and is detached from the inferior border of the mandible along with a small attached portion of periosteum. The masseter segment is innervated by the fifth cranial nerve, and its site of origin from the malar arch makes it an ideal muscle to activate the static sling, since its direction of pull and action will elevate the corner of the mouth. This segment of muscle can then be rotated approximately 60° for insertion into the static sling.

In all cases in which static or active supports are used to correct facial nerve weakness, *overcorrection* to a slight degree is necessary to compensate for the amount of recurrent lag noted when healing is complete.

The use of an active temporal muscle–fascia transfer to activate paralyzed upper and lower eyelids has proved successful in restoring adequate but not perfect function to the eyelids. The procedure was originally described by Gillies.[15, 22, 23, 33] Meticulous attention to detail along with careful surgical technique is the important ingredient for a successful result in this procedure.

The temporalis muscle and fascia are exposed through a vertical temporal incision within the hair-bearing area. Parallel incisions are made in the superficial fascia from the level of the zygoma to the superior level of pericranial attachment of the muscle. Care must be taken to preserve the attachment of the temporal fascia to the superior edge of the muscle and pericranial tissue. The pericranium is incised 2.0 cm. above the level of muscle attachment and is then freed by lateral incisions slightly wider than the width of muscle to be used for the muscle–fascia transfer. This entire muscle segment is then carefully elevated off the underlying bone along with its intact neurovascular supply and peeled downward toward the malar arch. Only that length of muscle is elevated to allow for adequate rotation of the muscle–fascia segment into the lateral canthal area and eyelids. The remainder of the procedure involves splitting the attached temporal fascia longitudinally so that one fascia limb attached to muscle can be passed through the lower eyelid margin and the other can go through the upper eyelid margin. These two segments are then brought out through a medial canthal incision and are placed under sufficient tension to slightly overcorrect closure of the eyelids, at which point they are sutured to themselves as well as to the canthal ligament.

It is possible to pass these temporal fascia strips under the canthal ligament without injury to the lacrimal sac or duct. This provides for a more secure fixation of the fascia segments and less postoperative recurrent lid lag. The points to be carefully observed in this procedure are: (1) maintenance of continuity between temporal muscle and its fascial pericranial attachment; (2) adequate width of muscle along with its intact nerve and blood supply for rotation and transfer to a new position; (3) adequate support of upper and lower eyelid margins by careful subcutaneous placement of the fascia lata strips; and (4) careful maintenance of tension and suture fixation of the fascia lata strips in the medial canthal area. A temporary tarsorrhaphy is kept in place for four to six weeks while the transferred active temporal sling is allowed to heal in its new position.

## MYOMECTOMY

The paralyzed facial musculature resulting from loss of its facial nerve supply cannot be restored to perfect functional or aesthetic levels as compared with the normal side. The procedures described previously can restore a functional and aesthetically acceptable result. Further improvement can be gained by rhytidectomy procedures and in some cases by selective myomectomy.[24, 25] Rhytidectomy may augment static and active slings by utilizing a limited resection of soft tissue to further elevate the drooping cheek or brow. The myomectomy is used to selectively weaken the muscles of facial expression on the normal side and deemphasize the difference between normal and reconstructed areas.

## NERVE TRANSFER

Other methods of reconstruction following loss of facial nerve function involve transfer of functioning cranial nerve segments to the distal fibers of the transected facial nerve. The transfers often used are hypoglossal-facial nerves and spinal accessory-facial nerves anastomoses.[3, 19] The nerve transfers are successful to some degree but are often accompanied by unacceptable side effects with secondary deformities that impair patient function. The functional level obtained in most cases is not as good as that obtained by use of active muscle–fascia transfers or slings and nowhere near as good as the results obtained from nerve grafts or primary anastomoses. When the facial nerve has been transected, every effort should be made to reanastomose the transected segments when possible, aided by intraoperative magnification. When it is necessary to sacrifice segments of nerve because of tumor involvement, reconstruction by immediate nerve graft is the treatment of choice, if possible. When major segments or all of the peripheral branches of the facial nerve must be sacrificed in the ablative procedure, use of static and active muscle–facia transfers is indicated. These methods should be considered first before embarking on transfer of the hypoglossal or spinal accessory nerve trunk to innervate residual peripheral facial nerve segments. The secondary defect of a drooping shoulder or tongue weakness and slurred speech should not be considered inconsequential.

## NERVE GRAFT

Autogenous nerve grafts should be used to replace missing segments of the facial nerve as the treatment of choice to provide the best results for restoration of facial nerve function on the affected side.[4] The great auricular and lesser occipital nerves are the usual donor graft structures and are

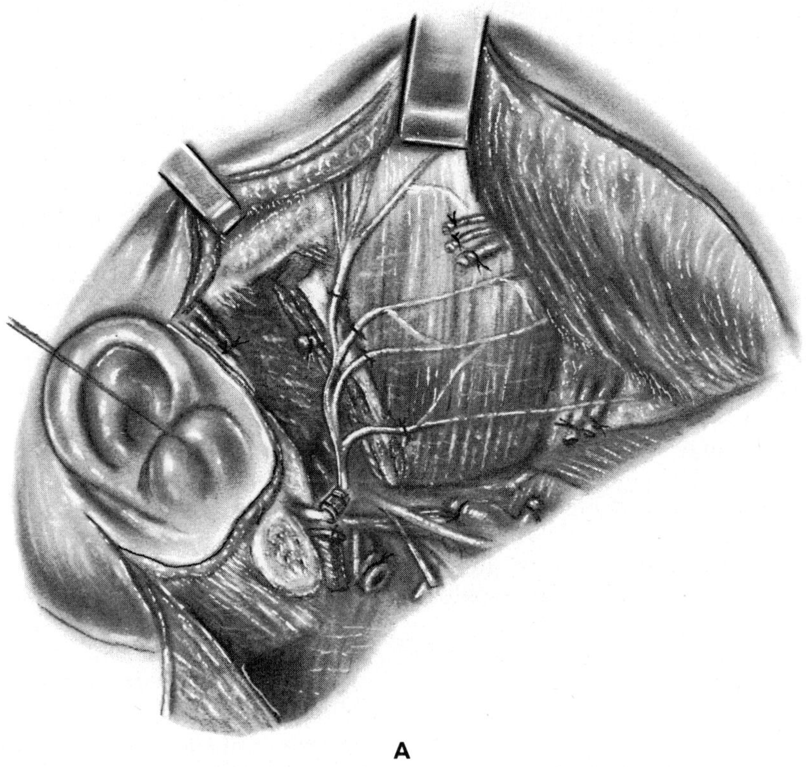


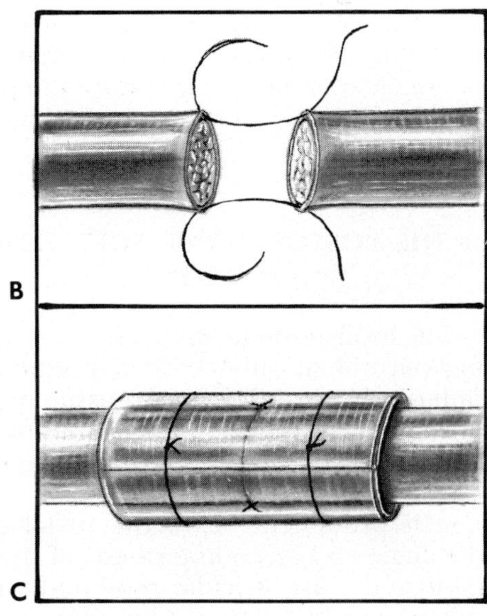


**Figure 14–12** *A,* The auricular nerve autograft is sutured in place to the proximal and distal stumps of the facial nerve. The graph should rest on the tissue bed to enhance vascularization and nourishment. It should not be tented across the defect but rather intimately follow its contours. *B,* The epineurium of the severed facial nerve, its branches and the graft are sutured to each other using #10–0 silicone-coated silk or nylon sutures with the aid of the operating microscope. *C,* Silicone, tantalum, polyethylene and millipore sheaths have been advocated by some surgeons to shield the nerve juncture between the main trunk and graft. It is possible that such shields may interfere with the mesoneural revascularization, and a meticulous microanastomosis remains the basic requirement. (From Rankow, R. M., and Polayes, I. M.: Diseases of the Salivary Glands. Philadelphia, W. B. Saunders Company, 1976.)

found adjacent to the surgical field of parotid surgery.[5, 29] Microanastomoses of the nerve graft to the transected facial nerve trunk and its branches have resulted in acceptable return of function in most cases in which meticulous technique has been used. The distance that the segment of nerve graft must bridge the severed nerve elements is the determining factor in the final result. The time element between reinnervation and degeneration of motor end plate segments within the muscle is the limiting factor to the degree of success in this procedure (Fig. 14–12).

Increasing experience gained with the use of the operating microscope in microvascular and microneural anastomoses involving free flaps, which may include both nerve and muscle segments, will most probably open up new and improved methods of restoring facial nerve function. Although theories explaining reinnervation of denervated facial muscle by neurotization through fifth nerve fibers have been proposed, they have not been proved.[26, 27, 37] Further proof of neurotization must be documented before the reinnervation of mimetic facial muscles can be credited to transfer of trigeminal motor segments. The autogenous denervated free skeletal muscle–tendon grafts described by Noel Thompson are interesting but still experimental.[35, 36] It is emphasized that the best chance for preserving normal facial muscle function is to preserve the integrity of the intact facial nerve or to immediately restore the severed facial nerve by direct neurorrhaphy or nerve graft.

## THE POSTOPERATIVE SOFT TISSUE "HOLLOW"[33]

The local aesthetic deformity accompanying parotid or submandibular gland excision consists mainly of a soft tissue deficit in the area of resection characterized by a hollow or depression covered by normal skin. The depressed area following parotid excision is prominent below the earlobe, over the angle and ascending ramus of the mandible in the preauricular zone outlining the site of parotid excision. The submandibular defect created by excision of the submandibular gland consists of a hollow in the digastric triangle. Although the aesthetic deformity in many patients may be minimal, it can be quite marked in others when compared with the normal facial contours of the opposite side. This is especially so in the "full-faced" patient. Dermal fat grafts have been used to fill out this hollow. Resorption over a period of time markedly reduces the cosmetic effect of the original graft, however.

Use of a composite pedicle flap (or myocutaneous flap) based on the mastoid area of the neck, "de-epithelialized" and rotated as a composite dermal pedicle flap under the depressed existing skin flap, can effectively fill out the concavity created by excision of the parotid gland. In most cases, the donor defect from the neck can be closed primarily. The very same flap can be elevated, "de-epithelialized" and rotated as a dermal composite flap into the digastric hollow created by a previous submandibular gland resection. The donor area of the upper neck can usually be closed primarily along the original line of incision used for the submandibular gland resection.

It is also possible to fill the submandibular hollow by use of a dermal fat pedicle flap developed at the time that a patient's "double chin" is reduced. Such a procedure provides the patient with reduction of a redundant chin while allowing use of the redundant fat as a dermal fat pedicle to be rotated posteriorly into the digastric hollow. In all cases, care must be taken not to injure the underlying branches of the facial nerve and the vascular supply to the pedicle. The rotated dermal composite flap is sutured to the margins of the hollow by absorbable Dexon #5-0 sutures and tacked along its edges to the undersurface of the overlying skin flap with the same absorbable suture material. This prevents shifting of the pedicle and distortion.

## EXTRAORAL AND INTRAORAL TISSUE LOSS[33]

Occasionally, loss of composite through and through soft tissue following resection of the parotid or submandibular gland from a previously irradiated area may result in a large orocutaneous fistula. This defect can be closed by several methods. Use of a neck-shoulder tube pedicle flap based on the mastoid-occipital area or a sternomastoid myocutaneous flap, however, is effective in bringing added blood supply to the area of radiation along with sufficient bulk of tissue to build out cheek contours. The distal pancake of this tube pedicle, when surfaced with a skin graft, provides lining for the mucosal surface of the defect while the intervening composite pedicle supplies the external skin surface of the cheek along with the bulk of fat and muscle, if necessary, to restore adequate cheek contour. At the same time, the remaining tube pedicle can be opened out, "de-epithelialized" and inserted beneath the original parotidectomy skin flap to fill out any remaining concavity as well as to provide added blood supply to the overlying irradiated tissues.

Major loss of the soft palate and glossopalatine arch may result in speech deficits as a complication of ablative surgery for tumors involving the minor salivary glands of the soft palate. The severity of this complication should not be underestimated, since it can interfere with the patient's livelihood and his or her return to society as a functional human being. Use is made of a lateral posterior cervical pedicle flap brought in to form a temporary oral cutaneous fistula at the angle of the mandible and joined to the remaining soft palate as well as to the ipsilateral glossopalatine arch. A superiorly based pharyngeal flap can be elevated at the same time to line the nasal surface of this pedicle flap. Skin grafts may also be used to complete that part of the flap's nasal lining not covered by the pharyngeal flap. It is necessary to determine the exact sites where the pharyngeal flap and skin grafts will be needed in order to provide nasal surface coverage of the entire transferred cervical pedicle flap. It is also important to attach the nasal lining to the pedicle flap before joining the oral surface of pedicle tissue to the remaining edges of the palate. Other sources for pedicle flap transfer to restore lateral pharyngeal wall, floor of the mouth, tongue or palate include the forehead, nasolabial and deltopectoral flaps.

## SALIVARY FISTULAS

Smaller salivary fistulas following parotid or submandibular surgical procedures often arise because the major salivary gland duct is obstructed and the normal egress of salivary fluid cannot occur. This fluid then accumulates proximal to the point of obstruction and eventually finds its way through the area of least resistance, namely, the area of surgical intervention or trauma. A drainage tract in the line of incision may arise at or through any point of weakness in the overlying skin flap. Sialography can be helpful in ascertaining the patency and competence of the major salivary ducts and often can pinpoint the site of obstruction. In the case of a segmental parotidectomy, postoperative accumulation of salivary fluid is common and usually subsides within two to three weeks, often requiring intermittent aspiration. When a definite salivary fistula persists several weeks or months after surgery, re-exploration of the site of surgery is indicated. Major duct transection may be found at the time of exploration, and this can be repaired over a Silastic catheter passed through the duct and secured at the oral opening by a #5-0 nylon suture. The duct is repaired by fine periductal #6-0 Dexon. The overlying fistula is closed by total excision of the fistulous tract and layer closure of the skin defect.

Small- to medium-sized oral cutaneous salivary fistulas through the cheek may be closed by use of both the skin margins at the common mucosal cutaneous opening of the fistula and the mucosal lining of the fistula. The skin surface of the communication can be incised, thus creating incontinuity flaps around and attached to the entire margin of the mucosal surface that can then be turned into the depth of the defect and sutured together, thereby closing the oral surface with skin and attached mucosa. The raw subcutaneous surface of this defect can then be covered by a cervical tube pedicle flap or rotation of a local composite cheek flap.

There are many methods being devised, such as free microvascular and myocutaneous flaps, that can also satisfactorily restore areas of soft tissue loss. Precise knowledge of the axial, cutaneous and myocutaneous blood supply, as well as of the limitations of random pattern flaps, must be understood by all surgeons involved in reconstructive surgery. The microanastomosis of a free flap adds a new dimension to restoration of major head and neck defects by enabling transfer of composite segments, including nerve, muscle, bone and cartilage. The future will most probably add even greater and more sophisticated techniques to the armamentarium of the reconstructive surgeon.

## Bibliography


1. Adams, W.: The use of masseter, temporalis and frontalis muscles in the correction of facial paralysis. Plast. Reconstr. Surg., *1*:216, 1947.
2. Brown, J. B., McDowell, F., and Fryer, M. P.: Facial paralysis supported with autogenous fascia lata. Ann. Surg., *127*:858, 1948.
3. Colman, C. C., and Walker, J. C.: Technique of anastomosis of the branches of the facial nerve with the spinal accessory for facial paralysis. Ann. Surg., *131*:960, 1950.
4. Conley, J. J.: Facial nerve grafting in treatment of parotid gland tumors. New techniques. Arch. Surg., *70*:359, 1955.
5. Conley, J. J.: Facial nerve grafting. Arch. Otolaryngol., *73*:322, 1961.
6. Converse, J. M.: Deformities of the eyelids and the orbital and zygomatic regions. *In* Kazanjian, V. H., and Converse, J. M. (eds.): Surgical Treatment of Facial Injuries. 3rd ed. Vol. 1. Baltimore, Williams & Wilkins Co., 1974, p. 628.
7. Converse, J. M.: Early treatment of facial injuries. *In* Kazanjian, V. H., and Converse, J. M. (eds.): Surgical Treatment of Facial Injuries. 3rd ed. Vol. 1. Baltimore, Williams & Wilkins Co., 1974.
8. Conway, H.: Muscle plastic operations for facial paralysis. Ann. Surg., *147*:541, 1958.
9. Eddey, H. H.: Parotid calculi. Aust. N.Z.J. Surg., *39*:225–231, 1970.
10. Eddey, H. H.: Recurrent parotitis and associated calculus, cyst or tumor. Med. J. Aust., *2*:581–585, 1969.
11. Foote, F. W., and Frazell, E. L.: Tumors of major salivary glands. Cancer, *6*:1065, 1963.
12. Freeman, B. S.: Facial palsy. *In* Converse, J. M. (ed.): Reconstructive Plastic Surgery. Philadelphia, W. B. Saunders Co., 1964.
13. Frey, L.: Le syndrome du nerf auriculotemporal. Rev. Neurol., *30*:97–104, 1923.
14. Friedman, W. H., and Pomarico, J. M.: The intratympanic correction of the Frey syndrome. Arch. Surg., *108*:366–368, 1974.
15. Gillies, H. D.: Experience with fascial lata grafts in the operative treatment of facial paralysis. Proc. Roy. Soc. Med., *27*:98, 1934.
16. Gordon, A. B., and Fiddian, R. V.: Frey syndrome after parotid surgery. Am. J. Surg., *132*:54, 1976.
17. Gore, D. O., Annamunthodo, H., and Harland, A.: Tumors of salivary gland origin. Surg. Gynecol. Obstet., *119*:1290, 1964.
18. Hobsley, M.: Amputation neuroma of the great auricular nerve after parotidectomy. Br. J. Surg., *59*:735–736, 1972.
19. Kessler, L. A., Moldover, J., and Pool, J. L.: Hypoglossal facial anastomosis for treatment of facial paralysis. Neurology, *9*:118, 1959.
20. Levy, D., Remine, W., and Devine, K.: Salivary gland calculi, J.A.M.A., *181*:1115, 1962.
21. Lowman, R. M., and Cheng, G. G.: Diagnostic roentgenology. *In* Rankow, R. M., and Polayes, I. M. (eds.): Diseases of the Salivary Glands. Philadelphia, W. B. Saunders Co., 1976, pp. 54–98.
22. Masters, F. W., Robinson, D. W., and Simons, J. N.: Temporalis transfer for lagophthalmos due to seventh nerve palsy. Am. J. Surg., *110*:607, 1965.
23. McLaughlin, C. R.: Permanent facial paralysis. Lancet, *2*:647, 1952.
24. Niklison, J.: Contribution to the subject of facial paralysis. Plast. Reconstr. Surg., *17*:276, 1956.
25. Niklison, J.: Facial paralysis; moderation of nonparalyzed muscles. Br. J. Plast. Surg., *15*:379, 1965.
26. Owens, N.: Preliminary report on development of neuromuscular functions by masseter muscle transplantations. Plast. Reconstr. Surg., *6*:491, 1950.
27. Owens, N.: Surgical treatment of facial paralysis. Plast. Reconstr. Surg., *7*:61, 1951.
28. Rankow, R. M.: Surgical decisions in the treatment of major salivary gland tumors. Plast. Reconstr. Surg., *51*:514–523, 1973.
29. Rankow, R. M.: An Atlas of Surgery of the Face, Mouth and Neck. Philadelphia, W. B. Saunders Co., 1968.
30. Rankow, R. M., and Mignogna, F.: Cancer of the sublingual gland. Am. J. Surg., *118*:790–795, 1969.
31. Rankow, R. M., and Polayes, I. M.: Diseases of the Salivary Glands. Philadelphia, W. B. Saunders Co., 1976, pp. 233–237.
32. Rankow, R. M., and Polayes, I. M.: Diseases of the Salivary Glands. Philadelphia, W. B. Saunders Co., 1976, pp. 311–313.
33. Rankow, R. M., and Polayes, I. M.: Diseases of the Salivary Glands. Philadelphia, W. B. Saunders Co., 1976, pp. 270, 327–330.
34. Rubin P., and Holt, J. F.: Secretory sialography in disease of the major salivary glands: Am. J. Roentgenol., *77*:575–598, 1957.
35. Thompson, N.: A review of autogenous skeletal muscle grafts and their clinical applications. Clin. Plast. Surg., *3*:349–403, 1974.
36. Thompson, N.: Treatment of facial paralysis by free skeletal muscle grafts. *In* Transactions. International Congress of Plastic and Reconstructive Surgery. 5th ed. New York. Appleton-Century-Crofts, 1971, p. 66.
37. Thompson, H., and Pollard, A. C.: Motor function in Abbe flaps. Br. J. Plast. Surg., *14*:66, 1961.

# 15 COMPLICATIONS OF NECK SURGERY

*Paul H. Ward*
*Herman A. Jenkins*

## PENETRATING WOUNDS OF THE NECK

The complex structure of the major vessels, nerves and important functional organs, such as the larynx, trachea, pharynx, esophagus and spinal column, are subject to many complications as a result of penetrating wounds in the neck. Complications encountered may be immediate or late and are related to injury of the *major vessels, digestive tract, respiratory tract* and *neurologic structures* coursing near or through the area. Many patients with injury to the major vessels of the neck and thoracic inlet die from massive exsanguinating hemorrhage or respiratory obstruction before reaching the emergency room. If the hemorrhage has been controlled with pressure, the next priority is the establishment of an airway by means of endotracheal intubation or tracheostomy. The latter is more appropriate if injuries are extensive or if there is massive transoral hemorrhage. A tracheostomy allows packing of the pharynx, if it is necessary for temporary control of intraoral bleeding.

The instruments most frequently responsible for penetrating wounds of the neck are knives, missiles (low- and high-velocity), steering wheels, dashboards, glass and wire cables. Knowledge of the type of instrument may provide some indication of the damage and complications that one may expect to encounter. For instance, a knife blade usually follows a straight course, and, if it is still in place, radiographs taken in two planes may provide information as to its location and the structural injury it may have inflicted (Fig. 15–1). High-velocity missiles (fired from high-powered rifles) cause massive injury to structures within their path and to surrounding tissues. Bones are shattered, vessels are penetrated and adjacent soft tissues are severely contused. The pathway of low-velocity bullets (fired from hand guns) may be diverted by the spine, mandible and other bones, by tissue planes and sometimes even by major vessels and their surrounding sheaths. Shotgun wounds are of intermediate velocity and produce multiple-entry sites with massively disrupted wounds (Fig. 15–2). High-velocity missiles often exit from the body; low- and intermediate-velocity missiles usually remain embedded in the soft tissues or bone.

The subsequent complications and eventual outcome are frequently predetermined at the time of injury. Often, however, impending and iatrogenically induced complications may be avoided with proper diagnostic assessment, appropriate surgical intervention, when indicated, and careful observation. Experience has proved that, unless there are signs and symptoms of significant structural injury to the major vessels, neurologic system or airway and digestive passages, careful evaluation and observation is the safest course of action. Routine exploration of all penetrating wounds of the neck has been advocated by Ashworth and his associates (1971),[1] Fogelman and Stewart (1956),[5] Sinkler and Spencer (1958)[13] and Yoder and Merck (1969).[19] The low mortality rate of 3 per cent and the small number of negative explorations (12 per cent) reported support the more conservative approach.[7-9, 11, 14] The high risk of anesthesia in patients who are in precarious states can thus often be avoided.

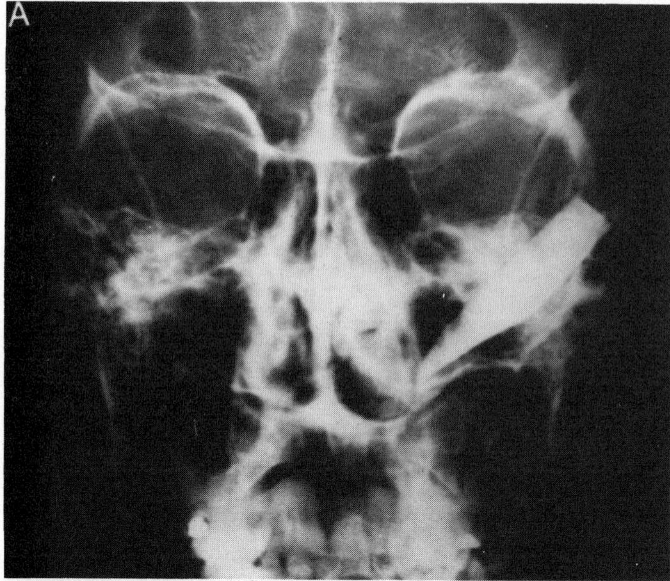


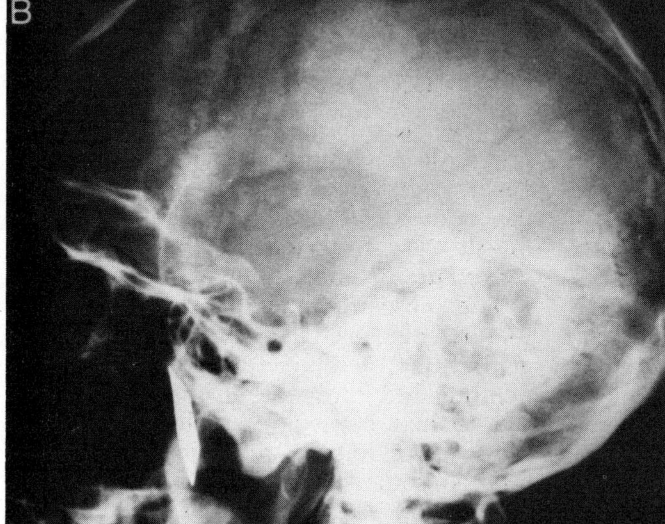


**Figure 15–1** Anteroposterior (*A*) and lateral (*B*) x-rays of knife blade in place. All major vessels were missed, and the patient was aware only of the entrance wound.

Exploration of the neck is mandatory when major vessel injury is suspected owing to the following: active hemorrhage, history of hemorrhage with hypotension, expanding cervical hematoma, extensive intraoral bleeding, chylous leakage, bruit, absence of pulses in extremities, progressive neurologic defect (due to compromised cerebral circulation), widening of the parapharyngeal space or mediastinum or airway compression. When these signs and symptoms are absent but vascular injury is suspected, arteriography and venography should be performed. Demonstration of arterial or venous damage, thrombosis or fistula or aneurysm formation calls for exploration.[3] Definitive diagnosis and treatment of the complications are approached by ligation of injured veins and arteries except for the common and internal carotids, which are repaired primarily when possible. Inclusion of vascular instruments in the surgical instrument set-up is mandatory for good preoperative preparation (Fig. 15–3). If the internal carotid injury is located at the base of the skull, ligation may be the only feasible method of control. It is generally recognized that ligation of the internal carotid

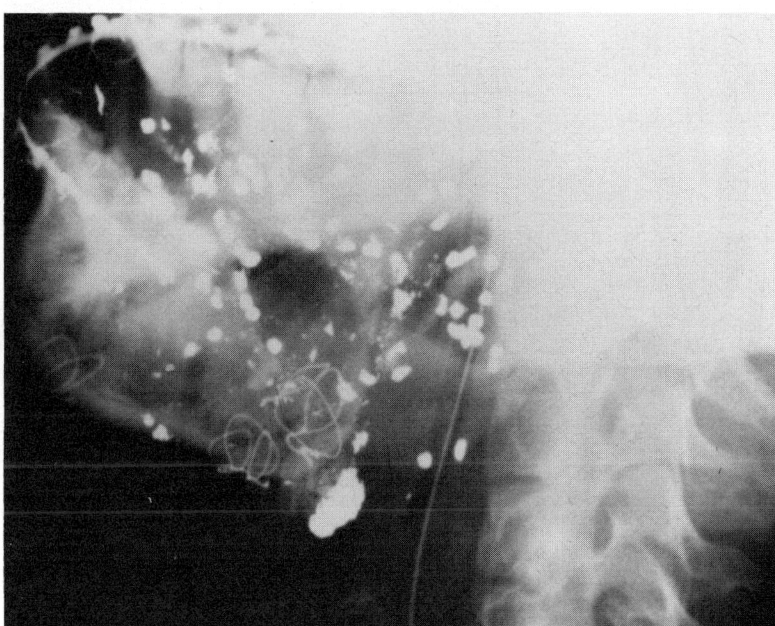

**Figure 15–2** Lateral x-ray with head tilted, showing repair with internal wiring and intermaxillary fixation of massive disruption of the mandible caused by shotgun wound. Note extensive residual metal foreign bodies, none of which penetrated major vessels or nerves.

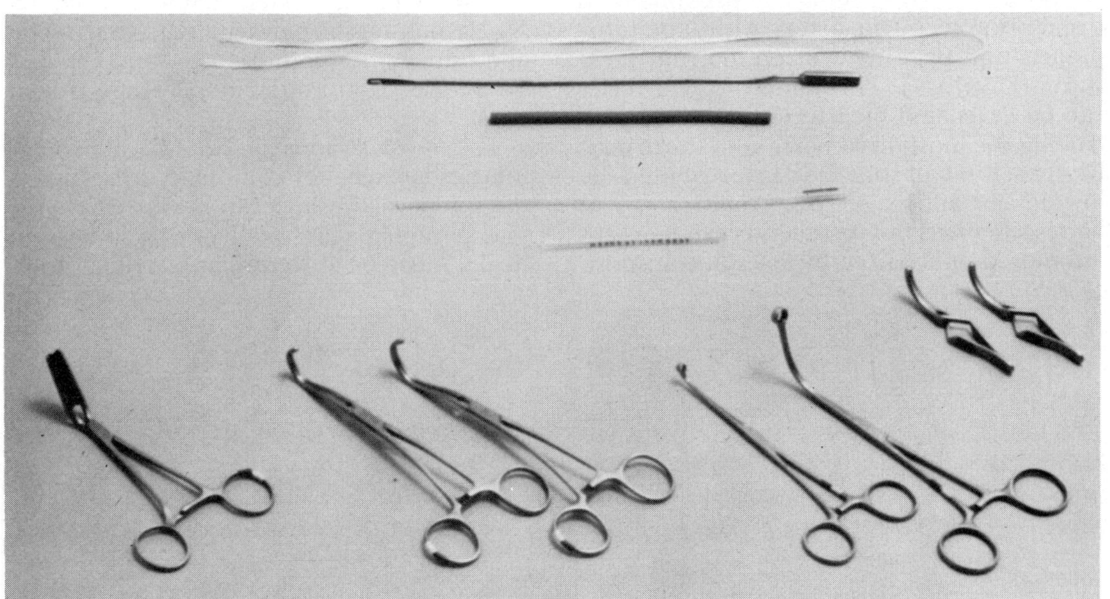

**Figure 15–3** Fogarty, Derra, Javid and Bulldog vascular hemostats, tape-rubber tourniquets and silicone internal shunt catheters.

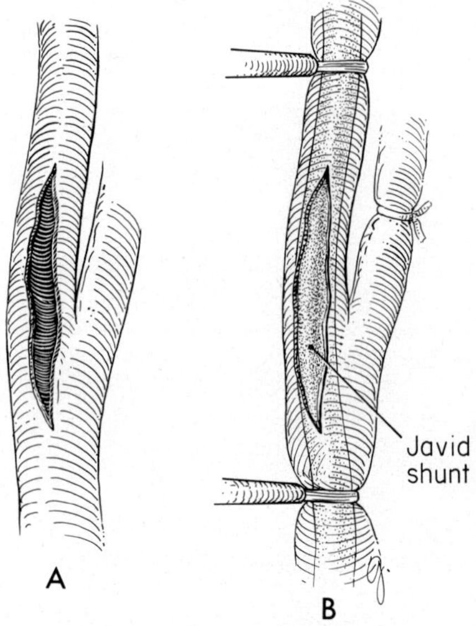


**Figure 15–4** Illustration of internal shunt in common and internal carotid arteries for continued perfusion of blood to the brain during vascular repair, end-to-end anastomosis or vein grafting.

artery will produce a hemiparesis in one third of the cases and a mortality rate of around 10 per cent. Contrary to common belief, the risks of hemiparesis are much greater in younger than in older people, who have developed more collateral circulation. Damage to the carotid arteries can be repaired after controlling the proximal and distal portions of the artery with tape tourniquets and placement of an internal Javid shunt (Fig. 15–4). Thrombus of the arteries can be evacuated by arteriotomy after controlling the most distal portion of the artery. Re-formation of the clot is prevented by low-dosage anticoagulants. Aneurysms can be resected and the vessel ends can be reanastomosed or repaired by arterial transposition or grafting. Arteriovenous fistulas can be doubly clamped with Derra or Satinsky vascular clamps and divided, and the defects in the vessels walls are sutured. Local injury to the arterial walls is repaired by achieving hemostasis with Derra clamps and transversely suturing the defect to diminish the reduction in lumen diameter (Fig. 15–5). Hematomas are evacuated and drained, and, since the wounds are contaminated, broad-spectrum antibiotic coverage is instituted.

The most serious of cervical neurologic injuries is partial or complete transection of the spinal cord, which can produce hemiplegia, paraplegia or quadriplegia. These injuries must be differentiated from similar

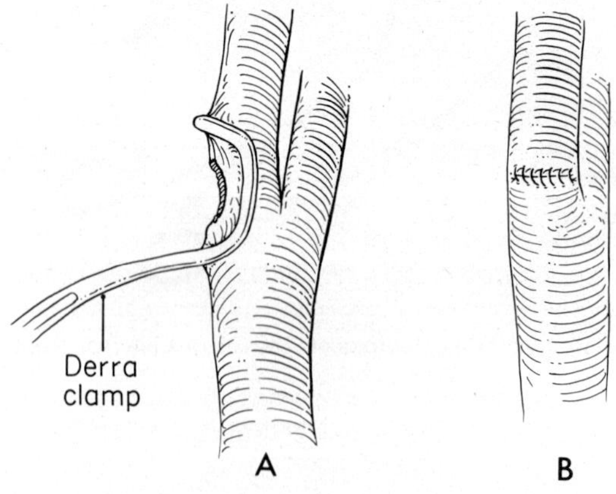


**Figure 15–5** Demonstration of the techniques of application of Derra clamp and repair of perforated vessel.

central nervous system damage resulting from penetrating wounds of the skull and major vessel injuries. Supportive treatment to prevent further injury to the spinal cord is indicated. Injuries to the IX, X and XII cranial nerves and sympathetic chain are relatively frequent and alone are not life-threatening; they often call attention to possible vascular injury in proximity to the respective nerves. During exploration, repair of these nerves may be attempted; however, regeneration of the most important nerve, the vagus, rarely results in effective reinnervation of the larynx.[16, 17] Likewise, repair of the brachial plexus should be attempted. Permanent defects persist, however, in 35 per cent of patients with injuries to the base of the neck.[9]

Penetration of the air and food passages requires exploration and repair except in the oropharynx and nasopharynx. Injury to the structures is evident from aphonia or dysphonia, respiratory obstruction and stridor, dysphagia, hemoptysis, saliva in the wound and a positive dye test or dye contrast study. Early exploration with primary closure and wound drainage may prevent the serious late complications of infection, abscess, mediastinitis, fistula and formation of strictures. Foreign bodies (e.g., metal and other debris) are removed if easily accessible, but extensive exploration with the risk of further tissue damage is not warranted. These patients often will spontaneously extrude pellets and lead particles for many years. Minor festering of these areas of extrusion is of little consequence. Development of an abscess or mediastinitis requires exploration and drainage.

## DEEP NECK INFECTIONS FOLLOWING HEAD AND NECK SURGERY

Infection of the neck following head and neck surgery is almost always secondary to an infected hematoma or may occur in heavily radiated patients in whom large flaps with compromised blood supply are overwhelmed by *Pseudomonas* or other gram-negative organisms. Rarely do these infections spread to the deep neck spaces, since they usually have been obliterated during radical surgery for laryngeal, pharyngeal or oropharyngeal tumors. In addition to hematomas, other contributing causes may be excessive blood loss without replacement, diabetes or other debilitating diseases.

Infections with abscess formation usually take several days to develop and more frequently occur in patients whose oral or pharyngeal cavities have been entered. Clinical features suggesting an infection or impending abscess formation are spiking fever, chills, malaise, weakness, presence of swelling or edema suggestive of underlying hematoma or serum accumulation under healing flaps, increased pain, thready pulse and increased respiratory rate. The presence of fullness sometimes with fluctuation underlying the skin flaps calls for immediate action. Failure to incise or reopen the wound and drain the serum or infected hematoma may result in further undermining and elevation of the flaps, with flap necrosis, spread of infection, exposure of major vessels and possible carotid blow-out. Spread of the infection into the pretracheal, retropharyngeal or prevertebral spaces may lead to fulminating mediastinitis. Septicemia results from invasion of the organism into the bloodstream and may in turn produce many life-threatening complications, such as bacterial endocarditis, meningitis, brain abscess or microabscesses in various other organs of the body.

Local wound breakdown may produce an oral, pharyngeal or esophagocutaneous fistula. The preferred solution for these serious complications is prevention. During surgery, dual hemostat application and division and ligation of the vessels with an appropriately fine suture using square-knot ties will diminish latent bleeding. Attention to wound cleansing and meticulous control of all bleeding vessels by irrigation of the wound with physiologic saline at the completion of the surgical resection may do little to remove bacteria but are of great value in removal of small clots in untied or inadequately cauterized vessels. Any residual bleeding from noncontrolled open vessels can be clamped and cauterized or tied.

Careful inverting suture closure of the oral, pharyngeal and esophageal mucosal edges with reinforcement of the suture line may diminish or prevent leakage of saliva into the wound. In recent years, the use of suction evacuation drainage of the wounds has considerably decreased the accumulation of blood under the flaps. Good subcutaneous tissue approximation and skin closure facilitate the creation of negative wound pressure and the collapse of the overlying skin flaps against the wound bed, with elimination of dead space. Successful use of the suction drainage requires attention to details, with immediate connection of the trap to suction in the operating room, recovery room, intensive care room and patient's room until a wound seal allows application of the negative pressure trap. A pressure dressing is not required if the wound suction is properly attended to; however, a good, evenly applied pressure dressing may be a safer back-up measure for the first day or two. A nonfunctioning, obstructed suction drainage may provide a false sense of security and an ineffectively applied pressure dressing may serve to cover up an accumulating hematoma. The absence of drainage or the presence of excessive suction drainage or excessive seepage of blood through the dressing calls for inspection of the wound. If significant hematoma is present, immediate reopening of the wound, evacuation of the hematoma and control of bleeding vessels under sterile conditions diminish the incidence of subsequent wound infections. The gentle, meticulous handling of tissues, use of fine suture material and closure of dead space also contribute to proper healing without the complication of wound infections.

The use of pre-, intra- and postoperative antibiotics whenever the oral cavity, pharynx, larynx or esophagus has been opened, particularly in heavily irradiated patients, is important in preventing infections. This judicious treatment of the contaminated wound should be directed toward the most likely culprits, streptococci and staphylococci, and consists of adequate parenterally administered therapeutic doses of broad-spectrum antibiotics.

In heavily irradiated patients, it is prudent to achieve wound closure without tension. This may sometimes mean removal of a segment of mandible to allow collapse of the tissues and closure of the mucosal margins without tension. The use of a pedicle flap (e.g., forehead or deltopectoral) may facilitate healing by bringing in additional blood supply and preventing tension upon suture lines. In other heavily irradiated patients and where extensive surgical removal of large tumors has been performed, the planned creation of a pharyngostome serves to prevent fistula formation, with leakage of saliva into the wound and dissection and undermining of the skin flaps. The pharyngostome, if small, may be allowed to close spontaneously or can be closed later with a local or regional pedicle flap.

Should any of the signs and symptoms of wound infection develop, immediate blood cultures, drainage of the wound with packing or insertion of a soft rubber drain and reapplication of gentle-pressure dressings are indicated. The principle of drainage is to evacuate and prevent the reaccumulation of blood or serum as well as to prevent further dissection of the skin flaps from their bed. Should there be infection in any unopened deep neck spaces, the skin flaps must be reopened widely enough to allow adequate dissection, evacuation and insertion of a drain into these spaces (e.g., pretracheal, retropharyngeal and prevertebral). When the carotid sheath space is involved, arteritis is produced. Exposure of the carotid artery beneath a necrotic flap requires immediate coverage with a vascular pedicle graft to prevent blow-out. Any significant bleeding from these infected wounds may be considered a "signal" of pending carotid blow-out and calls for exploration and ligation if necrosis of the carotid wall is evident. The risks of neurologic sequelae from ligation of the arteries must be accepted. At exploration, the dissection must be carried caudally along the common carotid and cephalically along the external and internal carotids until healthy vessel wall is encountered and can be successfully ligated.

Carotid blow-out is a disastrous emergency often resulting in fatality unless someone close to the patient responds appropriately. Pressure must be applied directly over the artery until bleeding is controlled (Fig. 15–6). The person applying the pressure should call for help and no effort should be made to find the bleeding site or to apply a hemostat, since this only results in further loss of blood. The operating room is alerted, an intravenous line is started and blood for typing and cross-matching is drawn. The patient and bed are rolled to the operating room. Only after adequate preparation

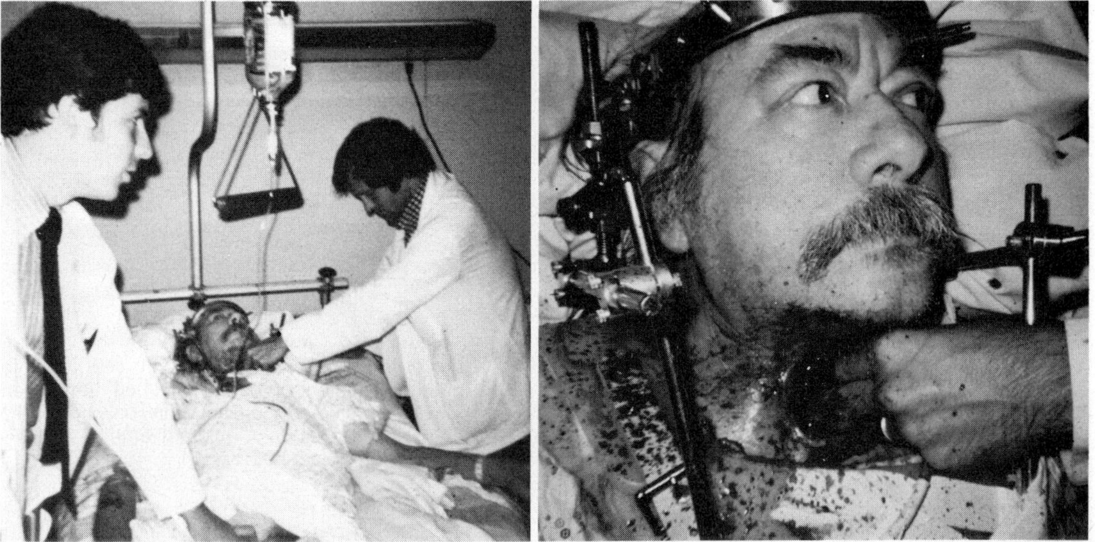

**Figure 15–6** Appropriate response to a carotid blow-out. Direct pressure is applied over the artery and assistance is called for to alert the operating room, start an intravenous line and take the patient to the operating room in his bed. Release of the pressure and definite exploration take place only after volume restoration and adequate preparation in the operating room.

(lighting, instruments, suction, blood volume replacement and adequate personnel for assistance) is the pressure released, the wound explored and the carotid vessels ligated. Hemiparesis remains a high possibility, but prevention of shock with maintenance of adequate perfusion of the brain through the opposite internal carotid artery diminishes the risk.

## COMPLICATIONS OF REPAIR OF PHARYNGOESOPHAGEAL (ZENKER'S) DIVERTICULUM

Zenker's diverticulum is generally considered to be a pulsion diverticulum occurring between the oblique and transverse fibers of the inferior constrictor muscle. This potentially weakened or congenitally deficient triangular area, known as Killian's triangle, receives the major portion of the pressure from a bolus of food passing from the hypopharynx into the esophagus just prior to the relaxation of the transverse circular (cricopharyngeal) muscle fibers. The diverticulum forms as the mucosa pushes through the weakened area and gradually enlarges as a true herniation as the muscle layer is thinned out and left behind. Surgical resection of the diverticulum and repair may result in the well-recognized complications of *stricture, abscess, fistula, reoccurrence* and *damage to the superior and recurrent laryngeal nerves*.[6, 16, 17]

*Stricture* of the hypopharynx and esophagus occurs as a result of removing excessive mucosa. Traction upon the mucosal diverticulum while dissecting the residual muscle fibers from its wall distorts the mucosal lumen. If particular care is not exerted, removal of excessive mucosa can produce a narrowed stenotic lumen. If the mucosal margins are inadequately approximated, accompanying infection ensues. Excessive fibrosis and scarring of the bed can produce further stricture of the narrowed area (Fig. 15–7).

Prevention of stricture by meticulous attention to details is superior to treatment of this complication. The preoperative or intraoperative introduction of a large (36–40 French) mercury bougie or an esophagoscope into the lumen of the upper esophagus facilitates identification of the appropriate area for amputation of the sac. The mucosal and muscular repair is easily accomplished prior to removal of the previously introduced intraluminal instrument.

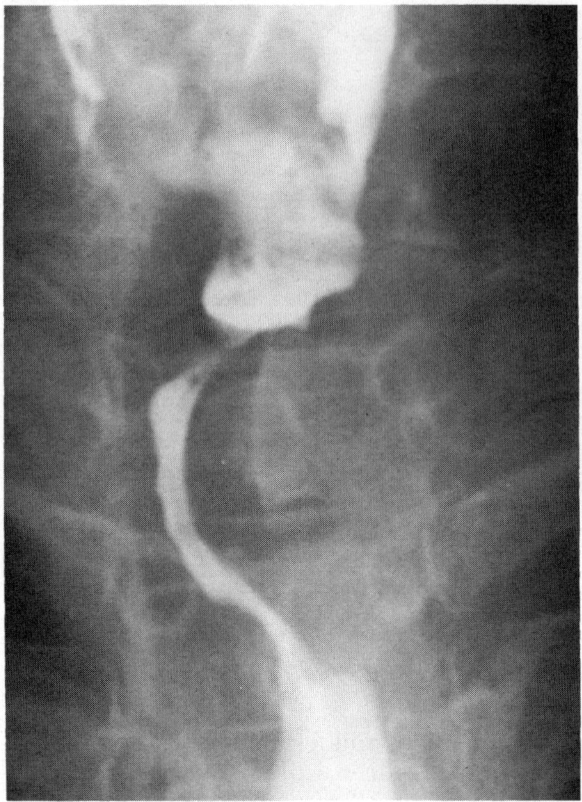

**Figure 15–7** Anteroposterior x-ray showing stricture of the esophagus following abscess formation (note indentation of barium-outlined lumen) and scarring. The lumen could be dilated only up to a #20 French bougie. Abscess required surgical drainage.

Entry of the esophagoscope or the bougie into the esophagus is sometimes difficult because the diverticulum may be large and the upper esophageal opening appears as a small orifice on the anterior wall.

Unless an extreme amount of mucosa has been removed, most strictures following repair of a Zenker's diverticulum can be treated by serial dilatations with mercury or other commonly used bougies. The dilatations are initially performed every several days, then weekly, every two weeks, monthly, and so on, increasing the time intervals until the desired lumen size is maintained without narrowing between dilatations. Severe strictures may require re-exploration and revision with Z plasty of the mucosal flaps or reconstruction of the esophagus with rotating deltopectoral skin flaps. If the stricture is several centimeters in length and cannot be managed successfully with dilatations or reconstruction with local tissues, then resection and colon replacement may be required.

Abscess and fistula of the esophagus are usually accompanied by inflammation of the surrounding tissues. Inadequate mucosal closure can allow the leakage of saliva and bacteria into the surgical wound, resulting in cellulitis, mediastinitis and abscess and fistula formation. The occurrence of any or all of these complications requires surgical drainage and appropriate antibiotic coverage in addition to maintenance of positive nitrogen balance and hydration by means of a feeding tube or a gastrostomy. Most of these latter complications heal without sequelae when so managed. An occasional permanent fistula with multiple abscess tracks or even a pharyngocutaneous sinus tract may persist, however. These require re-exploration, meticulous excision of the epithelial-lined tracks and reclosure of the freshened esophageal wall. The reinforcement with a vascularized muscle pedicle flap fashioned from the sternocleidomastoid or strap muscles facilitates healing.

Fistula formation is prevented by meticulously closing the mucous membrane with a running inverting suture and reinforcing it with interrupted sutures. Further support can be achieved by approximation of the stretched oblique muscle fibers and, if indicated, a pedicled prevertebral fascial or strap muscle graft. The transverse circular fibers of the cricopharyngeal muscle, presumably partially responsible for the formation of the diverticulum, are divided by an extramucosal cricopharyngeal myotomy.

*Reoccurrence* of the diverticulum as a complication takes place in 3 to 5 per cent of cases following resection and repair of a Zenker's diverticulum (Fig. 15–8). This complication is probably due to one or a combination of technical errors, such as performing an extramucosal myotomy to alleviate the obstruction, failure to remove adequate mucosa, or failure to adequately reinforce the defect.

Controversy exists as to the importance each of these factors plays in the reoccurrence. Persistence of a small diverticulum after inadequate resection certainly supports the third as a primary cause. If an extramucosal cricopharyngeal myotomy has been performed, the small residual sac may fail to enlarge significantly, and the patient may remain asymptomatic. The importance of removing the obstruction receives strong support from the concept upon which the endoscopic treatment of Zenker's diverticulum is based.[4] The tissues (including the cricopharyngeal muscle) between the diverticulum and the esophagus are divided transendoscopically. Posthealing cineradiography shows the barium passing freely from the diverticulum into the esophagus even though the diverticulum persists. A 7 per cent reoccurrence rate is reported, but repeated transendoscopic operations are simpler than reoperations through an external approach. Combinations of incomplete resection, inadequate repair and persistent obstruction would certainly appear to enhance reoccurrence. Prevention of reoccurrence is accomplished by avoidance of the technical errors described by giving meticulous attention to mucosal resection (de-

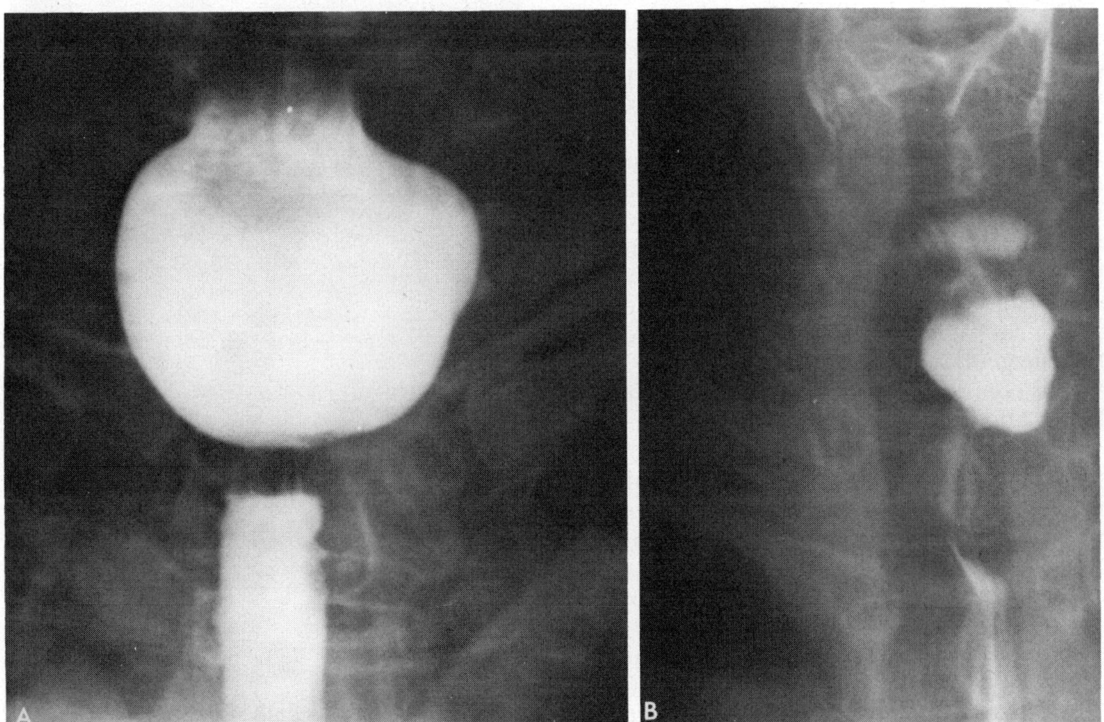


**Figure 15–8** Anteroposterior preoperative (*A*) x-rays of barium swallow and postoperative (*B*) residual or reoccurrence of Zenker's diverticulum.

scribed under stricture), extramucosal removal of the obstructing muscle and good mucosal repair with muscle reinforcement.

Damage to the recurrent and superior laryngeal nerves is not infrequent and may result from surgical trauma, retraction or devascularization. This complication of thyroid surgery is often passed off lightly unless the patient must use his voice professionally or both recurrent nerves are involved. The initial hoarseness is attributed to intubation or endoscopic trauma by those unable to visualize the larynx. Fortunately, the transient paralysis disappears and movement of the vocal cord returns. Even in most patients with permanent unilateral paralysis, compensation is achieved by the opposite vocal cord crossing the midline to obtain glottic closure. The problems encountered by paralysis of the recurrent and the external branch of the superior laryngeal nerves may be significant.[17] Paralysis of either of these nerves may terminate the career of the professional singer or speaker.

*Bilateral recurrent* nerve paralysis is a less common but much more severe complication, resulting in serious airway obstruction and calling for immediate tracheostomy. The voice may be fair after the patient awakens in the morning because the flaccid cords are near the midline. Severe inspiratory and expiratory stridor is highly indicative of bilateral nerve paralysis, and confirmation can be made by mirror examination of the larynx. Bilateral paralysis is a disaster requiring tracheostomy and subsequently arytenoidectomy, arytenoidopexy or nerve muscle pedicle grafting.[10, 16, 18]

Damage to the external branch of the superior laryngeal nerve can be prevented if the surgeon is aware of its location and avoids compressing it between the retractor blade and the thyroid alae of the larynx. The recurrent nerves are sometimes adherent to the walls of the sac, particularly when the sac is large. Preoperative endoscopic packing of the diverticulum with tracheostomy tape pushes the esophagus and trachea anteriorly, allowing identification of the posterior lateral aspect prior to the dissection of the sac. This area of the sac can be grasped with impunity, and, by cutting down to the mucosa and thereafter keeping the dissection immediately adjacent to the mucosa, the splayed out adventitia, muscle fibers and adjacent recurrent laryngeal nerve can be separated from the sac with less chance of damage to the nerves. When the diverticulum is large, traction may cause trauma to the opposite right recurrent nerve or may so distort its course that it can be injured during the dissection. The incidence of permanent nerve injury is probably even higher than the 3 per cent reported in the literature. Meticulous attention to surgical anatomic detail is essential if these complications are to be minimized.

Finally, a rare, unpleasant surprise and

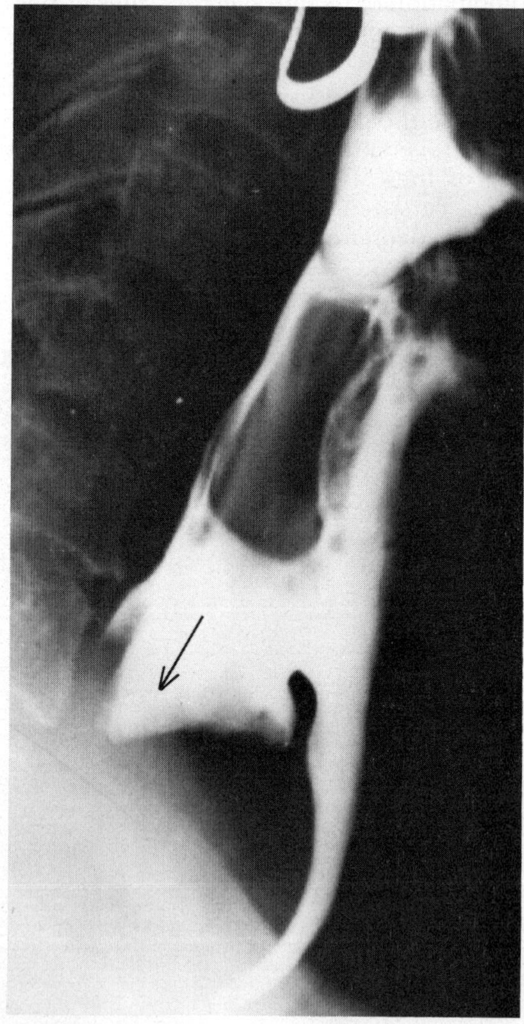

**Figure 15–9** Lateral x-ray of barium swallow showing large diverticulum that only partially filled (arrow). Endoscopy and biopsy revealed an epidermoid carcinoma arising within the diverticulum.

complicating factor may be encountered in the form of a carcinoma inside the diverticulum (Fig. 15–9). Awareness of the possible occurrence of such a lesion enables the surgeon to properly inform and prepare the patient preoperatively for wider resection and radical neck dissection, if indicated.

## PERFORATION OF THE CERVICAL ESOPHAGUS

Traumatic perforation of the cervical esophagus can occur as a complication of penetrating wounds of the neck, endotracheal intubation, esophageal intubation, ingested foreign bodies, endoscopy and bougienage. Cervical emphysema is usually the heralding sign. Pain in the neck and back, rapid pulse, elevated temperature and general toxicity indicate the onset of surrounding cellulitis and paraesophageal and mediastinal abscess formation. The perforation of the esophagus through a penetrating neck wound is usually accompanied by trauma and injury to other important structures and is an indication for exploration of the neck and repair. This was discussed earlier in the chapter.

Perforation of the pharyngoesophagus during hastily attempted peroral intubation has become a much more frequent occurrence with the increase in resuscitative sophistication. Most resident physicians are currently trained to establish an airway by rapid insertion of an endotracheal tube. Even in experienced hands, difficulties under these circumstances are encountered. The visualization of the landmarks of the larynx may be inadequate because of poor positioning, secretions and excessive movement from the external cardiac massage. Normally systematic and safe intubation may thus degenerate into blind thrusts of the tube toward the larynx. Endotracheal tubes, particularly when equipped with stylets, are potentially lethal weapons, capable of penetrating the delicate mucosa of the hypopharynx and cervical esophagus. Perforations, even in the hands of an experienced anesthesiologist, can occur during difficult intubation.

Experienced endoscopists have expressed concern over the potential hazards for perforation during emergency intubation when the emergency resuscitation crew blindly thrusts a tube into the esophagus, inflates a balloon and then ventilates the patient. There are surprisingly few reports of perforations from this device, however; the authors are aware of three cases of this complication. The paucity of reports probably does not represent the true incidence, since many of these patients die before reaching the hospital or are ill or injured to such an extent that perforations are overlooked and heal spontaneously.

The most frequent complication of esophagoscopy is perforation of the esophagus, which can also occur when a bronchoscope or a laryngoscope is forcefully introduced past the laryngeal lumen into the hypopharynx and cervical esophagus. Reverence and respect for the danger of these instruments increase with experience. Even highly skilled endoscopists periodically experience this disastrous complication.[12]

It is generally agreed among endoscopists that large tears or perforations require surgical exploration, drainage and repair. This is unequivocally true with perforations of the esophagus below the thoracic inlet. There is more confusion concerning the treatment of smaller perforations and in particular those located in the cervical area. Adherence to a "conservative" approach requires considerable experience and good judgment.[2, 12, 15]

Small perforations are a frequent complication of laryngoscopy, bronchoscopy and esophagoscopy, as manifested by an overall incidence of cervical emphysema in the range of 40 to 50 per cent as revealed by x-ray. Most of these cases go unrecognized, and those in which the emphysema is noted are treated by withholding oral intake and administering intravenous fluids and antibiotics for 24 to 48 hours. This conservative regimen for the treatment of small mucosal perforations has been successfully followed many times without complication. The abundant blood supply and rapid healing of tissues in the head and neck are probably responsible for the success of this type of management.

The diagnosis of the perforation is sometimes made during endoscopy. If a traumatic perforation is not recognized but is suspected, ingestion of radiopaque (iodinized) material or thin barium will facilitate identification and possibly give some indication of the size of the tear. Failure to demonstrate the leak of the contrast medium does not necessarily rule out the presence of a perforation. When a larger tear is recognized, it is most judiciously managed by immediate exploration of the neck with approximation and repair of the mucosa, just as is so successfully accomplished following radical surgery. The wound is drained, and rapid, uncomplicated healing is the rule. Immediate repair carries a much lower morbidity and mortality rate than does any attempt to perform primary closure several hours after secretions have entered the tissues and infection has become established.

If, after conservative management, a paraesophageal or mediastinal abscess develops, immediate exploration and drainage through a collar incision (or, if indicated, a thoracotomy) are performed; good drainage must be established. A nasogastric feeding tube can be inserted gently or a gastrostomy may be performed. Continued withholding of oral intake, use of expectoration or suction aspiration of saliva and continuation and increase in appropriate antibiotic coverage are essential.

Prevention of esophageal perforation is much preferred to the treatment of this often disastrous complication. Even in emergency situations, an awareness of the anatomy and of the delicate nature of the esophagus should engender sufficient respect that instrumentation of any variety is performed with maximum gentleness.

## Bibliography


1. Ashworth, C., Williams, L.F., and Byrne, J.J.: Penetrating wounds of the neck: Re-emphasis of the need for prompt exploration. Am. J. Surg., *121*:387–389, 1971.
2. Boyd, D.P., and Whittmann, C.J., Jr.: Some principles in treating perforations of the esophagus. Surg. Clin. North Am., *51*:567–574, 1971.
3. Calcaterra, T.C., and Holtz, G.P.: Carotid artery injuries. Laryngoscope, *82*:321–329, 1972.
4. Dohlman, G., and Mattson, O.: The endoscopic operations for hypopharyngeal diverticula. Arch. Otolaryngol., *71*:744–752, 1960.
5. Fogelman, M.J., and Stewart, R.D.: Penetrating wounds of the neck. Am. J. Surg., *91*:581–596, 1956.
6. Holinger, P.A., and Schild, J.A.: The Zenker (hypopharyngeal) diverticulum. Ann. Otol. Rhinol. Laryngol., *78*:679–688, 1969.
7. May, M., Lee, C., Sapote, P., et al: Penetrating wounds of the neck: Selective exploration, a study of 100 cases. Trans. Am. Acad. Ophthalmol. Otolaryngol., *75*:496–509, 1971.
8. May, M., Chaudaratana, P., West, J. W., et al: Penetrating neck wounds: Selective exploration. Laryngoscope, *85*:57–75, 1975.
9. May, M., Tucker, H., and Dillard, B.: Penetrating wounds of the neck in civilians. Otolaryngol. Clin. North Am., *9*:361–391, 1976.
10. Montgomery, W.W.: Surgery of the Upper Respiratory System. Arytenoidectomy. Philadelphia, Lea and Febiger, 1973, pp. 445–558.
11. Shirkey, A.L., Beall, A.C., and DeBakey, M.E.: Surgical management of penetrating wounds of the neck. Arch. Surg., *86*:955–963, 1963.
12. Simpson, J. S., Ruff, T., and Fearox, B.: Esophageal perforation during esophagoscopy in children. Ann. Otol. Rhinol. Laryngol., *83*:725–728, 1974.
13. Sinkler, W. H., and Spencer, A.D.: The importance of early exploration of vascular injuries. Surg. Gynecol. Obstet., *107*:228–234, 1958.
14. Stein, A., and Seaward, P.D.: Pentrating wounds of the neck. J. Trauma, 7:238–247, 1967.
15. Talbot, J.H.: Conservative management of esophageal perforations. J.A.M.A., *193*:537, 1965.
16. Tucker, H.M.: Human laryngeal reinnervation. Laryngoscope, *84*:769–779, 1976.
17. Ward, P.H., Berci, G., and Calcaterra, T.C.: New insight into superior and recurrent laryngeal nerve paralysis. Ann. Otol., *86*:724–736, 1977.
18. Woodman, D.G.: A modification of the extralaryngeal approach to arytenoidectomy for bilateral abductor paralysis. Arch. Otolaryngol., *43*:63–65, 1946.
19. Yoder, R.L., and Merck, D.E.: Innocuous appearing stab wounds to the neck. Is exploration always indicated? South. Med. J., *62*:113–115, 1969.

# 16 COMPLICATIONS OF TONSILLECTOMY AND ADENOIDECTOMY

*John D. Donaldson*
*Sylvan E. Stool*

Tonsillectomy and adenoidectomy are among the most frequently performed surgical procedures. Although considered by many to be a minor procedure, they carry a significant risk in both the child and the adult. The death rate from the procedure has been estimated to occur between 1 in 3000 and 1 in 27,000.[14] In the United States, this translates to between 40 and 350 deaths per year. The morbidity rates are impossible to calculate; they are obviously many times greater than the mortality rate. In some cases, the patient may receive an excellent surgical procedure but mismanagement of the complications results in prolonged morbidity and mortality. Many of the complications may be prevented by careful preoperative evaluation and attention to details of surgical technique. Even in the most carefully selected patient, who receives the best operative procedure, some complications will invariably occur, and these must be treated promptly and vigorously.

## PREOPERATIVE ASSESSMENT

The major concerns of preoperative assessment are the presence of airway obstruction, inflammation and the possibility of bleeding disorders.

### The Airway

One of the frequent indications for tonsillectomy and adenoidectomy is the presence of airway obstruction. This is usually manifested in the child by mouth breathing, snoring and, occasionally, difficulty in swallowing. In severe cases, airway obstruction may result in cardiovascular abnormalities with development of cor pulmonale. When patients present with severe airway obstruction, the physician must evaluate not only the local condition but also the cardiovascular status and correct any evidence of failure prior to the surgical procedure. Evaluation of airway obstruction by assessment of the size of the tonsils in relationship to the airway and evaluation of the degree of adenoid hypertrophy can be accomplished by physical and radiographic examinations. Lateral cephalometric films are helpful in assessing the degree of nasal obstruction and the location of the adenoid pad.

In recent years, there has been an increased interest in the relationship of tonsil and adenoid hypertrophy to the sleep apnea syndrome.[10] These children and adults develop respiratory obstruction during sleep and have cardiovascular abnormalities secondary to this respiratory obstruction. It is extremely important when the surgeon is contemplating an operative procedure that this be evaluated, since it is necessary to advise the anesthesia staff and the parents that there may be prolonged morbidity. Although it is not a complication of adenoidectomy and tonsillectomy, the hesitancy to perform the procedure may result in prolonged respiratory obstruction with subsequent cardiovascular complications, making the procedure ultimately more hazardous.

Examination of the mouth and the relationship of the mandible to the airway is extremely important in preoperative assessment of the possibility of airway obstruction. The presence of orthodontic appliances should be noted, as these appliances may interfere with the administration of anesthesia and performance of the surgical procedure. There is a possibility that such appliances may be dislodged and aspirated or ingested during the procedure.

Examination of the palate for its length, mobility and the presence of a submucous cleft should be part of every preoperative assessment. If there is any question regarding the speech mechanism, consultation with a speech pathologist may be advisable. It also may be appropriate to advise the parents of this finding.

### Inflammation

One of the frequent major indications for tonsillectomy and adenoidectomy is recurrent inflammatory disease. Inflammatory disease may occur very rapidly in children and result in an increase in morbidity of the procedure. Preoperative assessment for acute inflammation is necessary since the child may become ill within a few hours before the procedure is performed. In general, it is wise to try to eliminate as much of the acute inflammatory disease as possible and to avoid surgery during episodes of acute sore throat or nasopharyngitis in order to avoid the increase in capillary bleeding and bacteremia secondary to manipulation.

### Bleeding Disorders

Bleeding disorders are responsible for some of the complications of any surgical procedure. The methods of evaluation for bleeding disorders have been covered previously in the text (Chapter 5). A history of oozing from a dental extraction or similar procedures should alert the examiner to possible coagulation defect; history is one of the most important aspects of evaluation. In general, prothrombin time, bleeding time, partial thromboplastin time and platelet count are felt by most surgeons to constitute an adequate preoperative screening.[17] In some instances, evaluation for sickle cell disease may be indicated, especially in patients of African or Mediterranean descent. It is not unknown for an individual who appears to be in otherwise good health to have sickle cell crisis during the anesthetic and subsequent operative procedure.

## INTRAOPERATIVE COMPLICATIONS

### Anesthesia

It is important that the anesthesiologist evaluate the patient prior to the administration of premedication and anesthesia. In his evaluation, the status of the patient's airway should be noted and the general condition ascertained. This is important since many preanesthetic regimes are based on the patient's age; in children, however, it is extremely important that dosages of premedication be ordered according to weight. In children who have surgery for tonsil and adenoid hypertrophy, there is frequently an element of airway obstruction. Excessive premedication may depress respiration and the child may hypoventilate as a result. With the respiratory obstruction from the tonsils and adenoids superimposed, he may become hypoxic. In those cases in which there is marked respiratory obstruction, the anesthesiologist should omit the narcotic or hypnotic premedication or else provide constant monitoring for the sedated child.

In recent years, it has become the custom in most hospitals to use endotracheal intubation as the preferred route of anesthetic administration for tonsillectomy and adenoidectomy. The reasoning for this is that it provides better control of the airway and prevents aspiration of blood and secretions. There are institutions where insufflation anesthesia has been used for a number of years, and, in skilled hands, this is probably still an acceptable method of anesthesia. Whichever method of delivery of anesthetic agents is chosen, the surgeon and anesthesiologist must provide a patent, secretion-free airway. We prefer to use the RAE tube in conjunction with a McIvor-Sorenson mouth gag. This tube is preformed in a V shape, so that after placement it is centered over the tongue, held in place with the tongue blade and connected to a BAIN circuit over the chest. It is then firmly secured to the chin and the tongue, leaving the surgeon good visibility without moving the endotracheal tube from side to side. This arrangement prevents accidental displacement or kinking of the tube.

As with all patients under general anesthesia, the body functions must be continuously monitored. The minimum requirements are a precordial stethoscope and a blood pressure cuff. Most institutions now provide electronic monitoring of the patient's core temperature, since sudden and precipitous rises in temperature may occur, indicating malignant hyperpyrexia. All inhalation anesthetics are known to trigger this in susceptible individuals, with the combination of succinylcholine and halothane most frequently implicated numerically.[3] When core temperature is seen to rise precipitously, the operation should be terminated immediately and therapeutic measures should be instituted.[16]

Electrocardiographic monitoring is an excellent adjunct to the use of the precordial stethoscope and should be used whenever possible. It aids in rapid diagnosis of most of the dysrhythmias encountered when operating in the mouth using a suspension mouth gag. The digital readout provided by most modern cardiac monitors, together with the continuous visible tracing, provides instant reference for rate, rhythm and other abnormalities.

An intravenous infusion should be established in all tonsillectomy patients during the procedure, and it is probably wise, but not essential, to maintain this infusion overnight following the surgery. The intravenous is required for the administration of medication and fluid during surgery and may be used to supplement oral intake to maintenance levels postoperatively. If there are complications during the immediate postoperative period, fluid replacement will not be delayed because of difficulty in starting an intravenous infusion in a child who is in vascular collapse.

## Hemorrhage

Hemorrhage is the most frequent intraoperative complication of adenoidectomy and tonsillectomy. The surgeon must conscientiously monitor the amount of blood lost during the procedure, including an estimate of the amount of blood on the sponges. He must be aware of the patient's total blood volume as calculated in relation to the patient's weight. Multiplication of the patient's weight in kilograms by 70 or 80 milliliters will usually give an approximate volume in children. In general, a 10 per cent loss will cause concern; a 15 per cent blood loss should initiate replacement. The easiest way to reduce blood loss is to perform only the indicated operation. At times, this may be an adenoidectomy or a tonsillectomy alone. This principle seems especially true in older children and adults, in whom adenoid hemorrhage is frequent.

There continues to be much debate over surgical methods, and it is likely that no one technique has distinct advantages over another, provided the dissection is relatively atraumatic and the removal of the lymphoid tissue is complete. A few aspects of surgical technique are important and should be observed. The posterior nasal septum should be guarded from trauma. Dissection should not proceed from one area to another without first attaining reasonable hemostasis in the dissected area. For example, removal of a second tonsil without controlling bleeding from the bed of the first by packing or suture does not seem prudent. If sutures are used, their placement should be such that the vascular and neurologic structures lateral to the fossa are not violated. Similarly, the creation of blind pockets within the fossa should be avoided if the pillars are closed with sutures. If topical or chemical cautery such as silver nitrate is used, the excess chemical should be neutralized before the patient swallows. Before the termination of the procedure, complete hemostasis should be obtained, the mouth gag should be relaxed and the patient should be allowed to swallow and the pharynx reinspected.

There has been considerable difference of opinion regarding the best methods of control of bleeding in the tonsillar fossa. It varies among those individuals who prefer using some type of pack with pressure, cautery, either chemical or electrical, and various suture techniques. A number of articles have been written praising or condemning each of these techniques.[13, 19] All methods are probably effective when used appropriately.

Nasopharyngeal hemorrhage after removal of adenoids may be due to incom-

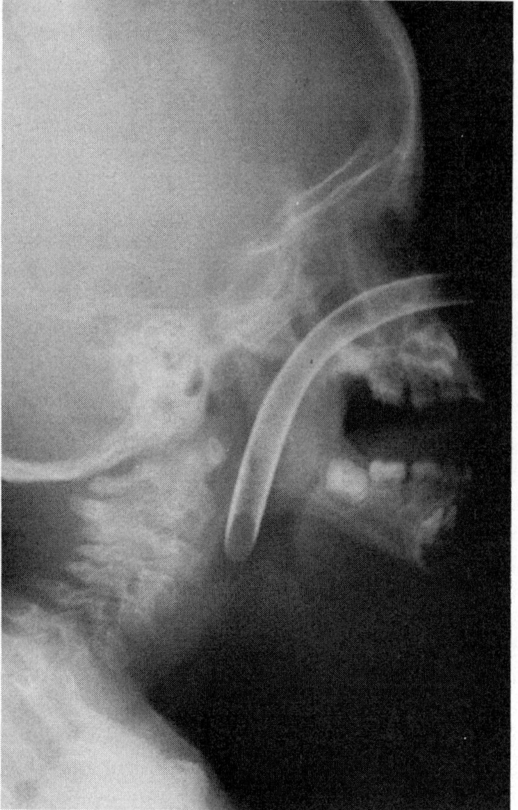

**Figure 16–1** Lateral radiograph of a patient with postnasal packing and a nasopharyngeal airway.

plete removal of lymphoid tissue or trauma to the nasal septum. Visual or manual inspection should be carried out to insure complete removal of all lymphoid tissue. If there is continuous blood loss from the nasopharynx, a posterior pack tailored to the location of the bleeding and the size of the nasopharynx should be inserted. The postoperative discomfort and airway obstruction may be relieved by the use of nasopharyngeal airway in conjunction with the packing (Fig. 16–1). This technique is of value in insuring the airway should there be swelling of the palate with subsequent increase in airway obstruction.

## Instrumentation

### DENTAL INJURIES

The use of muscle relaxants in conjunction with mouth gags is a boon to the surgeon. The combination may lead to inadvertent temporomandibular joint dislocation early in the procedure while the relaxant is still effective, however. Apart from minor postoperative discomfort, immediate recognition and reduction of the joint result in few sequelae.

The surface of the teeth may be damaged by the insertion of the mouth gag or, as previously mentioned, by injudicious use of the laryngoscope. This may be avoided by proper application of these instruments.

Primary teeth are frequently loose in the age group that undergoes tonsillectomy and adenoidectomy. In many instances, they should be removed prior to insertion of the mouth gag. Loose teeth may constitute a danger in the postoperative period, when they could be aspirated. Permanent teeth may be damaged during the operative procedure. This can occur in a number of ways. The most vulnerable patient is a child with a malocclusion characterized by overbite of the maxillary incisor teeth. The danger of damage is greatest when the incisors are first exfoliated because the peridontal membrane does not hold the teeth securely. Accidental pressure from the intraoral gag against these teeth may result in their removal. Should this accident occur, it is important that they be replaced promptly. If possible, a dentist should be consulted immediately. Under any circumstances, it is important that the tooth be kept moist. This can be accomplished by wrapping it in gauze soaked in saline. There is some difference of opinion among dentists as to whether a pulpotomy should be performed. If dental consultation is not immediately available, the tooth should be replaced in the socket and retained by either an acrylic splint or, if this is not immediately available, by wiring it to adjacent teeth.[5, 9]

Adults will immediately notice even the most minor chip on dental surfaces. Most of the smaller variety will respond to polishing by a dental colleague. Larger chips involving any portion of the tooth deep to the enamel require dental consultation and at least temporary capping.

### CARDIAC ARRHYTHMIA

Cardiac arrhythmia may occur during tonsillectomy and adenoidectomy. The arrhythmia may arise from vagal stimulation created by suspension of the mouth gag mediated through the superior laryngeal nerve. Carotid sinus stimulation may cause bradycardia. These generally are easily managed by the administration of appropriate blocking agents, such as atropine, and by deepening the anesthetic. Multiple ventricular contractions or bigeminy is suggestive of airway obstruction or hypovolemia. Again, the procedure should be suspended by relaxing the mouth gag and regaining control by correcting the deficiency. Malignant hyperpyrexia is also known to cause cardiac arrhythmias, probably secondary to acidosis. Occasionally, the simple maneuvers mentioned here do not resolve the problem, and the patient requires other medication, such as lidocaine. Hemostasis must be gained immediately, and the procedure should be terminated.

### PHARYNGEAL TRAUMA

Although the surgeon may be extremely competent, it is possible that during the instrumentation there may be trauma to the other structures of the pharynx. This can occur because of the effect of the suction used to remove blood or secretions being applied to tissue, resulting in marked postoperative edema. During intubation, if the patient is not satisfactorily relaxed, there may be trauma from instrumentation with the laryngoscope. In most instances, if the trauma is superficial, it results only in slight discomfort; however, it is possible that this pharyngeal trauma may lead to abscess formation in the retropharyngeal or lateral pharyngeal regions.

### EYE INJURIES

Since the surgeon is operating about the head, it is important to protect the eyes from drying and instrumentation. There is some controversy among surgeons as to whether the eyes should be taped shut or remain exposed so that the lids can be constantly visualized. The majority of surgeons doing tonsillectomy and adenoidectomy seem to prefer that the eyes have an application of inert ointment with tape applied to shut the lids.

**TABLE 16–1** SBE PROPHYLAXIS*

**The Following Should Be Given if Not Allergic to Penicillin:**

*One hour* prior to the procedure:
Penicillin VK 2.0 gm. by mouth
*Following the procedure*
Penicillin VK 500 mg. by mouth 4 times a day for the remainder of the day of the procedure and for the next 2 days
*For children less than 25 kg.*
Penicillin VK 500 mg. by mouth initially followed by 250 mg. 4 times a day
OR
*By injection if necessary*
Aqueous Penicillin G (30,000 units/kg) mixed with procaine
Penicillin G (600,000 units IM)
*Following the procedure*
Penicillin VK orally (same as above)

**The Following Should Be Given if Patient Is Allergic to Penicillin or Rheumatic Fever Prophylaxis**

Erythromycin 20 mg./kg. orally (maximum 1 gm.) 2 hours prior to the procedure followed by 10 mg./kg. (maximum 500 mg.) 4 times a day for the remainder of the day of the procedure and the next 2 days.

*Recommendation of the American Heart Association.

### BACTEREMIA

A number of studies have revealed that with operations in the mouth, such as extraction of teeth or tonsillectomy and adenoidectomy, there is usually a bacteremia. Despite the fact that in the healthy individual this usually results in very little morbidity, there are groups of patients who have cardiac or renal defects in whom bacteremia may result in carditis or nephritis. For this reason, it is important when operating on these patients that they be provided with adequate prophylaxis. The prophylaxis that is proposed by the American Heart Association for prevention of subacute bacterial endocarditis is shown in Table 16–1.

## IMMEDIATE POSTOPERATIVE PERIOD (0 TO 24 HOURS)

### Hemorrhage

In the first 24 hours following surgery, hemorrhage remains the most frequent complication. This problem is complex because the patient is not anesthetized. The younger child is apt to be crying and uncooperative. He may be vomiting blood and will be very apprehensive. Older children and adults may be unwilling to open their mouths so that the site of bleeding can be inspected.

This condition may become apparent either by the spitting out of large clots of bright red blood or vomiting large quantities of dark blood. The operative sites must be inspected in any patient in whom bleeding is evident. The formation of clots in the tonsillar fossa is indicative of a continuous oozing. Although one would imagine that a clot would stop the bleeding, maintenance or prolongation of this process is probably due to the anticoagulation effect at the edge of a clot.[2]

Minor bleeding can usually be managed without anesthesia. Inspection of the operative site with removal of the clot will often suffice. Topical vasoconstrictors, such as phenylephrine hydrochloride (Neo-Synephrine), ephedrine or epinephrine, may be effective. Tannic acid powder mixed into a paste with epinephrine and lidocaine has also been used for these minor hemorrhages. This paste is held on a sponge in the area of the hemorrhage for five minutes by the clock with the patient sitting forward. In general, it is important not to persist with these measures unless they are immediately effective.

Bleeding of a more severe nature or continued uncontrolled oozing is best managed by examination under general anesthesia. The anesthetic management of these cases is extremely difficult, but after careful suctioning and establishment of an intravenous route of medication, the patient can usually be intubated with a rapid sequence induction.[1] This involves inducing anesthesia with rapid-acting intravenous medications quickly followed by a depolarizing muscle relaxant. Applying cricoid pressure helps prevent regurgitation and rapid intubation. The tonsil and adenoid fossae can then be examined and hemostasis can be established. The patient must not be hypovolemic prior to the induction of this "crash technique." After intubation, a suction should be passed into the airway through the endotracheal tube. If blood is found, irrigation with sterile saline and suctioning

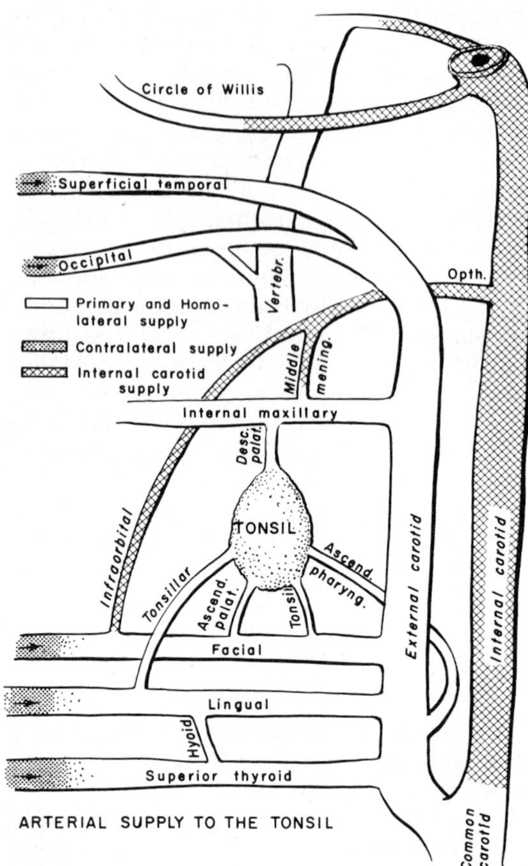


**Figure 16–2** The blood supply of the tonsil, showing the anastomosis between the contralateral external carotid artery and the homolateral internal carotid artery.

until clear should be carried out. Prior to termination of this procedure, the stomach should be emptied and a record made of the type and quantity of the contents.

There are a number of techniques that may be utilized to control this hemorrhage. If an isolated vessel is found to be the bleeding site, it may be ligated. Occasionally, areas may be controlled with electrocoagulation. In some instances, the bleeding may be rather generalized in the tonsillar fossa, and an alternate technique is to apply several layers of oxidized sponge, such as Surgicel, to the fossa, closing it with interrupted sutures by stitching the anterior and posterior pillars together. Occasionally, not one of these techniques is effective, and it is necessary to ligate the external carotid arteries. In ligating the external and carotid arteries, it is important that not only the main trunk be ligated but also the more peripheral branches, since the blood supply to the tonsil is both ipsilateral and contralateral with anastamoses (Fig. 16–2).

### FLUID MANAGEMENT OF POSTOPERATIVE HEMORRHAGE

The care of an acutely bleeding patient requires considerable judgment. Measurable losses of blood include blood lost during surgery, usually removed by suction. There frequently are hidden quantities of blood in the gastrointestinal tract. In a patient who exhibits signs of hypovolemic shock (low blood pressure, rapid steady pulse and peripheral vasoconstriction), the physician should assume that at least a 15 per cent depletion has occurred. Prompt treatment should be instituted. Blood should be obtained for cross-matching, and an intravenous with a large bore needle should be established. Fluid volume using isotonic solutions is then restored while awaiting the blood for replacement. In a child, monitoring of pulse and blood pressure before and after the rapid administration of 100 to 200 ml. quantities of lactated Ringer's solution provides an excellent guide to the effectiveness of fluid loading.

There is no substitute for blood. When it becomes available, it should be given to the volume of measured loss. Just prior to the administration of blood, a base line hematocrit and hemoglobin should be obtained. Blood for coagulation studies should be drawn. Whole blood or packed cells plus fresh frozen plasma should be used as required. Very rarely should unmatched blood be used unless there is a possibility of exsanguination. Serial hematocrits are obtained to monitor the progress of blood replacement.

The patient who has consistently low blood pressure and bradycardia may be suffering from a vagal reaction and appropriate therapy must be instituted. In some instances, it is felt that blood in the stomach or gastric distension may be the cause of the symptoms and signs.

A summary of fluid and blood loss in a four-year-old child having a post-tonsillectomy hemorrhage is shown in Table 16–2. The typical clinical picture is a child who exhibits the symptoms and signs of shock by appearing pale with cold extremities; the pulse rate would be elevated about 140 and blood pressure lowered to about 70/50.

Initial management while awaiting the cross-matched blood is to give ionic water, such as Ringer's lactate. Volume can be restored by rapidly giving up to 700 ml. intravenously and monitoring the pulse after every 200 ml. As the pulse rate drops and the blood pressure climbs, the intravenous fluid is slowed to maintenance rate. The whole blood is then given to measured loss when available. Careful monitoring of vital signs, urine output and perfusion is essential in all phases of fluid administration. Central venous pressure should be observed clinically or by direct measurement to prevent fluid overload, particularly during the administration of whole blood.

**TABLE 16–2** FLUID SUMMARY

Patient Weight: 20.2 kg.
Estimated Blood Volume: 1600 ml.
Daily maintenance requirement: 1500 ml.

| Losses | Fluid | Blood |
|---|---|---|
| NPO 12 hrs. | 750 ml. | – |
| Surgery | – | 120 ml. |
| Suctioning | – | 100 ml. |
| Vomitus (est) | 200 ml. | 200 ml. |
| Urine output | 200 ml. | – |
| Total loss | 1150 ml. | 420 ml. |
| **Replacement** | | |
| IV | 250 ml. | – |
| Oral | 200 ml. | – |
| Total Deficiency | 700 ml. | 420 ml. |

## Airway Obstruction

In the immediate postoperative recovery phase, the patient may develop airway problems related to bleeding directly into the airway. Swelling of the palate and uvula is not uncommon but usually does not endanger the patient, although a large uvula may cause discomfort and result in gagging.

Blood clots or swelling of the nasopharynx and nose may obstruct the patient's nasal airway. This is especially true in the presence of large tonsils after adenoidectomy without tonsillectomy. Patients with oral anomalies such as micrognathia or macroglossia are at higher risk if they develop nasopharyngeal obstruction.

Bleeding into the retropharyngeal or lateral pharyngeal spaces may be severe enough to pose a threat to the airway. These conditions are usually the result of trauma from the mouth gag. This may also occur when the tonsillar fossae are closed beneath a tight suture line and bleeding occurs in the closed fossae.

The management of airway obstruction may be simple or extremely complex and, therefore, must be individualized. Obstruction due to swelling of the palate or nasopharynx may be treated with the insertion of a nasopharyngeal airway. This should be done in the operating room under carefully controlled circumstances. A soft rubber nasopharyngeal tube may be inserted if the obstruction is of mild degree. If the patient awakens, the tube may be removed, and, although there is some slight danger of trauma to the adenoid fossa, usually as the patient has regained his reflexes, this will not constitute a serious problem.

The swelling in the retropharyngeal space may not be apparent for a few hours postoperatively, and in any patient with progressive obstruction and in whom there is difficulty with swallowing, hematoma should be suspected. The patient may be examined and, if the diagnosis is made, should be intubated. If swelling is severe, a tracheotomy should be performed and the hematoma should be evacuated.

Swelling of the tongue is not uncommon after tonsillectomy. This is probably due to the venous occlusion by the application of a mouth gag and usually is not severe. Occasionally, the child will experience pain in the tongue postoperatively, and massive edema can occur, resulting in respiratory obstruction. This is especially likely to happen if the child has chronic hypoxia or hypercarbia (Fig. 16–3). Treatment usually requires a nasopharyngeal airway to bypass the obstruction. If this is not effective, tracheotomy must be performed after reintubation.

## Neurologic Complications

Fortunately, neurologic complications are rare. Cases have been reported of bilateral vocal cord paralysis due to injury to the vagus nerve following application of nasopharyngeal packing. There have been case reports of blindness following the injection of steroids into the tonsillar fossa during the operative procedure. Lingual nerves and glossopharyngeal nerves have been sectioned.

## Neuromuscular Complications

Swallowing problems are very frequent after tonsillectomy and adenoidectomy. The etiologic factor is obvious, since there has been trauma to the muscles involved with swallowing. Usually, this complication can be considered a consequence rather than a complication of the surgery. On occasion, however, the swallowing problem is extremely severe and necessitates analgesics and, occasionally, treatment with intravenous fluid replacement. There is some difference of opinion as to whether analgesics such as aspirin should be used because of their anticoagulation effect. In the past, gum containing aspirin has been used; however, this is probably not warranted. If the child is encouraged to swallow and maintain fluids, these problems are usually rather transient. An infrequent neuromuscular complaint is neck pain following surgery in Rose's position when the neck has been hyperextended and the head has not been supported.

Velopharyngeal insufficiency following tonsillectomy and adenoidectomy is not an infrequent occurrence. If the patient was carefully evaluated preoperatively to eliminate the possibility of submucous cleft of the palate, the velopharyngeal insufficiency is usually transient and of very little consequence.[11] Parents should be warned preoperatively that this may occur, that it usually is of little consequence and that only in rare instances does it persist. The hypernasality may be due to the fact that sufficient tissue was removed to permit air escape by an untrained palate. On swallowing or speaking, the child does not achieve velopharyngeal closure until such time as the palate develops full excursion.

Bacteremia secondary to manipulation of the tonsil and adenoid tissue, as previously stated, does result in an occasional complication. If a patient should remain febrile, it is

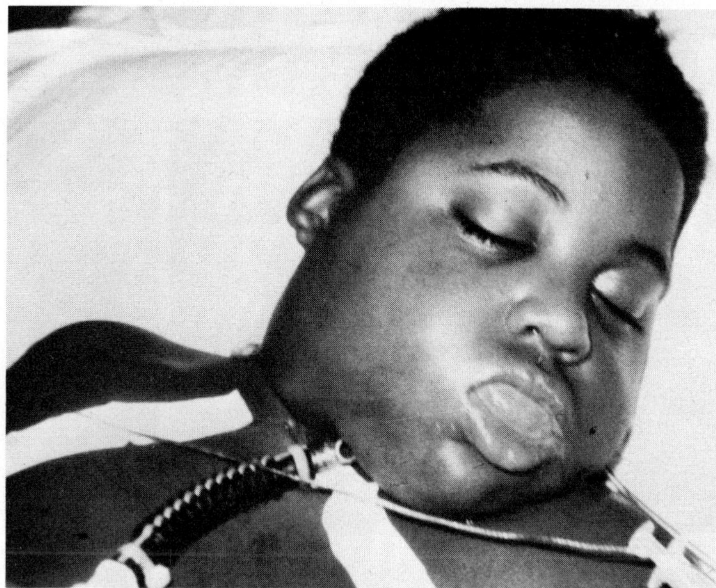

**Figure 16–3** This child developed massive swelling of the tongue after tonsillectomy. Tracheotomy may be necessary to provide an adequate airway in such circumstances.

necessary to obtain blood cultures and institute appropriate therapy.[4, 7, 18]

## INTERMEDIATE COMPLICATIONS (1 TO 14 DAYS)

### Hemorrhage

Bleeding into the operative area 7 to 14 days after surgery is termed secondary hemorrhage and appears not to be uncommon. The etiologic factor is unknown, and the incidence has been reported as between 2 and 8 per cent. Characteristically, the patient has a completely uneventful postoperative course until he suddenly begins to bleed. Hemorrhage at times may be very transient and inspection of the operative sites often may reveal no obvious cause. If there is considerable bleeding, however, the management of this condition does not differ significantly from that in the immediate postoperative period. It is important that even if the bleeding has ceased spontaneously, base line hemoglobin and hematocrits be obtained, since the child may be anemic from a slow but continuous ooze. In general, it is probably wise to hospitalize for 24 hours any child who has postoperative bleeding.

In some instances, postoperative bleeding may be major and is probably due to the erosion of a major vessel in the tonsillar fossa as the area necroses following application of sutures or cautery.[8] As the sutures dissolve, there is a foreign body reaction in the wall of the vessel, with sudden and massive hemorrhage. The management of this complication is adequate blood replacement, establishment of an airway and exploration of the bleeding site. Occasionally, it is necessary to ligate the external carotid and its branches.[15]

### Otitis Media

Otalgia is a common complaint following tonsillectomy and is due to referred pain from the tonsillar fossae. Some patients do develop acute otitis in the week following adenoidectomy. This is probably secondary to obstruction of the eustachian tube from postoperative swelling. When this occurs, treatment usually consists of analgesics. If the tympanic membrane is bulging, myringotomy may be necessary, and antibiotics appropriate for the age should be administered. One of the possible etiologic factors in the development of otitis media has been the fact that large adenoids that may have

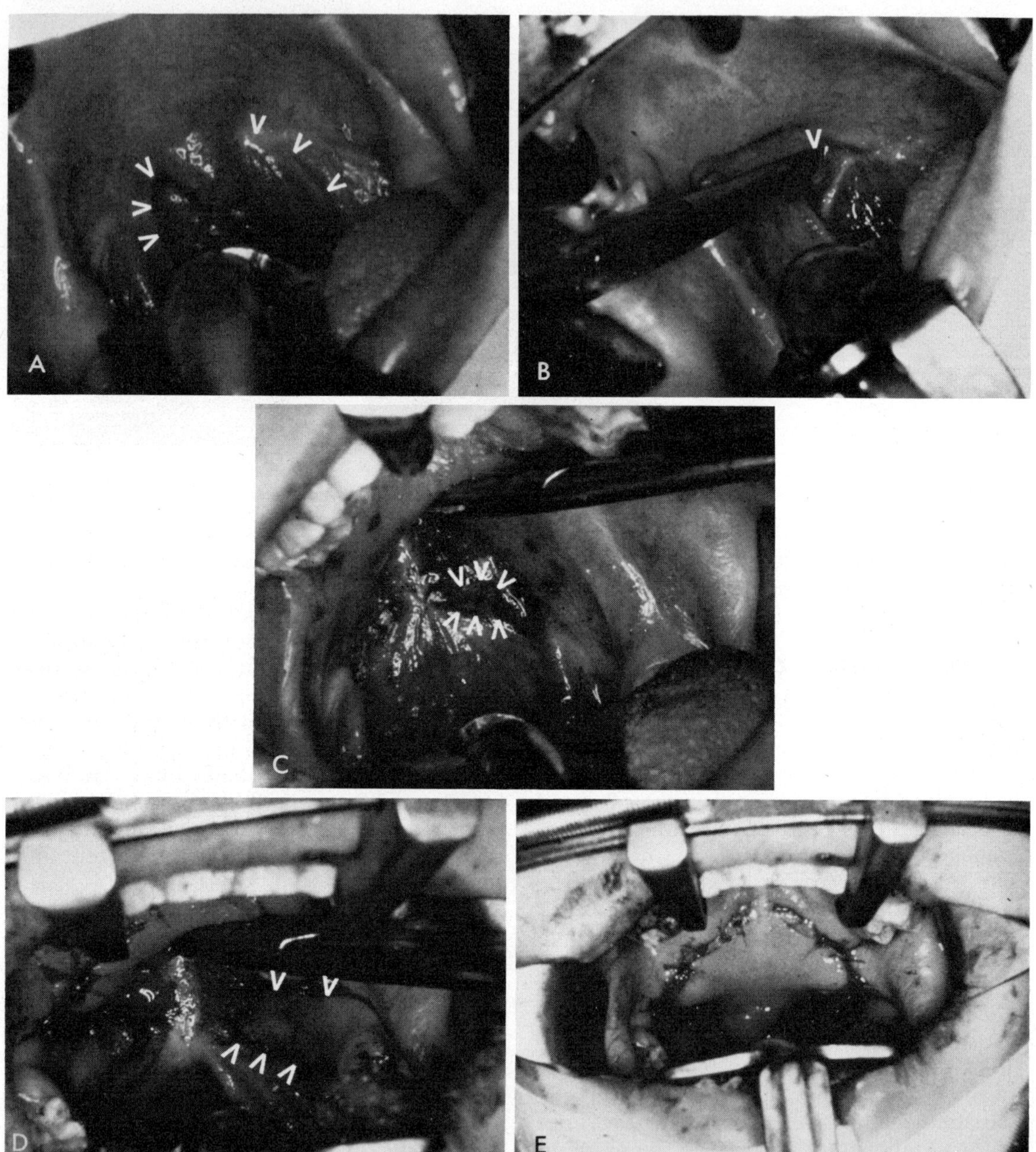

**Figure 16–4** *A,* Intraoral photograph of a child with postoperative nasopharyngeal stenosis. V's indicate the anterior pillar. *B*, The tip of a hemostat has been inserted into the nasopharyngeal opening, indicated by the V. *C*, The adhesion between the palate and posterior pharyngeal wall has been opened. The raw area of the posterior wall is indicated by V's. *D*, A flap has been rotated from the soft palate mucosa into the pharynx. The flap is indicated with V's. *E*, The donor site on the soft palate is closed with interrupted sutures.

been protecting an overpatulous eustachian tube preoperatively, permit reflux into the middle ear after removal.

### Velopharyngeal Incompetence

Many children continue to demonstrate a hypernasal voice with or without nasal regurgitation. In the intermediate postoperative period, it is usually not necessary to begin the medical therapy, since a large percentage of these patients will spontaneously improve once the splinting of the palate and the velopharyngeal musculature has ceased.

## LATE COMPLICATIONS (AFTER 14 DAYS)

### Hemorrhage

Late hemorrhage is uncommon; however, it has been known to occur, with fatal consequences. Hemorrhage of this kind is usually due to separation of a slough in the tonsillar fossa that exposes a major vessel. It usually must be handled expeditiously to avoid disastrous consequences. This is accomplished initially by applying local pressure, usually with an instrument and a tonsillar sponge. Following this, the site should be inspected and, if necessary, specific vessels are ligated.

### Airway Obstruction

Nasopharyngeal stenosis is a rare complication of tonsillectomy and adenoidectomy, and many times the cause is obscure. A surgeon who has performed hundreds of procedures without this complication may incur this problem without obvious change in technique. The symptoms are usually hyponasal speech, nasal obstruction, snoring and mouth breathing. Treatment of this condition requires surgical reconstruction.[12] This can usually be accomplished with Z plasties or local flaps (Fig. 16–4). The insertion of an obturator may be warranted.

Hypopharyngeal stenosis is another uncommon consequence of the tonsillectomy. It usually is manifested by progressive dysphagia and subsequent airway obstruction. Examination reveals a band stenosis in the hypopharynx at the base of the tongue and lower pole of the tonsil. This, if it is mild, may be treated with local injection of steroids; however, if it is severe, Z plasties and local flaps may be necessary. In some instances, construction of obturators that are attached to the teeth may be necessary.

### Velopharyngeal Insufficiency

This condition may persist with or without normal palatal function. Evaluation of the speech coupled with dynamic radiology will delineate the extent of the problem. Speech therapy aims at closing small gaps by inducing lateral pharnygeal closure. Persistence of velopharyngeal insufficiency in spite of good lateral movement may require any one of a number of available surgical techniques. A small gap may be treated by Teflon injection of the posterior pharyngeal wall; a larger space will require management with a pharyngeal flap or more extensive procedure.

### Psychologic Complications

There have been a few studies that indicate that surgery in young children results in some psychologic problems. Although it is difficult to preoperatively identify the patient in whom this might occur, it may be at least in part obviated by adequate preparation of the child for surgery.[6]

### Middle Ear Effusions

Middle ear effusions may persist following adenoid surgery. This may occur if there is sufficient scarring in the region of the eustachian tube that results in occlusion of the tube. On occasion, the removal of an obstructing adenoid mass will uncover a patulous eustachian tube with resultant reflux into the middle ear.

### Bibliography


1. Allen, T. H., et al.: The bleeding tonsil — anesthesia for control of hemorrhage after tonsillectomy. Anesth. Intensive Care, *1*:517–520, 1973.
2. Beck, W. S.: Hematology. Cambridge, Mass., MIT Press, 1973, lectures 20–23.

3. Britt, B. A., and Kalow, W.: Malignant hyperthemia: A statical review. Can. Anaesth. Soc. J., *17*:293–315, 1970.
4. Buckheit, W. A.: Brain abscesses complicating head and neck infections. Trans. Am. Acad. Ophthalmol. Otolaryngol., *74*:548–554, 1970.
5. Dannenberg, J. L.: Pedodontic endodontics. Dent. Clin. North Am., *18*:367–377, 1974.
6. Davenport, H. T., et al.: The effect of general anesthesia, surgery and hospitalization on the behavior of children. Am. J. Orthopsychiatry, *40*:806–824, 1970.
7. Eneroth, C. M., et al.: Pseudoaneurysm of the internal carotid artery. A warning of a septic erosion. Acta Otolaryngol., *72*:445–450, 1971.
8. Gardner, J. F.: Sutures and disasters in tonsillectomy. Arch. Otolaryngol., *88*:551–555, 1968.
9. Heithersay, G. S.: Replantation of avulsed teeth. Aust. Dent. J., *20*:63–72, 1975.
10. Kravath, R. E., et al.: Hypoventilation during sleep in children who have lymphoid airway obstruction treated by nasopharyngeal tube and T & A. Pediatrics, *59*:865–871, 1977.
11. Mason, R. M.: Preventing speech disorders following adenoidectomy by preoperative examination. Clin. Pediatr., *12*:405–414, 1973.
12. McDonald, T. J., et al.: Nasopharyngeal stenosis following tonsillectomy. Report of six cases and their repair. Arch. Otolaryngol., *98*:38–41, 1973.
13. Papangelou, L.: Hemostasis in tonsillectomy: A comparison of electrocoagulation and ligation. Arch. Otolaryngol., *96*:358–360, 1972.
14. Pratt, L. W.: T & A: Mortality and morbidity. Trans. Am. Acad. Ophthalmol. Otolaryngol., *74*:1146–1154, 1970.
15. Sholehvar, J., et al.: Arteriography in post-tonsillectomy hemorrhage. Arch. Otolaryngol., *95*:581–583, 1972.
16. Snow, J. C., et al.: Malignant hyperthermia during anesthesia for adenoidectomy. Arch. Otolaryngol., *95*:442–447, 1972.
17. Thomas, G. K., and Arbon, R. A.: Preoperative screening for potential T & A bleeding. Arch. Otolaryngol., *91*:453–456, 1970.
18. Van Eyck, C.: Bacteremia after tonsillectomy and adenoidectomy. Acta Otolaryngol., *81*:242–243, 1976.
19. Williams, J. D., and Pope, T. H.: Prevention of primary tonsillectomy bleeding. Arch. Otolaryngol., *98*:306–309, 1973.

17

# COMPLICATIONS IN THYROID AND PARATHYROID SURGERY

*Oliver H. Beahrs*

Complications resulting in morbidity and mortality can occur during and after surgical procedures on the thyroid and parathyroid glands. These are better prevented rather than treated after occurrence. Complications will occur infrequently if the surgeon is fully knowledgeable about the embryology and anatomy of the thyroid and parathyroid glands. The anatomy of the glands and adjacent structures must be fully known to the surgeon so that there is no hesitation in distinguishing one structure from another, whether they are in their normal relationships or are in abnormal positions because of distortion produced by the pathologic process. The surgeon must also have the surgical procedure well thought out and planned in a stepwise fashion so that it can be carried out safely and with dispatch, using those techniques that reduce the chance of morbidity and keep mortality to an absolute minimum. The pathologic conditions likely to be encountered should be recognized or suspected on gross examination so that the operation can be tailored in such a way that the patient is neither overtreated nor undertreated, exposing him only to the problems inherently associated with the correct surgical procedure and thus offering him the best chance of eradication of his disease. When complications do arise, they must be recognized early so that proper management can be instituted to prevent worsening of the problems and to prevent mortality.

## ANESTHESIA

Although local anesthesia was used widely in the past, intratracheal anesthesia is preferable because it assures an adequate airway during the operation and largely eliminates the complications associated with airway obstruction during manipulation of the structures of the neck. In the presence of large goiters producing marked deviation or compression of the trachea, the airway can be obstructed during the induction of anesthesia and at the time of intubation. In these instances, the responsible surgeon should be in the operating room in case a tracheostomy needs to be done immediately.

## INCISION

A collar incision for thyroidectomy or parathyroid exploration must be placed so as to allow the best cosmetic result possible. An asymmetric, oblique (rather than transverse) and poorly closed incision is objectionable. The incision should be made in a transverse direction and should be bilaterally symmetric unless the surgical procedure dictates its extension to one side or the other. The skin flaps should be elevated beneath the platysma muscle. For the most part, this is an avascular plane and thus there will less likely be fixation of the flaps to the underlying structures. On closure, the platysma muscle should only be approximated so as to prevent dimpling of adjacent skin. The skin edges, as in any procedure, should be approximated carefully to prevent overlapping and an unsightly scar. Keloids will form in some patients but they will be less likely and less severe if the wound is closed well.

## EXPOSURE

The operative site must be well exposed if intraoperative complications are to be avoided. Whether division of the strap muscles is advantageous is a controversial question. By not doing so and by applying traction on them, exposure is excellent, tissues separate in normal tissue planes and bleeding from the operative site is partially controlled. Nevertheless, if injury to important structures is to be prevented, the surgeon should use the techniques he prefers to assure the best exposure possible, so that he is comfortable in carrying out the surgical procedure.

Early in the operation, after the thyroid gland is exposed, the trachea caudad to the isthmus should be exposed also. If obstruction develops during the operation, the trachea is then immediately available for tracheostomy, thus preventing morbidity from lack of pulmonary air exchange.

## RECURRENT LARYNGEAL NERVE

In some techniques of thyroid surgery, the recurrent laryngeal nerve is not routinely exposed. Today, this is not considered a satisfactory approach to prevent vocal cord paralysis. The safest technique for thyroidectomy or parathyroid exploration is always to expose the nerve when a lateralized procedure is undertaken and to expose both nerves when a bilateral resection is undertaken. The nerve extends from the mediastinum upward into the neck, in or near the tracheoesophageal groove, to go before, between the branches of or behind the inferior thyroid artery (Fig. 17–1). It then proceeds downward and enters the larynx in the thyrocricoid membrane. The nerve is best exposed lower in the neck and should be kept in sight during thyroidectomy. It may not always be necessary to expose the nerve beyond where it crosses the artery. At no time should sharp dissection or clamping of vessels be done near the nerve without having the nerve in sight. Once in about every 400 cases, the nerve on the right is not recurrent but passes directly from the vagus nerve to the larynx. This rare variation must be kept in mind if the nerve cannot be found in its usual location. The nerve should be handled carefully to reduce the chance of temporary paresis.

In a review of 574 consecutive cases of thyroidectomy, this technical approach to the recurrent nerve was found to have resulted in minimal dysfunction. Vocal cord paralysis was present in nine patients before thyroidectomy and was caused by previous surgery or the lesion present. In 10 patients, the nerve was sacrificed intentionally because of the gross findings — invasion of the nerve by tumor — at the time of operation. In 20 patients, however, paralysis of the vocal cords was present immediately postoperatively, although the nerve on the corresponding side was known to be anatomically intact; in all cases, the function of the vocal cord returned to normal in three months or less. In a previous review of cases, one patient had permanent paralysis of the vocal cords. If the surgeon constantly keeps the recurrent nerve in mind during each step of a thyroidectomy or parathyroid exploration, the incidence of iatrogenic nerve injury should approach zero.

In carrying out a partial lobectomy, the surgeon can more adequately leave undisturbed the parathyroid glands and the recurrent nerves. In total lobectomy or total thyroidectomy, however, the recurrent nerves must be dissected free of the tissue being removed and must be known to be anatomically intact. Likewise, parathyroid tissue must be carefully dissected free of the thyroid tissue, and its delicate blood supply must be preserved. Only because of proximity of cancer should parathyroid tissue be removed (Fig. 17–2).

If it is necessary to re-enter the neck within a short period after thyroidectomy (two weeks), the anatomic landmarks and structures will, in part, be obliterated by edema and inflammatory reaction. Blunt dissection in such a surgical field is much preferable to sharp dissection because there is less likelihood of injury to the recurrent

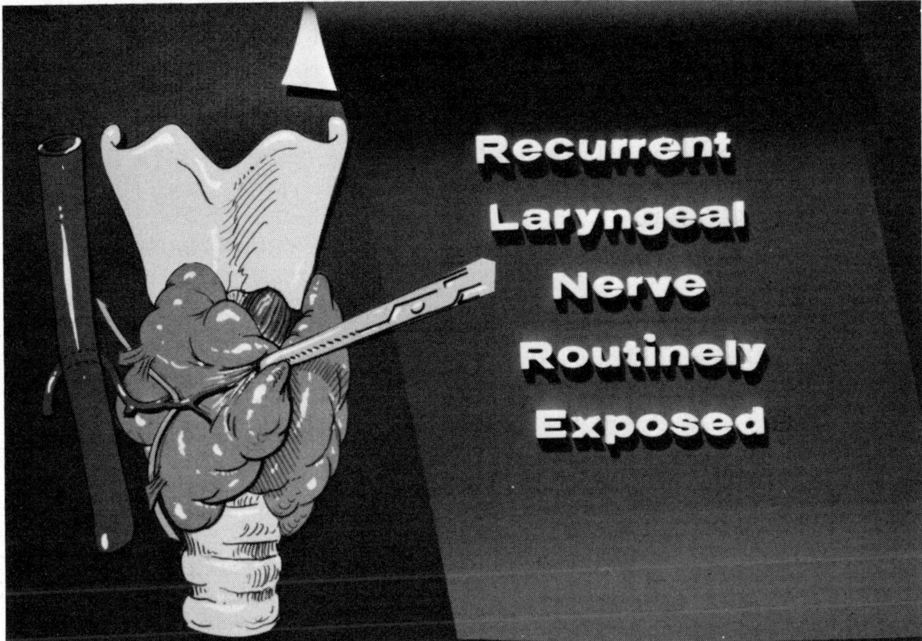


**Figure 17–1** The recurrent laryngeal nerve, diagrammatically illustrated, passes upward from the mediastinum in the tracheoesophageal curve, under, over or between branches of the inferior artery and finally into the cricothyroid membrane of the larynx. By exposing the nerve routinely in relationship to the normal anatomy or as distorted by pathologic change, iatrogenic injury can be avoided.

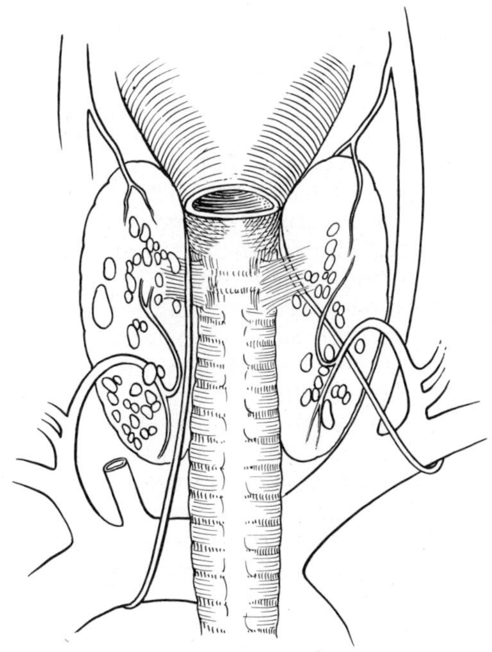

**Figure 17–2** This posterior view of the thyroid gland illustrates the typical locations of the superior and inferior parathyroid glands in relationship to the thyroid capsule and other adjacent anatomy. Atypical positions may be from the hyoid bone caudad into the mediastinum. In thyroid surgery, care must be taken to preserve parathyroid tissue and the blood supply to the glands if hypocalcemia and tetany are to be prevented.

laryngeal nerve, blood vessels and parathyroid glands. In general, the morbidity of secondary thyroidectomy is about twice that of the primary procedure.

On re-exploration of the thyroid gland much later (months to years), fibrosis is present and fine structures become much more difficult to identify. Sharp dissection often has to be used, and the risk of injury to the nerve or the parathyroid is considerably increased. It is often better to initiate the dissection away from the site of the primary operation until one can identify these nerves and then to proceed into the previous operative field.

## HEMORRHAGE

With proper tension on tissues, the use of traction and countertraction and appropriate pressure and exposure, uncontrolled bleeding should not occur. All bleeding points of the incision and deeper structures do not need to be ligated or fulgurated because most will thrombose in a minute or two. Other vessels are best ligated as they are approached, and this is easily done if the vascular anatomy is understood clearly. The thyroid ima vessels are first divided and ligated and next the middle thyroid vein. With the thyroid lobe pulled out of its bed, the inferior thyroid artery is lifted off the prevertebral fascia and, when seen alone, is ligated in continuity. If bleeding occurs, it should be controlled by finger pressure until the structures are clearly identified. Indiscriminately and blindly clamping in a pool of blood exposes many tissues to injury. The recurrent laryngeal nerve may be clamped. The sympathetic nerve can be injured, producing Horner's syndrome. The phrenic nerve is nearby and occasionally is injured. Without proper care, the major vessels and the vagus nerve may be in jeopardy. On the left side of the neck, the thoracic duct must not be forgotten; injury to it will result in a chylous fistula. (Most fistulas that have adequate drainage will close spontaneously.) Rarely is it necessary to pack or ligate the duct to control chylous drainage.

With the thyroid gland elevated, partially freed from its attachments and pulled caudad, the superior vessels are stretched; they can be felt easily and this is a safe time to clamp, divide and ligate them. In other techniques, the superior vessels are ligated earlier in the operation, when the thyroid is still in its bed. In these instances, clamping or ligating the vessels in a redundant position, higher in the neck in relationship to the larynx, puts the superior laryngeal nerve in jeopardy. The first approach does not require exposure of this nerve. It closely approximates the vessels and, with either approach, the presence of the nerve must be considered as the vessels are brought under control. Injury to this nerve leads to some alterations in the quality of the voice but not to obstruction of the airway.

Whether or not to drain a thyroidectomy or parathyroid exploration site is a controversial question. A ¼-inch soft Penrose drain, left in the thyroid bed and brought out through the midportion of the incision, is an excellent indicator of postoperative bleeding. It most often will decompress the oozing that might occur. It can be left in place for 24 to 48 hours and does not lead to other complications. Infection rarely occurs (1 case in 574). A Penrose drain will not suffice to evacuate major hemorrhage, however. If more than the "usual" amount of oozing is thought likely to occur, suction drainage is most beneficial.

If postoperative hemorrhage or tracheal obstruction is considered likely but there does not seem to be a need for a tracheostomy at the time of the operation, it is helpful to place a suture in the second tracheal ring and bring the ends out through the incision. This suture serves as an excellent guide to the site for tracheostomy, should that procedure become necessary postoperatively.

Hypoparathyroidism is a severe complication of thyroidectomy. The surgeon must be fully aware of the location of parathyroid tissue, taking special care to preserve it and its blood supply unless removal is essential to the treatment of the existing thyroid disease. The parathyroid glands are identifiable on gross inspection, and, although they are not routinely identified in thyroid surgery, one should be constantly watching for these glands. When one is seen, protect it. Because these small glands are closely adjacent to the posterior thyroid capsule, conservative thyroidectomy (consistent with treatment of the thyroid disease) should be done so that significant tetany does not occur. When partial or subtotal thyroidectomy is done, hypocalcemia can be expected in less than 1 per cent of cases (1 in 574 cases). When a total conservative or "narrow field" thyroidectomy is done, hypocalcemia will occur in about 4 per cent of cases; after a "wide field" or radical thyroidectomy, it is seen in about 40 per cent.

Interestingly, routine determination of serum calcium levels postoperatively has established that in about one fourth of cases the level decreases to slightly below normal. The patients are asymptomatic, and, within a week, the level returns to the normal range. This occurrence probably is caused by trauma to the glands or to their blood supply. It has been postulated that ligating the four main thyroid arteries will itself produce hypofunction of parathyroid tissue. Clinical experience shows that this is not uniformly true.

Should a parathyroid gland that has been inadvertently removed during thyroidectomy be implanted into other tissue? It seems reasonable to do so. A normal gland might be inserted into the sternocleidomastoid muscle or the subcutaneous tissue; it has been suggested that it be emulsified and injected into the venous system.

In parathyroid surgery, controversy currently exists as to the extent of parathyroid resection. The issue revolves around the question of whether parathyroid adenoma is in fact a reflection of hyperplasia. Those who believe that it is are performing subtotal parathyroidectomy, a 3½-gland resection, or total parathyroidectomy (implanting a portion of one gland). This approach leads to an occurrence of hypoparathyroidism of 10 to 20 per cent, which seems unnecessarily high.

Resecting one gland leads to a cure of the hyperparathyroidism in over 90 per cent of cases. No recurrence occurs. With this fact in mind, it is difficult to justify removing more than the one involved gland, except in obvious multiple gland involvement.

In the course of parathyroid exploration, if an obviously pathologic gland is encountered, it should be removed. Early in the exploration, a biopsy specimen should also be excised with care from one gland for histologic study. If normal-appearing glands are encountered as the dissection proceeds, none should be removed until all have been identified grossly or confirmed by biopsy, or both. If all glands are normal, a black silk suture should be left near each gland to aid in identification at a later date, if necessary.

Should hyperplasia be thought to be the pathologic process, then a 3½-gland resection should be done, leaving a remnant of one gland weighing no more than 100 mg. Total parathyroidectomy should not be done, as recommended by Paloyan and his associates[3] because of the severe complication of tetany, which in many instances is more difficult to control than the hypercalcemia of essentially asymptomatic hyperparathyroidism.

Because mediastinal exploration is a more formidable procedure than cervical exploration alone, it is usually reserved for a second operation rather than combining it with the neck operation.

When the mediastinum is explored secondarily, care should be taken to protect and preserve essential anatomic parts. The thymus gland, areolar tissue, fat and lymphoid tissue around the major vessels and pleura should be removed in the search for parathyroid tissue. If care is taken, no mortality or morbidity is associated with the procedure. Suction drainage should be used to aspirate serum, blood and exudate that might otherwise lead to complications.

Angiography for parathyroid localization is not indicated in primary cases because the diseased gland can be found by diligent search in 95 per cent of cases.[4] Angiography used for this purpose is time-consuming and costly and, most importantly, is associated with neurologic deficits in approximately 1 to 5 per cent of cases. Only in highly selected cases requiring secondary exploration should its use be considered. In such instances, the complications of the localization procedure are considered less threatening than those of the parathyroid disease.

Selective venous catheterization with multiple parathormone assays carries little morbidity but, in our experience, aided in localizing pathologic processes only in isolated cases. Nevertheless, its use should be considered in complicated cases in which parathyroid pathology was not found at the first operation.

## PNEUMOTHORAX

Rarely at thyroidectomy and occasionally at parathyroid exploration, the apical pleura may be injured or entered, resulting in a pneumothorax. This complication should be recognized immediately. Positive pressure anesthesia will keep the lung expanded and the air in the pleural space evacuated. Closure of the wound prevents recurrence. Rarely is it necessary to evacuate the pneumothorax in any other manner.

## POSTOPERATIVE HEMORRHAGE

The most serious postoperative hazard to the patient after thyroidectomy or exploration for parathyroid disease is hemorrhage. When bleeding occurs, the blood remains enclosed within a space in the midline of the neck below the strap muscles. Some blood may escape if the wound has been drained, but most does not. Pressure from the hematoma and continued blood accumulation builds up to the point at which the pressure causes collapse of the airway and, finally, obstruction. Because there is a margin of safety in the size of the lumen of the trachea, the seriousness of the situation is not always realized. Complete obstruction will occur quite rapidly, anoxia follows and irreparable damage is done in a manner of minutes. Death follows.

In cases of this magnitude, the wound must be opened immediately — in the patient's room or wherever he may be. Delay in order to transport the patient to the operating room should not occur. Opening the wound relieves the obstruction to the airway. Then the time can be taken to transport the patient, prepare for re-exploration of the operative site, control bleeding and close the incision again.

In such cases, edema of the airway will follow. Consideration should be given to doing a tracheostomy to assure no further problems with the airway postoperatively.

Complications of postoperative hemorrhage should occur in much less than 1 per cent of cases (1 in 574 cases).

## TRACHEOSTOMY

Tracheostomy should be done whenever there is a serious question about the adequacy of the airway. In large goiters, if the rigidity of the tracheal cartilages has been lost and tracheal collapse is possible, a tracheostomy should be done. If both recurrent laryngeal nerves have been traumatized or one or both have been sacrificed, a temporary tracheostomy can be a life-saving maneuver.

Certain pathologic conditions warrant tracheostomy, for example, cancer that has been incompletely resected, nerve destruction and anticipated postoperative radiation treatment. The need for an elective tracheostomy to prevent airway complications is present in about 1 per cent of cases (4 in 574 cases).

## TETANY

If the serum calcium level decreases to just below the normal range and the patient remains asymptomatic, treatment may not be required. If the patient develops symptoms, however, supplemental calcium must be given.

When hypocalcemia occurs (and if the patient is not achlorhydric), calcium carbonate, four teaspoons daily, is given. The dosage should be altered depending on results. If achlorhydria is present, calcium lactate dissolved in water is used. Patients should be observed over a period of months, and medication should be discontinued if the serum calcium levels remain in the normal range. If the hypocalcemic state is permanent, calcium must be given indefinitely. Vitamin D may be added to the regimen also.

## MYXEDEMA

Myxedema, or hypothyroidism, is not so much a complication of thyroid surgery as the end result of the pathologic process or the extent of surgery. Nevertheless, it does occur and does require treatment. The incidence after thyroidectomy for parenchymatous hypertrophy is 10 to 40 per cent, and after total thyroidectomy it is 100 per cent. In Hashimoto's thyroiditis, if left untreated, the incidence of myxedema would in time approximate 100 per cent also. The usual replacement therapy to maintain a euthyroid state is 2 to 3 gm. of desiccated thyroid extract or one of the synthetic preparations (e.g., 0.2 mg. sodium levothyroxine [Synthroid] ). Such medication completely replaces the normal thyroid secretion.

## INFECTION

Infection of neck wounds rarely occurs, especially after thyroidectomy (1 in 574 cases). When it does occur, the usual measures should be taken — adequate drainage, application of heat, use of antibiotics and reliance on the healing effects of time. Rarely is infection a serious problem.

## MORTALITY

Today, death after thyroidectomy or cervical exploration should be extremely rare (0 in 574 cases).[1] With such ancillary aids as intratracheal anesthesia, blood transfusions, antibiotics, suction drainage and well-trained surgeons, mortality is almost totally preventable. In 8972 cases previously reported,[2] the mortality rate was 0.1 per cent (1 in 1000 cases).

Several decades ago, thyroid storm led to mortality. Since the introduction of the use of iodine preoperatively by Plummer, in 1923, mortality from this complication is rarely seen. Antithyroid and other drugs are also now available to prevent this complication.

Although the comments made in this chapter relate primarily to thyroidectomy, they are all pertinent to cervical exploration for parathyroid pathology. As in any field of surgery, prevention of complications is the best and safest way to manage operative and postoperative problems. If they should occur early, recognition and prompt management are essential. Persistent morbidity and mortality are then held to a minimum.

## Bibliography

1. Beahrs, O. H.: Factors minimizing mortality and morbidity rates in head and neck surgery. Am. J. Surg., *126*:443–451, 1973.
2. Beahrs, O. H., Ryan, R. F., and White, R. A.: Complications of thyroid surgery. J. Clin. Endocrinol. Metab., *16*:1456–1469, 1956.
3. Paloyan, E., Lawrence, A. M., and Straus, F. H.: Hyperparathyroidism. New York, Grune & Stratton, 1973.
4. Satava, R. M., Jr., Beahrs, O. H., and Scholz, D. A.: Success rate of cervical exploration for hyperparathyroidism. Arch. Surg., *110*:625–627, 1975.

# COMPLICATIONS OF LARYNGEAL SURGERY

18

*Joseph H. Ogura*
*Stanley E. Thawley*

The practice of laryngeal surgery can be most satisfying in terms of successful results and patient gratification. To achieve a high percentage of success, laryngeal surgeons must be thoroughly knowledgeable about the various types of laryngeal pathology, preoperative evaluation, indications for each surgical procedure, technical aspects of each operation and postoperative care.

During surgery, certain postoperative problems may be anticipated, and prevention of complications should be attempted at the time of the procedure rather than postoperatively. It is always more difficult to correct problems in the postoperative period than to prevent them by selecting and using the proper surgical technique.

The first part of this chapter will discuss the various laryngeal operations and prevention of complications from a preoperative and intraoperative point of view. In the last part of the chapter, we will discuss each specific complication and its postoperative treatment.

## PREOPERATIVE AND OPERATIVE PREVENTION OF COMPLICATIONS

### *Laryngoscopy*

Laryngoscopy is the most common surgical technique employed for laryngeal lesions. The indications for laryngoscopy may be diagnostic or therapeutic. Many laryngeal lesions may be removed by laryngoscopy, including cysts, polyps, nodules and keratotic changes of the vocal cords. The only cancers adequately removed by laryngoscopic techniques are carcinoma *in situ* and superficially invasive carcinomas of the true vocal cords. All other cancers require more extensive laryngeal surgery.

#### INDIRECT LARYNGOSCOPY

Indirect laryngoscopy is performed using a head mirror for illumination and a laryngeal mirror for visualization. Lesions of the larynx may be removed by using angled instruments. This technique was performed frequently years ago but at the present time is not recommended because of the better control and precision of technique that is available with direct laryngoscopy.[10, 20]

#### DIRECT LARYNGOSCOPY

Direct laryngoscopy may be performed under either local or general anesthesia. Local anesthesia is usually attained with topical cocaine. The toxic dose of this drug must not be exceeded. Patients must be cooperative, and excellent rapport should be maintained prior to and during local anesthesia. Fear combined with poor anesthesia and surgical manipulations within the larynx may lead to laryngeal spasm with upper airway problems. In patients with large bulky lesions with a marginal airway, biopsy under local anesthesia without an endotracheal tube may lead to bleeding of the lesion, with loss of the remaining airway necessitating an emergency tracheotomy. These events must be anticipated preoperatively and adequate precautions of being prepared for an emergency tracheotomy must be taken. With direct laryngoscopy under general anesthesia, the endotracheal tube must be small enough to allow adequate visualization of the laryngeal structures. With large endotracheal tubes, the laryngeal anatomy may be distorted and the surgeon has a difficult time performing precision intralaryngeal maneuvers. At the time of laryngoscopy, malignant lesions are carefully mapped and recorded on a drawing for future reference (Fig. 18–1).

When removing lesions from the true vocal cords, the anterior commissure area should be maintained intact, if at all possible. Postoperative scarring in this area will lead to webs and secondary voice changes. Removal of lesions from the vocal cords must be done at a proper tissue depth. Inadequate superficial removal may lead to recurrence of disease, and specimens may be so small that pathologists are unable to adequately interpret them. True vocal cord lesions should be stripped from the cord, sparing the underlying vocal muscle. This produces a uniform surface that is inducive to a smooth re-covering by epithelium. If deep bites are taken out of the vocal cord and involve the vocal muscle, then uneven scarring and poor function of the vocal cord may result. During laryngoscopy, one must be careful not to exert great force on the upper teeth, since they may be loosened and fractured, requiring postoperative dental restoration.

Intralaryngeal manipulations may trigger a bradycardia via various nerve reflexes. We have found this to be especially true in chil-

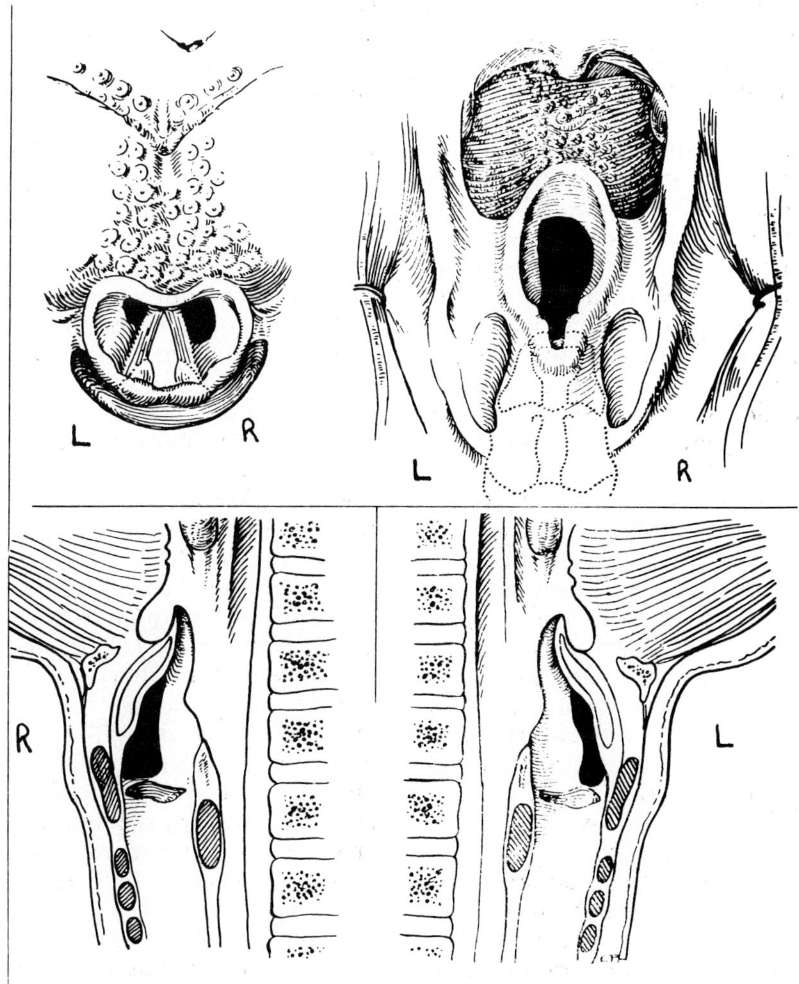


**Figure 18–1** Mapping of a typical supraglottic lesion.

dren when a great deal of laryngeal pressure is applied via the laryngoscope. This occurs more commonly with microlaryngoscopy, in which some of the laryngoscopes are larger than what would be used normally. The electrocardiograph of patients undergoing laryngoscopy should be monitored, and if any arrhythmias develop, the pressure exerted by the laryngoscope on the larynx must be reduced.

### LASER LARYNGOSCOPY

Laser laryngoscopy is a relatively new technique involving the microsurgical application of the $CO_2$ laser to laryngeal diseases. The $CO_2$ laser beam has a thermal effect on soft tissue. The water content is evaporated, rapidly producing destruction of the tissue. The amount of destruction depends on the power setting and the duration of exposure. The laser wound produces minimal bleeding and no visible postoperative edema. The laryngologist must be knowledgeable as to the amount of tissue destruction produced by the various power and time settings. This must be determined preoperatively in order to avoid excessive destruction of tissues. The subglottic area around the endotracheal tube must be packed to prevent the laser from hitting the endotracheal balloon and producing rupture of that structure. The surgeon must be careful to maintain the laser beam on the intralaryngeal structures and not allow it to go into the trachea. This is also prevented by the subglottic packing.[11, 19]

This technique is applicable to all lesions amenable to the direct laryngoscopic approach. If biopsies are taken at the same time, this must be performed first, and the base of the lesion may then be treated with the laser beam. For all patients who undergo direct laryngoscopy with surgical manipulation, voice rest is recommended for at least one week. This allows the vocal cords to be abducted, facilitating their rapid recovering by laryngeal epithelium. If patients do not rest their voice for an appropriate period of time, resultant scarring of the vocal cords may occur, with secondary voice changes. Patients also must not smoke during the recuperative period, as this further irritates the laryngeal epithelium and prolongs recovery time.

#### *Laryngofissure and Cordectomy*

This technique consists of splitting the thyroid cartilage in the midline and resecting the soft tissues on the side of the lesion down to the inner thyroid perichondrium. The midline is closed and the site of the resection forms a new pseudocord. This technique is applicable in early cordal cancer ($T_1$), which is limited to the membranous cord and does not involve the anterior commissure, the vocal process or the subglottic region. It cannot involve the ventricle, and the true vocal cord must be freely mobile.

Most modern laryngeal surgeons today feel that the procedure lacks versatility and tumor curability when compared to the more extensive technique of hemilaryngectomy. The reasons for the decline in its use are several: (1) the cure rates fell when the technique was extended to include lesions beyond the vocal cord, specifically those involving the anterior commissure; (2) the development of the hemilaryngectomy technique provided a wider margin of resection and increased security in removal of the lesion; and (3) the success of radiation therapy in treatment of $T_1$ lesions of the vocal cord has also discouraged the use of laryngofissure technique.

If the technique is performed on tumors with the proper criteria, it has a cure rate equal to radiation therapy and other more extensive laryngeal techniques. It has largely been supplanted by hemilaryngectomy and radiation therapy, however.

In terms of prevention of complications, the operation should be performed on those patients who have the correct indications, as stated previously. If these indications are extended, then complications of inadequate resection of tumors and recurrence of the cancer will occur. During the time of surgery, the midline thyrotomy must be closed in a secure fashion so that widening of the anterior commissure does not occur. Laryngofissure produces a hoarse voice, and the quality of the voice depends on the pseudocord that re-forms. Usually patients with a laryngofissure and cordectomy do not have the postoperative problems of aspiration, since the arytenoid is not disturbed. If the voice is excessively hoarse, with a great deal of air leakage through the glottic chink with phonation, then Teflon injected into the pseudocord may be attempted. This is difficult, since there is a great deal of scar tissue in this area. There is little space for Teflon, and the resulting contour of the pseudocord may be unpredictable and irregular.[4, 16]

### *Hemilaryngectomy*

This technique was initially used for carcinomas involving only the membranous true vocal cord. With more experience, the indications for this technique have been expanded. Glottic cancers that extend beyond the confines of the membranous true vocal cord, involving the arytenoid, anterior commissure, subglottis or opposite cord, have an increased incidence of local recurrence when treated by irradiation or by laryngofissure and cordectomy. Treatment with total laryngectomy improves survival rates but is unwarranted, since the present technique of hemilaryngectomy may be employed with cure rates comparable to those of the more extensive procedure.

At the present time, glottic lesions with the following characteristics may be adequately treated by hemilaryngectomy: (1) a true cord lesion that involves the anterior commissure, (2) a true cord lesion that extends to the anterior third of the opposite cord, (3) a true cord lesion that extends to the vocal process and the anterior and superior portions of the arytenoid and (4) a true cord lesion that extends to within 10 mm. subglottic. The involved true vocal cord may have limitation of mobility, but fixation of the true cord should not be present (Fig. 18–2).[3]

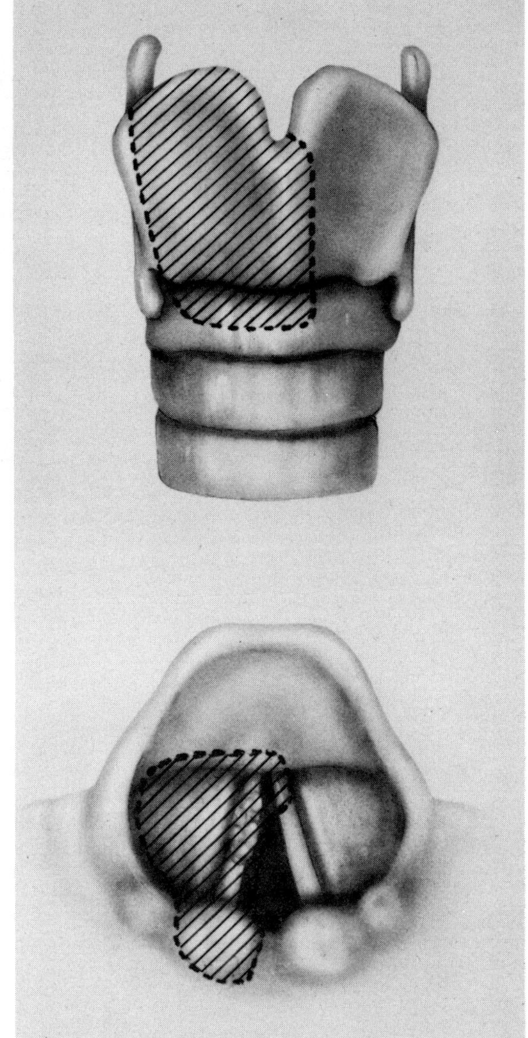

**Figure 18–2** Hemilaryngectomy — area that may be resected (shaded).

Hemilaryngectomy may be applied in selected cases of carcinoma of the true vocal cords following irradiation therapy. In these cases, the lesions must adhere to the following criteria: (1) the opposite cord must be free of tumor, although the anterior commissure may be involved; (2) the arytenoid, except for the vocal process, must be free of tumor; (3) subglottic extension should not exceed 5 mm.; (4) there should be no cartilage involvement; (5) the cord should not be fixed; and (6) the recurrent lesion should correlate with the original primary lesion prior to irradiation.[2]

Under general anesthesia, direct laryngoscopy is performed immediately prior to resection. This confirms the tumor extent and prevents errors in evaluating the tumor margins. A low tracheotomy with the resultant complication of innominate artery rupture must be avoided. At the time of surgery, most operative complications may be prevented by adequate exposure. An apron neck flap is elevated to the level of the hyoid bone. This is necessary because the epiglottis has to be sutured to the hyoid area during the closure procedure. Preserving the perichondrium is important since it is used in the closure. If this perichondrium is destroyed or severely lacerated, then the clo-

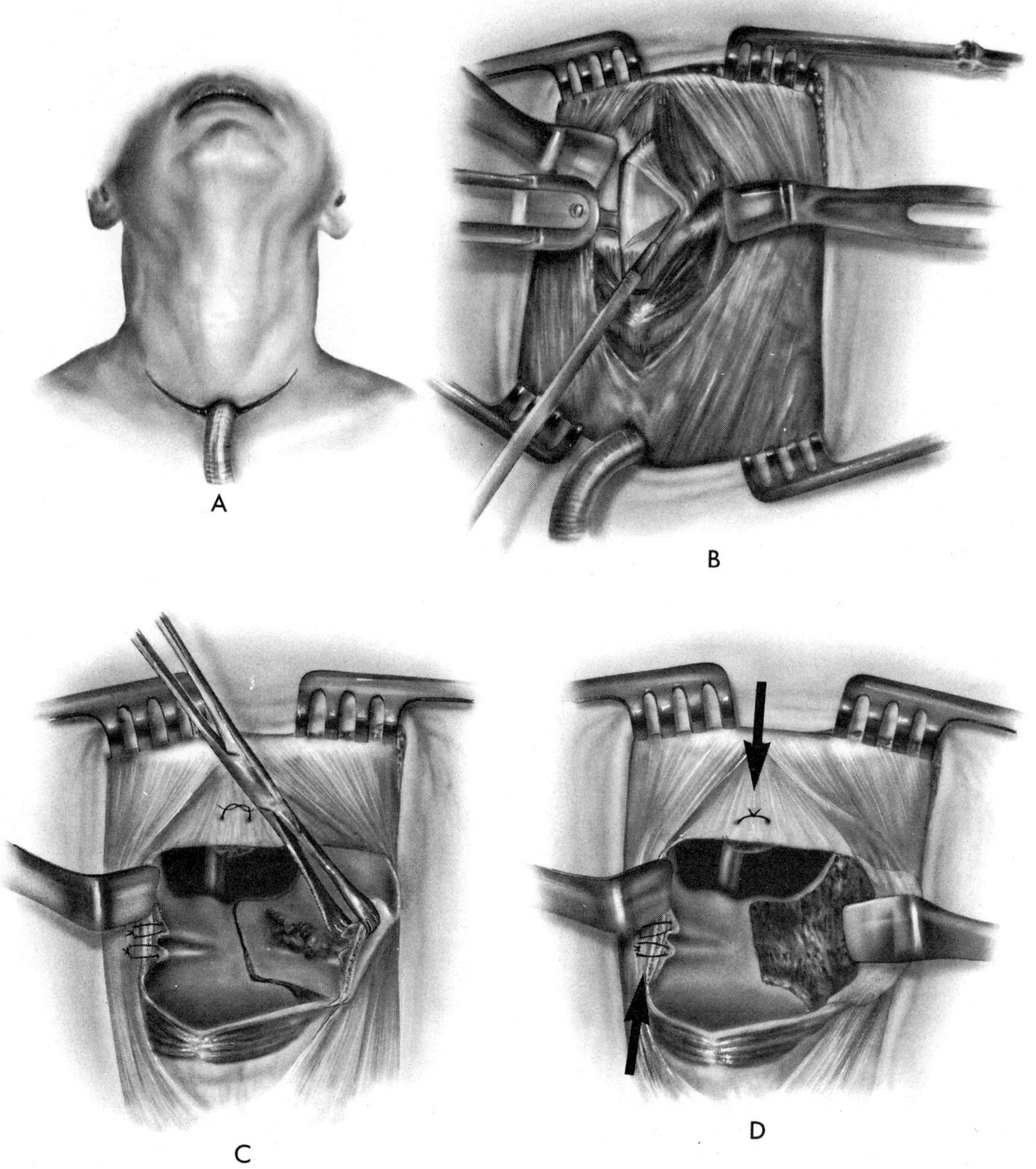


**Figure 18–3** Hemilaryngectomy. *A,* Tracheotomy and incision. *B,* Preservation of outer perichondrium. *C,* Anterior traction on specimen for exposure. *D,* Completed resection with suture of epiglottis to hyoid (upper arrow) and reattachment of remaining vocal cords (lower arrow).

sure is compromised (Fig. 18–3*B*). The thyroid cartilage cuts must be performed correctly by using an oscillating saw, and they must be in the correct position in order to adequately encompass the tumor. If they are incorrectly placed, complications will arise because the tumor will be transected, and recurrence may be expected. The location of the anterior cartilage cuts is determined by the position of the lesion. If the anterior commissure is not involved, the cut is made in the midline from the superior notch to the inferior border. If the anterior commissure is involved, the anterior cut is made 3 to 4 mm. from the midline on the noninvolved side. If the lesion involves the anterior commissure and the opposite anterior third of the cord, the anterior cartilage cut is made 4 to 5 mm. from the midline of the lesser involved side. The posterior cut is made 3 mm. from the posterior border of the thyroid ala on the involved side. This cut extends from the superior to the inferior thyroid margins, and great care must be taken that the cut is completely through the cartilage but does not involve the soft tissues. If the cut is incompletely performed as the specimen is being removed, it will be torn, with the likelihood of leaving tumor behind.

As the subglottic space is entered through the cricothyroid membrane anteriorly, one must be sure that the entrance is below the level of the tumor extent inferiorly. The superior portion of the anterior cricoid cartilage may be removed *en bloc* in order to insure an adequate inferior entrance to the subglottic airway. To adequately visualize the undersurface of the true vocal cords, the patient is placed in a Trendelenberg position and a headlight is used for visualization. Single hooks are then used to retract the cricothyroid membrane cuts laterally, and a Kelly clamp is placed posteriorly through the cricothyroid membrane cut and used to push the arytenoid cartilages laterally, thus separating the cords and allowing adequate visualization. Under direct vision, the cord is severed at the desired site anteriorly using a scalpel and the thyrotomy is completed. Maintaining adequate anterior tension on the specimen is important so that an inadequate resection is not performed (Fig. 18–3*C*). If the arytenoid is to be resected, adequate anterior tension on the specimen must be maintained while applying posterior pressure with right angle scissors in order to adequately resect the arytenoid. If this is not performed, an inadequate amount of specimen will be resected and recurrence of tumor will be likely. The arytenoid and cricoid may be left intact, depending on the location of the lesion. In order to prevent postoperative hematoma, the superior laryngeal vessels are suture-ligated and any other bleeding is controlled with cautery.

In cases involving resection of the arytenoid, sufficient bulk has to be placed posteriorly to prevent postoperative aspiration and to improve the quality of the voice. This is performed using a single pedicle sternohyoid or omohyoid muscle flap (Fig. 18–4). The muscle flap is brought through a perforation in the remaining perichondrium on the involved side or through the midline anteriorly. It is sutured posteriorly to the previously resected arytenoid area. If the arytenoid remains, a muscle flap is not necessary. If the arytenoid is resected without using a muscle flap, then an inadequate posterior glottic chink will result and postoperative aspiration and poor quality of voice will occur. This is a significant and debilitating complication and should be prevented at the time of surgery by correct surgical technique.

The detached epiglottis is sutured anteriorly to the perihyoid tissue with a # 2-0 chromic horizontal mattress suture (Fig. 18–3*D*). This allows the surgeon to visualize the glottic chink area postoperatively and is extremely important in terms of postoperative follow-up. If this is not performed, the epiglottis will flop inferiorly, limiting exposure and visualization of the glottic chink area, and the surgeon will be severely limited in terms of his ability to visualize the glottic chink in the office. Again, this is a postoperative complication that must be prevented at the time of surgery. The opposite true vocal cord is sutured to the anterior edge of the remaining perichondrium (Fig. 18–3*D*). This must be done in order to prevent postoperative shortening of the remaining true vocal cord and to avoid anterior glottic webbing. If this procedure is not performed, then shortening of the true vocal cord and glottic webbing will occur with a poor quality of voice.

If the anterior third of the opposite true vocal cord is resected, a tantalum keel is inserted anteriorly for 3 to 4 weeks. This prevents shortening of the lesser involved cord and also prevents anterior glottic webbing. If the tantalum keel is not used on these cases, anterior glottic webbing with reduction in total size of the glottic chink will occur, with resultant poor voice and perhaps a marginal airway for inspiration. The success of this procedure depends on the accurate preoperative assessment of the extent of the tumor and on limiting use of the procedure to those cases that fulfill the cri-

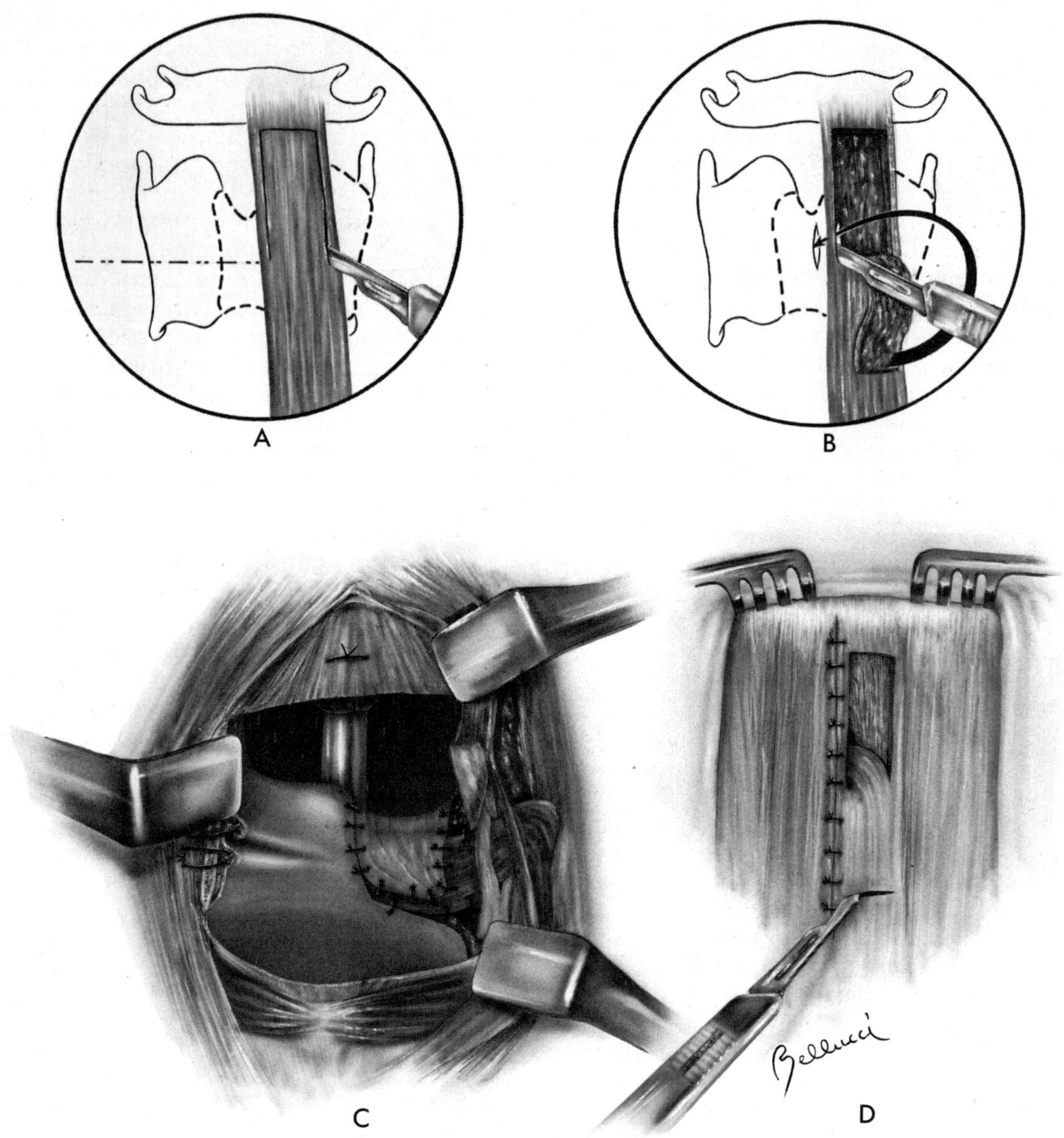


**Figure 18–4** Hemilaryngectomy — muscle flap reconstruction. *A,* Creation of sternohyoid muscle flaps. *B,* Mobilization of flap. *C,* Placement of flap to replace arytenoid bulk. *D,* Closure.

teria of resection. If this technique is extended beyond the limits of its indications, then tumor recurrence should be expected. At the time of surgery, adequate exposure is mandatory in order to visualize the tumor and thereby adequately resect it. Most postoperative problems may be prevented at the time of surgery by correct surgical technique in terms of resection and reconstruction.

### *Anterior Commissure Resection*

The anterior commissure technique of partial laryngectomy is employed for lesions of the anterior commissure that involve the membranous portion of both true vocal cords and extend below the level of the anterior commissure to a maximum of 1 cm. These lesions are distinguished from the more frequent glottic lesions that simply extend across the anterior commissure to involve only a few millimeters of the opposite cord. To insure adequate resection by this technique, the vocal process of the arytenoid must not be involved and the tumor cannot extend more than 1 cm. below the free edge of the true vocal cord.

The perichondrium is preserved in this procedure as it was in a hemilaryngectomy. Bilateral vertical thyroid cartilage cuts are made with an oscillating saw about 8 to 10 mm. from either side of the midline. Subperichondrial dissection is usually performed bilaterally, posterior to the anterior thyrotomy cuts. This allows conservation of portions of the thyroid ala but includes resection of the anterior portions of both true and false vocal cords bilaterally. It also includes excision of the thyroid cartilage in the anterior commissure, the site most likely to be involved with cancer. A tantalum keel is then placed with the phalanges extending over the thyroid ala bilaterally (Fig. 18–5). The keel extends posteriorly between the vocal processes but does not touch the cricoid posteriorly. If the keel is too long and touches the cricoid posteriorly, erosion in this area with infection and chondritis may be expected to occur. The keel is removed in 4 to 6 weeks, and the patient is decannulated in a few days. Again, to prevent complications, the correct indications for this procedure as stated previously must be used. If they are extended beyond the correct indications, inadequate tumor resection with tumor recurrences may be expected to recur. In all cases of anterior commissure resections, the keel must be used in order to prevent massive anterior glottic webbing with shortening of the remaining true vocal cords that results in a poor voice and an inadequate glottic chink.[8, 18]

### *Subtotal Supraglottic Laryngectomy*

Subtotal supraglottic laryngectomy is indicated for cancers of the epiglottis, false vocal cords and aryepiglottic fold. The epiglottic-aryepiglottic fold and false vocal cords are removed in the supraglottic resection (Fig. 18–6). This procedure may be extended to include one arytenoid cartilage, the vallecula and portions of the base of the tongue. The true vocal cords must be mobile, although there may be decreased mobility on the side of the lesion. Cartilage invasion is a contraindication. This may be ascertained by laminograms of the thyroid cartilage, xeroradiography (Fig. 18–7), and computerized axial tomography techniques. Preferably, the true vocal cords should not be involved with tumor; however, in some cases in which there is only superficial true vocal cord invasion, this may be included in the resection, with reconstruction of a new fixed cord. In lesions that involve the base of tongue and vallecula, the superior margin should be below the circumvallate papillae. Within the larynx, the resected margins may be close to the tumor; however, in the vallecula and base of tongue, the margins should be wider. If these preoperative indications for a supraglottic laryngectomy are not respected, then postoperative complications with tumor recurrence may be expected.

The basic technique in supraglottic surgery involves the resection of the supraglot-

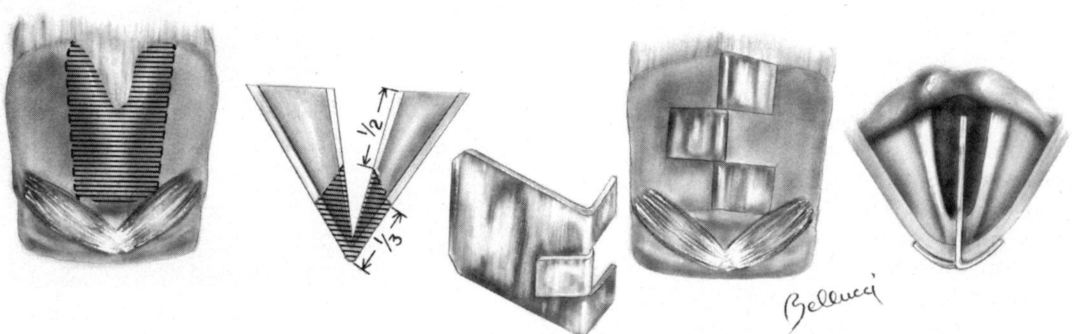


**Figure 18–5** Anterior commissure resection with keel placement.

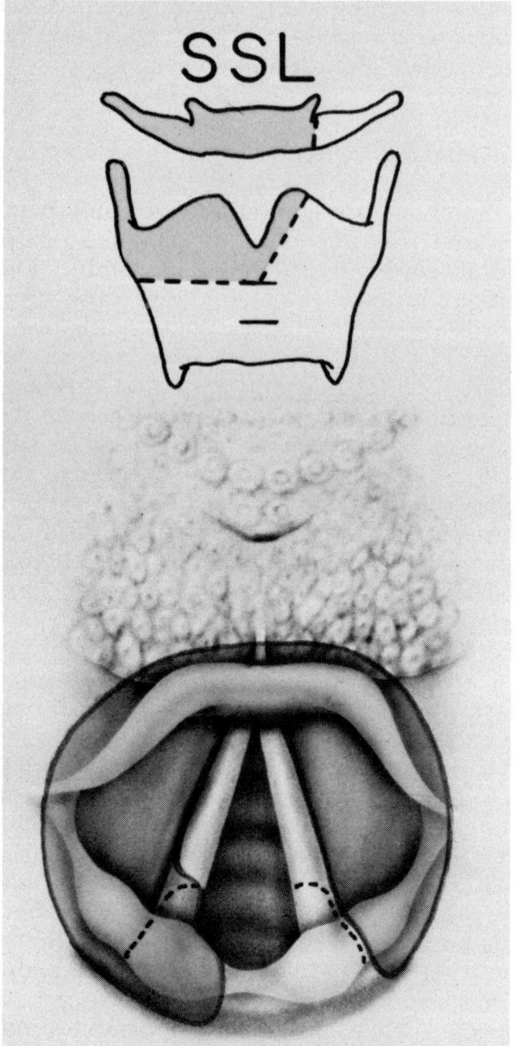


**Figure 18–6** Supraglottic laryngectomy — area that may be resected (shaded).

tic area, preserving the pre-epiglottic space, and, if indicated, a neck dissection encompassing the drainage site of the supraglottic area through the thyrohyoid membrane.

The thyroid perichondrium must be preserved intact, since this is the main tissue used in closure. The suprahyoid muscles are then incised along the superior edge of the hyoid bone extending from the greater cornu on the involved side to the lesser cornu on the uninvolved side. This step is important because this preserves the pre-epiglottic space into which tumor may have spread. If the lesion does not involve the vallecula, the mucosa underlying the superior hyoid cornu is pushed medially in order to preserve that area. The hyoid is transected using cartilage scissors at the lesser cornu on the uninvolved side. After the perichondrium of the thyroid cartilage has been elevated, a point is selected in the midline corresponding to the level of the vocal cords internally. This step is extremely important because correct cartilage cuts should be at the level of the ventricle. If the cartilage cuts are too superior, then inadequate inferior resection of the tumor may result. If the cartilage cuts are too inferior, they may extend below the level of the true vocal cord, which will be inadvertently resected in the specimen; if they are left intact, they will have no supporting cartilage. In the average male, the level of the vocal cords internally is a point midway between the inferior and superior thyroid margins. In the female or small male larynx, this point is at the junction of the upper third and lower two thirds of the thyroid cartilage. The mucosa un-

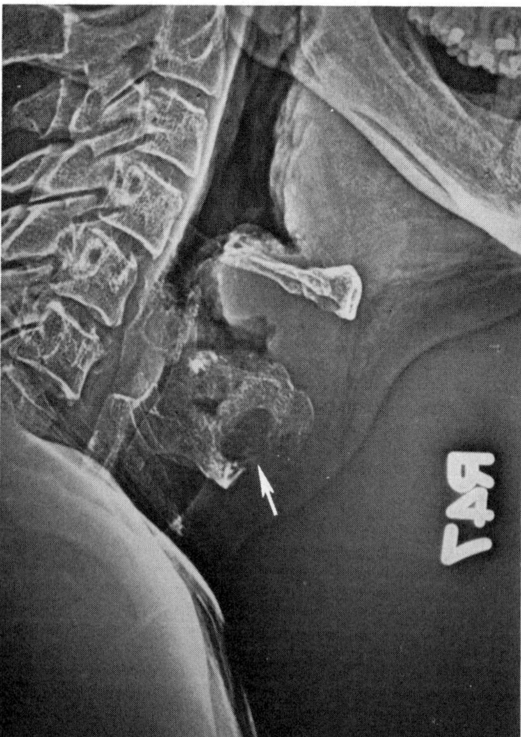

**Figure 18–7** Xeroradiograph demonstrating thyroid cartilage erosion (arrow) by cancer, contraindicating any conservation laryngeal surgery.

derlying the superior cornu of the thyroid ala is dissected and pushed medially to preserve pyriform fossa mucosa. This step is important because it preserves pyriform mucosa, which is quite helpful in terms of closure of the defect.

An oscillating saw is used to transect the cartilage, taking care not to cut the underlying tissues. The pharynx is entered through the vallecula or the pyriform fossa, depending on the location of the tumor. If the pharynx is entered at the incorrect position, the tumor may be transected at the time of entry. If only the false vocal cords and epiglottis are involved, the pharynx may be entered through the vallecula. If the tip of the epiglottis or vallecula is involved, the pyriform fossa is entered. If the tumor is on the epiglottis and false vocal cord, the superior margin is resected at the vallecula level. If the vallecula or base of tongue is involved, the margins have to be extended superiorly in order to encompass the tumor. Adequate musculature relaxation must be performed by the anesthesiologist to insure visualization during the resection. As the superior cut is made, a tenaculum is used to grasp the epiglottis, and superior and anterior traction is exerted for increased exposure (Fig. 18–8*A* and *B*). A single hook is placed on the aryepiglottic fold on the involved side near the arytenoid, and a clamp is used to push the opposite arytenoid laterally. This gives visualization of the tumor, the arytenoids and the glottic chink area. Adequate exposure is mandatory if precision cuts are to be performed.

Closure of the pharyngostoma is accomplished with interrupted #2-0 silk sutures approximating the preserved external thyroid perichondrium to the base of the tongue musculature. A mucosa to mucosa anastomosis is not accomplished. If the external thyroid perichondrium has not been preserved during the first steps of the procedure, then an inadequate, weak closure of the pharyngostoma will result and the incidence of fistulization increases postoperatively.[14] In selected cases with superficial extension onto the superior aspect of the true vocal cord on the involved side, the vocal cord may be resected with the specimen. This is commonly known as a three-quarter laryngectomy, and this should be planned preoperatively because the thyroid cuts are different. The cord is reconstructed by infractioning the superior part of the cartilage. This is held in place by sutures, and a mucosal flap is rotated to cover this infraction cartilage, thus reconstructing the true vocal cord on that side (Fig. 18–9).[12] A cricopharyngeal myotomy is performed prior to the closure of the pharyngostome; this is helpful in the postoperative prevention of dysphagia.

Complications may be prevented by using correct preoperative indications. During the time of surgery, there are a great number of technical steps that must be performed correctly in order to adequately resect the tumor and to reconstruct the larynx. If the limits of the operation are extended, then inadequate tumor resection will occur and tumor recurrence may be expected. If the operation is poorly performed, postoperative complications in terms of aspiration, fistula, infection, inability to decannulate and glottic insufficiency will occur.

### *Partial Laryngopharyngectomy*

Partial laryngopharyngectomy is indicated for isolated pyriform lesions or pyriform involvement from extension of a supraglottic tumor. The apex of the pyriform fossa should not be involved, since this necessitates a total laryngectomy. The true vocal cords should not be fixed. The resection includes the supraglottic area, the aryepiglottic fold, the arytenoid and indicated areas of the involved pyriform fossa (Fig. 18–10). The technique is similar to a supraglottic laryngectomy. The thyroid cartilage cuts are slightly different from the supraglottic cuts. The epiglottis may be split and the opposite false cord left intact. The pharynx is usually entered throught the vallecula or the opposite pyriform. The resection is similar to a supraglottic laryngectomy; however, more laryngopharyngeal wall is removed to encompass the pyriform lesion. The arytenoid is removed with this lesion, and the remaining true vocal cord must be fixed in the midline to prevent postoperative aspiration and also to improve the quality of the voice (Fig. 18–8*D* and *E*). The closure is the same as in a supraglottic resection except laterally, where a mucosa to mucosa closure is performed. This technique must not be extend-

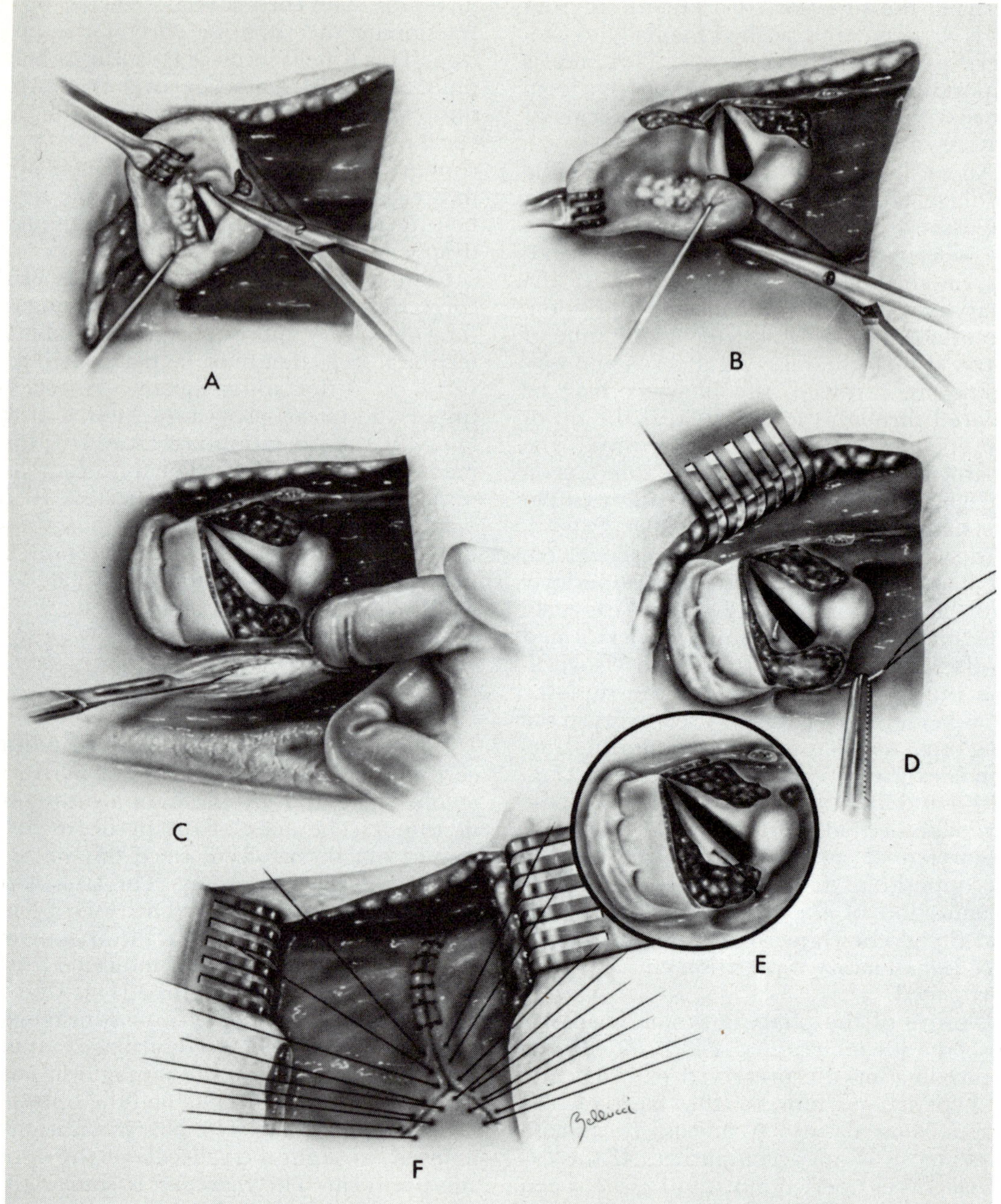


**Figure 18–8** Supraglottic laryngectomy. *A,* Excision of lesser involved side. *B,* Removal of arytenoid on involved side. *C,* Cricopharyngeal myotomy. *D,* and *E,* Suturing cord to cricoid, pulling cord medially. *F,* Complete closure.

ed beyond its indications. At the time of surgery, the apex of the pyriform fossa must be clear of tumor. One must not attempt to perform a partial laryngopharyngectomy by removing all of the pyriform fossa including the apex because a functional closure is impossible.

### *Total Laryngectomy*

Total laryngectomy is indicated for tumors that, because of their size or location, or both, are not amenable to more conservation types of laryngeal surgery. One should not perform a total laryngec-

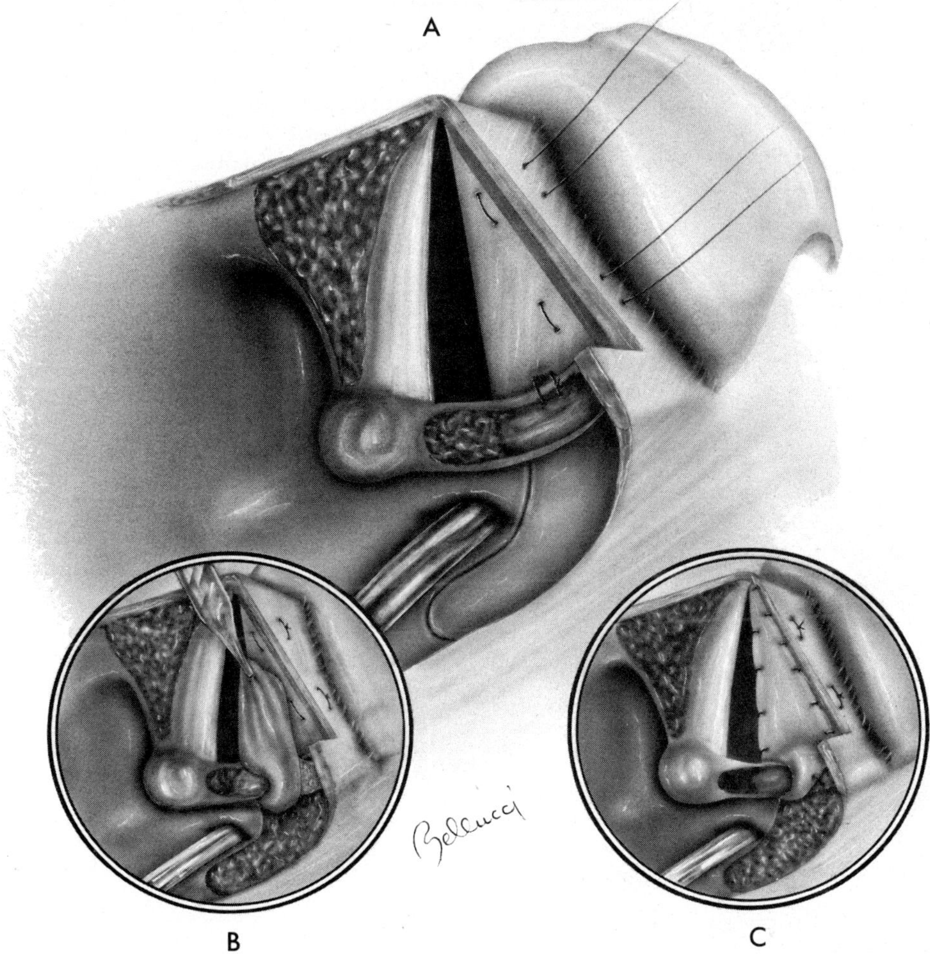


**Figure 18–9** Three-quarter laryngectomy. *A,* Infractioned cartilage segment. *B,* Mucosal flap rotated to cover cartilage. *C,* Reconstructed cord.

tomy for a lesion that can be encompassed by other larynx-sparing operations. An exception to this general rule is an elderly patient who perhaps has a supraglottic tumor that is resectable by supraglottic laryngectomy but is unable to tolerate the more strenuous postoperative course involved in partial laryngeal surgery because of poor general health and debilitation. In this type of patient, a total laryngectomy would be indicated even though the patient's lesion is amenable to conservation surgery.

If the tumor does not involve the pyriform areas, the mucosa underlying the superior cornu of the thyroid cartilage should be pushed off the thyroid cartilage medially in order to preserve the pyriform mucosa. This helps significantly in terms of closure. The failure to do this may result in resecting more mucosa than is actually necessary and may compromise the pharyngotomy closure, resulting in postoperative stricture. For endolaryngeal and pyriform lesions, the pharynx is entered in the vallecula and the resection is performed from superior to inferior. If the lesion involves the tip of the epiglottis and extends up into the vallecula and base of tongue, however, the trachea is entered first and the resection is performed from an inferior to superior manner. This allows excellent visibility in the superior

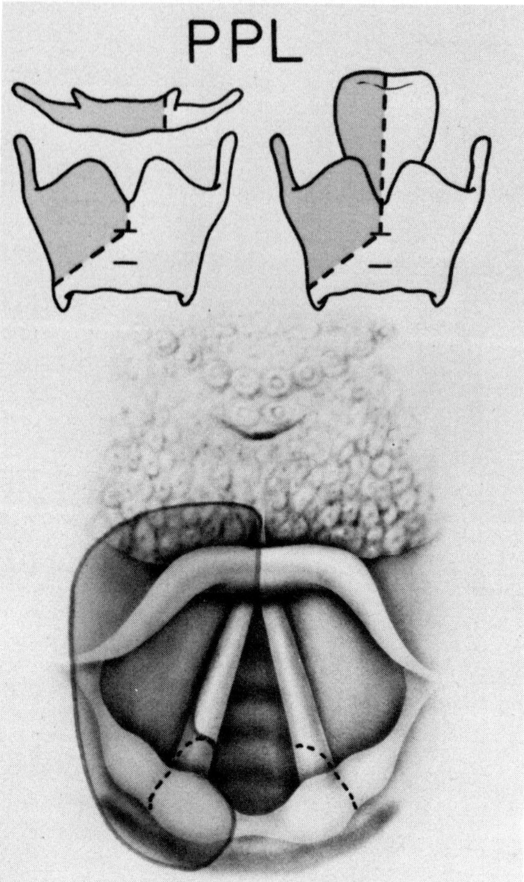


**Figure 18–10** Partial laryngopharyngectomy—area that may be resected (shaded).

area by having the remainder of the larynx out of the way and makes the resection of the tumor easier. If the resection is not performed in this manner for superior tumors, then one may inadvertently enter the pharynx through a tumor-bearing area and thus leave tumor behind at the time of surgery.

If the tumor involves the pyriform fossa and extends onto the lateral or posterior pharyngeal walls, adequate resection of this lesion may compromise a primary closure. If the patient has a large lesion in the hypopharyngeal area and the surgeon feels that his closure at the time of surgery will be compromised, then a chest flap may be used to facilitate this closure. Patients should be told preoperatively, so that one does not close the pharyngotomy with a primary closure and give the patient a very narrow neopharynx, producing a postoperative stricture with resultant dysphagia and inability to swallow. This problem must be anticipated preoperatively so that it may be adequately handled at the time of surgery and postoperative problems prevented.

Postoperative stricture of the tracheal stoma may be avoided by beveling the tracheotomy posteriorly in a superior fashion so that the surface area of the tracheal stoma is increased. It is helpful to cover all edges of the severed trachea with skin, since this decreases the postoperative crusting and occasional chondritis. Most tracheal stomas can be adequately created by suturing the trachea to the skin. Occasionally, the trachea has to be mobilized inferiorly in order to be attached to the skin. Mobilizing the trachea should be avoided, if possible, because during the mobilization the blood supply to that portion of the trachea may be compromised and that segment of the trachea may become necrotic, with resultant loss of the tissue and retraction of the remaining trachea down into the upper mediastinum.

## POSTOPERATIVE COMPLICATIONS

### *Infection*

Infection secondary to direct laryngoscopy procedure is rare and usually will not occur unless one is particularly vigorous and exposes a part of the laryngeal cartilage. With external laryngeal operations, the possibility for infection increases. The neck wounds are always drained, and this usually prevents localized infections secondary to small hematomas or seromas.

In the conservation types of laryngeal surgery in which cartilage cuts are performed, the possibility of chondritis always exists. It is important to preserve the outer thyroid cartilage perichondrium when performing hemilaryngectomy, supraglottic and partial laryngopharyngectomies. This covers the remaining thyroid cartilage, which has been exposed by the cuts, and will decrease the incidence of chondritis.

The incidence of chondritis is higher in patients who have received preoperative irradiation, especially in those patients who have received full course radiotherapy. We routinely place our patients on postoperative prophylactic, broad-spectrum antibiotics. If patients develop chondritis, the skin flap overlying the area of infection will become injected, and, commonly, the pharyngotomy suture line will break down, resulting in a pharyngocutaneous fistula. These patients have a characteristic odor, and it is noticeable when stepping into their room. Once chondritis is diagnosed, if the cartilage is exposed and visible in the fistula area, it may be debrided and the sequestrum may be removed (Fig. 18–11). If the fistula is small, it will usually close with time. Occasionally, the chondritis will respond to simple exteriorization of the fistula and continued antibiotic therapy without debridement of the cartilage. As in any surgery, the rate of infection is decreased by good postoperative care in terms of maintaining proper electrolyte balance, a proper hematocrit and correct management of any other associated medical problems, such as diabetes mellitus.

### *Wound Slough*

In a series of over 200 patients with laryngeal cancers treated with various types of laryngectomy procedures, only 4 per cent developed wound slough.[7] Wound slough problems vary from a superficial area of skin loss at the site of flap trifurcation to complete flap necrosis (Figs. 18–12 and 18–13). This complication is reported to result from excessive tension on wound margins, lack of adequately based flaps, traumatic handling of the tissues and damage to subdermal vessels. High doses of radiation, hematoma and infection may also contribute to this complication. Care must be taken in planning skin incisions for laryngectomy procedures. They must be placed properly to insure adequate blood supply to the base of the flap. This is especially true in patients who have received full course radiotherapy. Skin flaps should include platysma muscle unless there is tumor involvement. If the skin is involved with the tumor or if the overlying skin will obviously not survive, then resection of the skin in continuity with the specimen and chest flap coverage is performed (Fig. 18–14). Wound slough management includes conservative debridement with local wound care, split thickness skin grafting (Fig. 18–15) and flap reconstruction (Fig. 18–16), depending on the site and size of the tissue loss and the overall clinical setting.

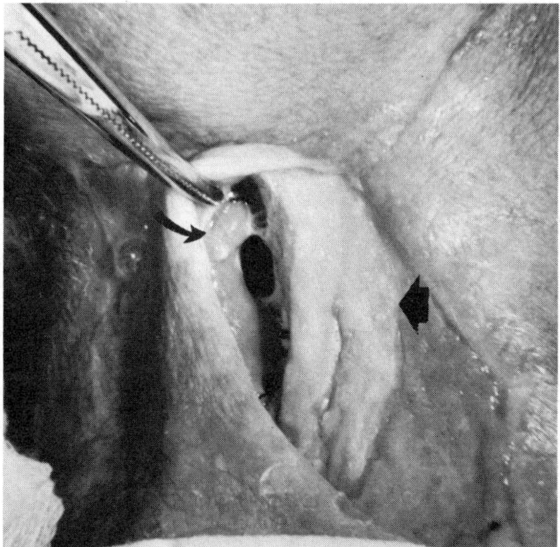

**Figure 18–11** Pharyngocutaneous fistula with exposed cartilage (small arrow) and dermal graft (large arrow) covering carotid artery.

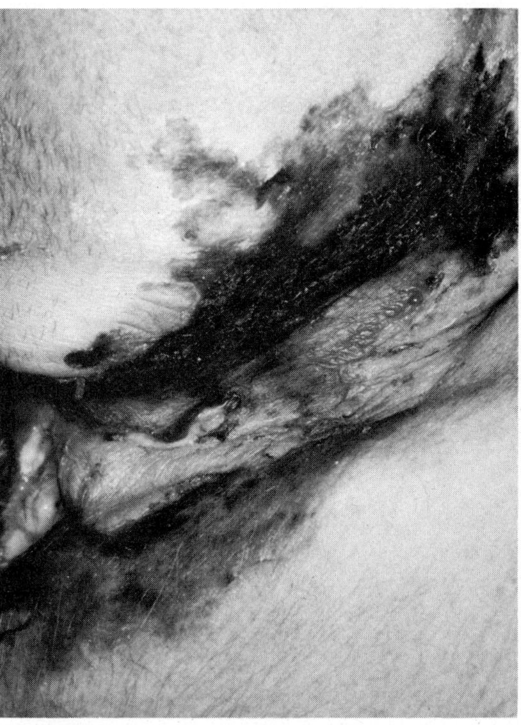

**Figure 18–12** Early necrosis of skin flap.

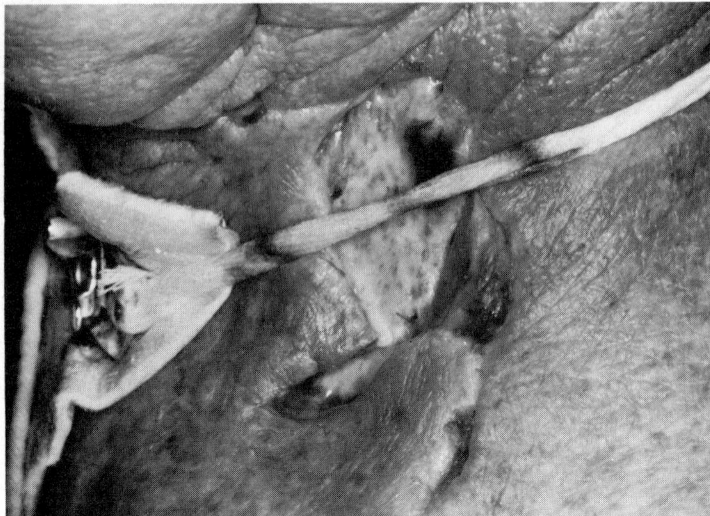

**Figure 18–13** Loss of full thickness of flap with exposure of dermal graft.

### *Fistula*

The incidence of fistula formation varies as to the size of the lesion, the dosage of preoperative irradiation, the presence of systemic disease, the operative technique and the failure of prior treatment modalities. Our overall incidence of postoperative fistula formation for subtotal supraglottic laryngectomy and radical neck dissection is

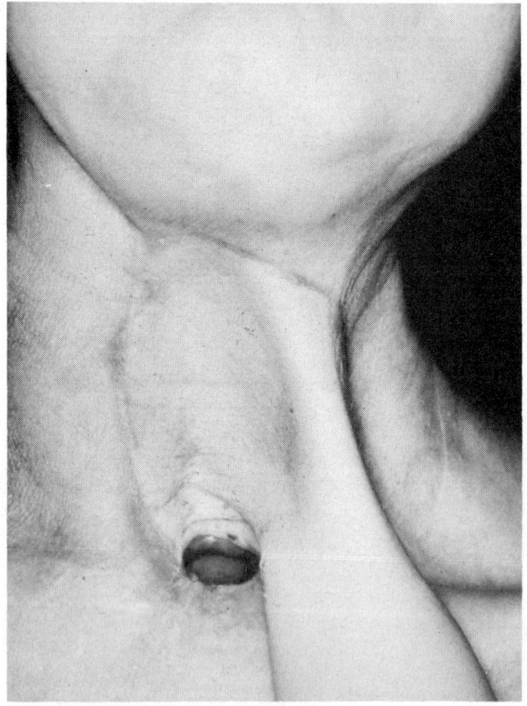

**Figure 18–14** Total laryngectomy with resection of overlying skin covered with chest flap.

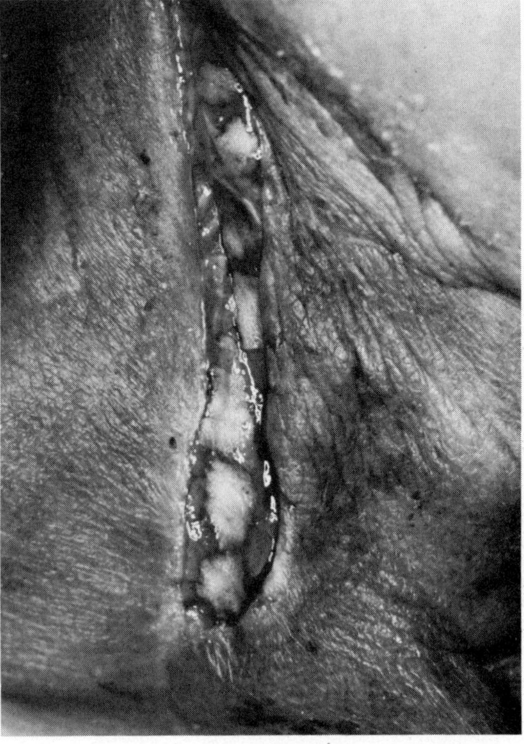

**Figure 18–15** Small area of skin loss grafted with split thickness skin grafting.

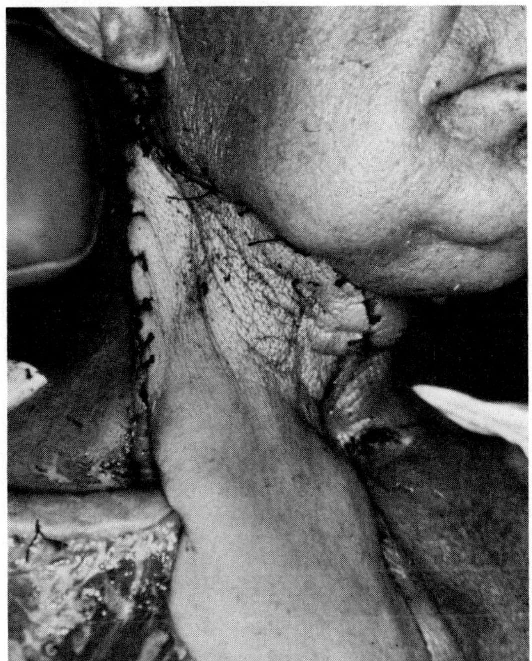

**Figure 18–16** Entire flap slough treated with full thickness chest flap.

8.3 per cent, and for partial laryngopharyngectomy and radical neck dissection is 20.8 per cent. This includes patients who had received no preoperative radiotherapy, those who had received both low and high doses of preoperative radiotherapy, those who were radiation failures and those who had had previous laryngeal surgery.

Preoperative identification of the high-risk patient likely to develop a fistula following a partial laryngopharyngectomy is predictable from certain factors. Large $T_3$ or $T_4$ tumors of the pyriform fossa are associated with a higher incidence of postoperative fistulas; tumor involvement of the lateral posterior pharyngeal wall markedly complicates primary closure of the neopharynx after extensive resection. Closure of the hypopharynx after a partial laryngopharyngectomy depends on the amount of mucosa remaining after primary tumor resection. When the lateral wall of the pyriform fossa remains, closure of the neopharynx can be accomplished without difficulty. The mucosa closure is compromised if the lateral and posterior pharyngeal walls are excised. As a result, closure may be under excessive tension, and necrosis and separation of the lateral pharyngeal suture line can occur. Some patients develop suture line abscesses that drain, leading to fistula formation. This may be secondary to the use of silk suture, especially in the lateral wall mucosa closure. For this reason, polyglycol suture material may be better, since it is an absorbable suture but remains long enough for healing to occur. If the patient has persistent carcinoma, this may prevent suture line healing, resulting in fistula formation.

The incidence of fistula formation is higher in patients who have received preoperative radiotherapy greater than 3000 rads. In general, patients with systemic disease, such as diabetes mellitus, will have a more complicated clinical course and may develop fistulas. Over 70 per cent of fistulas develop within three weeks after surgery. In patients with high-dose preoperative irradiation, therefore, decannulation and feeding is delayed longer than usual. This is done to encourage wound healing by not subjecting the neopharyngeal suture line to the stress involved in learning to swallow.

Fistulas present with injection of the skin overlying the lateral suture line of the neo-

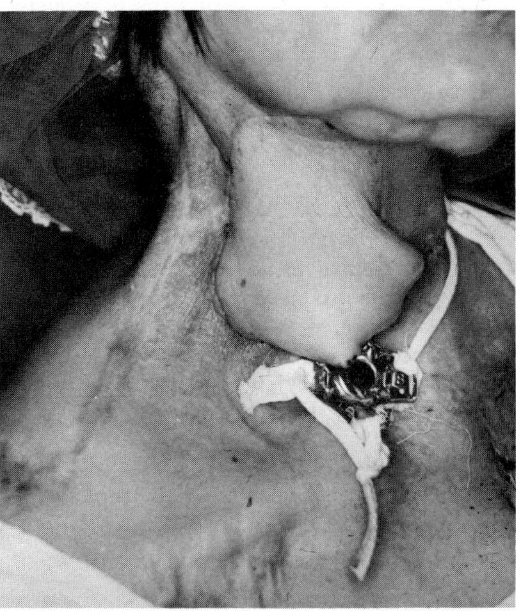

**Figure 18–17** Fistula closure using chest flap.

pharynx. The skin flap may become elevated secondary to extrusion of secretions beneath the flap. Any suspicious areas should be aspirated and drained. Once the fistula is diagnosed, it is exteriorized in order to prevent secretions from transversing the carotid artery and elevating the skin flap. It is exteriorized medial to the carotid artery to prevent rupture of that vessel. Local cleansing and treatment with Povidine-iodine is performed twice daily. A pressure dressing is applied to decrease dead space and facilitate sealing down of the skin flaps.[5]

Fistulas developing after supraglottic laryngectomy for smaller lesions will usually close spontaneously following local care and removal of any exposed necrotic cartilage and silk sutures. Those occurring after a partial laryngopharyngectomy for a large pyriform wall lesion do not close as readily and may require reconstruction using a chest flap (Fig. 18–17). Large fistulas may require bilateral chest flaps for closure (Figs. 18–18 and 18–19).[13] In cases with a tenuous closure at the primary resection, a small diverting pharyngostome may be used to attempt to prevent development of a postoperative fistula.

### *Stenosis*

Stenosis of the neoesophagus is occasionally seen after total laryngectomy. It occurs when too much of the mucosa is resected and primary closure is attempted. In cases in which a tight primary closure is predictable from the size of the lesion preoperatively, chest flaps should be considered to close the defect and reconstruct the esophagus. If this is not done, stenosis will most likely occur. If a stenosis of the neopharynx occurs following a total laryngectomy, repeated dilatations may be useful in allowing the patient to swallow. Some patients learn to do this daily in their homes. If a long stricture occurs, chest flap reconstruction is necessary.

Stenosis of the tracheal stoma may occur following a total laryngectomy. This may be prevented by beveling the remaining trachea posteriorly in a superior fashion so that the surface area of the tracheal stoma is increased. If tracheal stoma stenosis develops postoperatively, there are surgical procedures available for rotating small flaps at the edge of the tracheal stoma in order to enlarge the opening.

### *Glottic Insufficiency*

Glottic insufficiency refers to glottic closure that is inadequate for physiologic function. Glottic insufficiency may refer to a glottic chink that is too open (incompetent) or too closed (stenotic) for adequate function. Incompetent glottic insufficiency primarily affects deglutition and phonation, while respiration is usually adequate. Stenotic glottic insufficiency primarily affects the respiratory function, while phonation and deglutition may be normal. Postsurgical glottic insufficiency may present with problems of aspiration, inability to cough or strain, a weak voice or stenosis with stridor and respiratory distress. Incompetent glottic insufficiency is diagnosed by visualizing an inadequate glottic closure. These patients present with aspiration, recurrent pneumonia and poor voice associated with inability to close the glottic chink. Aspiration may be documented by cineradiographs of the swallowing mechanisms. Patients with stenotic insufficiency have respiratory distress, stridor and inability to decannulate the trachea. Commonly, these patients have a good voice and swallow adequately. Glottic insufficiency may be produced by recurrent carcinoma, and direct laryngoscopy with biopsy may be indicated.

The best way to treat glottic insufficiency is to prevent it from occurring. This is done by correct preoperative assessment of the tumor, selecting the right procedure and using correct surgical techniques in the resection and reconstruction process. The incidence of glottic insufficiency following partial laryngectomy is low. Specific areas excised are more important in determining functional ability than the size of the primary lesion. The arytenoid and base of tongue are the most important areas, and excision of these sites can lead to difficulty. Patients who have undergone full course irradiation therapy following partial laryngeal surgery can also be expected to have more problems. Patients with severe chronic lung disease may also experience postoperative difficulty. If the lung disease is severe, major

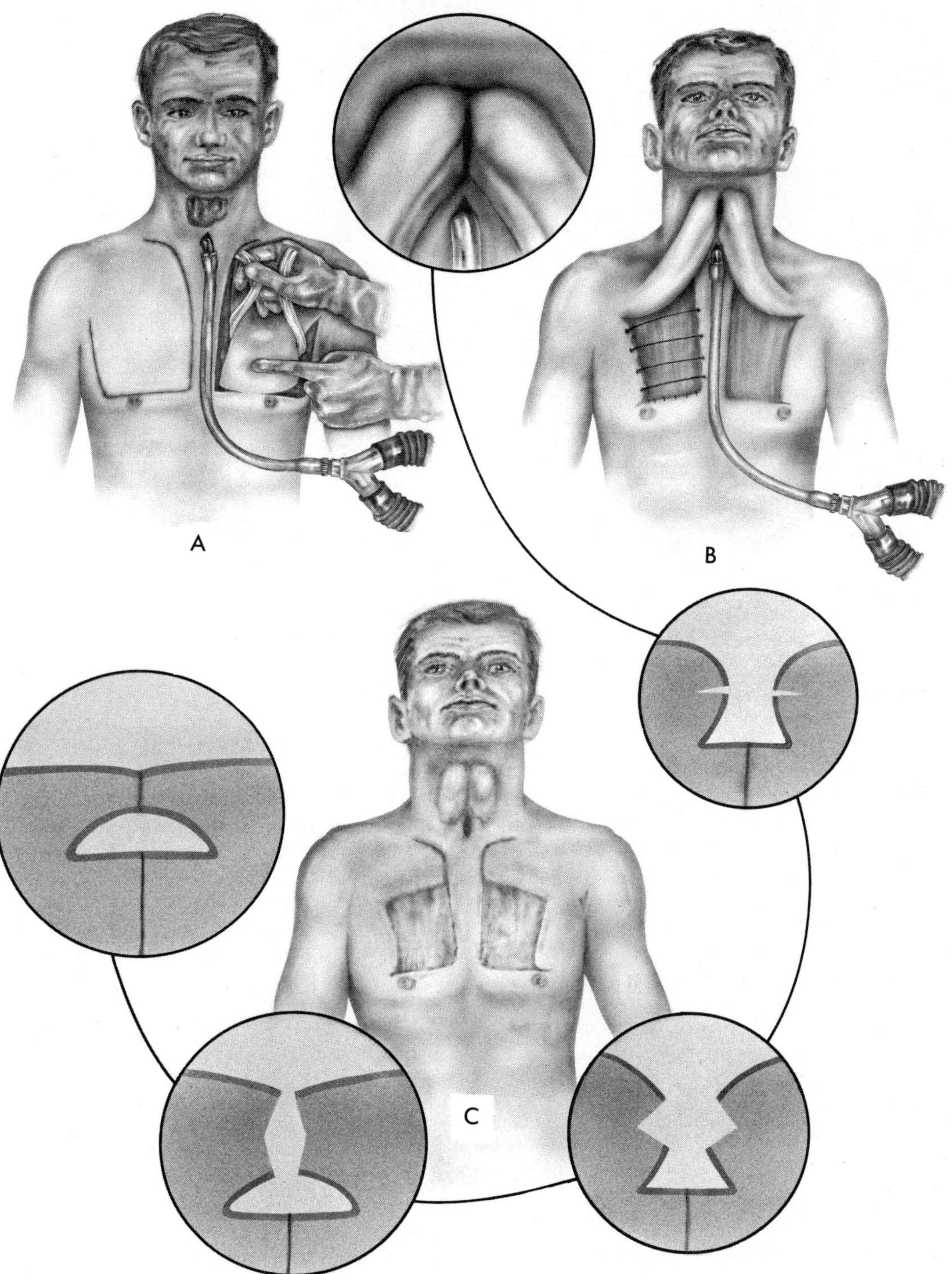


**Figure 18–18** Method of closing fistula using bilateral chest flaps.

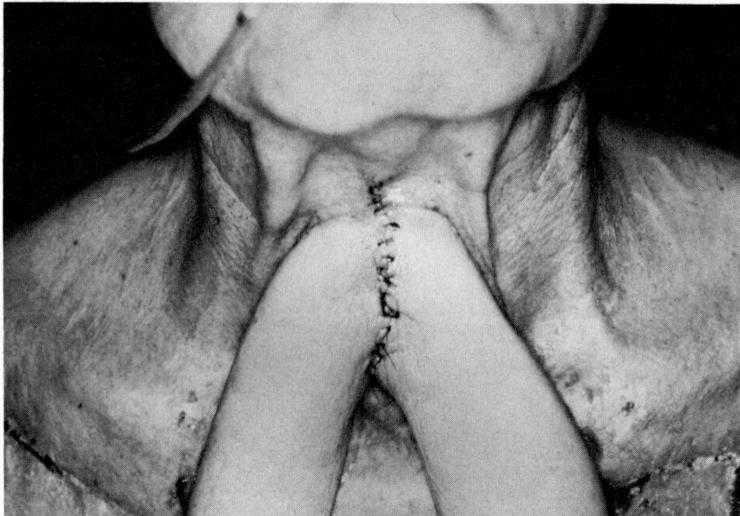

**Figure 18–19** Bilateral chest flaps in position for fistula closure.

conservation laryngeal resection should not be performed. Occasionally, patients with moderately severe chronic lung disease may receive intensive preoperative medical treatment in order to improve their pulmonary function, and these patients may tolerate their postoperative course.

Treatment of incompetent glottic insufficiency may include Teflon injection, muscle flap reconstruction, cartilage implants and, rarely, gastrostomy or conversion to total laryngectomy. Teflon injection is performed in the pseudocord; however, the technique is more difficult than in cases for injection of vocal cord paralysis. The pseudocord is scarred, there is little space for Teflon and the contour produced by the Teflon bulk may be unpredictable and irregular. Multiple laryngoscopies with several small injections may be more satisfactory than attempting to correct the insufficiency with one injection.

Muscle flap reconstruction of a cord uses the ipsilateral sternohyoid or omohyoid muscle. A thyrotomy is performed, the insufficient pseudocord area is elevated and the muscle flap is inserted through the thyrotomy area and sutured to the cricoid posteriorly. This is covered by a mucosal flap from the aryepiglottic fold or pyriform fossa. Thyroid cartilage implants may also be used for glottic reconstruction. A thyrotomy is performed, a subperichondrial pocket on the insufficient cord is created and a small wedge of cartilage is inserted. The mucosa is reapproximated, since it is important that the cartilage not be exposed.

Anterior glottic webs resulting from laryngoscopy techniques, external laryngeal procedures or trauma are treated with thyrotomy and insertion of an anterior commissure keel. A hyoid bone graft may be used anteriorly to lengthen the glottic chink (Fig. 18–20).

The three major requirements for adequate swallowing are closure of the glottic chink by the vocal cords, apposition of the larynx to the base of the tongue and a patent esophagus to avoid delay in passage of the bolus through the cricopharynx. A tight closure of the glottic chink by approximation of the true vocal cords is most important. It is not necessary that both cords function, but the remaining cord should be able to oppose the fixed or reconstructed opposite cord. Immediately following partial laryngeal surgery, there is almost complete obstruction of the glottic chink, which eliminates all of the major laryngeal functions. This swelling gradually resolves with time, and most patients are able to be decannulated and swallow within a period of three weeks. Patients unable to swallow or be decannulated after three weeks are discharged to their homes and given more time for their laryngeal function to return. Surgical procedures for glottic insufficiency are not performed before six months after surgery, and, in some cases, we wait as long as a year.

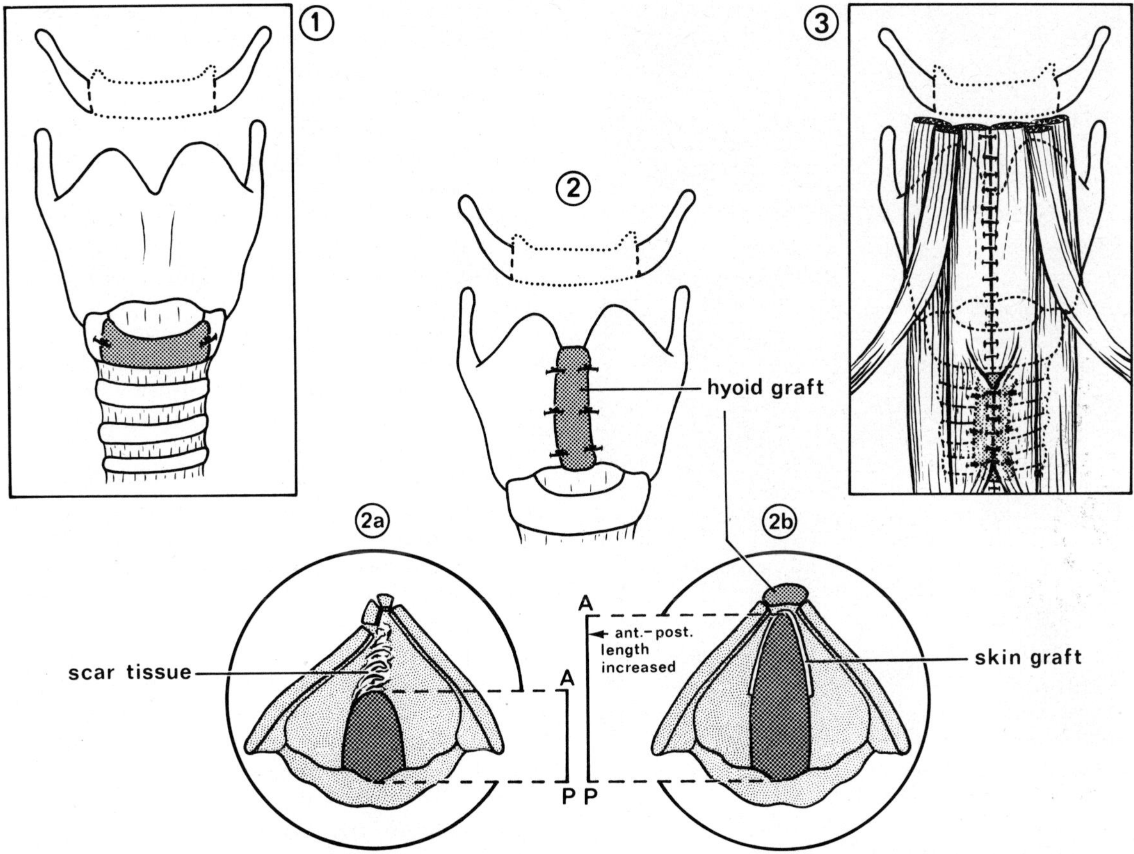


**Figure 18–20** Hyoid bone graft. *2,* Graft resected from mid-hyoid area. *2a,* Severe anterior glottic web with short glottic lengths. *2b,* Lengthening of glottis with hyoid graft and skin graft.

Despite the appearance of these functional problems, if they are recognized, diagnosed and adequately treated, return of laryngeal function is the rule rather than the exception.[17]

### *Dysphagia*

Dysphagia is commonly present in the immediate postoperative course of the patients, especially those with supraglottic resections and partial laryngopharyngectomies. As the patient practices with his reconstructed pharynx, dysphagia usually abates. Long-term dysphagia problems are more common in extended supraglottic resections when too much of the base of the tongue is resected. In spite of adequate closure and cricopharyngeal myotomy, the perichondria to muscle closure may impair the movement of the tongue posteriorly and inferiorly, impeding the bolus from entering the esophagus. One may surgically resect large areas of the base of the tongue, and surgical closure may be possible; however, reconstitution of swallowing function may be impossible.

### *Recurrent Cancer*

Most patients who undergo conservation laryngeal surgery with the correct indications will not develop a localized recurrent tumor. Its existence implies an inadequately performed initial surgical procedure. As stated before, the correct indications for conservation laryngeal surgery must be maintained, and, if these are extended, recurrences may be expected. The lesions must be accurately mapped preoperatively

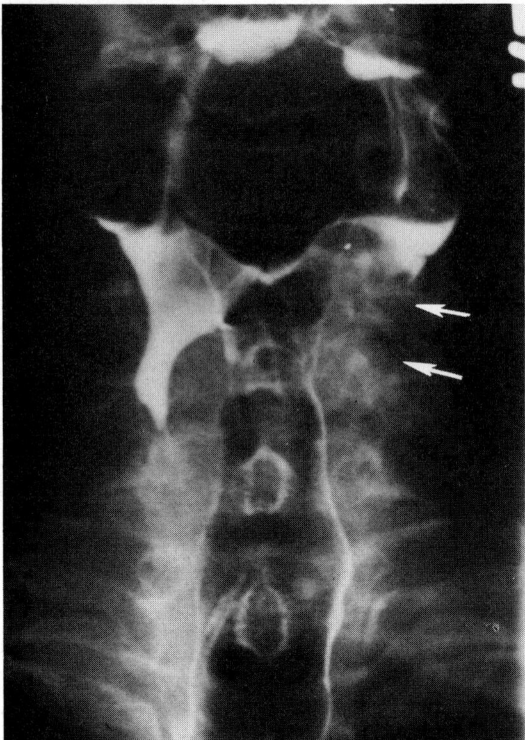

**Figure 18–21** Laryngogram demonstrating pyriform fossa obstructed with tumor (arrows).

using laryngograms (Fig. 18–21), xeroradiographs (Fig. 18–7) and direct laryngoscopy to prevent errors in judgment of tumor location. During the time of resection, the patient's larynx must be paralyzed so that adequate visibility is obtained. Use of single hooks and spreading with hemostats is important in the exposure. Use of a headlight is mandatory. The most common areas for positive margins are the anterior commissure, the posterior margin, the subglottic margin (in a hemilaryngectomy resection) (Fig. 18–22) and the superior margin (in a base of tongue and vallecular lesion). If the tumor involves the anterior commissure and also extends onto the opposite true vocal cord, one must be absolutely sure of the extent of the lesion before entering the larynx anteriorly. The anterior cartilage cuts must be properly placed, depending on the location of the lesion in the anterior commissure area. If this is improperly done, tumor transection and inadequate tumor resection will be the result. If the arytenoid is to be removed in a hemilaryngectomy resection, the specimen must be retracted anteriorly because posterior pressure is exerted with the scissors in order to remove the arytenoid. If this posterior pressure is not applied, the arytenoid has a tendency to retract posteriorly and one transects the specimen anterior to the arytenoid, producing an inadequate resection. If tumor extends subglottically but is in the limits of resection, the cricoid cartilage may be split anteriorly in order to insure an adequate subglottic margin.

Tumors in the base of tongue and vallecula area are treacherous for an inexperienced surgeon. With tumors in this area, the vallecula should not be entered, but the pharynx should be entered in the opposite pyriform fossa. The resection is extended superiorly and adequate visualization is achieved using this method. If a total laryngectomy is being performed, the resection should begin inferiorly in the trachea and extend up, assuring adequate visualization. The base of tongue area is probably the most common site for inadequate tumor margins. If recurrences occur following conservation laryngeal surgery, total laryngectomy is usually necessary.

Since recurrent cancer is such a significant problem, the surgeon must attempt to decrease the incidence of this complication by accurate preoperative mapping of the lesion, by performing the correct surgical

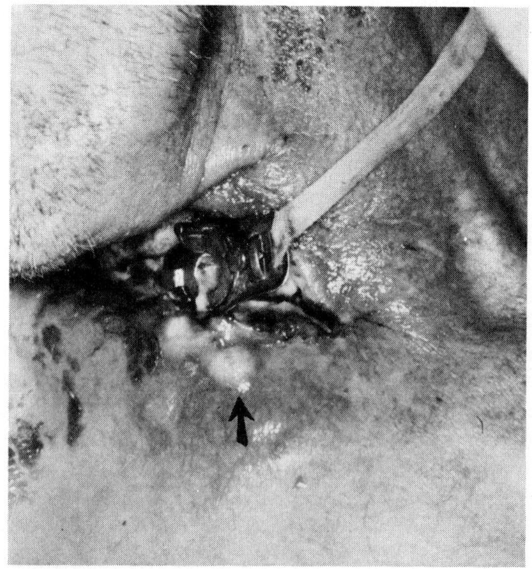

**Figure 18–22** Stomal recurrence from a positive subglottic margin (arrow).

technique with precision and by obtaining frozen sections during surgery for any questionable margin.

### *Hemorrhage*

Postoperative hemorrhage should be preventable at the time of surgery. The most common areas for postoperative hemorrhage are the base of the tongue and the superior laryngeal vessels. The base of the tongue is a very vascular area with multiple bleeding points. These should be controlled prior to closure. The superior laryngeal vessels should be suture-ligated at the time of resection. If the superior thyroid artery is transected, it should also be suture-ligated. These are the major areas of concern in terms of postoperative hemorrhage. If a neck dissection is performed in conjunction with a supraglottic, partial or total laryngectomy, then a dermal graft overlying the exposed carotid artery is necessary. This protects the artery, and, should a fistula develop postoperatively, carotid artery rupture will be minimized by the dermal graft protection. If the dermal graft is exposed to air, such as in a fistula, it will epithelialize and give skin covering and protection for the exposed carotid artery (Figs. 18–11 and 18–13). If carotid artery rupture does occur postoperatively, suture ligature of this vessel is necessary.

### *Voice Changes*

In almost all types of laryngeal surgery, voice changes will occur. Even with the simplest laryngoscopy techniques, the patient should be advised that voice changes may result. With simple stripping of the vocal cords at laryngoscopy, voice changes are usually minimal; however, they may be significant and can be catastrophic in singers. Usually with direct laryngoscopic techniques, the vocal cord is re-epithelialized quickly during the period of voice rest and there is vocal cord function and resultant good voice. Thyrotomies may produce anterior glottic webbing with resultant voice changes. Laryngofissure and cordectomy leads to formation of a pseudocord and, occasionally, anterior glottic webbing. This produces hoarseness with leakage of air during phonation and an airy type of voice. If deep musculature bites are taken during laryngoscopic techniques, inadequate function of the vocal cord may result secondary to trauma to the vocal muscle and voice changes may be the result. Patients who have had severe prolonged polypoid changes of the cords removed may experience voice problems, since these polyps may have performed a phonation function for years.

A study of postoperative partial laryngectomy patients has been performed to evaluate the quality of their voices. The three vocal parameters of breathiness, harshness and hoarseness were cross tabulated with the different types of surgical procedures performed — hemilaryngectomy, supraglottic laryngectomy and partial laryngopharyngectomy.[9] The supraglottic laryngectomy patients were least affected in terms of vocal breathiness; the partial laryngopharyngectomy patients were least affected in terms of vocal harshness. Hemilaryngectomy patients showed a significantly higher degree of vocal hoarseness than other patients. With surgical procedures that affect vocal cord adduction, as in the case of hemilaryngectomy and partial laryngopharyngectomy, a degree of breathiness will result in significant reduction in intelligibility of speech.

Surgical procedures that merely scar or affect the normal vocal cord vibratory pattern may only introduce hoarseness or harshness resulting in minimal effect on speech intelligibility. When a combination of breathiness and harshness with severe vocal effort occurs, the effect on speech intelligibility can be severe and extremely limit the listener's ability to understand the speaker. Patients who undergo partial laryngopharyngectomy procedures suffer the most severe consequence in speech intelligibility, and this is related to the amount of breathiness resultant from surgical resection. Hemilaryngectomy has the most significant affect on voice quality, with hoarseness affected the most. Ninety per cent of cases show a very satisfactory level of speech intelligibility independent of the type of conservation laryngeal surgery. The fact that over 80 per cent of patients report speaking effectively in most situations is a good indication that radical subtotal laryngectomy procedures can be performed without significant detriment to general speech intelligibility and communication effectiveness. Patients who have had supraglottic laryngectomies have minimal voice disorders since the vocal cords have not been disturbed, despite the fact that the entire supraglottis has been removed. Patients who have undergone partial laryngopharyngectomies will usually have one vocal cord fixed in the midline to prevent aspiration, and this consequently affects the quality of the voice. Of course, total laryngectomy patients have no voice and must either learn esophageal speech or use one of the multitude of vibrating devices available.

## POSTOPERATIVE CARE OF PATIENTS

### Supraglottic and Partial Laryngopharyngectomy

Patients must receive excellent tracheostomy care to prevent obstruction (Fig. 18–23). The patient is fed through a nasogastric tube for two to three weeks. Decannulation is accomplished about two weeks postoperatively or whenever the glottic chink is adequate. It is preferable to have the tracheal stoma almost closed before swallowing is initiated so that the patient may be able to build up pressure to assist in deglutition. Patients are started on foods of mixed consistencies; most patients do better with semisolids, such as puddings or mashed potatoes. Patients are encouraged to swallow hard rather than letting liquids trickle down slowly. Some patients learn to swallow quite rapidly, others are somewhat slower. The patient may need supplemental intravenous feedings for the first several days until oral intake is adequate. If aspiration persists, the nasogastric tube is reinserted and the patient is sent home for several weeks. Initiating and performing the act of deglutition following surgical resection requires strenuous activity, and elderly or debilitated patients may need extra time to gain weight and strength before deglutition is successful.

## LARYNGEAL TRAUMA AND STENOSIS

For the successful treatment of complications in laryngeal trauma, a fundamental understanding of the process of injury and its consequences is necessary. Laryngeal trauma may produce injuries involving the supraglottic, glottic and subglottic portions of the larynx, and various combinations of these areas. An accurate assessment of airway patency should be made as soon as possible. If a tracheotomy is not performed initially, these patients must be observed closely for the development of upper airway obstruction. The operative procedure employed for acute laryngeal injuries depends upon the type of injury.

### *Supraglottic Trauma*

These patients have usually received blunt trauma to the supraglottic portion of the larynx and will typically have edema or

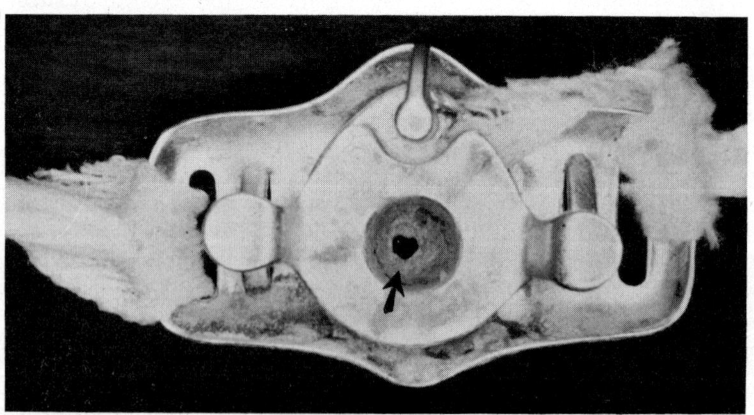

**Figure 18–23** Tracheostomy tube with almost complete obstruction of lumen (arrow). This is preventable with good nursing care.

hematoma, or both, involving the aryepiglottic folds and false vocal cords. The tissues in the supraglottic larynx are quite distensible and massive swelling with upper airway obstruction may occur quickly, necessitating a tracheotomy. There may be lacerations involving the epiglottis, and, occasionally, the entire supraglottis is avulsed with a posterior displacement. Laryngeal cartilage fractures may be present along with soft tissue trauma. If a fracture is present, a stent is applied. In severe injuries with avulsion of the entire supraglottic area, good results may be obtained by performing a completion supraglottic laryngectomy with removal of the false vocal cords and epiglottis. This repair is closed as a standard supraglottic laryngectomy, and we have found that this gives less scarring and more satisfactory results than attempting to reapproximate the supraglottis. If severe lacerations are present, massive supraglottic scarring may result with postoperative supraglottic stenosis. If an internal laryngeal stent is not used with fractures, then postoperative stenosis may occur. If laryngeal cartilage fractures are not present, internal stenting is usually not performed for supraglottic injuries.[15]

### Glottic Trauma

Glottic injuries usually involve a vertical thyroid cartilage fracture. This may displace cartilage into the laryngeal lumen. This injury is treated by a midline thyrotomy with exploration of the larynx, suturing all mucosal lacerations and applying a stent within the laryngeal lumen.

### Subglottic Trauma and Tracheal Separation

These injuries usually occur as a result of blunt trauma in the subglottic area. They present with swelling of the neck and progressive loss of airway. These injuries can be quite treacherous since on initial examination the severity of the injury may not be appreciated. If the trachea has been separated from the larynx or cricoid area, attempts at endotracheal intubation may be disastrous because the endotracheal tube may pass into the soft tissues in the subglottic area with total loss of airway.[1] This calls for immediate tracheotomy. Subglottic injuries may not have tracheal separation but may involve only fractures of the cricoid bone from external trauma. The cricoid cartilage may be fractured from a high tracheotomy. In all cases, these injuries must be explored, and realignment of the fractured cricoid with placement of an intraluminal stent must be accomplished. Failure to realign the cartilage fragments and to use a stent will result in postoperative subglottic stricturing of the trachea. Tracheal separation injuries should be explored, and the trachea should be reanastomosed (Fig. 18–24). With pure tracheal injuries, stents may or may not be used. Subglottic injuries must be evaluated carefully to insure that other pharyngeal or esophageal injuries are not present. These may be missed at the time of initial examination and result in infections and fistulas.

### Chronic Laryngeal Stenosis

The principles involved in the treatment of chronic laryngeal stenosis are dependent upon the location of the stenotic involvement.

#### SUPRAGLOTTIC STENOSIS

This usually occurs after supraglottic laryngeal trauma that has been unsuccessfully repaired initially. These patients not infrequently will have a good voice but an inadequate airway. The epiglottis may be bound to the posterior pharyngeal wall. The inferior vestibular area may be nearly closed by a mass of scar tissue almost obliterating the glottis. The upper portion of the thyroid ala may be displaced posteriorly secondary to blunt trauma. Supraglottic stenosis usually may be repaired by performing a supraglottic laryngectomy. This is closed by suturing thyroid perichondrium to the base of the tongue.

#### GLOTTIC STENOSIS

Glottic stenosis ranges from minimal to severe. Anterior glottic webbing may be treated by thyrotomy and placement of a McKnaught keel. With severe anterior glot-

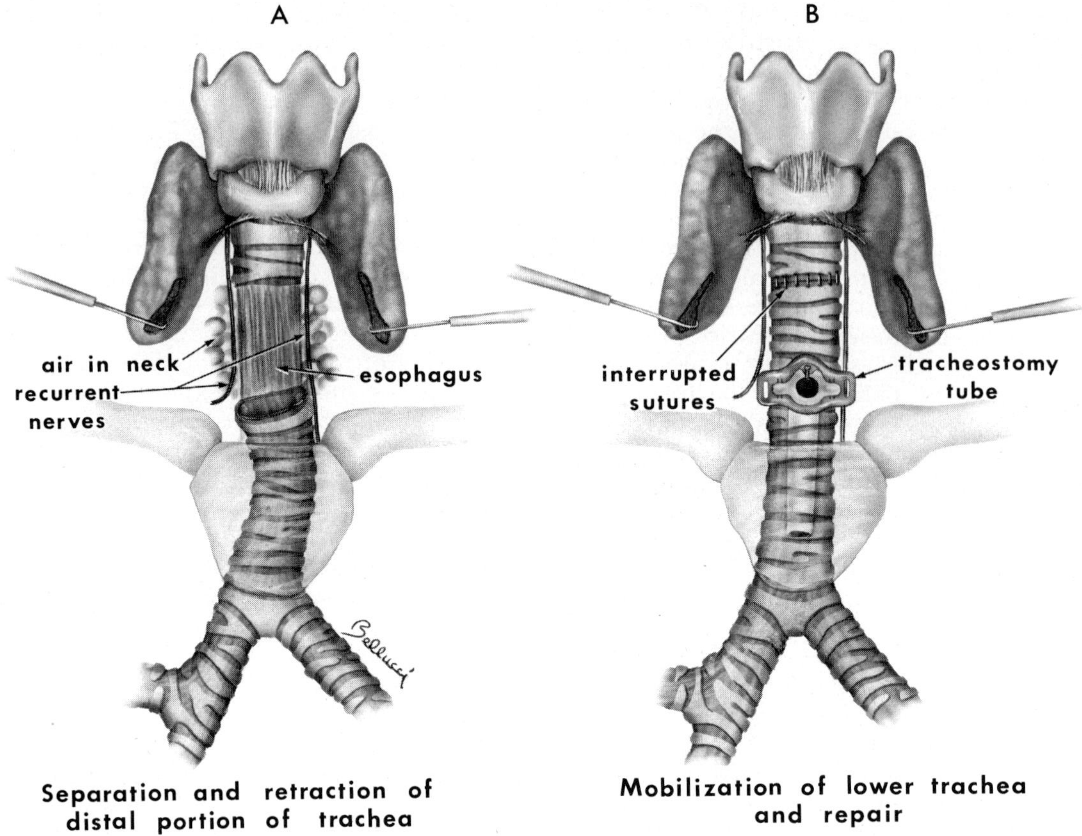


**Figure 18–24** Tracheal separation with reanastomosis. Note tracheostomy tube inserted below the separated area.

tic webbing, a thyrotomy with scar excision and skin grafting is performed. A hyoid bone graft wedged at the anterior commissure will increase the length of the glottis (Fig. 18–20).[6] Glottic stenosis with midline vocal cord fixation may be treated by a Woodman operation, in which the arytenoid cartilage is resected and the true vocal cord is lateralized. A Meurmann operation may be necessary to lateralize the true vocal cord. This consists of a thyrotomy and a submucosal resection of the true vocal cord and placement of a stent to lateralize the cord.

### SUBGLOTTIC STENOSIS

Subglottic stenosis may result from blunt injuries or from previous tracheostomies. It also occurs following long-term endotracheal tube maintenance. The exact location and length of the stenotic area must be ascertained via laryngograms and xeroradiograms (Fig. 18–25). Frequently, the stenotic area involves only the anterior tracheal wall. These may be repaired by a Schmieglow procedure, which consists of excising the scarred area and placement of a skin graft with a stent. If there is a great deal of deficient anterior tracheal cartilage, this procedure may be combined with a hyoid bone transplant to replace the anterior tracheal wall. If the stenotic area of the trachea is short with almost complete occlusion, a tracheal resection is indicated. Three centimeters is about the maximum length that can be safely resected; additional length may be obtained by severing the suprahyoid muscles, allowing the larynx and proximal trachea to drop down. If the true vocal cords are functional, great care must be taken to identify and isolate the recurrent laryngeal nerves and to avoid injury to the

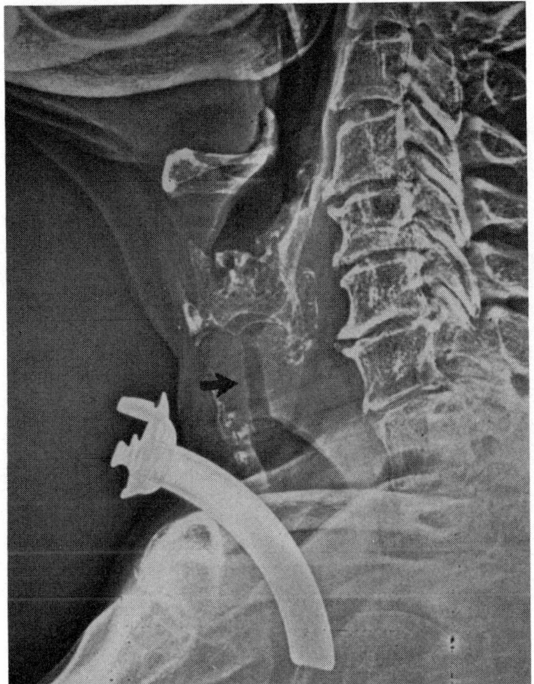

**Figure 18–25** Xeroradiograph demonstrating extent of subglottic stenosis (arrow).

structures. If the vocal cords are paralyzed and a sufficient airway does not exist, a Woodman procedure should also be done. Severe subglottic stenosis in the area of the cricoid may be treated by a resection of this area and a thyrotracheal reanastomosis. A hyoid bone graft may replace a crushed anterior cricoid cartilage. (Fig. 18–26). It must be re-emphasized that most tracheal stenoses involve the anterior tracheal wall, and a complete circumferential scar does not usually exist.

### *Bilateral Vocal Cord Paralysis*

Bilateral vocal cord paralysis is most commonly due to thyroidectomy. These patients usually have good voices but inadequate airways. There are several procedures available for lateralization of the true vocal cord, but we have found that the Woodman procedure performed properly gives the best results. The side (if any) most lateral is preferred. The steps involved in this operation

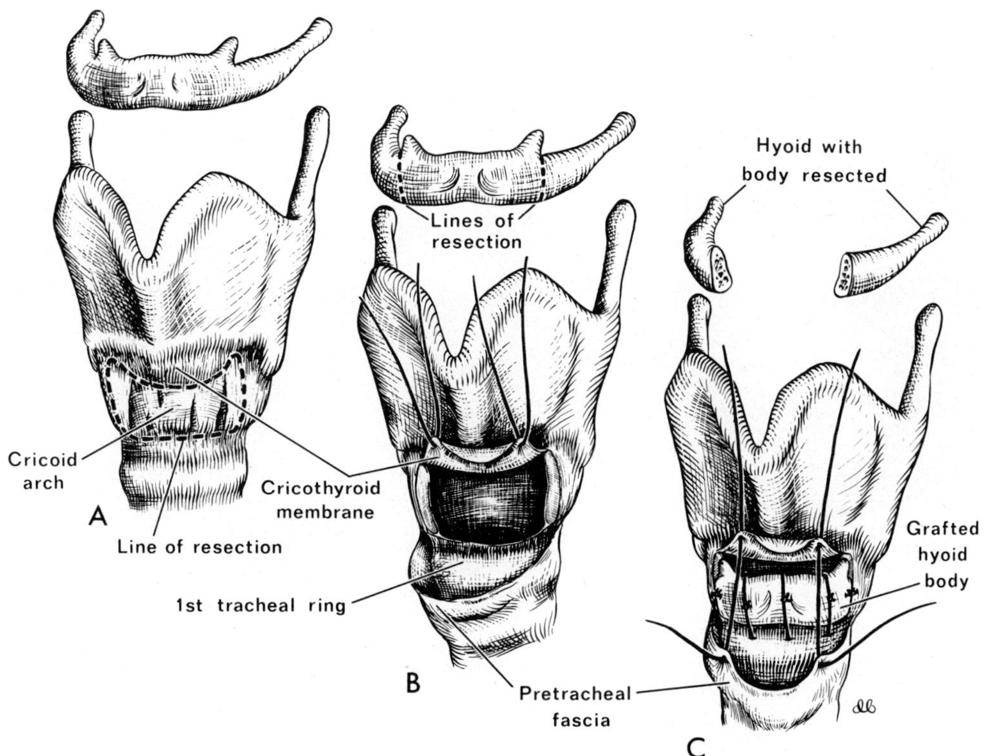


**Figure 18–26** *A,* Subglottic injury with crushed anterior cricoid arch. *B,* Resected anterior cricoid with area of hyoid to be used as graft. *C,* Grafted hyoid to reconstruct anterior cricoid arch.

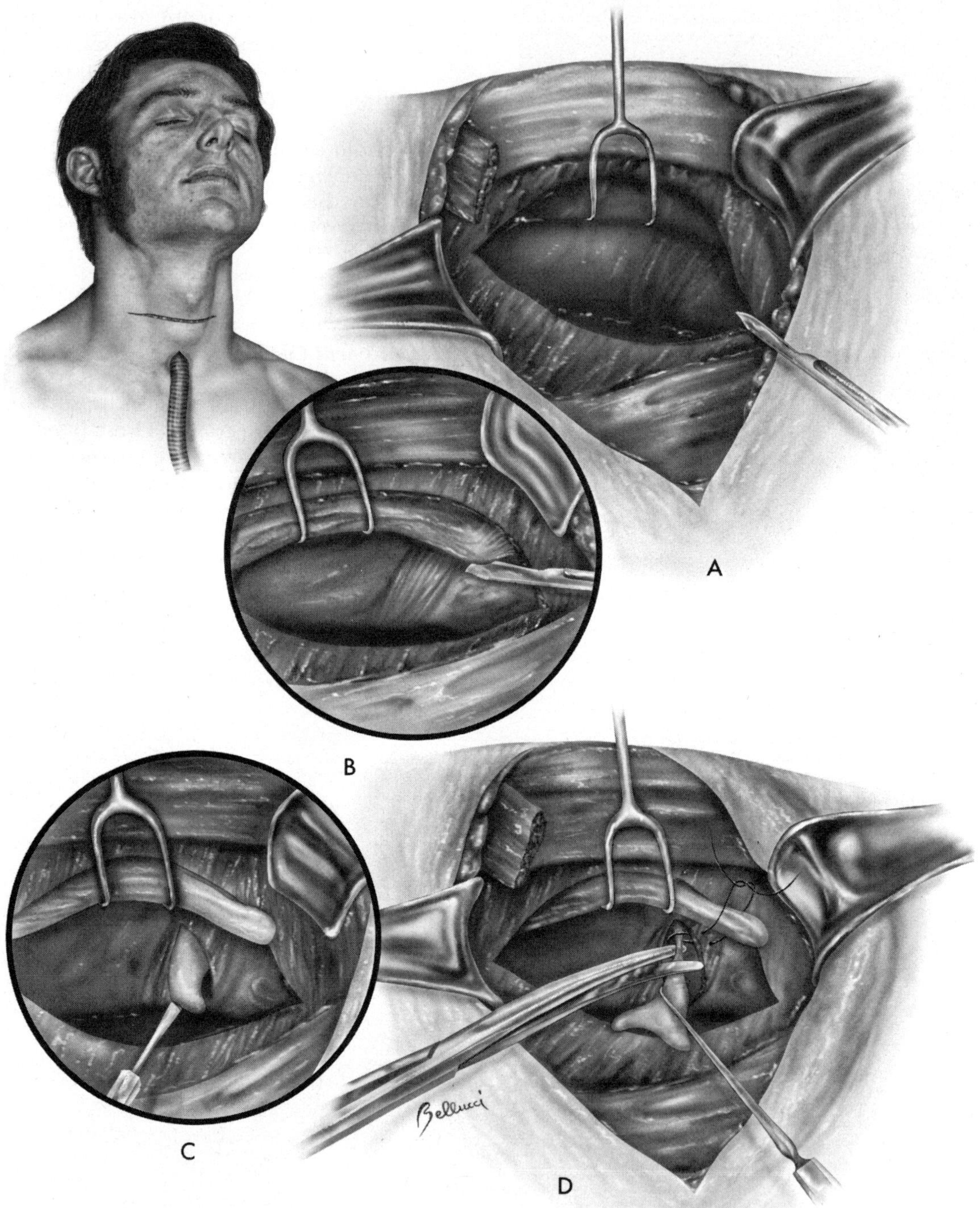


**Figure 18–27** Woodman procedure. *A,* Exposure of inferior constrictor. *B,* Removing muscle from larynx. *C,* Exposing arytenoid. *D,* Suture around vocal process of arytenoid.

are important in avoiding postoperative complications or failure of vocal cord lateralization resulting in an inadequate airway (Fig. 18–27). A large endotracheal tube placed into the laryngeal lumen is necessary to lateralize the cord during the time of surgery.

The inferior cricoid thyroid articulation must be separated. The inferior constrictor muscle is transected off the posterior margin of the laryngeal cartilage (Fig. 18–27*B*). The pyriform fossa is pushed medially away from the thyroid cartilage. The arytenoid is dissected free of its muscle attachments (Fig. 18–27*C*). A # 2-0 silk suture placed over the vocal process is then pulled laterally and attached to the lateral ala of the thyroid cartilage (Fig. 18–27*D*). The body of the arytenoid cartilage is resected, and, before the suture is tied in place an assistant looks through a laryngoscope and visualizes the glottic chink area to see if adequate lateralization has taken place. If it is adequate, the suture is tied in place. The placement of the stitch is the key to the operation. A tear in the mucosa with the first stitch leads to the complication of stricture of the posterior commissure. This occurs particularly if the first stitch is not around the vocal process before anchoring it to the lateral ala. If a stitch is placed and it slips, or a second stitch is placed because of improper position, the incidence of postoperative failure to lateralize the cords increases. A 5 to 6 mm. airway posteriorly is ideal.

## Bibliography


1. Alonso, W. A., Caruso, V. G., and Roncace, E. A.: Minibikes — a new factor in laryngotracheal trauma. Ann. Otol., *82*:800, 1973.
2. Biller, H. F., Barnhill, F. R., Ogura, J. H., et al.: Hemilaryngectomy following radiation failure for carcinoma of the vocal cords. Laryngoscope, *80*:249, 1970.
3. Biller, H. F., Ogura, J. H., and Pratt, L. L.: Hemilaryngectomy for $T_2$ glottic cancers. Arch. Otolaryngol., *93*:238, 1971.
4. Daly, J. F., and Kwok, F. N.: Laryngofissure and cordectomy. Laryngoscope, *85*:1290, 1975.
5. Dedo, D. D., Alonso, W. A., and Ogura, J. H.: Incidence, predisposing factors and outcome of pharyngocutaneous fistulas complicating head and neck cancer surgery. Ann. Otol., *84*:833, 1975.
6. Druck, N. S., Alonso, W. A., and Ogura, J. H.: Hyoid arch transposition. Trans. Am. Acad. Ophthalmol. Otolaryngol., *82*:175, 1976.
7. Gall, A. M., Sessions, D. G., and Ogura, J. H.: Complications following surgery for cancer of the larynx and hypopharynx. Cancer, *39*:624, 1977.
8. Kirchner, J. A., and Som, M. L.: The anterior commissure technique of partial laryngectomy. Clinical and laboratory observations. Laryngoscope, *85*:1308, 1975.
9. Klein, A. D., Wasserstrom, J., Sessions, D. G., et al.: Rehabilitation of partial laryngectomy patients. Trans. Am. Acad. Ophthalmol. Otolaryngol., in press.
10. Lillie, J. C., and DeSanto, L. W.: Transoral surgery of early cordal carcinoma. Trans. Am. Acad. Ophthalmol. Otolaryngol., *77*:92, 1973.
11. Lyons, G. D., Lousteau, R. J., and Mouney, D. F.: $CO_2$ laser laryngoscopy in a variety of lesions. Laryngoscope, *86*:1658, 1976.
12. Ogura, J. H., and Dedo, H. H.: Glottic reconstruction following subtotal glottic-supraglottic laryngectomy. Laryngoscope, *75*:865, 1965.
13. Ogura, J. H., and Dedo, H. H.: Repair of large pharyngostoma utilizing bilateral non-delayed regional pedicle flaps. Laryngoscope, *75*:588, 1965.
14. Ogura, J. H., and Mallen, R. W.: Partial laryngopharyngectomy for supraglottic and pharyngeal carcinoma. Trans. Am. Acad. Ophthalmol. Otolaryngol., *69*:832, 1965.
15. Ogura, J. H., and Mallen, R. W.: Trauma of the larynx. *In* Ballinger, J. J. (ed.): Diseases of the Nose, Throat and Ear. Philadelphia, Lea and Febiger, 1969, pp. 318–335.
16. Sessions, D. G., Maness, G. M., and McSwain, B.: Laryngofissure in the treatment of carcinoma of the vocal cord. Laryngoscope, *75*:490, 1965.
17. Sessions, D. G., Ogura, J. H., and Ciralsky, R. H.: Late glottic insufficiency. Laryngoscope, *85*:950, 1975.
18. Som, M. L., and Silver, C. E.: The anterior commissure technique of partial laryngectomy. Arch. Otolaryngol., *87*:42, 1968.
19. Strong, M. S.: Laser excision of carcinoma of the larynx. Laryngoscope, *85*:1286, 1975.
20. Stutsman, A. C., and McGavran, M. H.: Ultraconservative management of superficially invasive epidermoid carcinoma of the true vocal cord. Ann. Otol., *80*:507, 1971.

# TRACHEOSTOMY COMPLICATIONS

# 19

*John J. Conley*

## INTRODUCTION

Tracheostomy has developed from a surgical technique to relieve upper airway obstruction into a therapeutic facility in pulmonary physiology. Its essentiality has paralleled certain diseases and the development of new surgical techniques. It attained prominence in the 19th century in the management of diphtheria and croup. It was incorporated into the management of cancer of the larynx and pharynx and of trauma to the head and neck shortly after its advantages became apparent. Galloway (1943)[33] introduced tracheostomy to assist in the treatment of respiratory paralysis secondary to poliomyelitis. This application has become dramatically expanded to facilitate the management of not only those suffering from airway obstruction but also everyone who may develop airway obstruction, depressed pulmonary function, aspiration or unconscious states. Tracheostomy is also used as an adjunct to the new and evolving cardiopulmonary surgical techniques that require pulmonary toilet and respiratory control. It has become a prime mechanism in regulating pulmonary function in severe medical and surgical conditions.

New instruments have been developed to accommodate this broad therapeutic application. The original metal cannulas of various sizes and shapes had an inner tube that could be inspected and cleaned at any time and that was an essential part of the apparatus. Balloons were later applied to these tubes to make an airtight system. New products manufactured from synthetics were introduced to respond to developing techniques for pulmonary care in intensive care units.[7, 16, 34, 44, 55] Certain new tubes omitted the inner cannula. Smooth, nonadherent synthetics combined with constant high humidity, careful monitoring and suctioning reduced crusting in the tube and trachea and airway obstruction. In many instances, it was discovered that an oroendotracheal tube could be used in lieu of the tracheostomy.

This impressive expansion of technique, instrumentation and medical involvement carries with it an intrinsic risk outside the perimeters of the condition it is meant to alleviate. The operative mortality of individuals undergoing tracheostomy must therefore be divided into those who are undergoing extremely hazardous operations of which tracheostomy is only an ancillary part and those for whom tracheostomy is the prime operation. The mortality in the high-risk neurosurgical and cardiopulmonary cases ranges from 20 to 40 per cent. The mortality for tracheostomy as the prime operation varies from .5 to 3 per cent.[74] These variations can be explained by the different ages and conditions of the patients and by the urgency and the skill of the personnel involved. Elective tracheostomy is a much more favorable circumstance than waiting until the situation becomes an emergency. Elective and emergency tracheostomies are greatly assisted by inserting an oroendotracheal tube to control the airway prior to beginning the operation. In a broad review of the world's literature, Salmon (1975)[74] stated that some 2577 cases treated with tracheostomy for various conditions presented a 42 per cent mortality, whereas a group of 2818 cases had only 2.7 per cent mortality attributable to the tracheostomy itself. The mortality in children is slightly higher.

Hawkins and Williams (1976)[45] reported on 73 tracheostomies performed in children under three years of age. Operative complications developed in 14 per cent, and postoperative complications developed in 22 per cent. The most common complication was interstitial air, and the most deadly complication was obstruction of the cannula. The overall mortality of this group was 27 per cent. Only 5.5 per cent died as a result of the tracheostomy complication, however. Their paper highlights both the gravity of the basic condition for which the tracheostomy is done in children and the serious prognosis attached to that condition. It also emphasizes that tracheostomy in children still carries a significant mortality.

## INDICATIONS FOR TRACHEOSTOMY

There are two basic reasons to enter the trachea. The overriding indication is the relief of an anticipated obstruction or the emergent relief of a severe airway obstruction. In addition to the establishment of an adequate airway, tracheostomy may be introduced to support and control the ventilatory process for a broad list of medical and surgical conditions in which the normal respiratory physiology is depressed or handicapped to critical levels. These procedures are done electively or on an emergency basis. The airway is established by the oroendotracheal or the transtracheal route. A different set of instruments and techniques gain entrance to the airway system and then fulfill the purposes for which it was instituted. This combination of circumstances could not be expected to be devoid of complications and untoward results.

## TECHNIQUE

### Elective Tracheostomy

Once the decision regarding the necessity for tracheostomy has been made, it should be carried out on an elective basis.[3, 9, 24, 26, 38] This offers the best advantages to the surgeon and to the patient. Anesthetic techniques must be adapted to the circumstances governing the necessity for the tracheostomy. Most techniques are done under local anesthesia. There is, however, a definite role for oroendotracheal intubation in certain cases. Individuals who are excessively apprehensive or have a borderline airway problem, children and patients with short, thick necks who might present a technical problem are all potential candidates for intubation prior to tracheostomy. When possible, tracheostomy under local anesthesia should be done just prior to the beginning of a major cancer resection in the orolaryngopharyngeal areas. This eliminates the awkwardness of the anesthetic tube from the operative field and reduces the incidence of stomal recurrence. Some tracheostomies are done at the end of a major resection if the airway has become compromised. Patients with trismus present a special problem, in that oral entry is prohibited. In children, this is solved with adequate preoperative sedation and general anesthesia by mask technique while the tracheostomy is being done. In adults, a nasoendotracheal tube may be introduced under local anesthesia, or the surgeon may proceed directly with the tracheostomy. One per cent lidocaine (Xylocaine), without adrenalin, is used for infiltration, and 2 per cent lidocaine is injected into the tracheal lumen just prior to entry.

Different age groups require special considerations. Children present a delicate and diminutive anatomy and a dependency upon the tube.[4, 20, 21, 28] Their clinical problems are often desperate. They respond by instinct to these situations by crying, struggling and gasping, all of which complicate tracheostomy. Their incidence of complications is increased. There is a limited selection of tracheal tubes, and their tissues melt away rapidly from a poor fit and constant pressure. Decannulization is frequently insecure because of dependency on the tube and inability to test patency with the tube in position. At the other end of the spectrum are those who are old and infirm, with chronic lung disease and who are frequently aided, in a basic way, by tracheostomy.

The architecture of the neck and trachea can present problems in tracheostomy.[46, 48, 57] Short thick necks, rigid cervical spines, inability to extend the head, hypertrophy of the thyroid gland, calcification of the trachea or tracheal malacia, displacement of the trachea and abnormal position of great vessels in the root of the

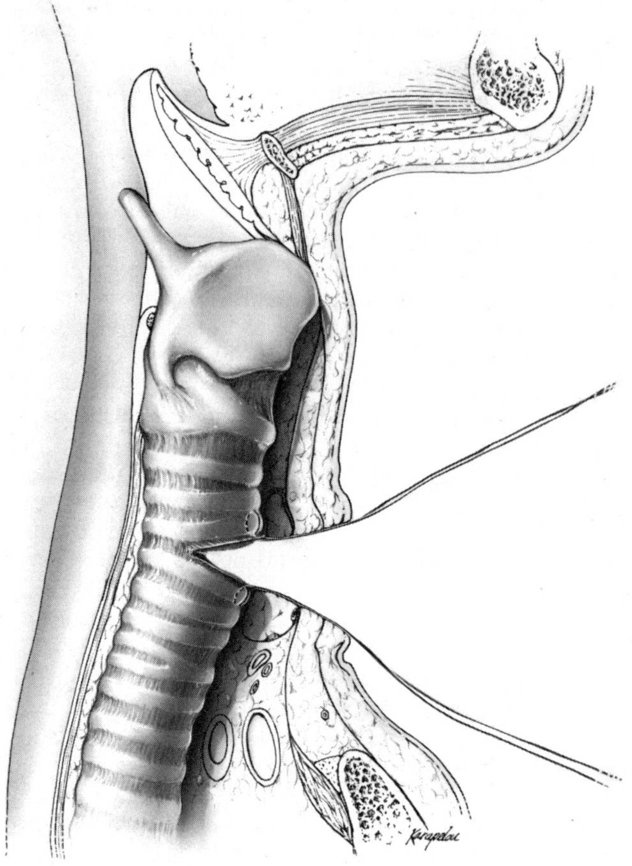

**Figure 19–1** Intracartilaginous incision between 3rd and 4th rings with long silk sutures to stabilize the segments for tube changing.

neck add danger to the technique. None of these abnormalities prohibit tracheostomy, but all need evaluation in advance and consideration for some modification of the routine. Oral or nasal intubation under local anesthesia may be very helpful.

There have been many debates about the position of the incisions in the skin of the neck and in the trachea. The vertical incision in the skin gives the best exposure to the trachea, but the horizontal incision gives the best aesthetic effect and the best design to accommodate other planned incisions in the neck. The horizontal incision is used in most instances. Incisions in the trachea include horizontal intercartilaginous, vertical cartilaginous, cruciate, superior and inferior tracheal flap incisions and the removal of a square or circular segment of trachea. The ones that disturb the anatomy of the trachea the least have proved to be the best. If the trachea is incised only once, there is no infection or hematoma and the patient is decannulated within a week, there is little danger of a tracheal complication or stenosis. If there are repeated tracheostomies done over an interval of years by various techniques, causing excessive scarring or infection or in the presence of irradiation, the possibility of tracheal stenosis is markedly increased. This author has recently operated on a patient who had had 19 previous tracheostomies without complication or stenosis, attesting to the fact that, within certain limits, the trachea has an exceptional capacity for spontaneous rehabilitation. This permits strong voices for and against almost all of these different incisional techniques. There is some consensus, however, that the vertical incision in the trachea is preferred in children. Lulenski and Batsakis (1975)[54] compared the inferiorly based tracheal flap with a vertical incision in 26 dogs and concluded that the inferiorly based tracheal flap was superior for preservation of the tracheal lumen and also for the healing at the stoma. It is generally agreed that individuals who have repetitive tracheostomies, a tracheal flap created or an excision of a part of the wall of the trachea and those who have to go on a respirator have a higher incidence of tracheal stenosis. It seems reasonable to state that a minimal disturbance to the tracheal architecture offers the best chance to avoid stenosis. We have used the horizontal intercartilaginous incision at the 2nd to 4th tracheal rings and have not seen a tracheal stenosis in 30 years.

Most complications are derived from the tube and the postoperative care.[66, 77, 84] After the trachea is identified and incised, it is stabilized with hooks to permit the entrance of an endotracheal anesthetic tube or a tracheostomy tube. This is the first act of trauma. A cuffed anode tube is the most suitable appliance for general anesthesia. The selection of tracheal tubes is governed by the requirements of the operation. In an uncomplicated tracheostomy, a noncuffed silver or plastic tube is the least troublesome. If it is necessary to protect the lower trachea and lungs from aspiration or hemorrhage, a plastic tube with an inner cannula and a built-in cuff is preferred. If the patient requires controlled ventilation, a Portex type of tube is satisfactory. These tubes should have a high-volume, low-pressure cuff system.

The postoperative nursing care for an uncomplicated tracheostomy requires proper humidification and suction. The nursing care for a cuffed tube on a ventilator is highly specialized and should not be delegated to an untrained or inexperienced attendant. This critical situation should have the supervision of the inhalation service.

### Emergency Tracheostomy

Emergency tracheostomy can be a harrowing experience for all concerned, and it is to be avoided whenever possible by the decision to do an elective tracheostomy. There are instances of trauma, foreign bodies, airway obstruction from neoplasia and respiratory failure that dictate immediate entrance into the trachea. When possible, the insertion of an oroendotracheal tube is the best first step in preparing for tracheostomy. This may not be realistic outside, or indeed even inside, a hospital facility, and the surgeon must then open the trachea in a forthright manner under this situation of stress. This act may be associated with mouth-to-mouth breathing and external cardiac massage.

The safest and easiest point of entrance is the cricothyroid membrane. This section of anatomy is thin, relatively avascular, positioned subglottically and usually above the isthmus of the thyroid gland. Ingenious devices have been invented to meet this crisis, but they are rarely available at the critical moment. Entrance is accomplished with what is available to cut the skin and membrane, to control the localized bleeding and to open into the airway. Scalpel, scissors, hemostat, razor blade and penknife have all been used successfully. There is, of course, increased danger to the cartilage and the recurrent laryngeal nerves and of infection. After the cricothyroid membrane has been opened, a tube inserted and the patient's condition stabilized, one can reassess the situation and proceed with lowering the tracheostomy to the 3rd tracheal ring. There is a danger of stenosis if the tube is permitted to remain above the cricoid cartilage.[49, 69]

## THE TUBE

It is unrealistic to expect one type of tube to satisfy all of the requirements of tracheal cannulization.[7, 14, 15, 16, 19] The variations range from the anatomic changes that one finds from infancy to old age; the gross differences between the short, fat neck and the long, thin neck; the differences in size and position of the trachea; flexible necks and those stiffened by arthritic processes; and all types and conditions of diseases for which the procedure of tracheostomy is being done. No single tube could fulfill all of these requirements. It is more realistic to appreciate that there are selections of tubes and that these are expected to change as new concepts of treatment and new materials enter the pic-

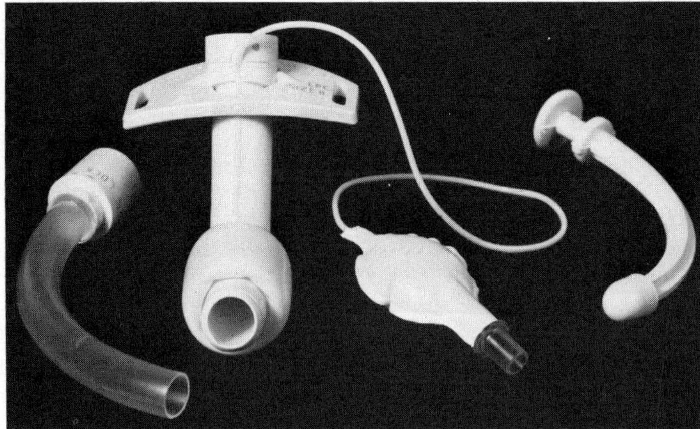

**Figure 19–2** Low-pressure, soft-cuffed Shiley tracheostomy tube with pivotal neck flange and inner cannula.

ture.[31, 55, 78, 82, 85] The original tubes were designed by prominent specialists in this field. Jackson, Tucker, Holinger all contributed their concepts as to the curve of the tube, the essentiality of the inner cannula and the fabrication in silver. Within the past 10 years, however, a new family of tracheostomy tubes has come into this specialty, of which Portex, Rush and Shiley are very popular. They have been designed from synthetic material, a majority have no inner cannula and many have a built-in, prefabricated cuff at the tip. Some of these tubes were designed specifically to serve new purposes in ventilation.[13, 34, 44, 52, 60, 68] The greatest accommodation comes from a pivotal neck plate, a semirigid outer tube and inner tube, a recessed inflation tube with a cuff that is built into the tube, a pressure indicator balloon and a standard 15 mm. connector at the head so that it may be adapted to ventilatory apparatus. A tube that is smaller than the trachea is desirable so that the patient will have an auxiliary air passage. This is, of course, not possible in infants because the cannula almost always fits rather snugly in the smaller tracheas.[30, 37, 45, 47]

The simplest tube is usually the best tube when the primary purpose of tracheostomy is to relieve tracheal obstruction. This is a tube with an inner cannula that has the correct size and shape to fit into that particular trachea. If the tube is used for the purposes of ventilation or protection from aspiration in addition to the establishment of an airway, then a

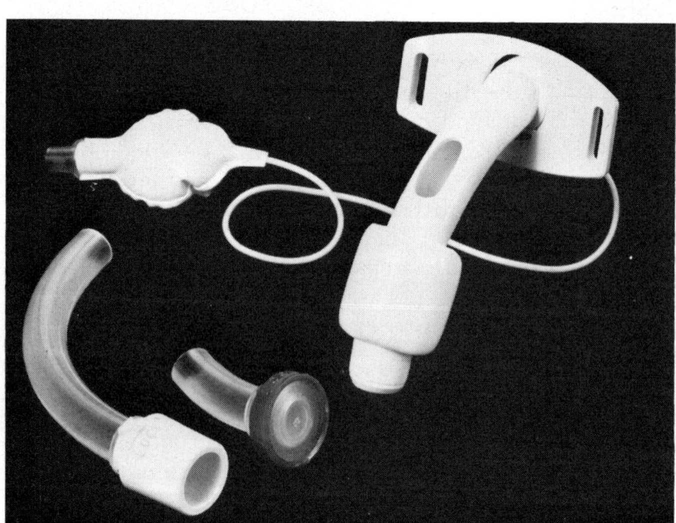

**Figure 19–3** Shiley speaking tube.

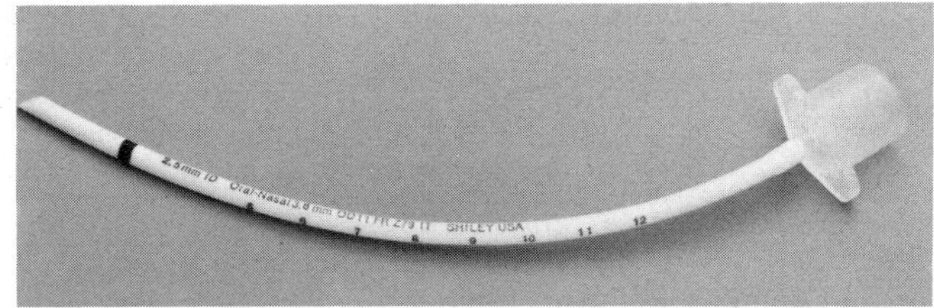

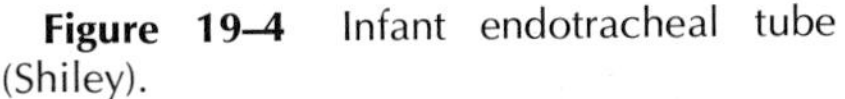
**Figure 19–4** Infant endotracheal tube (Shiley).

cuffed tube with or without an inner cannula is necessary. This would be a Portex or Shiley type of tube. Short tubes will become dislodged from the trachea upon coughing. Long tubes will impinge upon the carina or anterior wall of the trachea. Inflexible tubes do not mold in the trachea, and tubes without a mobile shield will cause pressure on the skin of the neck or trachea. It is therefore necessary to select the tube ideal for that particular tracheal wound and the purpose that it must service.

## COMPLICATIONS

The literature is replete with documentation of the pernicious effects of prolonged intubation, the cuffed tube, its association with the ventilator and the special problems encountered in children.[1–85]

McEwen (1880)[59] reported on the endotracheal tube and its traumatic effect on the larynx. He also proposed suggestions for modifying the tube and reducing the incidence of trauma and complications. This process of modification and the adaptation of new tubes is still going on. It is now fully appreciated that there is no such item as the ideal endotracheal tube that is completely free of causing complications in all instances. Hengerer, Strome and Jaffe (1975)[47] reported on the injuries to the neonatal larynx from long-term intubation. They state that, although more infants are being saved by this technique, there has been a marked increase in laryngeal defects. They propose a soft tube that is physiologically adequate. The tube should be tapered and create as little pressure as is necessary to make the respirator effective. They emphasize the importance of hydration to prevent drying of the membrane and drying of secretions in the tube. They stress constant supervision of the larynx over the period of intubation. They quote a dozen authors who have had complications from prolonged intubation, thus documenting the relatively high incidence, the immediate dangers and the prolonged effect. McCullough and Whytehead (1976)[58] state that tracheostenosis following assisted ventilation is now recognized as a major complication of tracheostomy when cuffed tracheostomy tubes are used. They emphasize the importance of the use of the correct tube with a regulated amount of air in the cuff under careful and constant supervision. Hawkins and Williams (1976)[45] reported on 73 tracheostomies performed in children under the age of three years. Fourteen per cent of these developed operative complications, and 22 per cent developed postoperative complications. Twenty-seven per cent of the patients died. About 22 per cent of these deaths were due to the patient's disease, whereas only 5 per cent were due to the tracheostomy technique itself. Aass (1975)[1] reviewed 79 patients who had undergone tracheostomy or long-term intubation. He discussed tube occlusion, dislocated tube, bilateral pneumothorax, one fatal innominate arterial hemorrhage, atelectasis, prolonged hoarseness and radiologically verified tracheal stenosis in 12 per cent of the 43 long-term surviving cases. Schloss (1972)[76] emphasizes the increase in laryngeal and tracheal complications following prolonged intubation. He outlines the causes, the incidence and the treatment. Tucker and Silberman (1972)[83] have reported on the special problems encountered in tracheostomy in children with suggestions on their control and treatment. Rabuzzi and Reed (1971)[73] emphasize the occurrence of intrathoracic complications in tracheostomy in children, detail the signs and symptoms and suggest ways of reducing this complication.

## Finding the Trachea

The identification of this vertical midline air tube that is an extension of the larynx is influenced by the physiognomy of the neck and the basic condition of the patient. Operations on individuals with short, fat necks are the most difficult since the trachea is buried deeply, requiring greater exposure and more manipulation of the tissues. Long, thin necks with prominent thyroid cartilages are ideal for rapid exposure and tracheal identification. Gross enlargement of the thyroid gland will cover the upper trachea, present additional bleeding and require transection of the isthmus in order to visualize the site of cannulization. The right angle retractors that are used for exposure may be placed too deeply on one side and dislodge and conceal the trachea beneath the retractor. If the trachea is very soft, it will be compressed with retraction unless special care is taken. The trachea may be deviated to one side or compressed by a mass displacing it in an abnormal position. The anatomy in children and infants is diminutive and delicate. Some individuals cannot extend the head and neck, thus reducing the presentation of the trachea.

The basic condition determines whether the procedure will be done under local or general anesthesia and whether it is under elective or emergency conditions. The vast majority of tracheostomies are done under local anesthesia. It is much simpler for the surgeon, however, to perform this operation with an oroendotracheal tube in position, and this is pertinent and desirable. When there is any question of airway obstruction or the possibility of surgical difficulty, an oroendotracheal tube should be inserted so that the tracheostomy can be carried out under safe and controlled circumstances.[1, 6, 11, 18]

## Hemorrhage

Hemorrhage during the operative phase may be encountered from the anterior jugular vein and thyroid gland. The thyroid isthmus is usually retracted superiorly to the opening in the trachea. Occasionally, it may be displaced inferiorly or transected and moved laterally. Bleeding of these vessels is controlled by #3-0 silk ties or #3-0 chromic catgut transfixions. There is a slight danger of severe hemorrhage from inadvertent injury to the right common carotid artery where it crosses the low trachea at the root of the neck and also of possible damage to the innominate artery when dissection is attempted in a very low position in the neck. Hemorrhage from these vessels requires immediate digital compression, opening the wound to expose the vessel adequately, possibly resecting a segment of clavicle and then suturing, patching, grafting or ligating the involved vessel. This complication can be avoided by identifying the trachea at the 2nd or 3rd ring and keeping the dissection in the tracheal fascia. The most serious type of hemorrhage occurs from one week to two months after tracheostomy and is the result of erosion of a major vessel by the tracheal tube or cuff.

## Subcutaneous Emphysema

This complication causes considerable concern but is rarely fatal when associated with tracheostomy alone. With tracheostomy, it is precipitated by the forceful in-

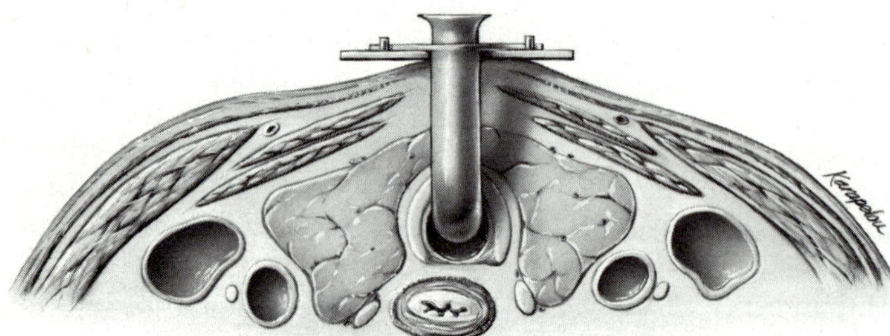

**Figure 19–5** Proper size and correct curve of cannula in the trachea with no pressure on the posterior wall.

jection of air from an opening in the airway system into the subcutaneous tissues. It may also connote serious airway abnormalities when associated with blunt or penetrating trauma to the neck or chest, continuous ventilatory support, percutaneous cannulation and surgery in the root of the neck.

A combination of factors causes a diversion of exhaled tracheal air through the tracheostomy into the superior and deep fascial spaces at the neck.[22, 56, 81] An overly large incision in the trachea; depression of the superior flap of the trachea above the incision, causing obstruction to excision; obstruction to the egress of air by glottic or pharyngeal obstruction; a tube that is partially obstructed or diverts air into the soft tissues of the neck; too tight a closure of the subcutaneous tissue and skin about the tracheostomy tube, causing a ball-valve effect; and excessive coughing may all contribute to subcutaneous emphysema. Air is forced into the loose fascial spaces of the neck by pressures high enough to open them, secondary to mechanical obstructions to its free escape about or in the tracheostomy tube. The continuous injection of this air mass forces it along the fascial spaces. The emphysema may be localized in the neck alone, but it can be forced to spread to the top of the scalp, eyelids, face, chest, abdominal wall, mediastinum and pericardium. It has not been documented that it produces serious pressure on the heart, lungs or mediastinum.

Subcutaneous emphysema secondary to tracheostomy is diagnosed by the sensation of crepitus to touch, localized swelling and characteristic roentgenography. It usually occurs within the first day and is usually self-limited to five to seven days unless the precipitating factors persist. It may be associated with a low-grade fever, mild localized cellulitis and a localized feeling of discomfort secondary to stretching and expansion of the skin. The precipitating factors of tight tissue closure or an improperly fitting tube are corrected immediately. The vast majority of these patients are already on antibiotics. Precautions must be taken to see that the tracheostomy tube is not dislocated on the basis of the swelling in the neck.

### Pneumothorax and Pneumomediastinum

(See Chapter 3.)

### Infections

Even though the tracheostomy may be done under sterile conditions, it is a matter of only a few hours until the area is grossly contaminated by the unsterile hands of the patient or his attendants, secretions from the oral cavity, suction tubes, instruments, dressings, bedclothes and the general environment. In addition to local wound contamination and infection, there is the increased hazard of contamination in the ventilatory system, in the intensive care unit and in the apparatus used to support the patient. The organisms are usually mixed, containing *Staphylococcus, Streptococcus, Pseudomonas aeruginosa, Escherichia coli* and oral cavity flora.[8, 72] The patient is routinely covered with antibiotics postoperatively, which helps to protect the local area and pulmonary system as the regional fibrous tissue barriers and local immunities develop.

Great advances in local hygiene have been made to protect the tracheostomy system, the ventilatory system and the necessary equipment. These advances include the use of disposable sterile gloves and sterile suction catheters for each suctioning procedure in the trachea. This routine hygienic act may appear wasteful, and certainly is not necessary for every patient. It is impossible, however, at this stage of management, to determine who is susceptible to a *Pseudomonas* septicemia on the basis of tracheal contamination and who is not. This is a significant step away from the days when the suction catheters were lying on the bed or on bedside tables or slipping to the floor and were used by hands that had been in contact with bedpans, toilet activity and other serious infections. Prophylaxis, therefore, is the best counteraction to infection. When infection occurs in the neck wound, which is quite unusual, it is usually indolent, producing mild cellulitis and granulation tissue. This wound is, fortunately, an open wound with adequate drainage. The most serious aspects of the infections about the tracheostomy is their possibility of infecting the trachea, lungs and mediastinum. *Pseudomonas* has proved to be the most troublesome organism and requires specific antibiotic treatment.

### Necrosis

This is one of the most serious complications associated with tracheostomy and results primarily from focal pressure followed by secondary infection. The pressure is derived from an oversized tracheostomy tube, an improper curve of the tube, an impingement of the tip of the tube or the pressure of a balloon on the tube.[5, 17, 31, 35] The effect of this pressure begins as an ulcer in the wall of the mid- or low cervical trachea. If the pressure is constant and protracted, it causes a penetration of the necrotic process. Previous irradiation, low-grade infection and poor physiological status exaggerate the condition. This may lead to necrosis of the trachea with subsequent stenosis or tracheoesophageal or tracheoarterial fistula. There has been a remarkable increase in these complications since the advent of the cuffed tube and mechanical ventilation. The greatest input into the literature on complications of tracheostomy and controlled ventilation has dealt with the difficulties encountered with tubes, cuffs, ventilating apparatus and the personnel assigned to supervise them. If the patient survives the immediate complications that may result from necrosis, he may later be confronted with possible tracheal stenosis. It is therefore essential that the regulation of pressure in the cuffed tube in the intensive care unit or on the ward receive the most careful attention. The responsibility for this should be assigned to an experienced and trained person. This is the most important single fact in reducing the incidence of this type of complication. Any sign of bleeding, pain or obstruction should receive immediate investigation and remedial action by the elimination of the pressure factors; careful inspection of the ulcer, with a decision to permit the ulcer to heal by secondary intention or to excise it and attempt a primary repair; protection of the great vessels with a muscle flap, if that is deemed necessary; and the elimination of or change in the position of the ventilatory apparatus.

### Scabs and Crusts

Tracheostomy alters the basic physiology of the larynx and trachea in the normal patient and in the patient with chronic pulmonary disease. It places the vocal cords at rest and replaces the filtered, warm and humidified air with dry, cold air directly into the trachea. This latter alteration causes a drying of tracheal and pulmonary secretions and aspirants and an interference with the ciliary capacity to move the mucous blanket, and thus causes a production of thick, tenacious mucus, scabs and crusts. This basic interference with the movement of the ciliary blanket, the perpetuation of the drying process, is one of the most serious aspects in the postoperative course of tracheostomy. This sequence of events leads to infection, obstruction, atelectasis and pneumonia if not corrected. If the situation is not controlled, the scabs increase in size, with the result that they are difficult or impossible to cough out or even remove by suction. This defeats the very purpose of the tracheostomy, which is to provide an adequate and safe airway, and can lead to asphyxiation, cardiac arrest and death. It is therefore imperative, in dry climates and particularly in rooms that have a dry heating system, to adapt an effective regime of humidification and aspiration.

There are many methods of supplying humidification in the postoperative tracheostomy. These services are usually provided by an inhalation therapy group that has special training in ventilatory therapy.[25, 27, 32, 53, 59] In most institutions, the Puritan mask placed over the tracheostomy tube supplies both oxygen and humidity in the immediate postoperative period. Eight to 10 liters per minute of 40 per cent oxygen is bubbled through a container of water and passed into the perforated mask over the tracheostomy tube, where it is mixed with air as it is inspired. The primary purpose of the tracheostomy in these cases is to provide an assured airway, and,

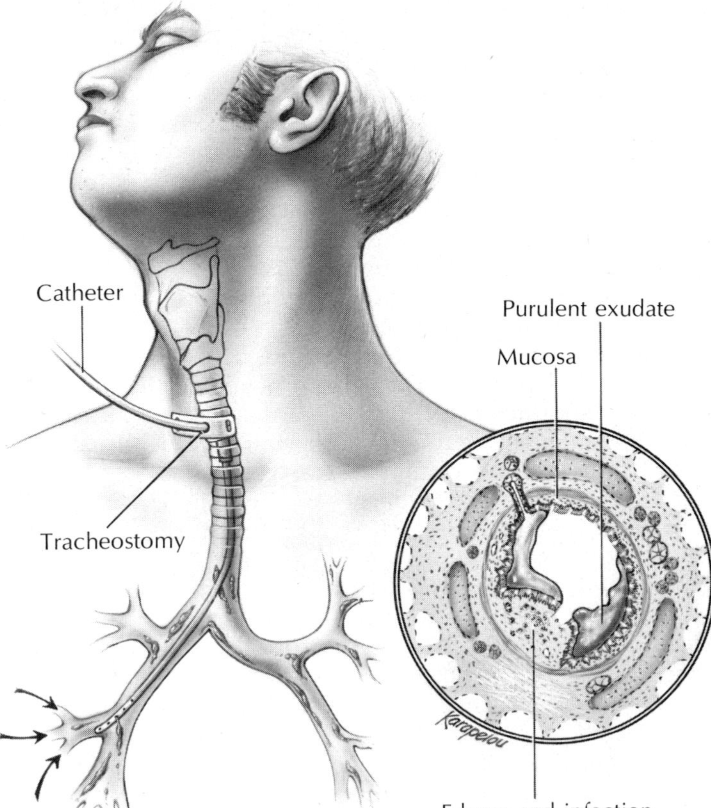


**Figure 19–6** Tracheobronchial pathology and the necessity for effective tracheal suction and humidity.

in the vast majority of cases, controlled ventilation and specific aerosolized medications are not indicated. When the patient is transferred back to the ward, the high humidification is continued with or without the oxygen. Suction is applied as needed with a sterile, disposable, smooth-tipped catheter and sterile gloves. Many of these patients aspirate the oropharyngeal secretions and, consequently, have an excessively wet trachea. There is a constant, slow weaning process over the weeks in preparation for decannulization or the trip home under the patient's own supervision. It is during the weaning process that special attention should be paid to the formation of scabs, since the trachea may not have successfully adapted to its new dry environment. There are many different methods of humidifying the air and many different solutions that can be aerosolized in a therapeutic program. This is not ordinarily a part of the management of the tracheostomy patient. The size of the humidified droplet, however, has considerable importance in that the droplet has to be less than 3 microns in order to escape the effect of gravity. One can attain a concentration for the particles of droplets of 100 to 1000 in one cc. of gas, depending upon the need and the condition. It is important, particularly in children, to calculate the size of the particle, the number of particles and the amount of fluid absorbed directly into the lung in a high-humidification program and to calculate this into the patient's fluid intake. The inhalation therapy department is well versed in an assortment of humidification techniques, embracing the jet aerosol, the liquid filtrate, the self-propulsion, the pass-over humidifiers, the bubble diffusion, the impeller nebulizer and the ultrasonic nebulizer. There is a list containing detergents, mucolytic agents (Mucomyst), ethyl alcohol, enzymes and sodium bicarbonate solutions to assist in mobilizing thick secretions. An auxiliary and simplified method of keeping the trachea moistened that may be carried out by the patient himself is the instillation of from 5 to 15 cc. of sterile saline solution intermittently. This wets the trachea, softens the secretions or scabs, causes a strong cough reflex and can be carried out at home without elaborate equipment. As the weaning program advances, the patient is aware that all dry heat in his room should be turned off and that an effective humidifier should be at his disposal. Upon discharge from the hospital, he should be prepared to manage the tube and the humidification by himself. If this regime cannot be carried out and the patient forms large crusts that cannot be coughed out through the tracheostomy tube, an emergency situation is precipitated that is handled by having the patient cough the crust out through the tracheostomy wound or up into the mouth. In some instances it may be necessary to insert a bronchoscope to clean out the trachea and bronchi. One encounter with a large tracheal plug convinces the patient and the doctor of the value of high humidity and diligent tracheal toilet.

## Changing the Tube and Decannulization

Changing a tracheostomy tube can be a harrowing experience. All difficult tracheostomies and those demanding early change should have a heavy silk suture in the upper and lower segments of the tracheal stoma in order to assure the best control for re-entry. On the whole, there is no need for frequent changing of these tracheostomy tubes. Some institutions insist on having the tube changed on the first postoperative day and frequently throughout the ensuing weeks. It takes at least three days for an established tract to be formed by the tube, and any changing prior to this might precipitate collapse of the tract and the wound upon coughing, gagging or inspiration. It is well recognized that the tubes become coated with mucus and dried blood and may be a nidus for infection. It is, however, much more dangerous to have a young resident change an essential tracheostomy tube on the first postoperative day without specific knowledge of the tracheal technique used, with no control over the tracheal stoma with silk sutures and with no assistance. Failure of re-entry may prove fatal. The hazards of this premature activity are compounded in infants and in patients with short, fat, thick necks and a very deep tracheal stoma. This author had occasion to treat a patient who had worn a silver tracheal cannula for 35 years without ever changing it. There was no recognizable harm to his tracheostoma, but the cannula was severely eroded and disintegrating. Under ordinary circumstances, changes on a weekly basis should prove adequate.

The permanent removal of the tracheal cannula is governed by the fact that it has completed its service to the patient, that the airway is adequate, as tested by corking, and that the patient can swallow without aspiration. The lungs should be clear. It is wise to cork the tube for one or two days before removing it. This is, of course, not possible in children because of the small diameter of the trachea in comparison with the diameter of the cannula. If there is any question, the tube should remain in position even though it may be corked most of the time, until the competency of the airway is established by endoscopy and tomographic examination.

## Vocal Cord Paresis

Unilateral or bilateral vocal cord paralysis may arise from inadvertent injury to the recurrent laryngeal nerves during an emergency tracheostomy and with reconstruction of the trachea in the presence of extensive scar tissue formation. A paresis is a conceivable, but not to be expected, complication in elective tracheostomy with severe deviation of the trachea to one side. It is usually not recognized during the operation.

There is no corrective treatment necessary if the voice and airway are adequate. Often the voice is of such good quality that the patient is actually not aware of a vocal abnormality until he is instructed that he has a paralyzed cord. Vocal production, however, even with good quality, is somewhat limited because of the weakness of one side of the larynx, and this would be more apparent in an individual who uses the voice more frequently. If the voice is of poor quality in unilateral paralysis, it may be improved by Teflon injection into the area of the vocal cords and vocal rehabilitation. There are two surgical methods of rehabilitating the paralyzed cord. The most direct is a nerve graft approximated to the proximal and distal stumps of the lysed recurrent laryngeal nerve. An alternate method, which may be done simultaneously with the first, is the transplantation of a nerve-muscle graft from the descending cervical and ribbon muscles into the postarytenoid musculature in order to supply a new source of axonal sprouting for preservation of the muscle volume, its tone and some aberrant movement. None of these techniques are expected to give an absolutely normal voice but should cause enough improvement to rehabilitate the functional capacity of the organ. Bilateral vocal cord paralysis presents with a weak but good quality voice but an inadequate airway. The previous methods of rehabilitation may be employed, but, in long-standing cases, lateral transposition of one or two cords will solve the airway problem but cause additional breathiness and weakness of the voice.

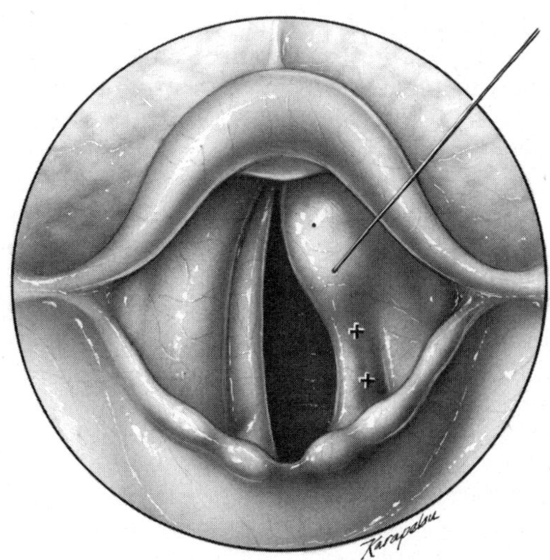

**Figure 19–7** Teflon injection into the anterior portion of the paralyzed cord to reduce breathiness and improve the voice.

### Stenosis

Tracheal stenosis has dramatically increased in the past 15 years.[23, 29, 36] The literature is replete with studies of the cause of this untoward event. There is little doubt that the majority of these stenoses came as a direct result of the use of the inflatable cuff on the oroendotracheal tube or the tracheostomy tube.[40, 58, 61, 67, 70, 71] One must appreciate, also, that tracheal stenosis can be caused by scar contracture resulting from an improperly placed incision, repetitive incisions, tracheal resections and trauma, tracheal infection and the effects of extrinsic pressure or organic disease about the trachea.

All larynges and tracheas sustain varying degrees of trauma upon either oral or endotracheal intubation.[50, 73, 79, 83] The vast majority of these injuries are mild and are associated with slight mucosal edema and injection. These ordinarily recover spontaneously in a few days. Moderate and severe injuries consist of increased edema and injection leading to ulceration and granuloma formation and, in some instances, delayed stricture contraction. Etiological factors are due to trauma at the time of intubation from the laryngoscope; the stylet; different types of retractors; incising the trachea at the wrong level or in the wrong direction; the type, size and position of the tube; and the duration of the intubation. Overriding all of these factors is the pressure created by the inflation of the balloon on the tube itself.

The mechanism of damage to the trachea following the use of the cuffed tube is an escalation in severity of the effects of the pressure of that tube. In the mildest instance, the cilia are destroyed. This may involve the mucosa, the submucosal structures, the capillaries and venules and then progress into the stroma and, finally, the tracheal cartilages. There is no specific volume of air that should be placed into the balloon; this is governed by the size of the trachea and the size of the tube and balloon entering the trachea. In most instances, 3 to 5 cc. of air are necessary to accomplish a seal. It is estimated that the pressure in the capillaries in the trachea is approximately 17 mm. Hg, and it is important that the mechanical part of the intubation mechanism does not compromise this physiological factor. The attempts to develop a safer tube have included the production of large volume, soft cuff with a self-regulating pressure system that does not permit the pressure to go over 30 mm. Hg and an external balloon control facility attached to the cuff to monitor the system. An absolute, complete seal is no longer desirable in the majority of these cases because of the inordinate pressure this sometimes applies to the mucosa. A slight leak upon "bagging" the patient increases the margin of safety. The fact that patients who have had to go on the respirator have a higher incidence of tracheal stenosis may be a direct derivative of the attempts to get a good seal.

Stenosis caused by other factors presents essentially the same clinical and anatomic picture associated with heavy scarring, contracture, collapse of the airway, granuloma[74] and a loss of supportive architecture.

The majority of the stenoses secondary to endotracheal manipulation appear within one to two months. Delayed stenosis has been seen as long as 60 years after tracheal diphtheria, with a gradual collapse and contraction at the level of the 4th, 5th and 6th tracheal rings and the appearance of a small granuloma. It is therefore possible that many of the individuals who have had subclinical injuries to the trachea in this generation will not manifest any degree of obstruction until decades have passed.

The treatment of stenosis is determined by its extent and its position in the trachea.[23, 29, 36, 80] Montgomery (1964)[63] and Grillo and Cooper (1969)[41] have established a comprehensive surgical basis for its correction by resection of the involved tracheal stenosis, release and mobilization of the trachea and then direct approximation. Montgomery[64] has also used the Silastic "T"-tube extensively in tracheal rehabilitation with considerable success. The application of these concepts has led to the resolution of the majority of these severe tracheal problems. When direct approximation of the trachea is not realistic, one may consider free composite auricular grafts, mucous membrane grafts and the use of regional skin flaps in single or multiple stage techniques. Stenting is required

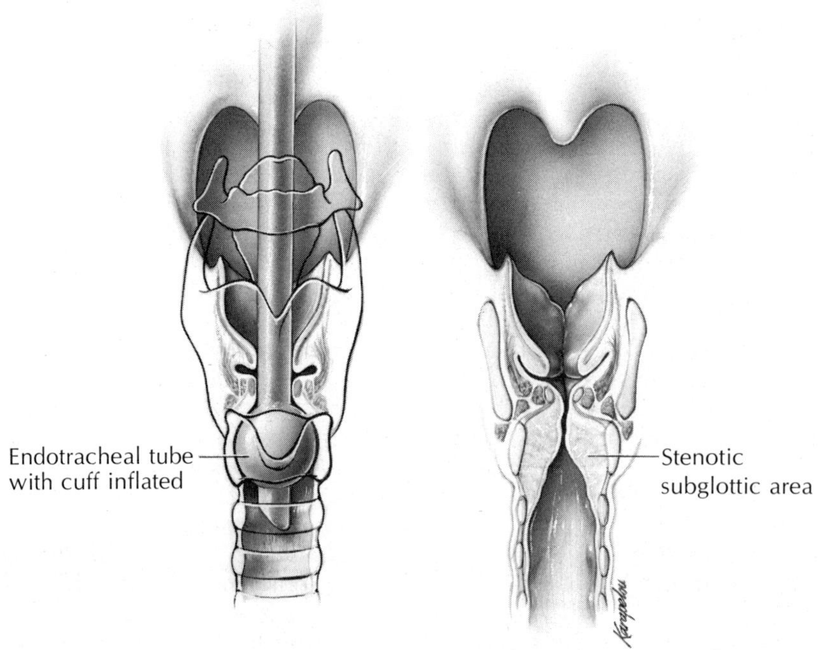


**Figure 19–8** Pressure from the endotracheal cuff ultimately producing the subglottic stenosis.

in all free graft reconstructions and is essential in molding when regional flaps are employed. The key to the technique of direct approximation is the release of the larynx or the hyoid laryngeal complex superiorly so that these structures may be displaced inferiorly without undue tension to close the gap in the trachea.[62-65] This, basically, consists of the release of the muscles and tendons that elevate the larynx and trachea. One may close a gap of 5 cm. in the trachea by this type of release. Additional inferior tracheal release can be accomplished intrathoracically when that is necessary.[40-43] The approximated segments of trachea are held together with nonabsorbable suture material that is positioned about the tracheal cartilages but does not enter the tracheal lumen. These sutures are therefore submucosal. Special attention is given to the recurrent laryngeal nerves and the parathyroid glands. The postoperative airway is maintained either by a low tracheostomy or by an oral endotracheal tube. All of these patients have some difficulty in swallowing postoperatively, but this usually clears spontaneously within a week. This direct approach to tracheal stenosis has reduced the usefulness of repetitive dilatations, steroids and piecemeal resections, which were rarely effective even in the most favorable situations.

## Tracheoarterial Fistula

This tragic complication occurs in about 0.4 per cent of tracheostomies.[7] It is associated with the improper positioning of the tube against the vessel or an improper curve and length to the tube or is secondary to pressure from a cuff.[5] The complication is almost always fatal,[11, 12] with only 4 long-term survivors reported in the literature.[1, 4, 9] Reich and Rosenkrantz[10] reported the first survivor in 1968. One of the essential prophylactic maneuvers in tracheostomy is to evaluate the position of the innominate artery by digital pressure. The position of the right common carotid artery should also be evaluated, as its position in crossing the lower portion of the trachea may vary.[2] Indeed, in some instances, it may be at the root of the neck. Tracheal fenestrae that are too low permit a long tracheal tube to rest almost directly over the artery. A low vertical incision in the trachea associated with tracheal tube pressure is conducive to erosion. The tip of the tube may be curved in such a way as to gouge its way through the anterior wall of the trachea into the artery. Any repair of the trachea at the site of the artery requires protection by an intervening muscle flap.[3] The use of the cuff on the tracheostomy tube or endotracheal tube for ventilatory purposes may contribute to an erosion at this site.

A significant warning sign prior to exsanguinating hemorrhage is slight bleeding from the vessel anywhere from three days to three weeks prior to the catastrophic hemorrhage.[8, 13] This bleeding must be analyzed carefully as to whether it may be a prodromal sign of innominate artery rupture. The trachea should be investigated endoscopically after the patient has been cross-matched and prepared for prophylactic ligation. Under general anesthesia in the operating room, the stoma is explored gently with the finger. If there is an erosion of the anterior tracheal wall, this necrotic area should be inspected and then excised and the innominate artery evaluated. If the artery is not affected, the deficient trachea may be directly approximated and a tube is inserted at a higher level. If the artery is compromised, even to the slightest degree, or if bleeding has been precipitated by the surgical investigation, then the bleeding is immediately controlled at this moment by clamping, digital pressure or transfixion of the innominate artery. The left carotid pulse rate should be checked digitally and, subsequently, by angiography.[6, 7, 8]

When the innominate artery ruptures unexpectedly on the ward, the patient is usually dead from exsanguination and asphyxiation before anyone can give assistance. If a knowledgeable person is available at this moment, the bleeding may be controlled by inserting the finger into the neck and compressing the innominate artery against the anterior wall of the chest. Controlling this type of bleeding with gauze packing is usually unrealistic because of inaccessibility for positioning the packing and the intra-arterial pressure working against it from the proximal segment of the innominate artery. Raskind and his coworkers (1973)[9] reported

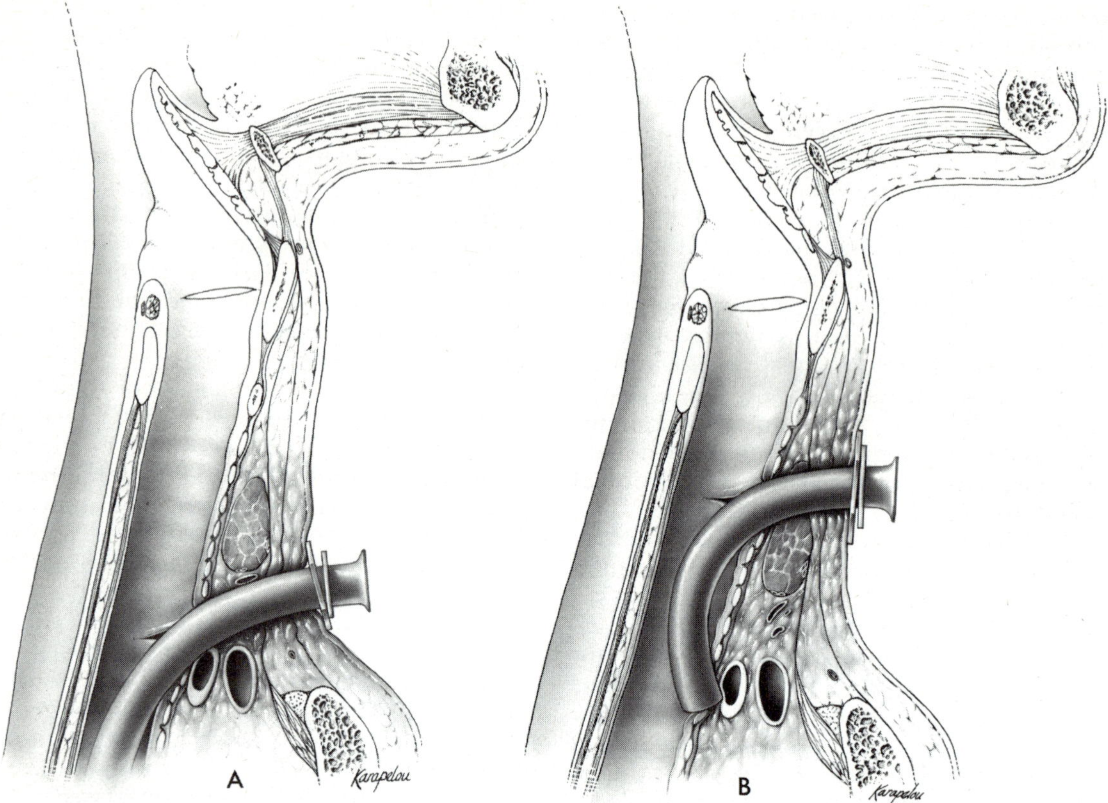


**Figure 19–9** *A,* Low tracheostomy with cannula compromising the subclavian artery (and vein). *B,* High tracheostomy with improper curve on the cannula compromising the subclavian artery.

such a case by a cervical approach and the use of a Week clip on the innominate artery. The airway was maintained and a cuffed endotracheal tube was placed inferior to the rupture. The right upper limb was cool and pulseless for approximately three weeks, but this recovered without complication. They proposed that this entrance through the neck was shorter and more direct and did not have the sequelae associated with thoracotomy. Thoracotomy, however, has a place in the management of these cases because it affords excellent exposure so that consideration can be given to artery repair or the institution of a bypass.[6, 7]

One must conclude that the primary improvement in the management of this complication will be the reduction of its incidence from approximately 0.4 per cent by prophylactic measures. It is expected that in such an area of concealment, and frequently without warning, this catastrophe will continue to prove fatal in the majority of instances.

## Tracheoesophageal Fistula

The introduction of each new surgical technique and device carries with it an intrinsic set of complications. The complication of tracheoesophageal fistula is associated in a small percentage with the introduction of the cuffed tracheal tubes. A review of 436 tracheostomy cases by Le Brigand and Roy (1966)[12, 13] revealed an 0.01 per cent incidence of tracheoesophageal fistula, 0.6 per cent tracheal stenosis, 0.5 per cent major hemorrhage and 1.5 per cent mortality associated with respiratory infection. Pearson (1971)[20] found that 21 per cent of his patients who had tracheal injuries and were supported by cuffed tracheal tubes and ventilatory assistance developed tracheal stenosis. Indeed, the incidence of tracheoesophageal fistula from cuffed tracheal tubes is likely to be higher than has been reported. Over 46 cases of tracheoesophageal fistula have been reported since Munck's report in 1961[17] This serious complication is not always easy to diagnose and requires definitive treatment for a successful outcome.

There are two significant factors contributing to the production of tracheoesophageal fistula.[1–10] Combined, they cause necrosis of the posterior wall of the trachea and the anterior wall of the esophagus, thus creating a fistula. This comes about as a result of an overinflated or improperly fitting tracheal cuffed tube, causing pressure on the posterior wall of the trachea against the indwelling nasogastric tube in the esophagus.[26] The tissue between these two points of contact and pressure is eroded. The fistula can occur in the absence of a nasogastric tube, but in the vast majority of instances they are coupled. There is a direct relationship, according to Mulder (1969),[16] with the duration of the intubation process. He found the incidence to be 18 per cent at seven days and 65 per cent at 30 days or more. Positive pressure ventilation is a significant contributory factor.[21, 24] The majority of the patients requiring nasogastric tube feeding, ventilatory support and cuffed tubes are cachectic and biologically depleted and often have some degree of pulmonary sepsis.[14, 15, 18, 19]

The diagnosis is made clinically by violent coughing associated with food ingestion, chronic coughing associated with the swallowing of saliva and, occasionally, air escaping into the hypopharynx. This is tested with methylene blue, the passage of catheters, radiologic investigation and endoscopic procedures. Thomas (1973)[22, 23] reviewed 46 cases of tracheoesophageal fistula caused by cuffed tracheal tubes. He felt the information on 30 cases was sufficient for a critical analysis. Eight of these 30 documented patients recovered, and all were treated by surgical closure. Six other patients survived and were cured without operative repair, apparently attaining a successful spontaneous closure. They, however, are not included in the 30 documented cases, since the criteria for diagnosis were not sufficient. It is recognized that the diagnosis of tracheoesophageal fistula may be difficult and obscure and require considerable effort.[27] As soon as the diagnosis is confirmed, however, the patient is gotten into the best physiological condition and the fistula is approached through a lateral cervical incision. The involved section of trachea and esophagus are identified and mobilized. The recurrent laryngeal nerves are protected. The esophageal defect is closed by direct approximation in two layers after resection of the slough. The suture line may be reinforced with a regional muscle cuff. The defect in the posterior tracheal wall is always larger than is suspected. The necrotic section of trachea is resected and, when possible, a direct approximation is carried out. If the gap is too broad, it may receive an autograph of trachea, fascia or regional muscle. Thomas reported that 11 patients had an operation for closure of a tracheoesophageal fistula and that eight survived.[23] This would present an operative mortality of 28 per cent. In contrast to this, all of the patients with a documented tracheoesophageal fistula who were not operated upon died. Four of the deaths were due to massive hemorrhage resulting from the erosion of a major vessel.[25]

Grillo, Moncure and McEnany (1976)[9] have presented a one stage treatment of the repair of tracheoesophageal fistula resulting from the pressure of a cuffed endotracheal tube in five patients. The pressure of the cuffed tube against the nasogastric feeding tube in the esophagus produced a localized fistula, but the pressure of the cuffed tube itself destroyed a larger area of trachea. In a single stage technique, they resected the scarred trachea and did a direct approximation. The esophageal fistula was repaired in layers. Transposed regional muscle flaps were used to support the esophageal repair. They also reported adaptations of this technique in two additional patients with fistulas resulting from direct trauma and sepsis. They reported good results in these seven cases, with no mortality.

## Bibliography

1. Aass, A. S.: Complications to tracheostomy and long-term intubation: A follow-up study. Acta Anaesthesiol. Scand., *19*:127, 1975.
2. Aberdeen, E., and Gover, W. J.: Endotracheal in-

tubation or tracheostomy. Lancet, *1*:436, 1967.
3. Acuna, P. T.: A simplified technique for tracheostomy. Ann. Otol. Rhinol. Laryngol., *75*:826, 1966.
4. Allan, T. H., and Steven, I. M.: Prolonged endotracheal intubation in children. Br. J. Anaesth. *37*:566, 1965.
5. Andersen, H. C., Elbrond, O., and Greisen, O.: Treatment of tracheal stenosis. J. Laryngol. Otol., *88*:615, 1974.
6. Arens, J. F., Ochsner, J. L., and Gee, G.: Long-term respiratory assistance with volume-limited intermittent cuff inflation. J. Thorac. Cardiovasc. Surg., *58*:837, 1969.
7. Auchincloss, J. H., Jr., Gilbert, R., and Mullison, E.: Self-inflating tracheostomy cuff of silicone for use as a mechanical aid to ventilatory support. Am. Rev. Resp. Dis., *97*:706, 1968.
8. Barge, W., and Slawson, K. B.: Infection: Experiences of an artifical ventilation unit. Br. J. Anaesth., *37*:574, 1965.
9. Bergström, O., and Diamant, H.: Mediastinal emphysema complicating tracheostomy. Arch. Otolaryngol., *71*:628, 1960.
10. Bryant, L. R., Trinkle, J. K., and Dubiler, L.: Tracheal damage from cuffed tracheostomy tubes. J.A.M.A., *215*:625, 1971.
11. Bryant, L. R., Trinkle, J. K., Mobin-Uddin, K., et al.: Tracheal cultures for infections in patients with tracheal tube intubation and using mechanical ventilation. Am. Surg., *38*:537, 1972.
12. Carroll, R., Hedden, M., and Safar, P.: Performance characteristics of intratracheal cuffs. Anesthesiology, *31*:275, 1969.
13. Chew, J. Y., and Cantrell, R. W.: Tracheostomy and decannulation — complications and their management. Arch. Otolaryngol., *96*:538, 1972.
14. Ching, N. P. H., Ayres, S. M., Paegle, R. P., et al.: Cuff volume and pressure contributing to tracheostomy tube damage. J. Thorac. Cardiovasc. Surg., *64*:402, 1971.
15. Ching, N. P. H., and Nealon, T. F., Jr.: New low-pressure high-volume tracheostomy cuffs for limiting intracuff pressure. N. Y. State J. Med., *74*:2379, 1974.
16. Christensen, K. T., and Duvall, A. J.: Tracheal stenosis from cuffed tracheal tube. Arch. Otolaryngol., *87*:279, 1968.
17. Conley, J. J.: Tracheal prosthesis for stenosis. Arch. Otolaryngol., *82*:433, 1965.
18. Cooper, J. D., and Grillo, H. C.: Evolution of ventilatory controls through cuffed tubes due to tracheal injury. Ann. Surg., *169*:334, 1969.
19. Cooper, J. D., and Grillo, H. C.: Change of composition and design of cuffed tracheal tubes to prevent damage and injury of the trachea. Surg. Gynecol. Obstet., *139*:1235, 1969.
20. Coppel, D. L., Bennett, E. J., and Ahlgren, E. W.: The prophylactic use of a nasotracheal tube in infants under three months of age. Surgery, *69*:354, 1971.
21. Davenport, H. T.: A perspective of long-term endotracheal intubation in children. Int. Anesthesiol. Clin., *8*:909, 1970.
22. Davis, H. S., Kretchmer, H. E., and Bryce-Smith, R.: Subcutaneous emphysema, a complication of tracheostomy. J.A.M.A., *153*:1156, 1953.
23. Dedo, H. H., and Fishman, N. H.: Laryngeal release with resection for tracheal stenosis. Ann. Otol. Rhinol. Laryngol., *78*:285, 1969.
24. Deverall, P. B.: Tracheal stricture following tracheostomy. Thorax, *22*:572, 1967.
25. Donnelly, W. H.: Endotracheal intubation. Arch. Pathol., *88*:511, 1969.
26. Durham, A. E.: On the difficulties and dangers of tracheotomy. Practitioner, *2*:212, 1869.
27. Dwyer, C. S., Krowenberg, S., and Saklad, M.: The traumatic effect of the endotracheal tube, and suggestion of tube modification. Anesthesiology, *10*:714, 1949.
28. Eckenhoff, J. E.: Endotracheal anesthesia for the larynx of the newborn. Anesthesiology, *12*:401, 1951.
29. Falbe-Hansen, J.: Treatment of tracheal stenosis in tracheotomized polio patients. Acta Otolaryngol., *45*:498, 1955.
30. Fearon, B., McDonald, R. E., and Smith, C.: Airway problems in children following prolonged endotracheal intubation. Ann. Otol. Rhinol. Laryngol., *75*:975, 1966.
31. Fishman, N. H., Dedo, H. H., Hamilton, W. K., et al.: Postintubation of cuffed tracheal tubes causing stenosis of the trachea. Ann. Thorac. Surg., *8*:47, 1969.
32. Freeman, G. R.: Comparative analysis of endotracheal intubation; its complications, prevention, and treatment. Laryngoscope, *82*:1385, 1972.
33. Galloway, T. C.: Tracheostomy in bulbar poliomyelitis. J.A.M.A., *128*:1096, 1943.
34. Geffin, B., and Pontopiddan, H.: Use of prestretched inflatable cuffs for reduction of tracheal damage. Anesthesiology, *31*:462, 1969.
35. Geffin, B., Grillo, H. C., Cooper, J. D., et al.: Post-tracheostomy stenosis. J.A.M.A., *216*:1984, 1971.
36. Gibson, R.: Etiology of intermittent positive pressure respiration following tracheostomy and repair of tracheal stenosis. Thorax, *22*:1, 1967.
37. Gibson, R., and Byrne, J. E. T.: Tracheostomy in the newborn. Laryngoscope, *82*:643, 1972.
38. Glas, W. W., King, O. J., Jr., and Lui, A.: Complications of tracheostomy. Arch. Surg., *85*:56, 1962.
40. Grillo, H. C.: Management of tracheal stenosis following assisted respiration. J. Thorac. Cardiovasc. Surg., *57*:52, 1969.
41. Grillo, H. C., and Cooper, J. D.: Endotracheal cuffed tubes causing tracheal damage. Surg. Gynecol. Obstet., *165*:1235, 1969.
42. Grillo, H. C.: Surgery of the trachea. Curr. Probl. Surg. 3–59, 1970.
43. Grillo, H. C., Cooper, J. D., Geffin, B., et al.: Minimal tracheal damage due to low-pressure cuff for tracheostomy tubes. J. Thorac. Cardiovasc. Surg., *62*:898, 1971.
44. Harrod, J. R., L'Heureux, P., and Wangensteen, O. D.: Severe respiratory distress syndrome treated with intermittent positive pressure breathing. J. Pediatr., *84*:277, 1974.

45. Hawkins, D. B., and Williams, E. H.: Tracheostomy in infants and young children. Laryngoscope, *86*:331, 1976.
46. Head, J. M.: Tracheostomy in management of respiratory difficulties. N. Engl. J. Med., *264*:587, 1961.
47. Hengerer, A. S., Strome, M., and Jaffe, B. F.: Injuries to the newborn larynx due to long-term endotracheal tube intubation. Consideration of a structural change suggested. Am. Laryngol. Assoc., *96*:46, 1975.
48. Hughes, M., Kirschner, J. A., and Branson, R. J.: Complication of a tracheostomy from the use of a skin-lined tube. Arch. Otolaryngol., *94*:568, 1971.
49. Jackson, C.: High tracheostomy and other causes of laryngeal stenosis. Surg. Gynecol. Obstet., *32*:392, 1921.
50. Johnson, J. D., Malachowski, N. C., and Grobstein, R.: Mechanical ventilation in the neonatal period. J. Pediatr., *84*:272, 1974.
51. Johnston, J. B., Wright, J. S., and Hercus, V.: Tracheal stenosis following tracheostomy — a conservative approach to treatment. J. Thorac. Cardiovasc. Surg., *53*:206, 1967.
52. Kamen, J. M., and Wilkinson, C. J.: Endotracheal tubes made with a new low-pressure cuff. Anesthesiology, *34*:482, 1971.
53. Lindholm, C.: Prolonged endotracheal intubation. Acta Anaesthesiol. Scand., *13*(Supplement 33):1, 1969.
54. Lulenski, G. C., and Batsakis, J. G.: Tracheal stenosis following tracheostomy. Am. Laryngol. Assoc., *96*:73, 1975.
55. Magovern, G. J., Shively, J. G., Fecht, D., et al.: Evaluation of controlled-pressure intratracheal cuff, clinically and experimentally. J. Thorac. Cardiovasc. Surg., *64*:747, 1972.
56. Marchetta, F. C., and Sake, K.: Pneumothorax occurring following radical neck surgery. Paper delivered at a meeting of the Society of Head and Neck Surgeons. Washington, D. C., March 30, 1959.
57. Meade, J. W.: Tracheostomy — complications and their management. N. Engl. J. Med., *265*:519, 1961.
58. McCullough, D. W., and Whytehead, L. L.: Tracheal stenosis. J. Otolaryngol., *5*:138, 1976.
59. McEwen, cited by Dwyer, C. S., Krowenberg, S., and Saklad, M.: The endotracheal tube: A consideration of its traumatic effect with a suggestion for the modification thereof. Anesthesiology, *10*:714, 1949.
60. McGinnis, G. E., Shively, J. G., and Magovern, G. J.: Endotracheal tubes using controlled-pressure occluding cuffs. Twenty-third Annual Conference on Engineering in Medicine and Biology, Abstract. 16.7, 1970.
61. Miller, D. R., and Sethi, G.: Causes and prevention of tracheal stenosis following prolonged cuffed intubation. Ann. Surg., *171*:283, 1970.
62. Montgomery, W. W.: Stenosis of the tracheastoma. Arch. Otolaryngol., *75*:62, 1962.
63. Montgomery, W. W.: Reconstruction of the cervical trachea. Ann. Otol., *75*:5, 1964.
64. Montgomery, W. W.: T-tube tracheal stent. Arch. Otolaryngol., *82*:320, 1965.
65. Montgomery, W. W.: Surgery of Upper Respiratory System. Philadelphia, Lea and Febiger, 1973.
66. Mulder, D. S., and Rubush, J. L.: Complications of tracheostomy. J. Trauma, *9*:389, 1969.
67. Murphy, D. A., MacLean, L. D., and Dobell, A. R. C.: Tracheal stenosis, a complication of tracheostomy. Ann. Thorac. Surg., *2*:44, 1966.
68. Nealon, T. F., Jr., and Ching, N.: Pressures measured in tracheostomy cuffs in tubes of ventilated patients. N. Y. State J. Med., *71*:1923, 1971.
69. Paloschi, G., and Lynn, R. B.: Observations on elective and emergency tracheostomy. Surg. Gynecol. Obstet., *120*:356, 1965.
70. Pearson, F. G., Goldberg, M., and daSilva, A. J.: Tracheostomy complicated by tracheal stenosis caused by cuffed tracheostomy tubes. Arch. Surg., *97*:380, 1968.
71. Pearson, F. G., and Andrews, M. J.: Stenosis of the trachea following cuffed tube tracheostomy: Its detection and management. Ann. Thorac. Surg., *12*:359, 1971.
72. Polk, H. C., Jr., Borden, S., and Aldrete, J. A.: Methods of prevention of pseudomonas infection in a surgical intensive care unit. Surg. Gynecol. Obstet., *177*:607, 1973.
73. Rabuzzi, D. D., and Reed, G. F.: Intrathoracic complications following tracheostomy in children. Laryngoscope, *81*:939, 1971.
74. Salmon, L. F. W.: Tracheostomy. Proc. Roy. Soc. Med., *68*:347, 1975.
75. Schlorf, R. A., and Duvall, A. J.: Postintubation granulomas of the larynx. Minn. Med., *52*:717, 1969.
76. Schloss, M. D.: Laryngeal and tracheal complications following prolonged intubation and tracheostomy. Can. J. Otolaryngol., *1*:135, 1972.
77. Shaw, H. J., Stylis, S. C., and Rosen, G.: Elective tracheostomy in head and neck tumor surgery. J. Laryngol. Otol., *88*:599, 1974.
78. Shelly, W. M., Dawson, R. B., and May, I. A.: Cuffed tubes cause for tracheal stenosis. J. Thorac. Cardiovasc. Surg., *57*:623, 1969.
79. Slater, E. A.: Endotracheal tube sizes for infants and children. Anesthesiology, *16*:950, 1955.
80. Sorensen, H. R., and Nielsen, P. A.: Circular resection of the trachea for strictures and tumors. Scand. J. Thorac. Cardiovasc. Surg., *5*:166, 1971.
81. Steir, M., Ching, N., Roberts, E. B., and Nealon, T. F., Jr.: Pneumothorax occurring during continuous pressure breathing support. J. Thorac. Cardiovasc. Surg., *67*:17, 1974.
82. Stetson, J. B.: Prolonged endotracheal tube intubation. Br. J. Anaesth., *40*:712, 1968.
83. Tucker, J. A., and Silberman, H. D.: Tracheostomy in pediatrics. Ann. Otol. Rhinol. Laryngol., *81*:818, 1972.
84. Watts, J. M.: Tracheostomy in modern practice. Br. J. Surg., *50*:954, 1963.
85. Way, W. L., and Sooy, F. A.: Endotracheal intubation and its histologic changes. Ann. Otol. Rhinol. Laryngol., *74*:799, 1965.

### Tracheoarterial Fistula

1. Biller, H. F., and Ebert, P. A.: Innominate artery hemorrhage complicating tracheostomy. Ann. Otol., *79*:301, 1970.
2. Fox, J. L.: Control of common carotid and innominate artery hemorrhage complicating tracheostomy. J. Neurosurg., *38*:393, 1973.
3. Grillo, H. C.: Surgical approaches to the trachea. Surg. Gynecol. Obstet., *129*:347, 1969.
4. Mathog, R. H., Kenan, P. D., and Hudson, W. R.: Delayed massive hemorrhage following tracheostomy. Laryngoscope, *81*:107, 1971.
5. Mulder, D. S., and Rubush, J. L.: Complications of tracheostomy: Relationship to long term ventilatory assistance. J. Trauma, *9*:389, 1969.
6. Myers, R. S., and Pilch, Y. H.: Temporary control of tracheal-innominate artery fistula. Ann. Surg., *170*:149, 1969.
7. Myers, W. O., Lawton, B. R., and Sautter, R. D.: An operation for tracheal-innominate artery fistula. Arch. Surg., *105*:269, 1972.
8. Myers, W. O., Lawton, B. R., and Sautter, R. D.: Axillo-axillary bypass graft. J.A.M.A., *217*:826, 1971.
9. Raskind, R., Glover, B., Arbegast, N. R., et al.: Control of hemorrhage from the innominate artery complicating tracheostomy through a suprasternal approach. Vasc. Surg., *7*:265, 1973.
10. Reich, M. P., and Rosenkrantz, J. G.: Fistula between innominate artery and trachea. Arch. Surg., *96*:401, 1968.
11. Schlaepfer, K.: Fatal hemorrhage following tracheostomy for laryngeal diphtheria. J.A.M.A., *82*:1581, 1924.
12. Silen, W., and Spieker, P.: Fatal hemorrhage from the innominate artery after tracheostomy. Ann. Surg., *162*:1005, 1965.
13. Utley, J. R., Singer, M. M., Roe, B. B., et al.: Definitive management of innominate artery hemorrhage complicating tracheostomy. J.A.M.A., *220*:577, 1972.

### Tracheoesophageal Fistula

1. Bargh, W., and Slawson, K. B.: Experiences with an artificial ventilation unit. Br. J. Anaesth., *37*:574, 1965.
2. Chapman, N. D., and Braun, R. A.: The management of traumatic tracheoesophageal fistula caused by blunt chest trauma. Arch. Surg., *100*:681, 1970.
3. Crosby, W. M.: Automatic intermittent inflation of tracheostomy tube cuff. Lancet, *2*:509, 1964.
4. Flege, J. B., Jr.: Tracheoesophageal fistula caused by cuffed tracheostomy tube. Ann. Surg., *116*:153, 1967.
5. Fleming, W. H., and Bowen, J. C.: Early complications of long term respiratory support. J. Thorac. Cardiovasc. Surg., *64*:729, 1972.
6. Geffin, B., cited by Cooper, J. D., and Grillo, H. C.: Evolution of tracheal injury due to ventilatory assistance through cuffed tubes: A pathologic study. Ann. Surg., *169*:334, 1969.
7. Georgiade, N., Maguire, C., Crawford, H., et al.: Practical considerations regarding tracheostomy. J.A.M.A., *160*:940, 1956.
8. Glas, W. W., King, O. J., and Lui, A.: Complications of tracheostomy. Arch. Surg., *85*:72, 1962.
9. Grillo, H. C., Moncure, A. C., and McEnany, M. T.: Repair of inflammatory tracheoesophageal fistula. Ann. Thorac. Surg., *22*:2, 112–119, 1976.
10. Harris, S. H., Jr., and deNiord, R. N.: Esophagobronchial fistula of 24 years' duration. J. Thorac. Cardiovasc. Surg., *54*:295, 1967.
11. Hedden, M., Ersoz, C. J., and Safar, P.: Tracheoesophageal fistulas following prolonged artificial ventilation via cuffed tracheostomy tubes. Anesthesiology, *31*:281, 1969.
12. Le Brigand, H.: Conclusion. Faudrait-il condamner la trachéotomie? Ann. Chir. Thorac. Cardiovasc., *6*:489, 1967.
13. Le Brigand, H., and Roy, B.: Fistules trachéo-esophagiennes après trachéotomie. A propos de quatre observations. Séance Du., 1966, p. 405.
14. Malmejac, C., Arnaud, A., Houel, J., et al.: Note à propos des fistules esotrachéales après trachéotomie. Ann. Chir. Thorac. Cardiovasc., *6*:483, 1967.
15. Martinez, L. R., and Kalter, R. D.: Extensive tracheal necrosis associated with prestretched tracheostomy tube cuff. Anesthesiology, *34*:488, 1971.
16. Mulder, D. S., and Rubush, J. L.: Complications of tracheostomy: Relationship to long term ventilatory assistance. J. Trauma, *9*:389, 1969.
17. Munck, O.: Mechanical ventilation for acute respiratory failure in diffuse chronic lung disease. Lancet, *1*:66, 1961.
18. Nicolas, F., Dupon, H., Guillon, J., et al.: Fistules trachéoesophagiennes après trachéotomie. Ann. Chir. Thorac. Cardiovasc., *6*:475, 1967.
19. Otteni, J. C., Morand, G., Tempe, J. D., et al.: Complications de la trachéotomie des fistules trachéoesophagiennes. Ann. Chir. Thorac. Cardiovasc., *6*:465, 1967.
20. Pearson, F. G., and Andrews, M. J.: Detection and Management of Tracheal Stenosis Ann. Thorac. Surg., *12*:359, 1971.
21. Stiles, P. J.: Tracheal lesions after tracheostomy. Thorax, *20*:517, 1965.
22. Thomas, A. N.: The diagnosis and treatment of tracheoesophageal fistula caused by cuffed tracheal tubes. J. Thorac. Cardiovasc. Surg., *65*:612, 1973.
23. Thomas, A. N.: Management of tracheoesophageal fistula caused by cuffed tracheal tubes. Am. J. Surg., *124*:181, 1972.
24. Toty, L., Hertzog, P., and Aboudi, A.: Cinq cas de fistules trachéoesophagiennes après trachéotomie. Ann. Chir. Thorac. Cardiovasc., *6*:471, 1967.
25. Utley, J. R., Singer, M. M., Roe, B. B., et al.: Definitive management of innominate artery hemorrhage complicating tracheostomy. J.A.M.A. *220*:577, 1972.
26. Von Schulthess, V. G.: Tracheostomy, Fortschr., Hals-Nas-Ohren-heilk., Vol. II. New York, S. Karger, A. G., 1964.
27. Wychulis, A. R., Ellis, F. H., Jr., and Andersen, H. A.: Acquired nonmalignant esophagotracheobronchial fistula. J.A.M.A., *196*:117, 1966.

# 20 COMPLICATIONS IN ENDOSCOPIC PROCEDURES*

*Gabriel F. Tucker, Jr.*
*John A. Tucker*

The complications resulting from endoscopic procedures range from such gross iatrogenic fatalities as massive hemorrhage and respiratory obstruction to the far more subtle failures to achieve either an optimal diagnostic examination or a therapeutic result. It is certainly in the best interest of the patient to consider all factors that may mitigate against such achievement.

## FACILITY FOR PERFORMANCE OF PROCEDURE

Optimum patient service can, of course, be given only if the procedures are performed in an area that is quiet, safe, free from distractions and completely equipped. In emergency situations, compromises may have to be made. The ideal facility is a specially equipped endoscopic operating room or at least an operating room equipped with the same safety facilities found within the general operating suite. Necessity may dictate that endoscopic procedures, especially emergency bronchoscopy, be performed in an intensive care unit. Although the advent of the fiber bronchoscope has led a number of people to perform endoscopic examination in less well equipped spaces, this cannot be condoned.

Especially dangerous is the practice of attempting to confirm the diagnosis of epiglottitis with a tongue blade at the bedside, on a house call or even in a physician's office or emergency room, said facility is not staffed and equipped to handle the emergency obstruction that might be produced by such meddlesome manipulation.

## ADMINISTRATION OF LOCAL ANESTHETIC

A local anesthetic should be administered only in a facility that allows for proper respiratory support and resuscitation in the event of untoward reaction. Furthermore, the atmosphere in which the local anesthetic is to be administered is most important. It should be recalled that the sedated patient may be easily confused and thus may misunderstand things happening in his surroundings. As such, the area reserved for the administration of local anesthetic should be free of extraneous stimuli. If one stops to listen in many operating rooms, there is, unfortunately, a modicum of small talk, chatter, jokes and so on that is not in the best interest of the pre-endoscopic patient. The increasing use of general anesthesia predisposes those involved to a lack of awareness of the sensibilities of the sedated, but somewhat receptive, patient. Especially important in this regard is a pattern of traffic flow that separates the pre- and posten-

*In accumulating material for this chapter, the members of the Philadelphia Bronchoscopic Club, the New York Bronchoscopic Society and the Committee on Bronchoesophagology of the American College of Chest Physicians were circularized. A number of most helpful replies were received. We are especially grateful for the extensive comments of Drs. Arthur Olsen and Paul Holinger.

doscopic patients who cough. Such patients may well increase the apprehension of the patient.

Complications incident to the administration of local anesthetic are in general thought to be due to overdose; idiosyncratic reactions are indeed rare, are thought to be of anaphylactic nature and, as such, said to be caused by even minimal amounts of the drug. The only protection against such idiosyncrasy seems to be the initial administration of a minimal amount of any given agent, waiting several minutes to be sure that no untoward reaction is occurring. The interdiction against the use of tetracaine (Pontocaine), which is also a major component of Cetacaine, in patients known to be asthmatic is usually followed. The reaction in this situation may not so much be anaphylactic as precipitative of an acute asthmatic episode.

## OVERDOSE REACTIONS

Overdose reactions depend primarily on the total amount of the drug in the circulation that is available to work as a central nervous system stimulant. The amount in the circulation at any given time is, of course, proportional to the total dose administered, the rate of administration and the rate of absorption. The rate of absorption is increased in highly vascular areas, inflamed areas and whenever the drug is instilled endotracheally. The toxicity of a local anesthetic agent is the same whether it is given endotracheally or intravenously.

The signs and symptoms of systemic toxicity are confusion, disorientation and apprehension. These are often associated with sweating, restlessness, hypotension and convulsions. The later fatal stage of such reactions is cardiac and respiratory depression. Barbiturates have been given to counteract such toxic effects; however, they may merely mask the symptoms and signs of central nervous system stimulation without affecting the dose of the anesthetic causing cardiopulmonary collapse.[16]

A crucial clinical judgment must be made in handling a patient who seems to become increasingly hyperactive as local anesthesia progresses. To assume that such hyperactivity calls for more and more local anesthetic may be to invite a fatal toxic reaction. The only safe course in such a situation is to cease administration of the anesthetic until it is absolutely certain that the patient's apprehensiveness is not due to the agent itself.

## THE OROPHARYNX

A light spray of Cetacaine is applied to the soft palate. This agent is a mixture of ethyl and butyl aminobenzoate and tetracaine. Because of the tetracaine content, it should be avoided in asthmatic patients. After such an initial spray, the patient should be observed carefully. The mucosa should be inspected for any sign of a local or systemic reaction. During this period, the mouth should be reinspected for loose teeth or dentures. Anesthesia is then applied to the fauces, especially the right posterior pillar and the plica triangularis. Special attention must be paid to anesthetization of the right upper alveolus and any portion of the oropharynx that may come into contact with the endoscope. Right upper edentia may at first glance be encouraging to the endoscopist when placing the instrument. If the edentulous gum is compressed by the endoscope against the bony alveolar ridge, however, it may become extremely uncomfortable for the patient. It should also be remembered that diffuse acute inflammation with hyperemia not only predisposes the mucosa to mechanical injury but also increases the rate of absorption of the anesthetic agent and the risk of toxic reaction.

## LARYNGEAL ANESTHESIA

Laryngeal anesthesia is obtained by direct instillation of the anesthetic agent under mirror guidance. The patient can easily be invited to hold his own tongue with the right hand while sitting upright on the side of the stretcher. (The use of a stretcher permits the quick placement of the patient in a supine position should he become faint.) A chair should not be used for local anesthesia. The position of the patient is similar to that used for other procedures involving mirror laryngoscopy: The patient's hips are back toward the wall, and he is bent forward at the waist with the cervical spine flexed and the occiput extended. This position is best explained to some patients as "like a race horse crossing the finish line." When the oropharynx is well anesthetized, one must, of course, be careful to avoid overheating the laryngeal mirror, since the well anesthetized palate may readily be burned, especially if such a mirror has been heated on an alcohol lamp. The Lukens syringe is filled from a medicine glass containing a measured amount of the agent to be used; the syringe itself is, of course, also calibrated for accurate fractionation of the dose applied. The tip of the cannula can be brought into contact with the undersurface of the epiglottis, and 0.25 ml. or so of the anesthetic agent is allowed to trickle into the larynx, without provoking cough. One can usually follow with a dropper-like technique, instilling the anesthetic agent drop by drop while the patient phonates ("e. . .e. . .e").

The use of such instillation to the absolute exclusion of swabs is recommended. Cotton swabs on a curved applicator not only stimulate the patient's hypopharynx but also can be grabbed by the partially anesthetized glottis and aspirated into the trachea.

Translaryngeal block (i.e., via the cricothyroid membrane) should not be used in the presence of laryngeal disease or in cases of hemoptysis; one disadvantage of this technique is that the larynx is not concurrently studied.

## THE USE OF GENERAL ANESTHESIA FOR ENDOSCOPY

Of prime importance are mutual understanding and cooperation between the anesthesiologist and the endoscopist. At no time should the operating requirements for either member of the team work to the detriment of the overriding necessity for a safe, functioning airway. This holds true not only for the obvious laryngeal and tracheobronchial problems but also for esophageal problems. Here, either party may interfere with the other by exerting pressure through the esophageal wall on the airway or by transmission of variations in intrapulmonary pleural pressure to the esophagus. If the endoscopist is to cooperate intelligently with the anesthesiologist, he must be well versed in respiratory physiology and the effects of the various general anesthetic agents and techniques. Pulmonary compliance, nitrogen clearance, carbon dioxide production, arterial $pO_2$ and the effects of vascular shunting in the unventilated lung should all be familiar matters to the endoscopist. There should be mutual agreement not only that the use of general anesthesia is indicated but also that it can be carried out safely. Conversely, general anesthesia may be contraindicated for endoscopic reasons or for general medical reasons. General anesthesia in the burn patient is particularly hazardous, since depolarizing agents are contraindicated.

## THE OXYGENATED LUNG

No matter what technique of anesthesia is selected, proper oxygenation is of prime importance. $PO_2$ levels below 60 and $pCO_2$ levels higher than 55 and lower than 20 require investigation and active treatment. Placement of the bronchoscope, suctioning, coughing, bucking and apnea quickly cause a decrease in oxygen concentration.

## NITROGEN CLEARANCE

Administration of pure oxygen in a nonrebreathing system for over seven minutes will clear over 90 per cent of the nitrogen from the normal lung. The oxygen content of the lung at the end of this time is enough to maintain the arterial $pO_2$ at normal levels or above for about five minutes (depending on metabolism and so forth). This in itself provides a large safety factor against serious complications.

## INSTRUMENTATION

The maintenance of an instrumentarium may involve complications that arise from overdoing attempts at maintaining absolute sterilization. The fundamental principle in sterilizing endoscopic instruments is to prevent the transmission of infection from one patient to the next. It is most practical, and state and not fully aerated, that the tracheot-

strument between use and to maintain them in a state of readiness and availability that is best described as only "surgically clean." Techniques that require that individual instruments be wrapped in plastic or paper bags may result in unnecessary delay in emergency procedure, and such wrapping also tends to bend forceps shafts so that they do not work smoothly.

## ELECTRICAL PROBLEMS

Since the Jackson teaching tradition has implied primarily the use of dry battery instruments, there has been little opportunity for high voltage in the use of American instruments. Switz and his colleagues,[19] however, recently reported the use of an American-made gastroscope that was powered by a transformer. This, in turn, led to two probable cases of electrocution. Sixty cycle alternating current is one of the most efficient fibrillating currents available. The delivery of an electrical conductor (connected to such a source) into the patient's mediastinum therefore creates an obvious potential for electrocution. The use of the newer fibroscopes, which carry no electrical conductors, will result in even greater safety, in spite of the fact that they are ultimately powered by 110 volt, 60 cycle current.

## TRACHEOTOMY[13]

The complications of a "rush," "crash" emergency tracheotomy are, of course, much greater than if an airway is previously established. The advantages of performing a tracheotomy over a previously placed bronchoscope were published by Tucker, Sr., in 1926.[21] With the development of endotracheal anesthesia, it has often become possible to relieve obstructions by the passage of an endotracheal tube. The principle herein elicited is that not only are such elements as haste and poor preparation eliminated but mechanical obstruction is also eliminated. Furthermore, one removes the pressure differentials across soft tissue that cause the veins to engorge and bleed more readily. Under respiratory stress, the pleural apices may herniate into the pretracheal space and even the posterior tracheal wall, and with it may cause the anterior esophageal wall to be pulled toward the tracheal lumen.

Proper placement of the head of the patient not only brings the larynx, and with it the trachea, out of the thoracic inlet but also brings the trachea forward. This makes the trachea more accessible and separates the desired site of incision from the vascular structures of the thoracic inlet.

In the performance of tracheotomy one should "know where one is going."[2] In dealing with an obese or tumorous neck, it is good to begin one's incision at an available landmark, such as the cricoid or even the thyroid notch if the cricoid is not available. In this regard, pretracheotomy soft tissue x-rays to demonstrate the relationship of the air column to the landmarks on the neck are of great value in dealing with the neck distorted by tumor. Visualizing a needle in the trachea via the bronchoscope or aspirating air and then cutting down on the needle as a guide to the lumen are at times valuable techniques.

A number of authors have suggested over the years that a horizontally placed incision is more conducive to a good cosmetic result. Such reasoning is probably fallacious in its assumption not only that the tracheotomy wound will be closed *per primam* but also that such transverse placement itself does not induce complications. Jackson, half a century ago, pointed out that the vertical midline incision was the safest way to avoid entering the paratracheal great vessels. It should also be noted that a transverse incision usually requires retraction in four directions instead of the conventional two, since the skin incision, if done transversely, must be held superiorly and inferiorly, whereas the dissection certainly should proceed in the vertical midsagittal plane and thus requires lateral retraction.

An incision that starts at the level of the cricoid or cricothyroid membrane and is carried inferiorly for 2 or 3 cm. toward the suprasternal notch is less apt to cause entrance into the vessels and pleural spaces at the root of the neck than the incision that is placed directly into the suprasternal notch. Note the innominate artery may be superior to the suprasternal notch; one should palpate for its presence prior to incision.

The high relation of the larynx and upper trachea to the cervical spine and their descent with age is known in general terms to most physicians. In other words, if one retracts the larynx vigorously with a hook in a pediatric patient, it is possible to enter the trachea as low as the 10th or 12th ring. On the other hand, in the senescent adult, it may require not only proper extension of the neck to place a hook under the cricoid but also further traction under the cricoid during the performance of the tracheotomy to bring the elderly trachea out of the thorax.

Dissection of the subcutaneous tissues should be confined to the midline. The first structure to be identified should be the inferior rim of the cricoid cartilage.

Davison[7] has emphasized the anatomic relationships wherein the thyroid capsule is formed from the decussation of the pretracheal fascia and the attachment of this pretracheal fascia to the inferior rim of the cricoid. By entering the pretracheal space at the level of the attachment of the thyroid isthmus to the inferior rim of the cricoid, one is able to avoid the troublesome ooze that is incident to an approach below the thyroid isthmus because of the presence of thyroid veins. This also makes available the superior rim of the thyroid isthmus, which can then be either retracted inferiorly or divided and ligated. The only complication inherent in this approach is the occasional presence of a pyramidal thyroid lobe that may have to be separately transected and ligated. Such a high approach to the pretracheal space does not in itself imply a high entrance site in the trachea. The dissection can be carried down in the relatively avascular pretracheal space to the 3rd or 4th tracheal ring, and then the trachea can be entered. The "L" shape of the Jackson tracheal hook is much less dangerous than the "J"-shaped hooks (often designed for use on the skin or for orthopedic purposes) that are occasionally encountered on tracheotomy sets.

A bronchoscope or even an endotracheal tube is of great value in the lumen of the trachea. The trachea can then be identified either by palpation or even transillumination, if necessary.

Jackson[10] pointed out the value of the operator's index finger in palpating for the "arteria trachea" or "rough artery," which indeed is the etymology of the term. Constant palpation with the index finger for identification of the trachea versus the great vessels is one of the greatest preventives against wandering into the paratracheal spaces (jugular, carotid hemorrhage or recurrent nerve trauma).

One must be especially aware of the possibility that over-enthusiastic assistance may capture the trachea under a retractor, resulting in the bringing of the carotid sheath directly into the wound. Jackson demonstrated the danger of entering the esophagus through the posterior tracheal wall; the use of a bronchoscope or an endotracheal tube not only relieves the negative pressure in the trachea but also provides protection for the posterior tracheal wall.

Once the trachea is opened, the anesthesiologist or assistant should be told that the tube is to be withdrawn *only to the superior rim of the tracheal incision.* It is *not to be* withdrawn completely *through* the larynx. The protection that this affords the airway is apparent if the operator has difficulty entering the trachea or placing a tracheotomy tube with an endolaryngeal airway. With the anterior tracheal wall freshly incised and the laryngeal airway obstructed by large tumor, subsequent urgent replacement of the endotracheal tube resulted in the passage of the endotracheal tube from the laryngeal and upper tracheal lumen through the previously made incision and into the anterior mediastinum. The failure to recognize this type of placement led to respiratory obstruction and the loss of the patient.

## Stomal Recurrence as a Complication of Tracheotomy

Keim and his coworkers[11] suggest that the performance of a tracheotomy for obstructive carcinoma may lead to recurrence in the permanently constructed tracheostome after resection. Experience at the Jackson Clinic (Norris, et al.)[14] suggests that the performance of the tracheotomy does not, in itself, cause stomal recurrence but that the tumorous recurrence is probably more properly related to the size of the initial tumor. To this end, it is suggested that tracheotomy be performed if a patient with an obstructing tumor presents in a dyspneic state and not fully aerated, that the tracheotomy be done at the level of the cricoid or first tracheal ring and that the site of the initial tracheotomy be resected in continuity with the larynx at the time of laryngectomy.

### Suture of the Tracheotomy Incision

Unless the tracheotomy incision gapes extensively, no attempt should be made to approximate the cut edges. Closure of the skin wound about the tracheotomy tube may result in *subcutaneous emphysema* that in turn may progress into the mediastinum and contribute to pneumothorax. As the patient coughs and raises his intratracheal pressure, air seeps from the trachea around the tracheotomy tube which is then prevented from egress at the cutaneous level and dissects subcutaneously.

#### DISLODGEMENT OF THE TRACHEOTOMY TUBE

Dislodgement is one of the most dreaded complications of tracheotomy, especially in the obstructed patient. It may be due to several factors.

**Discontinuity of the securing tape.** A square, or preferably a surgeon's, knot is much less apt to slip. Certainly no patient's life should depend on a bow knot. If a slotted tape is used, the slots must be parallel to the edge of the tape and in the midline; diagonally placed slots weaken the tape and may tear through. It has been suggested that this may be avoided by threading the tape in one slot and out the other.

**Slackening of the tape.** This may be due to slippage of a "granny" knot or failure to flex the neck at the time the tape is initially tied. Such slackening of the tape is especially dangerous since the tip of the tube may be merely dislodged from the trachea into the pretracheal space without being externally evident.

Treatment may be expedited by having a complete replacement tube available, by suturing the cut ends of the thyroid isthmus[21] or by placing silk sutures in the wound edges[8] and bringing lengths of such suture well out of the wound. Byork flap is advocated by Cantrell[4] as a means of preventing decannulation.

Suturing the tube in place may not only prevent its accidental dislodgement but may also impede the ready removal of an obstructed tube.

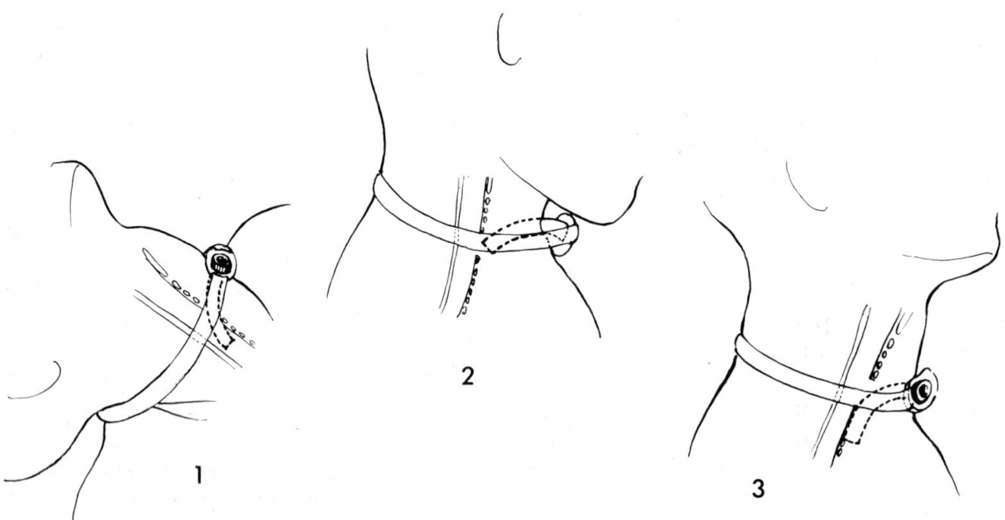


**Figure 20–1** "How to win the battle and lose the war." *1,* Tracheotomy tube in place (battle won). If tape is tied while neck is still extended, *2,* tape will be slack when neck is straight or flexed, *3,* permitting pretracheal dislodgement, which may be fatal if patient has no alternative airway (war lost). (Y. Yung, Temple Medical School, Department of Medicine. Illustrated for author.)

#### OBSTRUCTION OF THE TUBE

This may result from a dry atmosphere, thick secretions or a combination of the two. Use of proper humidification and a readily removable and cleanable inner cannula may avert such a complication.

#### DECUBITUS ULCERATION

Ulceration may be seen in unconscious or paralyzed patients if the tracheotomy tape has been tied in a knot placed in the midline over the prominence of the cervical spine.

### Post-Tracheotomy Bleeding

Venous bleeding is most often associated with a "low" approach in which the venous plexus inferior to the thyroid isthmus is injured. Packing and compression are of value in the immediate emergency. Arterial bleeding is also more commonly seen in the "low" approach and results in injury either to an anomalously high aortic arch or even to the innominate artery. Few textbooks emphasize the fact that as the trachea enters the thorax it tends to swing posteriorly, parallel to the dorsal curve of the upper thoracic spine. As such, pretracheal dissection may parallel the anterior tracheal wall rather than approach it. It has been observed that an extremely long metal tracheotomy tube can impinge against the pulse of the innominate artery and cause slow erosion of the innominate artery through the anterior tracheal wall.

## ENDOTRACHEAL INTUBATION

The most serious complication of endotracheal intubation is failure to provide an airway in the obstructed patient. This is seen most often in situations in which the larynx is obstructed, irritable and difficult to expose (i.e., epiglottitis). Ideally, if serious mechanical obstruction to the larynx is present, a rigid bronchoscope is used for intubation. The open bronchoscopic tube not only supplies a rigidity that may overcome the mechanical resistance of a pathologic obstruction but also permits the endoscopist to visualize the larynx and trachea.

Injuries due to endotracheal (intubation) tubes may be subdivided into two categories: those due to the cuff and those due to the tube itself.

Lindholm[12] has nicely illustrated the mechanics whereby the "memory" of a plastic tube tends to return it to its original straight shape and thus places pressure on the posterior endocricoid and posterolateral cricoarytenoid joints.

Injuries due to endotracheal cuffs are readily found at routine autopsy. They result from the pressure of the cuff against the tracheal mucosa and are more common in debilitated patients. The use of "soft" cuffs and devices applying less positive pressure to the ischemic mucosa of the trachea has lessened this complication.

Progressive distention and hyperinflation of the trachea is a rare complication due to overinflation of the endotracheal cuff. The most common complications are the result of mechanical irritation, ulceration, destruction, granulation, scarring and eventual stenosis.

## POST-TRACHEOTOMY ASPIRATION

Loss of the bechic blast may encourage post-tracheotomy aspiration because the expiratory air stream is diverted through the tracheotomy tube rather than upward through the larynx. This is most often seen in patients with laryngeal incompetence of either neurologic or surgical origin. It was pointed out many years ago that the valved inner cannula was of benefit not only in those patients with bilateral recurrent nerve paralysis, for whom the tube was designed, but also in the rehabilitation of laryngeal reflexes by supplying a physiologic expiratory laryngeal air stream.[21]

## FIBEROPTIC BRONCHOSCOPY

Suratt, Smiddy and Gruber[18] have recently surveyed, by way of a questionnaire, 48,000 bronchoscopic examinations, including 6300 biopsies. They reported 12 deaths and commented on potentially fatal complications. Their conclusions were as follows:

> Although fiberoptic bronchoscopic examination is a relatively safe procedure, deaths and other serious complications can occur. A careful

cardiovascular and pulmonary evaluation prior to bronchoscopic examination is essential. Blood gases should be obtained in most cases and certainly in all patients where hypoxia is suspected. Patients with cardiovascular disease should be monitored electrocardiographically; those with a $PaO_2$ of less than 70 mm mercury should receive supplemental oxygen. Sedatives and local anesthetics should be employed judiciously, particularly tetracaine. Resuscitative equipment must be readily accessible. Repeated use of biopsy brushes is hazardous, and a brush with a bent tip should be discarded. If a patient experiences pleuritic pain during a biopsy, the biopsy instrument should be withdrawn and re-inserted. Use of these simple precautions should minimize serious complications associated with fiberoptic bronchoscopic examination.

## COMPLICATIONS INCIDENT TO THE PERFORMANCE OF THE ENDOSCOPIC PROCEDURE

Mechanical injuries may result from the application of a mechanical *force* that is too large or misdirected or both. Misdirection of the instrument more laterally to contuse the faucial pillars or tonsillar fossae may occur if the patient is not sufficiently relaxed and compliant.

### GENTLENESS

One of the first points for insuring that undue force is not exerted is the use of the thumb and forefinger to grasp the tube of the endoscope. The "handle" is not a handle *per se.* It is, in fact, a support post for the light carrier and should be used for this purpose only. Grasping this support post in a pistol grip or engaging it with the operator's thumb makes it possible to apply much greater force along the axis of the tube than may be safe. An endoscope should never be advanced blindly. If the lumen cannot be seen under direct vision, it should be marked by a previously placed string or wire guide that, in turn, is followed. In some instances, great help can be obtained by the use of a fluoroscope to ascertain the position and direction of the tip of the endoscope. This is especially true of the flexible endoscopes that do not transmit to the operator a definite sense of the position of the flexible tip.

### TUBULAR VISION

*"Tubular vision,"* wherein the operator concentrates on the endoscopic image to the exclusion of an awareness of the relationship of the tube to the patient as a whole, is probably the greatest single cause of the misdirected application of forward propelling force to perforate the contralateral (usually left) pyriform fossa.

The novice may best be coached by an instructor who is at the left side or foot of the patient and can thus maintain a broad perspective as to the direction of the open tube and its relation to the whole patient. It is often found helpful to encourage the endoscopist to work with the contratubal eye open.

### INSTRUMENTAL INJURIES

Instrumental injuries may be classified by site; the instruments most likely to cause such injuries are as follows:

I. Nasal—fiber bronchoscopy
II. Oral
    A. Dental—all open tubes, especially laryngoscopes
    B. Faucial—all open tubes
III. Hypopharynx
    A. Undiagnosed lingual thyroid—may bleed profusely if traumatized by broad laryngoscope blade
    B. Pyriform—all open tubes, especially esophagoscope (anatomy of the cricopharyngeus and Zenker's diverticulum)
IV. Laryngeal
    A. Supraglottic—pediatric—laryngoscope
    B. Glottic
        1. Cordal—tubes and forceps
        2. Arytenoid—endotracheal tube
        3. Subglottic—pediatric bronchoscopy and endotracheal tube—posterolateral injury and posterior injury
V. Tracheal
    A. Anterior wall—tracheotomy site, granuloma and innominate pulse
    B. Posterior wall—sharp tube, tracheotomy tube, endotracheal tube and transtracheal needle
    C. Circumferential—cuff injury
VI. Bronchial—biopsy force and foreign body impaction

VII. Esophageal—biopsy, scope and dilators

### DENTAL INJURY

Sound teeth are rarely dislodged in the performance of an endoscopic procedure. Carious, loose, capped or deciduous teeth are more susceptible to injury. Pre-endoscopic examination should also include a search for permanent artificial bridges or even solitary teeth. Loose teeth should be extracted prior to elective endoscopy. Such teeth may not only be dislodged, but also be aspirated readily by the sedated patient, especially if the protective action of the larynx is diminished by local or general anesthesia.

The upper incisors and canines are the most at risk. Flexion of the cervical spine and extension of the atlanto-occipital joint will minimize the pressure needed to pass a straight tube over the dorsum of the tongue. Such an approach is probably required by the broad based Lynch and Jako laryngoscopes and by the Negus and Jesperg esophagoscopes.

Narrower instruments, such as the Broyles, Holinger and Tucker laryngoscopes and the Jackson bronchoscopes and esophagoscopes, may be placed over the plica triangularis. If the head is flexed laterally (the left ear toward the left shoulder) in the "hung" position, the bulk of the base of the tongue and upper alveolar prominence may be avoided.

The enamel of the teeth may be protected by

A. The use of dental compound of soft lead or a boxer's mouthpiece to protect the incisors in suspension laryngoscopy in which there is a considerable leverage against the upper teeth.
B. A folded gauze pad placed between the upper teeth and the endoscope.
C. Placement of the endoscopist's left hand so that the middle fingers guide the placement of the upper alveolus while the left thumb serves as the fulcrum against which the tube is balanced.
D. Laryngoscopes that are "C"-shaped in contradistinction to the anesthesiologist's instrument to permit application of a *lifting* force to the upper limb if the "C" minimizes pressure against the upper teeth. (The "L"-shaped scope may be lifted by gripping the handle tightly and supporting the tongue with a vertical thrust; this effort is mechanically disadvantageous and usually results in a "prying" motion in which the fulcrum is the upper teeth.)
E. The left side of the mouth, which may occasionally provide better access if the problem is limited to the right larynx, right lung or right hypopharynx.

Intubation laryngoscopes (with an open right side) should, of course, never be used on the left side of the mouth lest the lumen fill with the tongue and thus be totally obscured.

## HYPOPHARYNGEAL ("ESOPHAGEAL") PERFORATION

Perforation of the laryngopharyngeal mucosa proximal to the cricopharyngeus may be due to the lodgement of a sharp foreign body at this region of physiologic construction. It is also the most frequent site of endoscopic instrumental trauma (esophagoscopy, both rigid and flexible, bronchoscopy and even endotracheal intubation).[13]

### ANATOMIC POINTS

1. In the resting patient, the postcricoid laryngeal mucosa lies in contact with the posterior hypopharyngeal mucosa.

2. The cricopharyngeal sphincter is not a true sphincter but a muscular sling attached to the lateral aspects of the cricoid cartilage.

3. This pharyngoesophageal segment is normally closed and has only a potential lumen until the larynx is lifted forward, away from the cervical spine.

4. In patients with a Zenker's diverticulum, this "inferior constrictor" moves anteriorly with the cricoid, leaving a lumen behind the cricopharyngeus which leads only to the diverticular pouch. The lining of the diverticulum consists only of mucosa without muscular reinforcement and is especially susceptible to perforation. A number of precautionary steps will help to minimize the chances of such perforation.

### Pre-esophagoscopic X-rays

1. A "swallowing function" or "cervical esophagram" that demonstrates the cervical esophagus and cricopharyngeus well should be included. The contrast material should be sufficiently thick to distend this region fully.

2. Lateral soft tissue films of the neck are helpful to demonstrate not only soft tissue but also the subglottic airway and cervical spine.

3. All films should be available in the endoscopic room at the time the procedure is performed.

4. X-ray reports, verbal or written "GI series" and "esophagrams" or "barium swallows" that do not demonstrate the cervical esophagus are not acceptable substitutes.

5. Complete esophageal obstruction (high) is the only exception under which one should proceed.

6. The use of a barium-impregnated cotton bolus can drive a sharp foreign body through the esophageal wall and into the mediastinum.

### Mechanical Guidance

1. The use of a previously swallowed string as a guide is probably the safest technique, especially if a diverticulum is suspected. At least five feet of string should have been swallowed, sufficient to permit safe traction on the proximal end without dislodging the string. (Occasionally, the bolus of string itself has been reported to cause gastrointestinal complications.)

2. A nasogastric tube may often be followed esophagoscopically. The authors are aware of at least one case in which a Zenker's diverticulum was fatally perforated by a Levin tube.

3. Lumen finders — A spring mounted metal olive has been advocated[21]; it is to be preferred to a fine woven silk "filiform" bougie for such a purpose. The smaller filiforms, 6, 8 or 10 French, may actually be quite sharp and may in themselves perforate the mucosa. Such fine filiforms may double back outside the lip of the scope. If the scope is then advanced mistakenly, perforation may well ensue.

### Flexible Fiberesophagoscopy

The large square end of the fiberesophagoscope makes it difficult to introduce such an instrument blindly, since the cervical esophagus is seen only as the instrument is withdrawn. It is especially necessary to rule out cervical esophageal and hypopharyngeal pathology prior to flexible examination by the use of radiologic examination (esophagram, lateral neck barium swallow), and if these are not absolutely negative, direct inspection should be undertaken before the passage of a flexible instrument.

## FOREIGN BODY MANIPULATION

The most prevalent "complication" of foreign body management is impaction of the foreign object deeper into the tracheal bronchial tree. This, in turn, most likely results from a failure to understand and apply Jackson's dicta regarding the proper holding and manipulation of cannulated forceps. The forceps must be stabilized so that the open blades, once placed around the foreign object, are then closed by advancement of the cylindrical portion over the solid shaft rather than by the withdrawing of the shaft into the cylindrical portion. Such withdrawal results in a failure to grasp; conversely, reopening of the forceps after such withdrawal results in impaction.

General anesthesia, especially of the paralytic variety, has in recent years been responsible for degrees of bronchial impaction not noted by the generation of endoscopists who worked only with the awake patient.[22]

## ESOPHAGOSCOPY

In esophagoscopy, the anesthesiologist and endoscopist are no longer in competition for the same working space. Endotracheal anesthesia can usually be accomplished with ease. An endotracheal tube not only assures the anesthesiologist of a working airway but also prevents the endoscopist from compressing the trachea from behind. The act of intubation itself involves specific hazards and requirements, especially in cervical esophageal problems. It is often best to apply local anesthesia to the larynx and to intubate the patient with the aid of local anesthetic before proceeding to induction of general anesthesia. Placement of the endotracheal tube under mirror guidance may be often useful. Whether under mirror or direct guidance, placement of an endotracheal tube must be precise when cervical esophageal disease is present. Entrance of the endotracheal tube into the upper esophagus instead of the larynx is usually not considered a serious mishap by many anesthesiologists. The danger of serious damage to an esophagus that contains a tumor or a foreign body or to patients with a high level stenosis is quite apparent if the endotracheal tube is inadvertently placed through the cricopharyngeus muscle.

Another technique that must be used with caution in the presence of a cervical esophageal tumor mass or foreign body is that of exerting pressure on the anterior wall of the larynx to bring it into the view of the anesthesiologist's laryngoscope. Such pressure may bring the posterior tracheal wall forward with subsequent trauma to the posterior tracheal wall by the endotracheal tube.

Positive pressure respiration-inspiration is accomplished by increasing the endothoracic and pleural pressures with a consequent squeeze on the esophagus, which is opened through the endoscope to the atmosphere. This may be especially troublesome when one is dealing with tightly impacted foreign bodies or those that are irregular and whose points are imbedded in the esophageal wall. In such cases, it is incumbent on the anesthesiologist to make possible a more physiologic form of inspiration so that the esophagus will be opened by negative extraesophageal pressure.

## PEDIATRIC ENDOSCOPIC COMPLICATIONS

The normal anatomic limitation of the subglottic larynx as the smallest diameter of the main conductive airway in the child makes it difficult to decide whether subglottic edema, ulceration and even stenosis are purely due to the mechanical effects of an oversized bronchoscope or endotracheal tube or whether there may not have been underlying congenital or inflammatory pathology. It has been retrospectively postulated that some of the subglottic injuries seen in children and occasionally even in adults have been due to gas sterilization of the rubber endotracheal tube when the caustic sterilizing agent has been absorbed by the porous rubber and then released to damage the delicate tissue. Further complicating this problem is the poor circulation secondary to the child's basic congenital heart disease and so on. It is uniformly agreed that intubation *per se* is not an acceptable treatment for true croup when the inflammation is in the subglottic larynx. Conversely, current practice is tending toward the use of intubation in those situations in which the inflammation is purely supraglottic.[5]

## HYPOPHARYNGEAL HEMORRHAGE

Lesions of the pyriform sinus and hypopharynx, especially those involving the lateral wall, should be approached for biopsy with extreme caution. If possible, biopsy should be taken from anteromedial reflections (laryngeal surface) of the pyriform sinus. Involvement of the carotid artery itself or the superior laryngeal or superior thyroid vessels by tumor can precipitate hemorrhage if compounded by deep biopsy.

## BRONCHIAL HEMORRHAGE

Bronchial hemorrhage is uncommon as a complication of bronchoscopy *per se*. Preexisting massive bleeding may indeed be a contraindication to bronchoscopy unless the procedure is to be performed with an open tube in an operating room, where the main problem is deciding which side of the chest is to be entered. Bleeding sufficient to preclude the visual use of the endoscope is accepted as a contraindication to bronchoscopy.

Bleeding associated with bronchoscopy in most situations is found to have been associated more directly with the taking of a bronchial biopsy. The safest guideline is to attempt to limit one's biopsy to material that is already presenting in the bronchial lumen. Attempts to diagnose submucosal pathology (with the specific exception of the search for sarcoidosis in the mucosa just to the left of the carina) are indeed dangerous. Many endoscopists feel that the return of cartilage as part of the biopsy specimen is a suggestion that the technique may be too penetrating.

Although rarely seen in current practice, luetic aneurysm, if strongly suspected, may certainly be a contraindication. The fragility of aneurysmal walls as they erode a major bronchus may be such that the performance of even the gentlest procedure can cause a patient to drown in the outpouring of the cardiac output into the left bronchus.

## TRACHEOESOPHAGEAL FISTULA

As noted previously (p. 301), this complication may occur if the posterior tracheal wall is incised, and it may also be secondary to the blind use of a tracheal trocar or a late complication of an overly straight tracheotomy tube. More recently, this complication has been found to arise in patients for whom the only suspicion in the history is that of transtracheal aspiration. The mechanism of fistula formation in this particular case seemed to be osteonecrosis of the posterior plate of the cricoid, which apparently had been perforated by the needle placed through the cricothyroid membrane to obtain culture material.

Perforation of the tracheal wall has also been observed in misdirected insertion of a sharp obturator used with an infant tracheotomy tube. This complication has also been documented in the use of the Sheldon tracheotome, which deliberately employs a cutting obturator. The treatment of a perforation was emergent repair and drainage. Many of these conditions are now managed initially by large dose antibiotics.

## ESOPHAGEAL DILATATION

"Sooner or later all cases of stricture of the esophagus die of the bougie."[20] Perforation of the esophagus is indeed inevitable if it is approached as a "blind" procedure. The use of string, guide wire[3] or fluoroscopic assistance,[15] or a combination of these, may be helpful.

Retrograde dilatation utilizes the force of traction rather than pulsion.[25] Even this may result in "splitting" if too ambitious an attempt is made to dilate vigorously. In practice, it is probably safest to use no more than two or three consecutive "working" dilators.

Steroid therapy poses a dilemma that has not yet been fully resolved. If administered sufficiently early to prevent scar formation, such therapy prevents the occurrence of the scar, which in truth has probably protected the patient from the dilator. It is suggested that a patient's stricture not be dilated while he is on such a regimen. Those strictures that have occurred in spite of such a regimen should be approached with extreme care.

## MEDIASTINOSCOPY

Mediastinoscopy is a surgical endoscopic technique for examination and biopsy of the mediastinum. The term mediastinoscopy may indeed be misleading, however. The surgical application of the Carlens procedure is really a limited field operation.[6] The actual area for exploration is confined to the medial paratracheal area in the region of the superior and posterior portions of the middle mediastinum. The anterior, lateral and posterior mediastinal areas are not examined. The validity of this approach rests in the fact that peripheral lung lesions tend to drain toward the hilum, to the root of the lung, and from there up and about the paratracheal area.

Since the introduction of mediastinoscopy by Eric Carlens in 1959, a vast experience has been accumulated, with over 80,000 mediastinoscopies in the world literature. Approximately 60,000 of these are in European and Asian literature and 20,000 are in North American literature. This establishes mediastinoscopy as a valuable and safe procedure.

The main application of mediastinoscopy is the differential diagnosis of mediastinal adenopathy.

It has also been used in determining resectability in carcinoma of the lung. Respiratory carcinoma in the United States represents approximately 12.5 per cent of total cancer, cancer of the larynx being 2 per cent and of the lung approximately 10 per cent. Total salvage from cancer of the lung is quoted at 4 to 5 per cent in national experience. Of all patients who undergo thoracotomy for carcinoma of the lung, approxi-

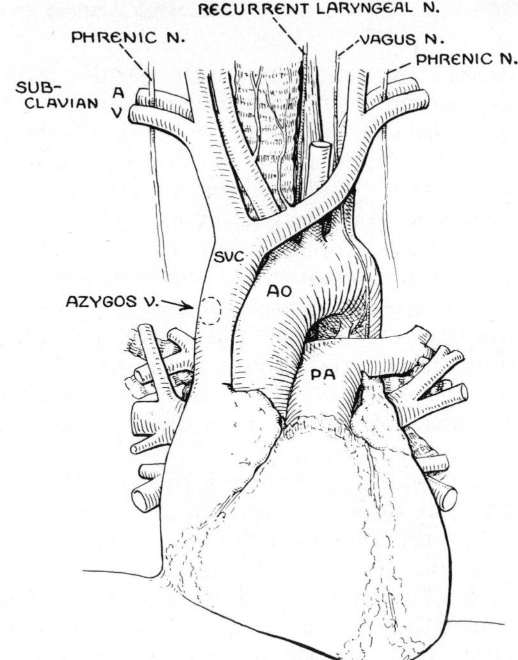


**Figure 20–2** Anterior view of the mediastinum (thymus not included). (Schenck, *Otolaryngology*, courtesy of W. F. Prior Co.)

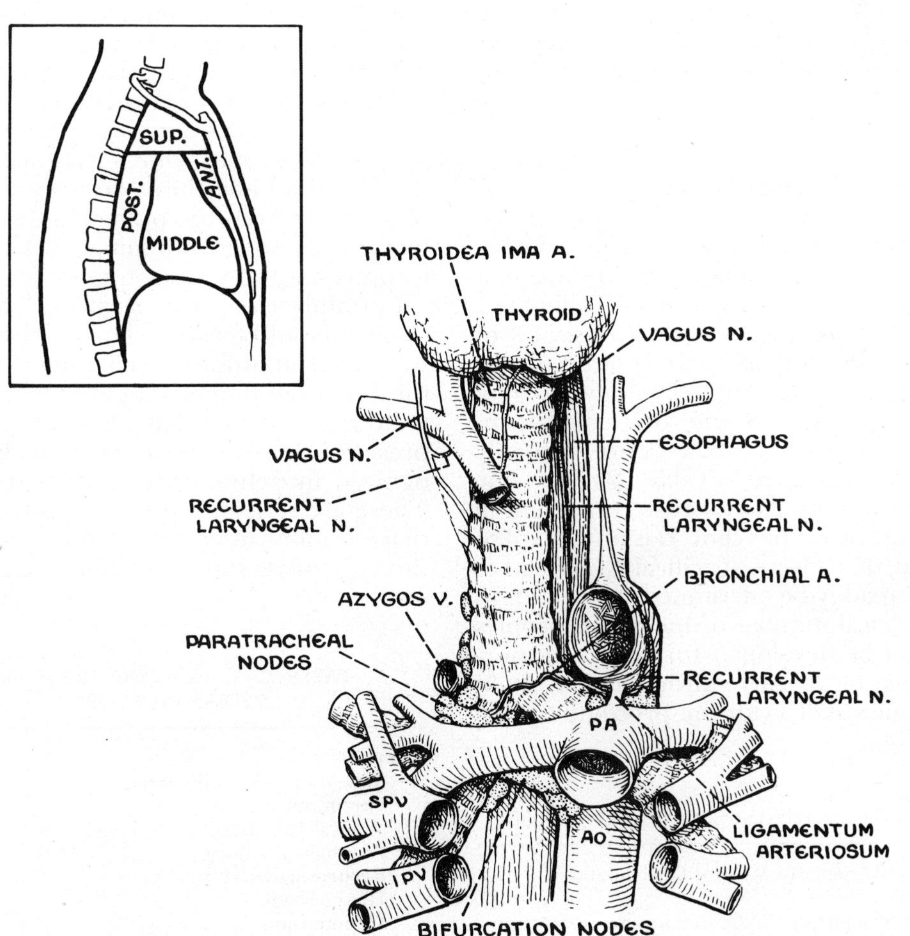


**Figure 20–3** Middle mediastinum. *Inset,* Sagittal section of the mediastinum. (Schenck, *Otolaryngology,* courtesy of W. F. Prior Co.)

mately 40 per cent undergo a "futile" thoracotomy, since only 60 per cent prove to be resectable. Mediastinoscopy is therefore intended as a prethoracotomy screening procedure. It should be noted that the differential diagnosis of mediastinal adenopathy and determination of resectability may be the result of the same observation.

Therapeutic considerations for mediastinoscopy are cardiac pacemaker implantation, thymus resection and radon seed implantation. Figures 20–2 and 20–3 illustrate the exceptional vascularity of the immediate paratracheal area.

Technically, the procedure of mediastinoscopy is done through an incision placed below the thyroid isthmus and above the innominate artery. The tissues are dissected in a blunt way to the pretracheal fascia. Through the natural tunnel of the investing fascia of the trachea, the mediastinum is then entered just posterior to the innominate artery. The paratracheal tissues are freed down to the level of the pulmonary artery.

## Complications

By careful attention to technique, the actual complication rate in mediastinoscopy is repeatedly less than 2 per cent. Table 20–1 represents a statistically compiled review of 1076 mediastinoscopies from three different authors and notably varying geographical areas.[26] Of the 1076 mediastinoscopies presented, 826 were actually statistically reviewed (Table 20–2). The complications in Table 20–3 represent a percentage of 1.7 per cent. It is important to note that there were specifically no deaths.

It can readily be envisioned that a significant statistical number of mediastinoscopies might not be developed for reporting purposes because of early difficulties in establishing one's skills with the procedure. Listed are the authors' own knowledge of complications that have been reported to them.

1. Biopsy of the innominate artery with severe hemorrhage and/or death.

2. Perforation of the esophagus with mediastinitis and fistula formation.

3. Biopsy of the pulmonary artery on two different occasions. One was associated with the use of an anesthesia laryngoscope. One patient in whom the pulmonary artery was biopsied survived with initial packing of the wound and later thoracotomy.

Certainly the most hazardous complication is that of bleeding. This can be avoided by careful attention to technique. The site of the proposed biopsy should first be aspirated to make certain that a blood vessel is not present. The greatest hazard has been recognized in defining the venous structures. These are thin-walled low pressure systems that are more subject to trauma. Included in this type of vessel may be the pulmonary artery.

**TABLE 20–1** MEDIASTINOSCOPIES PERFORMED

| | |
|---|---|
| Tucker — Hahnemann Medical College and Hospital | 400 |
| Ward — University of California, Los Angeles | 300 |
| Duval & Koop — University of Minnesota | 376 |
| Total | 1076 |

**TABLE 20–2** MEDIASTINOSCOPIES REVIEWED

| | |
|---|---|
| **Carcinoma of the Lung** | 446 |
| Number Positive | 190 |
| Per cent Positive | 42 |
| **Sarcoidosis** | 157 |
| Number Positive | 152 |
| Per cent Positive | 97 |
| **Miscellaneous Malignancies** | |
| Miscellaneous Metastatic | 5 |
| Head and Neck | 5 |
| Breast | 3 |
| Hodgkin's | 17 |
| Lymphoma | 10 |
| **Miscellaneous Nonmalignant** | 29 |
| Histoplasmosis | 6 |
| Tuberculosis | 13 |
| Total | 826 |

**TABLE 20–3** COMPLICATIONS OF MEDIASTINOSCOPY

| | |
|---|---|
| Per cent | 1.7 |
| Subcutaneous Emphysema | 2 |
| Pneumothorax | 4 |
| Wound Infection | 2 |
| Esophageal Injury | 0 |
| Recurrent Nerve Injury | 5 |
| Hemorrhage | 5 |
| Hypotension | 0 |
| Wound Hematoma | 1 |
| Deaths | 0 |

In bleeding from a low-pressure system, wound packing can be of life-saving assistance. Arterial bleeding is more difficult to control. The artery is more readily visualized, however, since it is a thick-walled high-pressure system. The value of the compressing finger should not be ignored simply because one is operating in a deep wound. The placement of a patient on a heart-lung by-pass machine after bleeding has been temporarily controlled in the presence of a major vascular injury gives stability to a situation that might otherwise be tenuous.

Carlens, in a series of 685 cases, listed only three significant complications: (1) paralysis of the right recurrent laryngeal nerve, (2) excessive bleeding from a tumor biopsy requiring thoracotomy and resection of the tumor in which the patient survived, and (3) one death on the third postoperative day from myocardial infarction.

Again, the statistical review of mediastinoscopy in the world literature points up the safety of this procedure, with complications being in the range of 1 to 2 per cent. Fatal complications are accurately recorded as less than one-half of one per cent.

## Bibliography


1. Adriani, J.: The Pharmacology of Anesthetic Drugs. Springfield, Ill., Charles C Thomas, 4th ed. 1962, p. 105.
2. Bordley, J. E.: Personal communication.
3. Bunker, T. G., and Carter, B. L.: A method for passing a string in esophageal stenosis cases. Trans. Am. Bronchoesoph. Assoc., *44*:28–31, 1964.
4. Cantrell, R. W.: Personal communication.
5. Cantrell, R. W., Bell, R. A., and Morioka, W. T.: Acute epiglottis. Trans. Pac. Coast Otoophthalmol. Soc., 1976.
6. Carlens, E.: Mediastinoscopy. Ann. Otol. Rhinol. Laryngol., *74*:1102–1112, 1965.
7. Davison, F. W.: Acute laryngotracheal infections in childhood. Otolaryngol. Clin. North Am., *1*:69–89, 1968.
8. Figi, F.: Tracheotomy: A study of 200 consecutive cases. Ann. Otol., *43*:178–192, 1934.
9. Goodman, L. S., and Gilman, A.: The Pharmacological Basis of Therapeutics. 2nd ed. New York, Macmillan Publishing Co., 1955, p. 239.
10. Jackson, D.: Bronchoscopy and Esophagoscopy. Philadelphia, W. B. Saunders Co., 1927, p. 392.
11. Keim, W. F., Shapiro, M. J., and Rosin, H. D.: Study of postlaryngectomy stomal recurrence. Arch. Otolaryngol., *81*:183–186, 1965.
12. Lindholm, C. E.: Prolonged endotracheal intubation. Acta Anaesth. Supplement *33*:1, 1970.
13. McGovern, F. H., Fitz-Hugh, G. S., and Edgemon, L. J.: The hazards of endotracheal intubation. Ann. Otol. Rhinol. Laryngol., *80*:556–564, 1971.
14. Norris, C. M., Tucker, G. F., Jr., Kuo, B. F., et al.: A correlation of clinical staging, pathological findings and five year end results in surgically treated cancer of the larynx. Ann. Otol. Rhinol. Laryngol., *79*:1033, 1970.
15. Norris, C. M., Tucker, G. F., Jr., and Woloshin, H. J.: Bronchoesophagologic application of recent advances in fluoroscopy. Ann. Otol. Rhinol. Laryngol., *80*:528–534, 1971.
16. Steinhaus, J. E.: Comparative study of experimental toxicity of local anesthetics. Anesthesiology, *13*:577–586, 1952.
17. Steinhaus, J. E.: Personal communication, June, 1976.
18. Suratt, P. M., Smiddy, J. F., and Gruber, B,: Deaths and complications associated with fiberoptic bronchoscopy. Chest, *69*:747–751, 1976.
19. Switz, D. M., Clarke, A. M., and Longacher, J. W., Jr.: Electrical malfunction at endoscopy. Possible cause of arrhythmia and death. J.A.M.A., *235*:273–275, 1976.
20. Trousseau A.: Biography of Armand Trousseau. J. Organotherapy, *11*:208–209, 1927.
21. Tucker, G.: Recent developments in peroral endoscopy. Surg. Gynecol. Obstet., June, 1926, pp. 743–752.
22. Tucker, G. F., Jr.: Anesthesia in peroral endoscopy, Otolarynogol. Clin. North Am., June, 1968, p. 37.
23. Ibid, pp. 55–56.
24. Tucker, J. A., and Silberman, H. D.: Tracheotomy. *In* Ferguson, C. F. (ed.): Pediatric Otolaryngology. Philadelphia, W. B. Saunders Co., 1972, pp. 1219–1230.
25. Tucker, J. A., Turtz, M. L., Silberman, H. D., et al.: Tucker retrograde esophageal dilatation 1924–1974. Ann. Otol. Rhinol. Laryngol., (Supplement 16) *83*:1974.
26. Tucker, J. A., Ward, P. H., Duvall, A. J., et al.: Mediastinoscopy Scientific Exhibit, AAOO, 1972.

# PREVENTION OF NUTRITIONAL COMPLICATIONS*

21

*Edward M. Copeland, III*
*Oscar M. Guillamondegui*
*Stanley J. Dudrick*

Malnutrition in patients undergoing head and neck surgery is primarily associated with advanced cancer in these areas. It is rare indeed that trauma, congenital abnormality and infection in these regions will precipitate a serious nutritional deficit. Patients with resectable or radiosensitive malignant lesions of the head and neck should be nourished adequately in order to promote optimal wound healing and to minimize the incidence and severity of catastrophic complications of surgery and radiotherapy.[3] A functional gastrointestinal tract is the best means of insuring normal digestion and assimilation of foodstuffs; however, the gastrointestinal tract is not always available for use. Delivery of adequate nutriments to the gut does not always result in rapid nutritional repletion because malnutrition may lead to anorexia, nausea and vomiting and to malabsorption and loss of enteral nutriments in the stool. Patients with head and neck malignancies often have a history of heavy alcohol intake, smoking and dietary indiscretions and may be protein-calorie malnourished at the time they develop an oropharyngeal malignancy. Such preexisting malnutrition may be potentiated by the cancer if it produces obstruction or pain on deglutition. Attention to nutritional status at the initial interview and appropriate dietary counseling and vitamin supplementation will result in nutritional rehabilitation of most patients. Other patients will require nasogastric tube feeding supplements prior to operation or radiation therapy. Rarely, a gastrostomy or jejunostomy feeding tube must be inserted to deliver nutriments to a normally functioning gastrointestinal tract. If time permits, restoration of good nutritional status may be possible by tube feeding maneuvers; however, nutritional rehabilitation via the gastrointestinal tract can be time-consuming, and the operative insertion of gastrostomy or jejunostomy tubes can impose an acute surgical stress upon the patient that will further delay nutritional repletion. Similarly, indwelling nasogastric tubes are unsatisfactory for long-term use because they often cause nasopharyngeal ulcerations and esophagogastric reflux around the tube. Nevertheless, short-term nutritional repletion of the moderately malnourished patient or nutritional maintenance of the previously healthy patient who cannot swallow is quite satisfactory via a nasogastric feeding tube. For those patients whose gastrointestinal tracts are unavailable for nutrient administration or who need rapid nutritional repletion in order to initiate antineoplastic therapy quickly, the technique of intravenous hyperalimentation (IVH), properly applied, has allowed appropriate cancer treatment to be administered and, in some cases, has been lifesaving.[4]

## TUBE FEEDINGS

A #16 or #18 nasogastric tube may be inserted through the external nares to lie

*Supported in part by National Institutes of Health Grant CA 16672

within the distal third of the esophagus. This supplementary feeding method satisfies the major nutritional requirements in the vast majority of patients and, when applicable, is by far the most expeditious. A small #8 pediatric feeding tube may be used; however, the patency of this tube is difficult to maintain if viscid feedings are to be administered. If the tube does not transverse the gastroesophageal junction, reflux esophagitis can be prevented because competency of the physiologic gastroesophageal sphincter is maintained. Every 10 to 14 days, the tube should be replaced and repositioned via the opposite nostril in order to prevent pressure necrosis of the nasal and nasopharyngeal mucosa. Most nasogastric tubes have markings spaced equal distances along the tube to allow proper positioning of the tip of the tube 30 to 35 cm. from the external nasal orifice (the gastroesophageal junction is 40 cm. from the nasal opening in the average adult male patient). Proper tube placement is important, and if difficulty in insertion is encountered or doubt about location of the distal end of the feeding tube exists, roentgenographic confirmation of tube location is indicated. Aspiration of the tube diet into the tracheobronchial tree can be especially dangerous in the malnourished patient who has depressed inflammatory and immunologic responses to infection and who does not have the ability to clear tracheobronchial secretions because of weak and ineffective respiratory musculature. The threat of aspiration can be obviated further by having the patient in the semi-Fowler's or upright position during feeding, by slow instillation of the tube feeding diet (best monitored by the patient, if possible) and by *not* feeding the patient while he is asleep.

Gastrostomy is rarely necessary today in surgery of the head and neck. In some circumstances, there may be the need to divert food preoperatively. An occasional patient can be cured or can receive radiation therapy, which leaves the patient's deglutitory function disabled permanently. In this situation, gastrostomy or jejunostomy tube insertion is preferred over long-term nasogastric or esophagogastric intubation (unless the patient, for some reason, has a permanent cervical esophageal stoma through which a feeding tube can be inserted intermittently). The gastrostomy tube has the advantage of being readily available and visible to the patient and easy to manipulate. The stomach may retain its role as a reservoir for foodstuffs, and the "dumping syndrome" that sometimes follows food administration is minimized. Likewise, the gastroesophageal sphincter remains intact, and esophageal reflux is minimal. Either a Janeway[9] or Stamm[10] gastrostomy is satisfactory. Both require a surgical procedure to construct, but only the former requires a surgical procedure to close, because it is essentially a gastric mucosa-lined conduit from the stomach to the anterior abdominal wall. The operation to fashion the Stamm gastrostomy may be done through a midline upper abdominal incision. A #30 to #36 mushroom catheter is inserted into the middle third of the stomach midway between the lesser and greater curvatures. The catheter is secured in place with two purse-string chromic catgut sutures and exits the abdominal cavity through a stab wound in the left upper quadrant 2 cm. below the left costal margin. The serosa of the stomach must be sewn securely to the parietal peritoneum around the catheter in order to prevent subsequent leakage of intragastric content and soilage of the peritoneal cavity. Performed properly, this operation has minimal risk even in the malnourished patient. If the stomach is unavailable for insertion of a feeding tube, a #12 to #16 French red rubber catheter can be inserted into the proximal jejunum 30 cm. from the ligament of Treitz. If jejunal feeding will be necessary for periods of months or years, the Maydl jejunostomy should be constructed.[1] This type of jejunostomy makes chronically implanted rubber feeding tubes unnecessary and provides a satisfactory small bowel feeding fistula through a jejunal Roux-en-Y limb, with the stoma sutured to the skin (Fig. 21–1).

Feedings may begin through a surgically prepared feeding fistula as soon as there is adequate wound healing and return of peristalsis. Initially, small amounts of glucose water or balanced salt solution should be introduced through the tube, and, if well tolerated, skimmed milk progressing to a milk base or water base blenderized or commercially prepared diet may be infused in amounts of up to 400 ml. every 4 hours. A similar program should be followed when

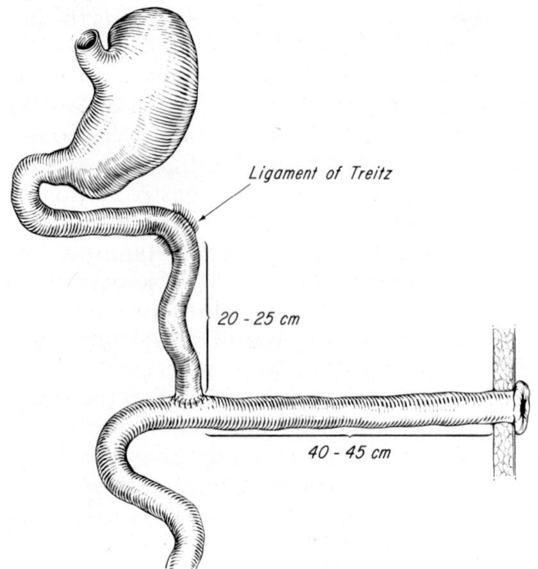


**Figure 21–1** Maydl jejunostomy. (From Copeland, E. M.: Nutritional Aspects of Cancer, *In* Hickey, R. C. (ed.): *Current Problems in Cancer,* September, 1976. Copyright © 1976, by Year Book Medical Publishers, Inc. Chicago. Used by permission.)

initiating feedings through a nasogastric tube. For example, if aspiration does occur with the initial feedings, glucose water or balanced salt solution will be readily absorbed across the bronchiole-alveolar surface without resultant pneumonia. An adequate blenderized diet is outlined in Table 21–1.[2] This diet provides 2765 kcal., 90 gm. of protein, 145 gm. of fat and 275 gm. of carbohydrate diluted in a volume of 3465 ml. The ingredients of this diet should be warmed, blended together in an electric blender, strained and administered at body temperature. The glass of formula should be stirred before pouring it into the feeding tube in order to suspend the solids. Coffee and citrus juices are not integral constituents of the formula but are given to simulate a more normal diet. Any excess formula may be refrigerated and served at body temperature within 24 to 48 hours. If the patient is unable to tolerate milk, two 12 oz. cans of Isocal can be substituted for the formula feeding, and a diet equal in caloric value but much lower in fat content can thereby be provided.

**TABLE 21–1** REGULAR TUBE FEEDING

| Suggested Daily Meal Plan |
|---|
| *Breakfast:* |
| 1 cup citrus juice (as orange, grapefruit or tomato) |
| Coffee, ½ ounce cream, 2 teaspoons sugar |
| 3 glasses *formula* containing 240 cc. each: |
| ½ cup warm strained cooked refined cereal (as farina, cream of wheat, cream of rice) |
| 1 cooked egg |
| 1½ cups warm milk |
| ¼ cup corn syrup |
| 1 tablespoon vegetable oil |
| ½ cup water |
| *Lunch and Supper (same):* |
| 1 cup juice |
| Coffee, ½ ounce cream, 2 teaspoons sugar |
| 3 glasses *formula* containing 240 cc. each: |
| 1 jar (3½ oz.) warm strained meat |
| ½ cup warm strained vegetable |
| 2 cups warm milk |
| 2 tablespoons vegetable oil |

(From Copeland, E. M.: Nutritional aspects of cancer. *In* Hickey, R. C. (ed.): *Current Problems in Cancer,* September, 1976. Copyright © 1976, by Year Book Medical Publishers, Inc., Chicago. Used by permission.)

## ELEMENTAL DIETS

Chemically defined, "elemental" diets consist primarily of mixtures of purified L-amino acids, glucose, short- or medium-chain triglycerides and baseline requirements of electrolytes, water and fat-soluble vitamins exclusive of vitamin K (Table 21–2). Almost complete absorption takes place in the proximal jejunum, and these diets may be used when terminal digestion is impaired due to either malabsorption or restricted absorptive surface area. These diets should be administered at one-quarter or

**TABLE 21–2** COMPARISON OF COMPOSITIONS OF CHEMICALLY DEFINED DIETS (per 1000 ml. of 25% solution)

| | Unit of Measurement | Vivonex* High Nitrogen | Vivonex* Standard | Flexical** |
|---|---|---|---|---|
| Calories | kcal. | 1000 | 1000 | 1000 |
| Carbohydrate | gm. | 210 | 226 | 154 |
| Amino acids | gm. | 75 | 22 | 22.5 |
| Nitrogen | gm. | 6.7 | 3.3 | 3.5 |
| Fat | gm. | 0.9 | 1.4 | 34.0 |
| Sodium | mEq. | 33.5 | 37.4 | 15.2 |
| Potassium | mEq. | 17.9 | 29.9 | 38.5 |
| Chloride | mEq. | 52.4 | 50.8 | 33.8 |
| Magnesium | mEq. | 9.6 | 16.0 | 14.4 |
| Calcium | mEq. | 13.3 | 22.2 | 25.0 |
| Osmolality | mOsm. | 844 | 500 | 805 |

*Eaton Laboratories; Norwich, New York
**Mead-Johnson Laboratories; Evansville, Indiana
(From Copeland, E. M.: Nutritional aspects of cancer. *In* Hickey, R. C. (ed.): *Current Problems in Cancer*, September, 1976. Copyright © 1976, by Year Book Medical Publishers, Inc., Chicago. Used by permission.)

one-half strength initially, until the small bowel adapts to the osmolar content and diarrhea ceases. When mixed at "full strength," these formulas provide approximately 1 kcal per ml. and have an osmolarity between 600 and 1200 mOsm. Disadvantages of the diets include nausea, vomiting and diarrhea even after a period of bowel adaptation. The diets also have an unappealing taste imparted to them by the contained amino acids. This taste can be masked partially by the addition of various flavoring agents; however, these agents significantly increase the osmolarity of the diet. Moreover, it is difficult to motivate many cancer patients to drink the diet or to instill it through a nasogastric tube because regurgitation produces a most unpleasant aftertaste. During administration of chemically defined diets, the urine should be checked routinely for glycosuria to insure that the administered glucose is being metabolized completely and not lost in the urine. If significant glycosuria occurs and sufficient water and electrolytes are not provided, hypertonic dehydration and hyperosmolar coma can result. Additional metabolic monitoring of the patient should include daily weights and strict intake and output measurements. Serum electrolytes, blood urea nitrogen and blood sugar determinations should be done every other day until the desired amount of diet is being tolerated.

## INTRAVENOUS HYPERALIMENTATION

There remains a group of patients who are resistant to standard nutritional supportive techniques. In 1966, Dudrick, Rhoads and Vars tested the hypothesis that concentrated intravenous nutriments would meet the caloric requirements of critically ill patients. These investigators initially fed beagle puppies exclusively by infusing a 30 per cent nutrient mixture composed primarily of glucose, protein hydrolysates, minerals, trace elements and vitamins via the superior vena cava.[6] The animals grew and developed normally for periods exceeding six months. From this experience, the technique of intravenous hyperalimentation was adapted for use in the human being.[7] Currently, intravenous hyperalimentation solutions are formulated by mixing 500 ml. of 50 per cent glucose with 500 ml. of 8.5 to 10 per cent crystalline amino acid solution. Each unit of IVH solution so prepared contains approximately 1000 calories and 6.8 to 8.0 gm. nitrogen and exerts between 1800 and 2400 mOsm of pressure. Electrolytes and vitamins must be added to these base solutions in sufficient quantities to correct existing deficits and to satisfy maintenance requirements. The usual electrolyte additives to solutions derived from protein hydrolysates are approximately 40 to 50 mEq. of sodium chloride, 20 to 40 mEq. of potassium chloride, 10 to 15 mEq. of magnesium sulfate and 15 to 20 mEq. of potassium acid phosphate per liter. The amino acids in commercially available amino acid products may be in the solution as the acetate, chloride or hydrochloride salts. These preparations are acidic, and infusion of solutions that contain large amounts of sodium or potassium, or both, as the chloride salt may result in hyperchloremic metabolic acidosis. Consequently, sodium and potassium should be added as the lactate, acetate, bicarbonate, acid phosphate or chloride salt, as directed by the patient's serum electrolyte concentrations and acid base status (Table 21–3). Calcium and phosphate must be added to commercially prepared amino acid solutions in order to maintain normal calcium and phosphorus metabolism. Hypomagnesemia will often occur within 10 to 14 days of intravenous hyperalimentation if sufficient quantities of this element are not added. Both fat- and water-soluble vitamins should be added to 1 liter of IVH solution daily, and vitamin K, folic acid and vitamin $B_{12}$ must be administered regularly and as necessary. Serum albumin concentration should be corrected to at least 3.5 gm. per cent by the daily administration of 12.5 to 50 gm. of albumin, which can be added directly to the IVH solution, and the hematocrit should be restored to normal by infusion of packed red blood cells.

Since several electrolyte mixtures must be added to the IVH solutions in the pharmacy, aseptic mixing under a laminar-flow, filtered-air hood is essential for optimum safety. These additives should be placed in the IVH solutions immediately prior to infusion so that current electrolyte requirements are satisfied. The solutions should be refrigerated immediately after preparation and administered within the next 24 hours.

**TABLE 21–3** USUAL COMPOSITION OF AMINO ACID SUBSTRATE SOLUTION

| | |
|---|---|
| 500 ml. 50% glucose plus | |
| 500 ml. 8.5% crystalline amino acids | |
| Additives: | |
| 40–50 mEq. | Sodium chloride |
| 20–30 mEq. | Potassium acetate |
| 10–15 mEq. | Potassium acid phosphate |
| 15 mEq. | Magnesium sulfate |
| 5 ml. | Multivitamins* (M.V.I.)** |
| 1 gm. | Calcium gluconate* |

*Added to only one unit of solution daily.
**M.V.I. — USV Pharmaceutical Corp. Tuckahoe, New York

In order to prevent thrombophlebitis secondary to the high osmolarity of the IVH solutions, a large diameter vessel must be catheterized. Our group has used the superior vena cava exclusively, and access to this vessel has been obtained preferably by infraclavicular, percutaneous catheterization of the subclavian vein. The external or internal jugular vein is acceptable for catheterization, but the catheter dressings are cumbersome and uncomfortable. Moreover, a catheter in these latter locations might interfere with the treatment plan for a head and neck malignancy. Antimicrobial ointment is placed over the catheter exit site, a sterile dressing is applied, tincture of benzoin is painted on the skin and water-repellent adhesive tape is placed over the dressing. In those patients with a draining pharyngocutaneous or tracheostomy stoma, a sterile plastic sheet is placed over the catheter dressing to minimize further the risk of contamination from stomal secretions. In those individuals who are to receive radiation therapy through a lower neck portal, the catheter skin entry site is placed outside the radiation field. No tape is applied to any skin of the neck or upper thorax that is included within the radiation portal in order to prevent skin bullae formation secondary to the tape. Accurate position of the catheter tip in the middle of the superior venal cava is documented roentgenographically prior to beginning the hypertonic hyperalimentation solutions. If the catheter has been directed into the internal or the external jugular vein, it should be removed and replaced; otherwise, thrombophlebitis usually will occur promptly.

The same registered nurse, assigned to the hyperalimentation team, assists with the insertion of each catheter, dismantles the catheter dressing three times a week, reprepares the skin around the catheter with a defatting agent and an antiseptic solution before reapplying the antimicrobial ointment and sterile dressing, changes the hyperalimentation delivery tubing and provides psychologic support for the patients. The hyperalimentation system consists of the IVH bottle or plastic bag connected to a pediatric microdrip set and a 30 inch extension tubing that inserts into the hub of the catheter. The catheter and delivery system are not used for administration of blood or blood by-products, central venous pressure monitoring, bolus drug administration or withdrawal of blood samples. Any manipulation of the delivery system results in increased frequency of catheter contamination. If simultaneous intravenous fluids other than IVH are necessary, they should be infused through a peripheral venous site, if possible. Simultaneous administration of other fluids through the IVH delivery tubing may be necessary, however, because malnourished patients often have very fragile peripheral veins, making peripheral infusion of these solutions impractical or impossible. At the termination of IVH, each catheter is removed and immediately cultured for aerobic and anaerobic bacteria and fungi. If the patient is febrile at the time of catheter removal, a blood culture is taken through the catheter and simultaneously from a peripheral vein. Inanition and malnutrition are two predisposing factors to bacterial and fungal septicemia. The need for rigorous aseptic management of the subclavian vein catheter is greatest in patients undergoing treatment for a head and neck cancer because they are malnourished, and secretions from pharyngocutaneous and tracheostomy stomas often continually contaminate the catheter dressings. Each febrile episode should be considered catheter-related, and if another source of fever cannot be identified, then the catheter should be incriminated empirically and removed. In order to prevent catheter contamination, dressings are changed as frequently as necessary, often twice daily. Intravenous hyperalimentation should not be reinstituted until 24 to 48 hours have elapsed after return of temperature to normal. Fever, *per se,* is not an absolute indication for discontinuing IVH. If an obvious source of infection is identified, it should be treated appropriately, and the catheter should be left in place. If the elevated temperature does not respond to reasonable treatment, the catheter should be removed. An absolute indication for removal of a subclavian venous catheter is a positive blood culture. The catheter should not be reinserted until blood cultures have been negative for at least 48 hours. Routine catheter changes have not been necessary in our experience, and the longest time that a single catheter has remained in place is 96 days.

Hypertonic IVH solutions should be delivered at a constant rate throughout each 24 hour period in order to promote optimum assimilation of the administered glucose, amino acids, minerals and vitamins. The rise in pancreatic insulin output in response to the infused glucose is not immediate, and blood sugar concentrations will gradually fall to normal throughout the initial 24 to 48 hour period. Fractional urine sugar concentrations should be determined every six hours, and, although glycosuria may be noted initially, it will usually disappear in 24 hours. Although 2000 to 3000 ml. of IVH solution can be given to many patients during the first day of nutritional repletion, these large dextrose dosages may result in hyperglycemia and excessive glycosuria in some patients and may lead to hypertonic dehydration and coma. These are serious complications of IVH delivery and must be prevented. Once the patient is capable of metabolizing 1000 ml. of IVH during a 24-hour period, the flow rate may be increased to 1000 ml. every 12 hours. Pancreatic islet cells again will need to adapt with an increased insulin output in response to the increased glucose infusion. Within the first three to five days of nutritional rehabilitation, the average adult will tolerate a daily ration of 3000 ml. of IVH. Manual regulation of the pediatric microdrip system usually is satisfactory for maintenance of a reasonably constant infusion rate. A widely fluctuating rate of delivery of IVH will be signaled by glycosuria, and a constant flow rate should be re-established. If glycosuria is encountered in a patient with continuously elevated blood sugar concentrations, either exogenous insulin must be supplied because the patient's capacity for metabolizing the administered glucose has been exceeded or the glucose delivery rate must be reduced. Our recommendation is that additional insulin should be added directly to IVH solutions rather than given subcutaneously. Although crystalline insulin adheres to the bottle and administration tubing, the amount of insulin lost in this manner is insignificant. If the insulin is in the IVH bottle and the infusion stops, insulin administration obviously also stops. If insulin has been administered subcutaneously and the infusion stops, marked hypoglycemia may result in potentially severe adverse clinical situations. Initial insulin dosages should be 5 to 10 units per 1000 ml. and increased gradually until blood sugar levels return to normal. IVH solutions should not be stopped suddenly because "rebound" insulin hypoglycemia or shock may occur. The pancreatic output of insulin does not cease immediately upon discontinuing the hypertonic glucose; consequently, if IVH is stopped abruptly, a relative excess of insulin will exist, and dangerously low blood sugar levels may result. We recommend that IVH be tapered over a 24- to 48-hour period prior to completely discontinuing it. If rapid tapering is necessary, this can be accomplished over a 4- to 6-hour period if a 10 per cent glucose infusion is given through a peripheral vein after IVH is stopped. One extreme note of caution is that prior to any general anesthetic, IVH must be tapered and discontinued because insulin hypoglycemia during anesthesia may go unrecognized and permanent brain damage can occur.

Patients should be weighed daily, using a metabolic scale. Accumulation of lean body mass should not exceed more than one-half pound per day following the initial 48 to 72 hours of rehydration, when weight may increase three to five pounds. After stabilization, if daily weight gain exceeds one pound per day, fluid retention must be assumed to have occurred, and either a diuretic should be administered or the delivery rate of IVH should be reduced. Serum electrolyte, blood urea nitrogen and blood sugar concentrations are determined every Monday, Wednesday and Friday. Serum albumin, magnesium, phosphorus, calcium, creatinine and liver function tests are determined weekly each Monday. A coagulation profile and complete blood count are obtained once weekly. All personnel who participate in the care of the patient should be familiar with administration of the IVH solutions. A pharmacist is usually designated as a member of the intravenous hyperalimentation team and serves as a liaison between the physicians, nurses and pharmacy. All pharmacy personnel, however, should be familiar with the formulation of the IVH solutions. A rehabilitation therapist should also be a member of the hyperalimentation team because active physical exercise is important for optimal nutrition and for rehabilitation of the musculoskeletal system. The team should make rounds each day and observe the patient's temperature, electrolyte balance, weight gain, adequacy of glucose metabolism, fluid intake and output and important physical findings. The results of these observations and determinations allow the team to predict the proper composition and quantity of IVH for each patient for each subsequent 24 hours.

## CLINICAL MATERIAL

Nutritional depletion is defined as a recent weight loss of 10 pounds or more of usual body weight, a serum albumin level of less than 3.4 gm. per cent and a negative reaction to a battery of recall skin test antigens. Patients with head and neck cancer may be malnourished because of prior dietary indiscretion, inadequate nutrient intake because of oropharyngeal obstruction and pain or concomitant illness that limits gastrointestinal absorption and assimilation. Previously healthy patients may be incapable of adequate enteral nutrition because of the malabsorption secondary to malnutrition imposed by prior radiation therapy, chemotherapy or surgery. To date, 70 patients (Table 21–4) with head and neck malignancies have received IVH in order to prepare, maintain or rehabilitate them nutritionally and metabolically so that surgery, chemotherapy or radiation therapy could be completed and tolerated with maximum safety and efficacy.

**TABLE 21–4** HYPERALIMENTATION IN HEAD AND NECK CANCER (70 Patients)

| *Indications for IVH* | *Number of Patients* |
|---|---|
| Perioperative support | 29 |
| Convalescent support | 10 |
| Radiation therapy | 9 |
| Chemotherapy | 16 |
| Enterocutaneous fistulas | 6 |

### *Perioperative Support*

Of the 29 patients who received IVH in the perioperative period, 19 had laryngopharyngectomy, 16 had radical neck dissection and 10 had thoracoacromial flap repair (Table 21–5). The average age of these patients was 61.1 years, and they required IVH for an average period of 36.6 days, during which they gained an average weight of 10.8 pounds. Intravenous hyperalimentation was used both pre- and postoperatively in 15 patients, the average weight gain was 11.3 pounds, and serum albumin rose from an average level of 3.23 gm. per cent to an average level of 3.46 gm. per cent. Hyperalimentation was used preoperatively for an average period of 16.1 days to promote adequate nutritional rehabilitation so that the extensive surgical procedure would be better tolerated and the maximum potential for wound healing would be provided. These patients required IVH for an average period of 20.3 days postoperatively until adequate nutrition could be maintained enterally.

### *Complications*

Catheter-related sepsis is the most frequent complication of intravenous hyperalimentation. In a recent review of the complications encountered in 406 consecutive cancer patients who received IVH at our institution, catheter-related sepsis occurred in only 2.3 per cent of patients.[2] Catheter-related sepsis was more common in patients treated for head and neck malignancies, however, because of the already mentioned frequency of catheter site contamination from pharyngostomy and tracheostomy stomas. Similarly, moist desquamation and superficial infection in the skin covering a radiation field often occurs and increases the chance of subclavian catheter contamination.

**TABLE 21–5** PERIOPERATIVE SUPPORT

| Operation | Number of Patients |
|---|---|
| Laryngopharyngectomy | 19 |
| Radical neck dissection | 16 |
| Thoracoacromial flap | 10 (1 bilateral) |
| Glossectomy | 3 |
| Mandibulectomy | 3 |
| Forehead flap | 2 |

**TABLE 21–6** COMPLICATIONS

| Catheter Culture | Blood Culture |
|---|---|
| *Candida tropicalis* | *C. tropicalis* |
| *C. tropicalis* | *P. mirabilis* |
| *Staphylococcus aureus* | *S. aureus* |
| Enterococcus and *Proteus mirabilis* | Enterococcus and *P. mirabilis* |
| *C. tropicalis* | Negative |
| Enterococcus | Negative |
| *Klebsiella pneumoniae* | Negative |
| *Serratia marcescens* | Negative |

No patients who received IVH as nutritional support during chemotherapy for head and neck malignancies had organisms grown from their catheters. Eighteen per cent of all catherers used in patients in the perioperative or convalescent support groups, however, were contaminated upon removal. Four of these patients had simultaneous positive blood and catheter cultures associated with sepsis (10.3 per cent) (Table 21–6). In two patients, a subsequent source of infection responsible for the positive blood culture was identified, but in the other two patients, the catheter was incriminated as the source of sepsis. Three of the nine patients who received radiation therapy had pathogenic organisms grown from their catheters, only one of these patients had a febrile episode and no patient had a positive blood culture. To date, no deaths or complications secondary to catheter-related sepsis have occurred; nevertheless, a constant vigil against catheter contamination must be maintained, and if proper aseptic technique is practiced, infectious complications can be minimized to our acceptable level.

Subclavian vein thrombosis occurred in one patient and was recognized by swelling of the arm ipsilateral to the subclavian vein catheter. The catheter was removed, edema resolved within seven days and heparin therapy was not necessary. One patient developed symptomatic hypophosphatemia, which was manifested by bizarre behavior. Symptoms resolved with the infusion of an appropriate dosage of phosphate (in this situation, calcium must also be infused to prevent a reciprocal fall in serum calcium).

## CONCLUSION

Attention to proper metabolic, physiologic and nutritional repletion and maintenance can minimize the complications from all modalities of oncologic therapy for head and neck malignancies. Inadequate nutritional status must be recognized, and proper treatment must be individualized for each patient. Those patients who require intravenous nutritional repletion should be admitted to the hospital, and IVH should be utilized preoperatively until weight gain has begun and muscular strength has returned. If the patient is to undergo an operation, IVH should be tapered and discontinued 8 to 12 hours prior to surgery and reinstituted 24 to 48 hours after operation. It should be continued until adequate enteral nutrition can be maintained by mouth or by feeding tube. With optimal nutritional rehabilitation, oncologic therapy can be safely recommended to a group of patients who might otherwise be denied possible curative surgical or radiation therapy because of the threat of major complications secondary to malnutrition and inanition.

## Bibliography


1. Brintnall, E. S., Dahm, D., and Womack, N. A.: Maydl jejunostomy. Arch. Surg., *65*:367–372, 1952.
2. Copeland, E. M., and Dudrick, S. J.: Nutritional aspects of cancer. *In* Hickey, R. C. (ed.):*Current Problems in Cancer,* Chicago, Ill., Year Book Medical Publishers, Inc., 1976.
3. Copeland, E. M., MacFadyen, B. V., Jr., MacComb, W. S., et al.: Intravenous hyperalimentation in patients with head and neck cancer. Cancer, *35*:606–611, 1975.
4. Copeland, E. M., MacFadyen, B. V., Jr., and Dudrick, S. J.: Intravenous hyperalimentation in cancer patients. J. Surg. Res., *16*:241–247, 1974.
5. Copeland, E. M., Souchon, E. A., MacFadyen, B. V., Jr., et al.: Intravenous hyperalimentation as an adjunct to radiation therapy. Cancer, *39*:609–616, 1977.
6. Dudrick, S. J., Vars, H. M., and Rhoads, J. E.: Growth of puppies receiving all nutritional requirements by vein. *Fortschritte der Parenteralen Ernahrung.* Symposium of the International Society of Parenteral Nutrition in 1966. Pallas Verlag, Lochham bei Munchen, West Germany, 1967.
7. Dudrick, S. J., Wilmore, D. W., Vars, H. M., et al.: Long-term total parenteral nutrition with growth, development and positive nitrogen balance. Surgery, *64*:134–142, 1968.
8. Hugon, J. S., and Bounous, G.: Elemental diet in the management of the intestinal lesions produced by radiation in the mouse. Can. J. Surg., *15*:18–26, 1972.
9. Martin, H. E., and Watson, W. L.: The original Janeway gastrostomy. Surg. Gynecol. Obstet., *56*:72–78, 1933.
10. Stamm, M.: A gastrostomy by a new method. Med. News, *65*:324–326, 1894.
11. Trier, J. S., and Browning, T. H.: A morphologic response of the mucosa of human small intestine to x-ray exposure. J. Clin. Invest., *45*:194–204, 1966.

# 22 COMPLICATIONS DUE TO ANTINEOPLASTIC DRUGS USED IN THE TREATMENT OF HEAD AND NECK CANCER

*Robert L. Capizzi*

Today, the role of chemotherapy in the treatment of cancer is changing. The use of systemic drugs is no longer considered only for the palliation of patients with advanced recurrent disease but is now included as a component of curative therapy when introduced shortly after surgery for those patients who are at a high risk for recurrence. The encouraging results of the preliminary clinical trials describing the combined modality management of osteogenic sarcoma[19, 34, 56] and breast cancer[9, 26] support this approach. The success of these programs, with the resultant wider use of chemotherapy, makes it imperative that all physicians be familiar not only with the therapeutic potential of these drugs but also with their toxic effects on the patient. This chapter will deal with the medical complications produced by antineoplastic drugs used in the treatment of epidermoid carcinoma of the head and neck.

All anticancer drugs interfere with some metabolic process in the tumor cell that eventually inhibits cell replication and causes cell death. Similar effects occur qualitatively in normal cells. With the drugs in current clinical use, however, the quantitative difference between the cytocidal effect on tumor versus normal cells is such that the tumor is destroyed and the host survives. Because of the low therapeutic index of most anticancer drugs, considerable experience must be brought to bear in offsetting host toxicity with tumor toxicity. Organs composed of cells with a rapid turnover rate, e.g., bone marrow, hair follicles and oral and gastrointestinal mucosa, are frequently affected and show the earliest signs of drug toxicity. If these organs are not affected to a profound degree, the toxic effects are usually reversible, and, since they are dose-related, their reoccurrence can be minimized by suitable dose attenuation. These acute toxicities usually do not result in any long-lasting debility. Certain drug toxicities, however, are the result of the cumulative drug effect on organs that do not have a high rate of cell turnover, e.g., liver, lung and heart. Toxic effects on these organs are insidious and frequently irreversible. Irreparable organ damage can only be prevented by anticipating such effects and discontinuing the drug with the first sign of drug toxicity.

Drugs effective in the treatment of head and neck cancer are listed in Table 22–1, along with the general drug classification to which these agents belong and their mechanism of action. In the treatment of head and neck cancer, the medical practice has been to reserve drugs for patients with advanced recurrent disease that is no longer amenable to surgery or irradiation. At this time, the patients are usually nutritionally deficient and debilitated, having lost considerable weight. Frequently, there are fistulous tracts and severe pain due to invasive tumor growth. It is in this setting that chemotherapy-induced tumor shrinkage has

**TABLE 22–1** DRUGS WHICH HAVE PRODUCED TUMOR REGRESSION IN HEAD AND NECK CANCER

| Drug | Chemical Class | Mechanism of Action |
|---|---|---|
| Methotrexate | Antimetabolite antifolate | Binds the enzyme dihydrofolate reductase |
| 5-Fluorouracil | Antimetabolite; false analogue of the natural pyrimidine uracil | Binds the enzyme thymidylate synthetase |
| 6-Mercaptopurine | Antimetabolite; false analogue of natural purine bases | Uncertain |
| Hydroxyurea | Miscellaneous | Binds the enzyme ribonucleotide reductase |
| Nitrogen mustard | Alkylating agent | Cross-linkage of DNA strands |
| Cyclophosphamide | Alkylating agent | Cross-linkage of DNA strands |
| Chlorambucil | Alkylating agent | Cross-linkage of DNA strands |
| Procarbazine | Miscellaneous | Uncertain |
| Vinblastine | Natural product; alkaloid | Inhibits mitosis |
| Vincristine | Natural product; alkaloid | Inhibits mitosis |
| Bleomycin | Natural product; antibiotic | DNA strand scission |
| Doxorubicin | Natural product; antibiotic | Intercalates into DNA strands |

occurred. When applied at this late date, chemotherapy usually does not contribute to meaningful increases in useful life span. It is hoped that the adjunctive use of drugs with surgery or radiotherapy, or a combination of the two, would improve future survival statistics. The earlier use of drugs in healthier subjects would also allow greater host tolerance to the side effects of chemotherapy.

## METHOTREXATE

Methotrexate (MTX) is perhaps the most effective single agent and has been most widely used in the treatment of advanced recurrent epidermoid carcinoma of the head and neck.[6] Its main mechanism of action is as an inhibitor of folic acid metabolism by inhibiting the folate-reducing enzyme, dihydrofolate reductase, which effectively removes the folate coenzymes from some very important steps in pyrimidine, purine and amino acid biosynthesis. Its cytotoxic effect on tumor and normal cells is generally believed to be the consequence of inhibition of DNA synthesis.[7] Leucovorin (Leucovorin; 5-formyl-5, 6, 7, 8-tetrahydrofolic acid; folinic acid; citrovorum factor) effectively bypasses this metabolic blockade and supplies the cells with the reduced folates necessary for these biochemical processes (Fig. 22–1). Leucovorin may effectively reduce or abolish the toxic effects of MTX if it is administered within 24 to 42 hours of MTX.[13, 43] This delayed administration of leucovorin optimizes the MTX effect by selectively rescuing the normal cells to a greater degree. The concomitant administration of leucovorin with MTX would effectively abolish the therapeutic as well as toxic effects of MTX.[27] Leucovorin is commercially available as a parenteral injection. This form can also be given orally if mixed in a suitable vehicle, such as juice or carbonated beverages. The usual dosage is 10 to 15 mg. per $M^2$ repeated at six-hour intervals. The frequency and duration of therapy with this antidote depends on the dose and blood level of MTX.

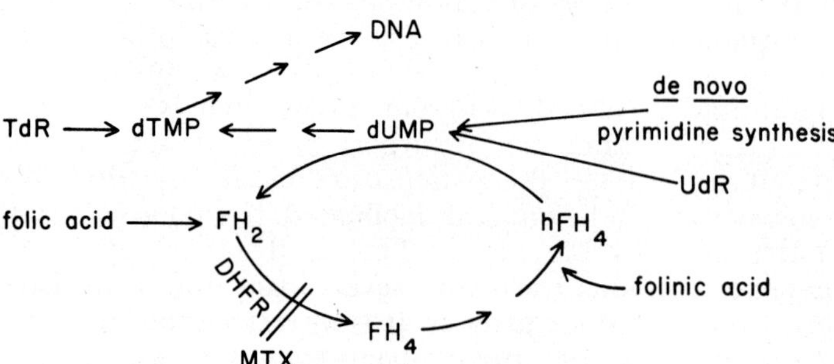


**Figure 22–1** Locus of action of MTX. $FH_2$ = dihydrofolate; DHFR = dihydrofolate reductase; $FH_4$ = tetrahydrofolate; UdR = deoxyuridine; dUMP = deoxyuridine monophosphate; dTMP = deoxythymidine monophosphate; TdR = deoxythymidine.

The largest percentage of an adminstered dose of MTX is excreted essentially unchanged in the urine. Because of this, renal function must be assessed prior to the initiation of therapy with MTX. This is most adequately assessed by the determination of the endogenous creatinine clearance; a reduction of the glomerular filtration rate should most appropriately be associated with a reduction in the dose of MTX or perhaps serve as a contraindication to its use. If the drug is intended to be used in a patient with compromised renal function, this should only be done where appropriate facilities exist for monitoring the blood levels of the drug so that the appropriate dose and frequency of leucovorin can be employed. The very high doses (gm./$M^2$) of MTX currently being employed in some medical centers may be associated with MTX-induced nephrotoxicity (vida infra), which in and of itself may delay the excretion of MTX and result in unexpected toxicity.

The dose of MTX most frequently employed in patients with recurrent epidermoid carcinoma of the head and neck is a weekly injection (I.M. or I.V.) of 40 to 50 per mg. per $M^2$. This is the usual starting dose for patients with normal renal function and may be scaled upward or downward depending on patient tolerance. In general, approximately one third of the patients will sustain a partial response; complete responses are infrequent.[6] The use of larger doses as a 24-hour infusion followed by leucovorin rescue has improved the response rate,[13] but this method of administration has a major drawback — the requirement of hospitalization — whereas with rapid intravenous injections, treatment can be carried out on an outpatient basis.

Normal organ toxic effects of MTX are dose- and schedule-dependent. Daily oral low doses of MTX (e.g., 5 mg. daily) are therapeutically the least effective method of drug administration and result in a high frequency of bone marrow suppression and oral and gastrointestinal ulceration. This method of drug use is not recommended. The smaller weekly parenteral doses, e.g., 30 to 40 per mg. $M^2$, are associated with minimal to no anorexia, nausea and vomiting. The incidence of this and other complications increases with the dose. Oral toxicity ranging from erythema and a burning sensation to isolated, white, painful patches to frank hemorrhagic necrosis is one of the most distressing problems that the patient may have to contend with. It usually begins three to four days after drug administration and reaches its peak 7 to 10 days later. The presence of isolated white patches one week after MTX administration should dictate a waiting period of another seven days. History of oral burning sensation, especially with the use of mint-flavored tooth pastes, or presence of moderate oral erythema is not an absolute contradiction to the administration of another injection of MTX but rather warrants attention to the dose. The frequency and intensity of mucositis may be increased in those patients with severe xerostomia secondary to extensive radiotherapy. It is also enhanced by the folate deficiency that most patients with advanced head and neck cancer are experiencing when MTX treatment is initiated. At times, mucositis can be so severe as to preclude any oral alimentation, thus necessitating hospitalization. With proper attention to dosage, renal function and hydration, this severe complication should rarely occur. The use of topical viscous lidocaine (Xylocaine) is of some help in alleviating the discomfort of mucositis. Oral ulceration may predispose the patient to the development of oral candidiasis; this should be looked for and appropriately treated. At times, mucositis may not be very evident in the oral mucosa, but the patient may complain of sore throat or the pain of esophagitis, which can be relieved by oxethazaine (Oxaine).

The frequency of ulceration of the mucosa of the gastrointestinal (GI) tract is fortunately much lower than oral mucositis. Moderate GI intoxication may be evidenced by frequent bowel movements or diarrhea. Severe toxicity may be manifested by a sloughing of the intestinal mucosa and a hemorrhagic enteritis. The rapid (i.e., less than one hour) infusion of large doses (i.e., larger than one gm./$M^2$) may be associated with cramping abdominal pain; this is avoided by extending the duration of infusion to two to three hours.

Oral mucositis frequently heralds the appearance of bone marrow suppression. After a single dose of MTX, marrow suppression usually reaches its nadir 7 to 10 days later, with full recovery within two to three weeks. The white cell precursors appear to be more sensitive to MTX than the erythroid precursors or megakaryocytes. Bone marrow examination after MTX treatment may reveal megaloblastoid features due to the drug-induced folate deficiency. All degrees of hematologic suppression may occur, ranging from mild leukopenia and thrombocytopenia to severe bone marrow hypoplasia predisposing the patient to severe infection or hemorrhage or both. These life-threatening complications can be treated with the appropriate use of antibiotics and blood component therapy (platelet and white cell transfusions).

It is well known that MTX is a potent immunosuppressive agent in animals and humans,[3] and it is well established that head and neck cancer patients are significantly immunosuppressed at the time of diagnosis.[24, 44] At the time at which chemotherapeutic management is usually entertained, the tumor burden is greater, nutritional status is poorer and weight loss has been excessive, all of which may accentuate the immune deficiency. The administration of an immunosuppressive agent to such a patient would not be the intended therapeutic plan. Most of the therapeutically effective drugs are significantly immunosuppressive, however, as noted in Table 22–2. The immunosuppressive potential of a combination of these drugs would be expected to be greater. Systematic studies in this regard re-

**TABLE 22–2** TOXIC REACTIONS TO DRUGS EFFECTIVE IN HEAD AND NECK CANCER

| Reaction | Drug |
|---|---|
| **I. Immediate** | |
| 1. Fever | Bleomycin |
| 2. Anorexia, nausea and vomiting | Methotrexate, 5-FU, nitrogen mustard, hydroxyurea, cyclophosphamide, procarbazine, doxorubicin, bleomycin |
| 3. Phlebitis; tissue necrosis if extravasates | Nitrogen mustard, doxorubicin, vinblastine, vincristine |
| **II. Early—Acute (i.e., within 1–14 days)** | |
| 1. Renal impairment | Methotrexate |
| 2. Oral and gastrointestinal ulceration | Methotrexate, 5-FU, bleomycin, doxorubicin |
| 3. Immunosuppression | Methotrexate, 5-FU, 6-MP, nitrogen mustard, cyclophosphamide, chlorambucil, procarbazine, doxorubicin |
| 4. Bone marrow suppression | Methotrexate, 5-FU, 6-MP, hydroxyurea, nitrogen mustard, cyclophosphamide, chlorambucil, procarbazine, vinblastine, doxorubicin |
| 5. Abnormal liver function | Methotrexate |
| 6. Syndrome of inappropriate ADH | Cyclosphosphamide, vincristine |
| 7. Skin rash | Methotrexate, 5-FU |
| 8. Constipation, paralytic ileus | Vinblastine, vincristine |
| 9. Disulfiram (Antabuse) effect after alcohol ingestion | Procarbazine |
| 10. Radiation recall | Doxorubicin, 5-FU, bleomycin |
| **III. Late—Acute (i.e., 2–4 weeks)** | |
| 1. Alopecia | Methotrexate, 5-FU, nitrogen mustard, cyclophosphamide, vincristine, vinblastine, bleomycin, doxorubicin |
| 2. Peripheral neuropathy | Vincristine |
| **IV. Early—Chronic (i.e., months to years)** | |
| 1. Hepatic cirrhosis | Methotrexate, 6-MP |
| 2. Hypersensitivity pneumonitis | Methotrexate |
| 3. Pulmonary fibrosis | Bleomycin |
| 4. Skin pigmentation and ulceration | Bleomycin |
| 5. Cardiomyopathy | Doxorubicin |
| 6. Sterility | Methotrexate, 5-FU, 6-MP, nitrogen mustard, CTX, chlorambucil, procarbazine |
| **V. Late—Chronic (i.e., years)** | |
| 1. Secondary neoplasms | Nitrogen mustard, cyclophosphamide, chlorambucil, procarbazine, doxorubicin |

main to be done, however. This significant complication might be reversed by the judicious use of immune adjuvants. Nevertheless, the choice, dose, scheduling and efficacy of such adjuvants are still in the research stages.

With the use of weekly doses of MTX, i.e., 40 to 50 or 200 to 500 mg. per $M^2$, with leucovorin rescue, skin toxicity in the form of a maculopapular eruption may occur in 10 to 20 per cent of patients. Biopsy of some of these lesions has shown a vasculitis.[13] A rare patient must sustain severe skin toxicity manifested as toxic epidermal necrolysis with a total sloughing of the skin. This complication usually accompanies very severe oral, gastrointestinal and bone marrow toxicity; fortunately this is seen very rarely.

MTX is a known hepatotoxin. Biochemical hepatic dysfunction occurs infrequently with low doses (30 to 60 mg./$M^2$)[42] and much more frequently with the very large doses (2 to 20 gm./$M^2$) employed in newer protocols.[33, 54, 56] The abnormal liver function tests do return to normal within a month. Biopsy of the liver while the liver function tests are abnormal has revealed focal necrosis and portal inflammatory reactions.[29] Long-term methotrexate therapy has been associated with cirrhosis.[67] Since most patients with head and neck cancer have a history of excessive alcoholic intake, the hepatotoxicity of MTX coupled with the hepatic effects of ethanol should be kept in mind.

Impairment in renal function is hardly ever observed with the small, weekly doses of MTX. The 2 to 10 gm. per $M^2$ doses, however, may cause a transient rise in BUN and serum creatinine or produce frank renal failure.[33] This nephrotoxic effect has been attributed to MTX crystalluria. (MTX is a weak organic acid that can precipitate in acid solutions such as urine.) This problem may be averted with proper hydration and alkalinization of the urine by the systemic administration of sodium bicarbonate.[53]

MTX may produce pulmonary toxicity that is more an idiosyncratic reaction than a dose-related toxic effect. The clinical manifestations include dyspnea, dry cough and fever. Acute nonspecific infiltrates are seen on the chest x-ray; most cases demonstrate linear and reticulonodular infiltrates predominately at the bases and mid-lung zones. Arterial blood gases usually reveal hypoxemia and hypocapnia, and pulmonary function tests may reveal a diminished diffusing capacity for carbon monoxide as well as a restrictive ventilatory defect. Biopsy of the lesions reveals nodules of noncaseating granulomas composed of plasma cells, lymphocytes and histiocytes in varying proportions with focal interstitial fibrosis. Cessation of therapy is associated with improvement in symptoms and roentgenographic abnormalities, usually within a month's time. There are reports of recovery even though the MTX was continued. Steroids do not appear to appreciably hasten the recovery. Rechallenge with MTX after the acute process has resolved has not produced a recrudescence of signs or symptoms.[61] A rare patient may have signs of panmesotheliitis, with pleuritis, peritonitis and pericarditis. This is also self-limiting and is not necessarily associated with other signs of toxicity. The extent and rapidity of alopecia is a function of dose and is uncommonly seen with the low-dose, weekly regimens.

## 5-FLUOROURACIL (5-FU)

Mediation of the toxic and therapeutic effects of 5-FU is believed to be the result of the irreversible inhibition of the enzyme thymidylate synthetase by a metabolite of 5-FU — 5-fluorodeoxyuridylic acid.[18] 5-FU is also catabolized to several metabolites; this catabolism occurs in many organs, most notably the liver. Thus, patients who have extensive replacement of hepatic parenchyma by tumor and abnormal liver function tests should receive an attenuated dose because of delayed catabolism.[51]

The initial clinical reports of 5-fluorouracil described daily injections of 15 mg. per kg. for 5 days followed by half dosage every other day until evidence of drug toxicity.[20] The full spectrum of 5-FU toxicity was seen with this regimen. The intravenous injection of the drug may be associated with a metallic taste and a generalized sensation of warmth. Anorexia and nausea with minimal vomiting may occur in the first week. This can usually be alleviated with antiemetics. During the first week, oral mucositis and diarrhea may also occur. The diarrhea is a reflection of gastrointestinal mucosal toxicity and should serve as an indication for stopping the drug, since GI toxicity can advance to severe sloughing of the intestinal mucosa. Manifestations of bone marrow suppression are seen in the second week as leukopenia and thrombocytopenia. Continued therapy under these circumstances can lead to drug-related deaths as a result of severe intestinal toxicity, infection and bleeding. This potentially lethal drug toxicity is clearly dose- and schedule-related. The five-day course of therapy is the most toxic. Since equivalent antitumor responses have been achieved with the weekly injection of 15 mg. per kg., this regimen is to be recommended. The weekly schedule allows better manipulation of dose, based on very early signs of drug toxicity, such as minimal mucositis or hematologic suppression.[30] It has been suggested that mild to moderate toxicity (chiefly bone marrow suppression) is necessary in order to achieve an antitumor effect.[51]

Uncommon nonlethal drug toxicity affects the skin with diffuse erythema, scaling, desquamation or bullous formation and alopecia.[37] Other less common toxicity is epistaxis unrelated to thrombocytopenia[1] and cerebellar ataxia.[51]

## 6-MERCAPTOPURINE (6-MP)

The precise mechanism of action of 6-MP is not fully understood; however, it does interfere with purine biosynthesis. The average dose is 2.5 mg. per kg. given as a single daily oral dose. The major dose limiting toxicity is bone marrow suppression, which usually occurs after weeks of treatment. This usually develops gradually, and the bone marrow usually recovers uneventfully within two to three weeks. The only other major toxicity of 6-MP is its effect on the liver. Both hepatocellular necrosis and intrahepatic cholestasis have been reported. These toxicities usually improve upon cessation of drug.[16, 47, 60]

## HYDROXYUREA

The chief mechanism of action of hydroxyurea is inhibition of the enzyme ribonucleotide reductase, an enzyme necessary in the conversion of ribonucleotides to the deoxyribonucleotide form utilized in DNA synthesis. The drug is usually given orally at a dose of 30 to 40 mg. per kg. per day in two to three divided doses. The acute toxicity may cause nausea and vomiting, which is well controlled with antiemetics. The toxicity of major concern is hematologic suppression, which usually recovers quickly upon cessation of therapy.[25, 64]

## NITROGEN MUSTARD

Nitrogen mustard's cytotoxic action is mediated by cross-linking DNA strands, thus inhibiting DNA replication. The drug is highly reactive in aqueous solution and consequently must be used immediately upon solubilization. It is given as a rapid intravenous injection, preferably through a running I.V. The usual dose is 0.4 mg. per kg. once every three to four weeks. It may cause an immediate toxic reaction with pain at the injection site and possible subsequent phlebitis and venous thrombosis. If the drug extravasates into subcutaneous tissues, it may produce a tissue slough. These reactions can be minimized if the drug is given through a free-flowing, rapidly running I.V. Nausea and vomiting begin in most patients within one to eight hours and usually last several hours. This effect is only minimally attenuated by antiemetics. It may be considerably lessened by giving the drug at bedtime after the combined use of antiemetics and heavy sedation so that the patient sleeps through the night. Hematologic suppression is dose-related and invariably occurs with the usual therapeutic dose (0.4 mg./kg.). Leukopenia and thrombocytopenia usually occur within 7 to 10 days, with complete marrow recovery within the next one to two weeks.[21, 36] The drug is immunosuppressive[28] and carcinogenic in animal species,[21] and thus the potential exists for secondary neoplasms occurring years after drug administration.

## CYCLOPHOSPHAMIDE (CTX)

CTX is an alkylating agent that is inactive in its native form and is activated in the liver by the mixed-function oxidase system of the smooth endoplasmic reticulum.[10] It is given in an oral dose of 100 to 200 mg. daily or as a single, large intravenous dose at 1 to 2 gm. per $M^2$ given once every three to four weeks. With the daily oral doses, minimal anorexia and occasional nausea and vomiting are seen. Anorexia and nausea with some vomiting occur with the larger, intermittent, intravenous therapy. This can be controlled to some degree with antiemetics and may be better controlled when the drug is given at bedtime after the combined use of antiemetics and sedatives. Unlike the parent alkylating agent, nitrogen mustard, the drug does not irritate the veins and does not cause thrombophlebitis.

CTX is extensively metabolized and the metabolites are predominantly excreted in the urine. A sterile cystitis may appear within a few days following the large intravenous dose or after several weeks to months of oral therapy. This is due to the irritative effect of the drug's metabolites on the bladder mucosa.[2,22,48] The patient may complain of a burning on urination, along with urgency, frequency and hematuria. Characteristically, the urine is sterile on culture, and cystoscopy reveals a hyperemic edematous bladder with multiple hemorrhagic areas. The cystitis usually subsides in four to five days after stopping the drug; rarely, it may persist for several months and may become secondarily infected. This unpleasant side effect may be obviated by sufficient oral or intravenous hydration, insuring a copious urine flow. Occasionally, this irritative phenomenon may progress to a severe hemorrhagic cystitis. This is usually self-limiting but has occasionally resulted in death.[4,32,39] The chronic effects of CTX on the bladder mucosa have been noted in an autopsy series of patients with leukemia. The long-term administration of CTX in this series was associated with a 25 per cent incidence of transmural fibrosis and submucosal telangiectasia.[35] Several cases of carcinoma of the bladder have been reported in patients with CTX cystitis.[65,68]

Alopecia is fairly common and begins to occur within the third week. The extent of the epilation is roughly proportional to the dose. Hematologic suppression is also dose-related, and the drug has a greater propensity for leukopenia than thrombocytopenia, although platelet suppression may be severe with the very large intermittent doses.[12,31]

Very large intravenous doses (50 mg./kg.) have been associated with a transient syndrome of inappropriate secretion of antidiuretic hormone.[22] This phenomenon has been autocorrectable within a few days. Cyclophosphamide is significantly immunosuppressive.[58]

## CHLORAMBUCIL

Chlorambucil is an alkylating agent that is effective orally. It is usually administered daily at a dose of 6 to 10 mg. in divided dosage. Its major toxicity is bone marrow suppression from which recovery rapidly occurs upon cessation of therapy,[48,57]

## PROCARBAZINE

The exact mechanism of action of procarbazine has not been clearly defined. Decreased synthesis of DNA, RNA and protein has been noted,[38] as well as intracellular formation of hydrogen peroxide with resultant oxidative damage to DNA.[5] The drug is administered orally at a dose of 200 to 300 mg. per day. Although initial nausea and vomiting may occur, this effect can be minimized by reduction in dosage, after which one may escalate to full dosage within one to two weeks. Antiemetics are of some help also. Hematologic suppression occurs and is dose-related. Since the drug is administered as a daily oral dose, the hematologic suppression may not be evident until a month has gone by. Stopping the drug enables full bone marrow recovery. Minimum to moderate alopecia and a mild maculopapular skin eruption have been reported. Central nervous system depression ranging from mild drowsiness to profound stupor has occurred as well as paresthesias of the extremities.[11,46,62] Procarbazine has produced a disulfiram (Antabuse)-like effect when patients have taken alcoholic beverages while on therapy,[46] a problem of some concern in patients with head and neck cancer.

## VINBLASTINE

Vinblastine is an alkaloid derived from the periwinkle plant, *Vinca rosea* Linn. Its cytotoxic effect is probably mediated through disruption of the mitotic spindle with a consequent metaphase arrest. It is given intravenously at a dose of 4 to 6 mg. per $M^2$ per week. Its major toxicity is pain at the injection site and chemical cellulitis if the drug extravasates. Mild nausea and vomiting rarely occur and stomatitis is not usually prominent. Its major toxicity consists of dose-related hematologic suppression, with full recovery within one to two weeks upon cessation of the drug.[69]

## VINCRISTINE

Vincristine is another plant alkaloid derived from the same source as vinblastine. Although it is structurally similar to vinblastine and probably has the same mechanism of action, the toxicity and therapeutic spectrum are different. At the usual dose of 1.4 mg. per $M^2$ given weekly, the predominant side effect is toxicity to the peripheral nervous system. Deep tendon reflexes are diminished or abolished almost routinely. Paresthesias in the fingers and toes are an indication for reduction in dosage and, if severe, an indication for temporary withdrawal of therapy, since the continued use of the drug under these circumstances produces foot or wrist drop, or both. Other neurotoxic manifestations are cranial nerve malfunction and constipation. While on therapy, patients should be advised to take stool softeners or mild laxatives. Large doses or continued therapy in the presence of moderate constipation may lead to a paralytic ileus. Return of gastrointestinal function may take weeks, and improvement in peripheral nervous system toxicity may take months. Alopecia is common. Significant bone marrow suppression is rare.[14, 59]

## BLEOMYCIN

Bleomycin is composed of a mixture of sulfur-containing polypeptide antibiotics isolated from *Streptomyces verticillus*. It inhibits DNA synthesis and produces single-strand breaks in DNA. Most reported studies have used bleomycin at a dose of 15 mg. per $M^2$ given intravenously or intramuscularly twice a week. Responses of greater than 50 per cent shrinkage of tumor occur in approximately 15 to 20 per cent of patients, and the duration of response is disappointingly short. The drug is well tolerated when given either intravenously or intramuscularly; only a rare patient has complained of pain at the injection site. Fifteen to 50 per cent of patients have had drug-induced fever occur within one-half to three hours of drug administration lasting one-half to eight hours. Fevers of 100 to 103° F. were common following the first dose, subsided spontaneously and were less common with subsequent doses. Four cases of severe hyperpyrexia, hypotension and cardiorespiratory collapse and death have been reported. All four of the patients had lymphoma, were not septic and had received high single doses (25 to 40 mg./$M^2$) of bleomycin.

Minimal anorexia and mild nausea and occasional vomiting have been noted in 10 to 15 per cent of patients. These complaints were most common with the initial injections and were self-limiting. Minimal to no hematologic suppression is produced, and, if it occurs, it is transient with full recovery despite continued therapy.

Alopecia has been reported in 10 to 40 per cent of patients, beginning approximately three weeks after initiation of treatment. Oral mucositis occurs in 20 to 40 per cent of the patients, first appearing in seven to nine days as pain and erythema and followed within two to three days by shallow necrotic ulceration. This propensity for mucositis is enhanced when bleomycin is given in combination with other drugs sharing in this toxicity.

Bleomycin is concentrated in skin and pulmonary tissue, and, consequently, these two organs show the most serious signs of bleomycin toxicity. The toxic effect on these organs is related to the cumulative dose. The skin lesions characteristically begin as erythema over pressure areas, such as elbows, fingertips, feet and so on, and then progress to painful ulceration. Hyperpigmented striae of the trunk are common.

Dose-related pulmonary toxicity, at times fatal, has been reported. Because of this, the drug should be avoided in patients with impaired pulmonary function, a problem to keep in mind for patients with head and neck cancer due to the high incidence of excessive cigarette smoking. Although pulmonary toxicity can occur with lower doses, it is more frequent with total doses in excess of 300 mg. The patients initially complain of dyspnea, tachypnea, and nonproductive cough and fine rales may be heard on auscultation. Chest radiographs are nonspecific, the most common finding being diffuse interstitial fibrosis. Pulmonary function tests (PFT's) should be obtained before starting therapy, especially in patients with a history of pulmonary disease or heavy smoking. The PFT's can be repeated serially, especially when the total dose is approaching 300 mg. The most consistent bleomycin-induced abnormalities have been a decrease in vital capacity and diffusion capacity. The microscopic changes that have been described include bronchiolar squamous metaplasia, proliferation of reactive macrophages, atypical alveolar epithelial cells, fibrinous edema and interstitial fibrosis. Steroids have not been of any value in reversing or attenuating bleomycin-induced pulmonary toxicity.[8, 52, 70]

## DOXORUBICIN (ADRIAMYCIN)

Doxorubicin is an anthracycline antibiotic derived from *Streptomyces peucetius* var. *caesius*. Its main mechanism of action is as an intercalator between the nucleotide bases of DNA. It has a wide spectrum of antineoplastic activity and is usually given as a single intravenous injection of 60 mg. per $M^2$ every three weeks. The drug should be given through a running I.V. since it has strong irritative properties for the veins. Care should be taken to avoid extravasation because of the strong vesicant properties of the drug that result in a slowly healing chemical cellulitis. Nausea and vomiting occur within hours of drug administration and can usually be attenuated with antiemetics. Oral mucosal ulceration and bone marrow suppression occur between the first and second week and last for 7 to 10 days. Alopecia begins to occur between the third and fourth week.[49, 63, 66]

Of major concern is the potential cardiac toxicity of doxorubicin. A number of transient EKG abnormalities are seen at various cumulative dosages and consist of sinus tachycardia, ST segment depression, T wave flattening and occasional premature ventricular contractions. These have been observed during or shortly after intravenous administration and in the course of chronic treatment. Discontinuation of treatment has resulted in a return to normal EKG. These reversible abnormalities do not necessarily predict the more serious cardiac complication — intractable congestive heart failure — which is the result of a diffuse cardiomyopathy. The electrocardiogram of these patients shows diffuse low voltage, and autopsy examination of the heart reveals decrease in the number of cardiac muscle cells, degeneration of the remaining myocardial cells, loss of contractile substance, mitochondrial swelling and intramitochrondrial dense inclusion bodies. The occurrence of this lethal cardiac toxicity is dose-related and is seldom seen at cumulative doses less than 500 mg. per $M^2$, although cardiac toxicity may occur at lower doses, especially in patients with antecedent heart disease or who may have had mediastinal irradiation.[40, 41, 50] Serial measurements of the systolic time interval have been suggested as a way of diagnosing early doxorubicin-induced cardiac toxicity;[55] however, the utility of this approach has been questioned.[50] Doxorubicin has been shown to induce a radiation recall reaction in previously irradiated tissues, producing enhanced skin reactions, mucositis, pneumonitis and possibly enhanced cardiac toxicity.[15, 23]

## REGIONAL INFUSION

Several agents, most notably MTX and 5-FU, have been infused through the catheter placement in the arterial supply of a tumor. This approach is attractive from a theoretic point of view, in that relatively higher concentrations of the drug would be delivered to the tumor that would then be diluted in the systemic circulation. Further advantages might accrue if the drug is rapidly excreted or metabolized to inactive byproducts. This would ideally result in a greater tumor destruction with relatively less patient toxicity. Despite the fact that some studies indicate that this method of drug delivery produces superior results compared to the usual systemic route, the exper-

**TABLE 22–3** COMPLICATIONS UNIQUE TO INTRA-ARTERIAL INFUSION OF DRUGS IN HEAD AND NECK CANCER PATIENTS

| |
|---|
| Catheter displacement and leakage |
| Localized severe stomatitis |
| Local edema |
| Hemorrhage |
| Slough |
| Cerebrovascular accident |

tise required of the physician, the inconvenience of hospitalization for the patient and the complications unique to the procedure (Table 22–3) significantly reduce the benefit to risk ratio, making this an unpopular method of treatment.

The complications detailed on the preceding pages are the effects of single drugs on normal organs. There is, however, significant precedence for using combinations of drugs. Various combinations have produced superior results over single agents in advanced neoplastic disease, such as acute lymphoblastic leukemia of childhood, Hodgkin's disease, diffuse histiocytic lymphoma and several others. As a result of this, the possibilities for combining drugs are now being explored in patients with head and neck cancer. These regimens would be expected to have not only an additive effect for the individual agents on an organ but also a synergistic effect as a result of drug–drug interactions. An understanding of the basis for these combinations and the pharmacologic interaction of drugs would be of help to the physician caring for the patient.

## Bibliography


1. Ansfield, F. J., Schroeder, J. M., and Curreri, A. R.: Five years clinical experience with 5-fluorouracil. J. A. M. A., *181*:295–299, 1962.
2. Bagley, C. M., Bostick, F. W., and DeVita, V. T.: Clinical pharmacology of cyclophosphamide. Cancer Res., *33*:226–233, 1973.
3. Berenbaum, M. C., and Brown, I. N.: Dose-response relationships for agents inhibiting the immune response. Immunology, 7:65–71, 1964.
4. Berkson, B. M., Lome, L. G., and Shapiro, I.: Severe cystitis induced by cyclophosphamide. J. A. M. A., *225*:605–606, 1973.
5. Bernies, K., Kofler, M., Bollag, W., et al.: The degradation of DNA by new tumor inhibiting compounds: The intermediate formation of hydrogen peroxide. Experientia, *19*:132, 1963.
6. Bertino, J. R., Boston, B., and Capizzi, R. L.: The role of chemotherapy in the management of cancer of the head and neck: A review. Cancer, *36*:752–758, 1975.
7. Bertino, J. R.: The mechanism of action of the folate antagonists in man. Cancer Res., *23*: 1286–1306, 1963.
8. Blum, R. H., Carter, S. K., and Agre, K.: A clinical review of bleomycin — a new antineoplastic agent. Cancer, *31*:903–914, 1973.
9. Bonnadonna, G., Brusamolino, E., Valagussa, P., et al.: Combination chemotherapy as an adjuvant treatment in operable breast cancer. N. Engl. J. Med., *294*:405–410, 1976.
10. Brock, N.: Pharmacologic characterization of cyclophosphamide and cyclophosphamide metabolites. Cancer Chemother. Rep., *51*:315–325, 1967.
11. Brunner, K. W., and Young, C. W.: A methyldydrazine derivative in Hodgkin's Disease and other malignant neoplasms. Ann. Intern. Med., *63*:69–86, 1965.
12. Buckner, C. C., Clift, R. A., Fefer, A., et al.: High dose cyclophosphamide for the treatment of metastatic testicular neoplasms. Cancer Chemother. Rep., *58*:709–714, 1974.
13. Capizzi, R. L., DeConti, R. C., Marsh, J. C., et al.: Methotrexate therapy of head and neck cancer: Improvement in therapeutic index by use of leucovorin rescue. Cancer Res., *30*:1782–1788, 1970.
14. Carey, R. W., Hall, T. C., and Finkel, H. E.: A comparison of two dosage regimens for vincristine. Cancer Chemother. Rep., *27*:91–96, 1963.
15. Cassady, J. R., Richter, M. P., Piro, A. J., et al.: Radiation–adriamycin interactions: Preliminary clinical observations. Cancer, *36*:946–949, 1975.
16. Clark, P. A., Hsia, Y. E., and Huntsman, R. G.: Toxic complications of treatment with 6-mercaptopurine. Br. Med. J., *1*:393–395, 1960.
17. Coggins, P. R., Ravdin, R. G., and Eisman, S. H.: Clinical evaluation of a new alkylating agent: Cytoxan (cyclophosphamide). Cancer, *3*:1254–1260, 1960.
18. Cohen, S. S., Flaks, J. G., Barner, H. D., et al.: Mode of action of 5-fluorouracil and its derivatives. Proc. Nat. Acad. Sci. U.S.A., *44*:1004, 1958.
19. Cortes, E. P., Holland, J. F., Wang, J. J., et al.: Amputation and adriamycin in primary osteosarcoma. N. Engl. J. Med., *291*:998–1000, 1974.
20. Curreri, A. R., Ansfield, F. J., McIver, F. A., et al.: Clinical studies with 5-fluorouracil. Cancer Res., *18*:478, 1958.
21. Dameshek, W., Weisfuse, L., and Stein, T.: Nitrogen mustard therapy in Hodgkin's Disease. Blood, *4*:338–379, 1949.
22. DeFronzo, R. A., Braine, H., Colvin, M., et al.: Water intoxication in man after cyclophosphamide therapy. Ann. Intern. Med., *78*:861–869, 1973.
23. Donaldson, S. S., Glick, J. M., and Wilbur, J. R.: Adriamycin activating a recall phenomenon

after radiation therapy. Ann. Intern. Med., *81*:407–408, 1974.

24. Eilber, F. R., Morton, D. R., and Ketcham, A. S.: Immunologic abnormalities in head and neck cancer. Am. J. Surg., *128*:534, 1974.
25. Fishbein, W. N., Carbone, P. P., Freireich, E. J., et al.: Clinical treatment of hydroxyurea in patients with cancer and leukemia. Clin. Pharmacol. Ther., *5*:574–580, 1964.
26. Fisher, B., Carbone, P., Economou, S. G., et al.: L-phenylalanine mustard (L-PAM) in the management of primary breast cancer. Report of early findings. N. Engl. J. Med., *292*:117–122, 1975.
27. Goldin, A., Venditti, J. M., Kline, I., et al.: Eradication of leukemic cells (L1210) by methotrexate and methotrexate plus citrovorum factor. Nature, *212*:1548, 1966.
28. Green, D. M.: The effects of nitrogen mustard [methyl bis (B-chloroethyl) amine HCL] on the immunological responses of the rabbit. I. The effects of nitrogen mustard on the preliminary response to bacterial antigen. Br. J. Exp. Pathol., *39*:192–198, 1958.
29. Hersh, E. M., Wong, V. G., Henderson, E. S., et al.: Hepatotoxic effects of methotrexate. Cancer, *19*:600–606, 1966.
30. Horton, J., Olson, K. B., Sullivan, J., et al.: 5-Fluorouracil in cancer: An improved regimen. Ann. Intern. Med. *73*:897–900, 1970.
31. Host, H., and Nessen-Meyer, R.: A preliminary clinical study of cyclophosphamide. Cancer Chemother. Rep., *9*:47–50, 1960.
32. Hutter, A. M., Bauman, A. W., and Frank, I. N.: Cyclophosphamide and severe hemorrhagic cystitis. N. Y. State J. Med., *69*:305–309, 1969.
33. Jaffe, N.: Recent advances in the chemotherapy of metastatic osteogenic sarcoma. Cancer, *30*:1627–1631, 1972.
34. Jaffe, N., Frei, E., Traggis, D., et al.: Adjuvant methotrexate and citrovorum factor treatment of osteogenic sarcoma. N. Engl. J. Med., *291*:994–997, 1974.
35. Johnson, W. W., and Meadows, D. C.: Urinary bladder fibrosis and telangiectasia associated with long term cyclophosphamide therapy. N. Engl. J. Med., *284*:290–294, 1971.
36. Karnofsy, D. A.: Nitrogen mustards in the treatment of neoplastic disease. Adv. Intern. Med., *4*:1–77, 1958.
37. Kennedy, B. J., and Theologides, A.: The role of 5-fluorouracil in malignant disease. Ann. Intern. Med., *55*:719–730, 1961.
38. Kreis, W.: Studies on the mechanism and reaction mechanism of methylhydrazine derivative in BDF, P815-leukemic mice. Proc. Am. Assoc. Cancer Res., 7:39, 1966.
39. Lawrence, H. J., Simone, J., and Aur, J. A.: Cyclophosphamide-induced hemorrhagic cystitis in children with leukemia. Cancer, *36*:1572–1576, 1975.
40. Lefrak, E. A., Pitha, J., Rosenheim, S., et al.: Adriamycin cardiomyopathy. Cancer Chemother. Rep., *6*:203–208, 1975.
41. Lefrak, E. A., Pitha, J., Rosenheim, S., et al.: A clinicopathologic analysis of adriamycin cardiotoxicity. Cancer, *32*:302–314, 1973.
42. Leone, L. A., Albala, M. M., and Rege, V. B.: Treatment and carcinoma of the head and neck with intravenous methotrexate. Cancer, *21*:828–837, 1968.
43. Levitt, M., Mosher, M. B., DeConti, R. C., et al.: Improved therapeutic index of methotrexate with leucovorin rescue. Cancer Res., *13*:1729–1734, 1973.
44. Lundy, J., Wanebo, H., Pinsky, C., et al.: Delayed hypersensitivity reactions in patients with squamous cell cancer of the head and neck. Am. J. Surg., *128*:530–533, 1974.
45. Masterson, J. G., Calame, R. J., and Nelson, J.: A clinical study on the use of chlorambucil in the treatment of cancer of the ovary. Am. J. Obstet. Gynecol., *79*:1002–1007, 1960.
46. Mathe, G., Schweisguth, O., Schneider, M., et al.: Methyl-hydrazine in treatment of Hodgkin's Disease. Lancet, *2*:1077–1080, 1963.
47. McIlvanie, S. K., and MacCarthy, J. D.: Hepatitis in association with prolonged 6-mercaptopurine therapy. Blood, *14*:80–90, 1959.
48. Melner, A. N., and Sullivan, M. P.: Urinary excretion of cyclophosphamide and its metabolites: Evidence for the existence of an active cyclic metabolite. Cancer Chemother. Rep., *51*:343–345, 1967.
49. Middleman, E., Luce, J., and Frei, E.: Clinical trials with adriamycin. Cancer, *28*:844–850, 1971.
50. Minow, R. A., Benjamin, R. S., and Gottlieb, J. A.: Adriamycin cardiomyopathy — an overview with determination of risk factors. Cancer Chemother. Rep., *6*:195–201, 1975.
51. Moertel, C. G., Reitemeier, R. J., and Hahn, R. G.: Fluorinated pyrimidine therapy of advanced gastro-intestinal cancer. Gastroenterology, *46*:371–378, 1964.
52. Pascual, R. S., Mosher, M. B., Sikand, R. S., et al.: Effects of bleomycin on pulmonary function in man. Am. Rev. Resp. Dis., *108*:211–217, 1973.
53. Pittman, S. W., Parker, L. M., Tattersall, M. H. N., et al.: Clinical trial of high dose methotrexate with citrovorum factor — toxicologic and therapeutic observations. Cancer Chemother. Rep., *6*:43–49, 1975.
54. Pratt, C. B., Roberts, D., Shanks, E. C., et al.: Chemical trials and pharmacokinetics of intermittent high dose methotrexate–leucovorin rescue for children with malignant tumors. Cancer Res., *34*:3326–3331, 1974.
55. Rinehart, J. J., Lewis, R. P., and Balcerzak, S. P.: Adriamycin cardiotoxicity in man. Ann. Intern. Med., *81*:475–478, 1974.
56. Rosen, G., Suwansirikul, S., Kwon, C., et al.: High dose methotrexate with citrovorum factor rescue and adriamycin in childhood osteogenic sarcoma. Cancer, *33*:1151–1163, 1974.
57. Rundles, R. W., Grizzle, J., Bell, W. N., et al.: Comparison of chlorambucil and myeleran in chronic lymphocytic and granulocytic leukemia. Am. J. Med., *27*:424–432, 1959.
58. Santos, G. W., and Owens, A. H., Jr.,: A comparison of the effect of selected cytotoxic agents on

the primary agglutinin response in rats injected with sheep erythrocytes. Bull. Johns Hopkins Hosp., *114*:384–401, 1964.

59. Selawry, O. S., and Hananian, J.: Vincristine treatment of cancer in children. J. A. M. A., *183*:741–746, 1963.
60. Shorey, J., Schenker, S., Suki, W. N., et al.: Hepatotoxicity of mercaptopurine. Arch. Intern. Med., *122*:54–58, 1968.
61. Sostman, H. D., Matthay, R. A., Putman, C. E., et al.: Methotrexate-induced pneumonitis. Medicine, *55*:371–388, 1976.
62. Stolinsky, D. C., Solomon, J., Pugh, R. P., et al.: Clinical experience with procarbazine in Hodgkin's Disease, reticulum cell sarcoma and lymphosarcoma. Cancer, *26*:984–990, 1970.
63. Tan, C., Etcubanas, E., et al.: Adriamycin—an antitumor antibiotic in the treatment of neoplastic disease. Cancer *32:9*–17, 1973.
64. Thierman, W. G., Bloedow, C., Howe, C. D., et al.: A phase 1 study of hydroxyurea. Cancer Chemother. Rep., *29*:103–107, 1963.
65. Wall, R. L., and Clausen, K. P.: Carcinoma of the urinary bladder in patients receiving cyclophosphamide. N. Engl. J. Med., *293*:271–273, 1975.
66. Wang, J., Cortes, E., Sinks, L. F., et al.: Therapeutic effect and toxicity of adriamycin in patients with neoplastic disease. Cancer, *28*:837–843, 1971.
67. Weinstein, G., Roenigk, H., Maibach, H., et al.: Psoriasis-liver-methotrexate interactions. Arch. Dermatol., *108*:36–42, 1973.
68. Worth, R. H. L.: Cyclophosphamide and the bladder. Br. Med. J., *3*:182, 1971.
69. Wright, T. L., Husley, J., Korst, D. R., et al.: Vinblastine in neoplastic disease. Cancer Res., *23*:169–179, 1963.
70. Yagoda, A., Mukherji, B., Young, C., et al.: Bleomycin, an antitumor antibiotic. Ann. Intern. Med., *77*:861–870, 1972.

# 23 COMPLICATIONS OF RADIATION THERAPY FOR CANCER OF THE HEAD AND NECK

*Manuel Lederman*

## INTRODUCTION

The majority of patients suffering from cancer will at some stage of their disease be either submitted to or considered for radiotherapy. This wide use of radiotherapy should, in part, be regarded as an index of its success as a therapeutic agent, but indirectly it also reflects the paucity of reliable methods available for treating cancer.

Historically, radiotherapy is as old as this century and, in its first thirty years, was used purely empirically, with not infrequent disasters to both patient and radiotherapist. The next decade saw the successful solution of the physical problems connected with dose measurement, and it was thus possible to put treatment on a rational basis upon which clinical experience could be built. The post-war decades continued the remarkable technical advances in apparatus and the production of radioactive isotopes for clinical use, and in recent years, apparatus and techniques have reached a high degree of refinement, so much so that further progress in this direction is not to be expected outside the experimental laboratory.

## TECHNIQUES OF RADIOTHERAPY

There are two main technical methods of using radiant energy in the treatment of malignant disease: external and internal.

### *External Application*

This technique necessitates the use of special apparatus capable of producing either x or gamma radiations, which are part of the electromagnetic spectrum, or of emitting nuclear particles, such as electrons and neutrons.

A cobalt-60 unit is the most common source of high-energy gamma radiation, having the advantages of being a robust, all-purpose apparatus, relatively inexpensive to purchase and maintain and capable of providing a beam of irradiation equivalent to three million volt (3 Mev.) x-rays. Its disadvantages are that only a limited number of patients can be treated daily and the radioactive source decays at the rate of 1 per cent per month, needing replacement every three years.

In busy departments, where a large number of patients have to be treated daily, a linear accelerator emitting x-rays at an energy of 4 to 18 Mev. has much to recommend it. It is a more expensive piece of equipment than a cobalt unit, is physically and mechanically more sophisticated but does have more maintenance problems. Linear accelerators have become standard equipment in most large radiotherapy departments.

Although x- and gamma rays, however produced, have similar physical and biologic properties, there are other forms of radiant energy that are already in or about to enter into routine clinical use. There are, in particular, two so-called nuclear particles, electrons and neutrons, that can be put to clinical advantage because of their physical and biologic differences from x and gamma irradiation.

#### ELECTRON BEAM THERAPY

The usual source of electrons is a betatron, which can produce either electrons or x-rays at energies ranging from 18 to 42 Mev. Although the ultimate biologic effects of electrons are similar to those of x-rays, the physical distribution of their energy within the tissues differs, in that a relatively sharply circumscribed maximum effect can be produced, allowing the concentration of irradiation within a neoplasm and so sparing normal adjacent tissue. When the normal tissue to be spared happens to be the eye, the cerebrospinal axis, the buccal cavity or the bone marrow, the advantages of electrons are evident. Malignant disease of the head and neck, breast and skin provides important scope for electron beam therapy.

#### NEUTRON THERAPY

Neutrons of 6 Mev. energy suitable for clinical use can be obtained from a cyclotron, and their physical distribution in the tissues is similar to that of 250 kv. x-rays.

Although there may be no apparent physical advantage to neutrons over ordinary x-ray therapy, they do possess two biologic advantages of importance: (1) the relative anoxia of neoplastic tissue is less of an adverse factor with neutron therapy than with x-ray therapy and (2) the biologic effects of neutrons on mammalian cells are irreversible, and there is thus a negligible recovery factor from any damage inflicted by the irradiation.[5] Neutrons were first used in the treatment of malignant disease over thirty years ago,[16] with somewhat disastrous results.[17] Interest has been revived in recent years, and neutron therapy trials have been undertaken with encouraging results.[2]

Other particulate forms of irradiation of possible clinical importance exist and are being investigated, e.g., protons, alpha particles and negative pi mesons, but their use has not yet passed beyond the experimental stage.

### *Internal or Local Techniques*

When a tumor is limited in size and accessibility, it can often be successfully treated by the local application of radioactive materials: e.g., implantation of a tongue cancer; placed into the cavity of an organ, e.g., the uterus; or introduced systemically by injection or ingestion.

The systemic use of radioactive isotopes in the treatment of cancer has proved disappointing, and, apart from tracer investigations and the treatment of thyrotoxicosis by iodine-131, they seem to have little future in therapy as the discovery of suitable isotopes capable of selective and adequate concentration in diseased tissue is proving to be elusive.

By contrast, considerable progress has been made in the technique of implantation and intracavitary treatment. The radium sources that have hitherto been widely used can be replaced by radioactive cesium ($^{137}$Cs), cobalt ($^{60}$Co), tantalum ($^{181}$Ta), gold ($^{198}$Au) or iridium ($^{192}$Ir). The advantages of the newer isotopes are as follows: they are relatively inexpensive, they can be selected for use for individual patients because of some special physical property, protection is easier and an afterloading technique can be used. This last term means that metal or plastic containers suitable for retaining or guiding the necessary radioactive sources can first be placed in position in the patient, the physical accuracy of the treatment can be verified and the radioactive materials can subsequently be inserted. In this way, exposure of personnel is reduced to a minimum and accuracy of treatment greatly increased.

The implantation of radioactive materials has a useful but limited application in head and neck cancer. The sites most suitable for an implant as a primary method of treatment are the anterior two thirds of the tongue, the floor of the mouth and the buccal mucosa, including the angle of the mouth. As a palliative procedure, a large fixed metastatic mass in the neck can be implanted with plastic tubes containing radioactive gold, iridium or tantalum wire, whereas a small inoperable mass can be easily implanted with radioactive gold grains. Implantation is a simple and economic way of dealing with $T_1$ lesions in the sites mentioned before, but it should not be used as a primary method of treatment for $T_2$ to $T_3$ lesions or any lesion that cannot be encompassed by a single plane implant. Above all, implantation of a primary lesion should be avoided if bone involvement or operable cervical lymph node metastases are present.

In the author's view, the natural history of cancer of the head and neck is such that it is a mistake to concentrate on the primary site to the exclusion of the neck, since a clinically node-free neck cannot be equated with a cancer-free neck. Because of the prognostic gravity of neck node metastases and the high risk of their development in stages other than $T_1NO$, it has long been the author's custom to advise as the initial method of treatment simultaneous *en bloc* external irradiation of the primary site and the regional lymph node areas, even where the neck is clinically node-free. Patients undergoing this form of *en bloc* irradiation receive 5400 rads in five weeks, and thereafter, if the response is satisfactory, treatment to the primary site is continued to full dosage by external radiation with suitable technical modification. If, however, after completion of this dose the response of the primary is unsatisfactory, the treatment is stopped and the residuum is implanted or excised one month later, depending on circumstances.

This policy of routine elective irradiation of the node-free neck is not practiced when the primary tumor arises in one of the following sites:

1. The skin, including the pinna and external nose
2. The lip
3. The paranasal sinuses, including the hard palate
4. The glottic or subglottic regions of the larynx
5. Lesions limited to dorsal mucosa of tongue
6. $T_1NO$ lesions of lateral margin of tongue in elderly or unfit patients unable to tolerate neck irradiation

In sites 1 to 5, the natural history of the disease is such that the probability of the patient with a clinically free neck having macroscopic deposits or developing palpable lymph node metastases appears to be less than 20 per cent; under these circumstances, an expectant or observation policy relative to the neck is justifiable.

A routine elective neck irradiation policy of the kind outlined clearly restricts the scope of implantation to its use as a supplement to external irradiation.

## PURPOSE OF RADIOTHERAPY

In the treatment of malignant disease, radiation may be used for cure, for palliation or as an adjunct to surgery.

There are very few forms of cancer that cannot be treated by radiotherapy, but the cancers that can be properly termed "radiocurable" are, in fact, few in number. In the head and neck, they are composed of cancers arising from accessible regions, namely the skin, lip, buccal cavity and larynx. The inaccessible cancers of the body cavities, namely intracranial, intrathoracic and intra-abdominal neoplasms, still as a rule defeat the radiotherapist, although recent technical improvements have increased the salvage rate of this group.

### *Curative Treatment*

The curative treatment of cancer by radiotherapy is a serious undertaking, and the patient should never be given the impression that radiotherapy is an easy alternative to surgery. Although there is no immediate mortality or mutilation, a curative course of treatment may throw a heavy burden on the patient, since it is long and tedious, accompanied by constitutional disturbances and considerable local discomfort and is not without risk of complications. It is important that patients be given a full and clear picture of all that the treatment entails at the outset.

## THE EFFECTS OF RADIATION ON THE TISSUES

Ionizing radiation is a nonspecific irritant, and the response provoked in normal tissues is an inflammatory one possessing all the classic characteristics of such a process. This tissue response to radiation is termed a reaction, and its onset is usually preceded by a latent period of some 10 to 14 days and its termination is evidenced by a return to normal within a period of one month after completion of treatment; i.e., a radiation reaction is reversible. When a tissue heals after radiotherapy but does not return completely to normal, e.g., the skin remains hairless and depigmented or the mucous membrane is atrophic, glazed and dry, such changes can be regarded as acceptable and unavoidable sequelae. Should healing take place and, after a period of six months or more, some unexpected or undesirable events occur, e.g., perichondritis or bone or skin necrosis, then such events must be regarded as complications and means should be found for their avoidance.

### *The Skin*

The skin is the most commonly treated tissue in the body, since its irradiation is inevitable when external beam therapy is employed. In the early days of radiotherapy before the adoption of scientific units of doses, the skin changes after treatment by the relatively low-energy radiation available were so marked and followed such a regular pattern that the skin erythema was used as an index of dose (erythema dose). With modern supervoltage and megavoltage equipment, the maximum dose is achieved below the skin surface, which is thus "spared" many of the changes customarily seen in a previous era.

Classically, the reaction seen in the skin resembles that seen after exposure to any thermal, chemical or bacterial irritant; i.e., there is a phase of erythema followed by one of desquamation of surface epithelium, the desquamation being either dry or moist depending on the intensity of the irritant. Using standard methods of protracted fractionated radiation, there is usually a latent period of 10 to 14 days before skin changes become apparent, and, once started, they build up during the course of treatment, usually becoming maximum towards the end. Healing should take place three to four weeks after the termination of treatment, although pigmentation or subcutaneous edema, if marked, may take longer to settle down. Although the basic pattern of the skin reaction is similar in all patients, the precise response is influenced by certain factors other than the physical ones associated with treatment.

**Skin pigment.** Although the dark-skinned patient does not tolerate irradiation better because of the presence of pigment, the reaction is modified by the absence of an erythema and an increased degree of pigmentation of the treated area prior to desquamation. In contrast, the fair-haired, light-skinned patient with minimal skin pigment is less tolerant of radiation, and reactions tend to be brisker and moist desquamation readily occurs. In these patients, a guide to the tolerance of the skin to radiation is given by the patient's known tolerance or intolerance to sunlight.

**Age.** In the elderly patient, the thin atrophic "senile" skin that is often found does not tolerate radiation well. In contrast, moist desquamation is rarely seen in children.

**Hormonal factors.** It is said that patients suffering from hyperthyroidism show a brisker reaction than do normal euthyroid patients. This observation has little practical significance.

**Scars.** The presence of extensive scars following either burns or operations on the face or neck, e.g., block dissection scars, influences the reaction, since an avascular cicatrix may not show an erythema. Because the reaction and healing are dependent on the integrity of the blood supply, such modified skin is more likely to be damaged by radiation than comparable normal skin.

**Skin grafts.**[14] The wide use of reconstructive procedures following radical surgery for head and neck cancer often presents the radiotherapist with problems in postoperative radiation. Although it is customary to regard grafted skin as less tolerant to irradiation, experimental work by Grise and coworkers[4] on pigs subjected to full and split thickness grafts resulted in the following conclusions:

1. Fresh grafts reacted earlier and more vigorously than did normal skin, and recovery was slower.
2. Split thickness grafts tend to react less vigorously than full thickness grafts.
3. The intensity of the reaction was

found to be inversely proportional to the quality of the radiation, and fractionation seemed to help recovery.

4. Irradiation should not be begun immediately after grafting.

They emphasized that grafted skin reacts and recovers from radiation differently than does normal skin, the differences depending on the stage of union of the graft. They recommend allowing a period of three to four weeks for a "good take" before embarking on postoperative irradiation.

### SITE

Difference in epidermal thickness, the presence of moisture, warmth and exposure to friction may all render the skin less tolerant to irradiation. In the head and neck, the areas where these factors operate are the supraclavicular region and the neck, generally below the "collar line," the retroauricular sulcus, the suboccipital and temporal regions and the angles of the mouth, nose and inner canthus.

### SEQUELAE

The extent to which irradiated skin may return to a normal appearance after a curative course using modern super- or megavoltage apparatus is often surprising. Although depigmented, atrophic telangiectatic scars are relics of the days of orthovoltage therapy, there is a tendency after high energy irradiation for the production of subcutaneous edema, which may persist for some time.

Epilation and loss of function of the sweat and sebaceous glands occur but may not be permanent.

### COMPLICATIONS

**Chronic subcutaneous fibrosis and edema.** These can be seen 6 to 12 months after a severe moist reaction when, apart from atrophic skin changes, there is progressive fibrosis of the subcutaneous tissue that may compress vessels draining fluid from the skin and so produce edema of the skin. Despite the fact that the patient is conscious of the presence of a fibrotic mass, few symptoms are produced and no clinical action is either available or indicated.

**Radionecrosis (Fig. 23–1).** Radionecrotic ulceration may appear a year or more after treatment, usually when a severe skin reaction has occurred. The precipitating causes may be trauma, infection or exposure to extremes of temperature. These lesions are characterized by their indolence and painfulness. Analgesics, systemic antibiotics and topical steroid application may ultimately result in healing, although the risk of further breakdown is ever-present. Surgical excision and grafting may in the end become necessary.

**Chronic radiodermatitis.** This is rare after modern therapeutic radiation but was seen in the earlier part of this century after occupational exposure to radiation by workers and in patients suffering from nonmalignant dermatologic lesions, which were customarily treated by repeated small doses of soft radiation over a long period of time. There are marked differences between the effects of long-term repeated exposure to low doses of radiation and the changes seen after a single course of curative radiation for cancer. In the former case, the changes seen may be hypertrophic in character, with the epidermis becoming thickened, hyper-

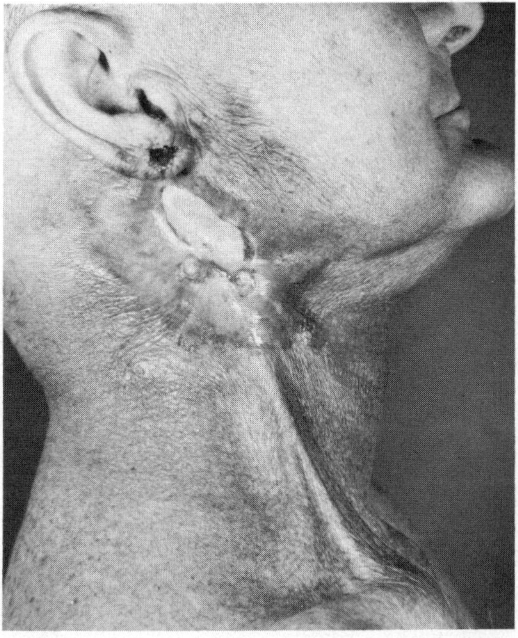

**Figure 23–1** Recurrence in block dissection scar after radiotherapy, showing poor response of the tumor and radionecrotic slough in the upper end of the scar.

keratotic and epilated. Alternatively, the skin may become atrophic and thinned, with telangiectatic vessels and the tendency to permanent superficial ulceration. Chronic radiodermatitis is associated with an increased incidence of skin carcinoma.

### *The Mucous Membranes*

The mucous membranes of the mouth, pharynx and larynx are less tolerant to irradiation than the skin, and hence this may act as a limiting factor to the amount of radiation that a patient can support. The reactions occuring in the mucous membrane are basically similar to those occurring in the skin; i.e., there is an inflammatory response preceded by a latent period of 10 to 14 days, during which very little may happen except that the mucous membrane begins to get rather dry and becomes red and glazed and the tongue papillae become red and prominent. Thereafter, the mucous membrane becomes edematous and patches of yellowish membrane appear on the irradiated mucosa, apparently scattered in a haphazard manner.

The yellowish membrane so produced is termed a "radiation membrane," radiation mucositis or radioepithelitis and appears only after the surface epithelium has desquamated. This membrane may appear on the ulcerating surface of a tumor within 24 hours of irradiation, or, if a biopsy is performed prior to irradiation, a patch of membrane will appear on the biopsy site immediately after treatment is begun. Apart from the ulcerated tumor surface, on which the early appearance of radiation membrane is termed a "false membrane," the normal intact mucous membrane shows a true radioepithelitis in certain selected sites before becoming confluent. The sites in the buccal cavity first affected are on either side of the base of the uvula, the lower alveololingual sulcus, the cheek and soft palate.

If teeth are present and abrade the tongue, membrane appears at the site of abrasion and outlines the teeth in shape (Fig. 23–2). The dorsum of the tongue, the hard palate and the alveolar ridges, where there is practically no submucosa, become involved belatedly. In the case of the pharynx and larynx, there is no selective site of onset of membrane formation, the latter appearing in a patchy fashion within the treated area and becoming confluent with increasing dosage.

As the mucosal reaction develops, so do its associated symptoms, which are usually pain, dryness, loss of taste, viscidity of the saliva and difficulty in mastication, dyspha-

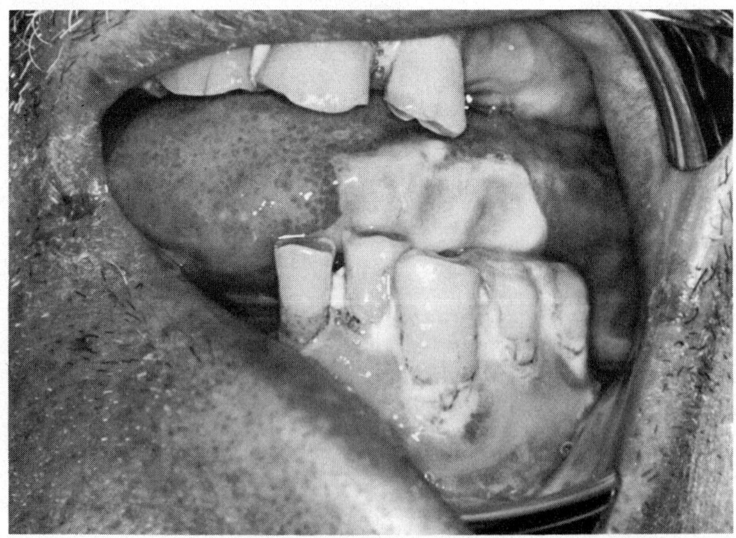

**Figure 23–2** Thick membranous reaction on tongue in contact with teeth. The teeth are outlined by the membrane.

gia or huskiness, depending on the anatomic territory being irradiated. These symptoms and signs tend to reach their peak at about the fifth week of treatment and thereafter wane. The mucositis disappears within a fortnight after treatment, although the mucosae may remain red and somewhat edematous.

The production of an intense mucositis is not as essential to cure as was once believed; on the contrary, a mucositis can be controlled up to a point and a patient's discomfort thus much diminished without worsening the prognosis.

It is remarkable how patients tolerate the discomforts provoked by a severe mucosal reaction, provided remedies for relief of symptoms are employed, such as analgesics, antibiotics and topical anaesthetics (Mucaine or Benzocaine), and the nutritional status maintained.

There are two special areas in the head and neck where severe mucosal reactions must be avoided at all costs.

#### THE LARYNX

A severe reaction accompanied by edema, when provoked in a larynx already partially obstructed by neoplastic infiltration or proliferation, may totally obstruct the airway and so endanger the patient's life.

#### THE ORBICULARIS ORIS

A severe reaction involving the anterior third of the buccal cavity is one of the most dangerous of all the tissue reactions that can be provoked by irradiation in the head and neck region. A patient can be helped to overcome a severe reaction in the larynx, oropharynx or nasopharyngeal region by tracheotomy or intubation, but when a severe reaction involves the anterior third of the tongue and the mucous membrane lining the orbicularis oris sphincter, a patient's suffering may become intolerable and incapable of relief by nasogastric intubation, since this is the most sensitive part of the buccal cavity and has functions other than those related to mastication and deglutition. A severe reaction in this area in the elderly, in debilitated patients and particularly in diabetic patients can prove fatal and must be avoided at all costs.

## EFFECTS OF RADIATION ON BONE AND CARTILAGE

Growing bone and cartilage are markedly affected by irradiation, the changes being at their most striking with the long bones and vertebral column, where arrest or retardation of epiphyseal growth takes place with resultant deformity. Flat bones are also affected, and, in the case of the skull, "spoon defects" or hollowing of the bone appears where irradiated bone shows diminished growth while the surrounding unirradiated bone continues to grow at its normal rate.[1, 13]

Fortunately, cancers of the head and neck are rare in children, the tumors usually seen in this region being the lymphomata and the special tumors of the eye and orbit. In the author's experience, it is rare to see serious bone deformities in the head and neck region following the irradiation of childhood tumors, even after full doses (5000 rads or more) are given, as is the case in the rhabdomyosarcomas. Asymmetry of the jaw, deformity of the nasal bones and delay in appearance of dentition are the usual acceptable complications that may occur in the long-term survivors. Irradiation-induced neoplasms are discussed elsewhere.

In contrast to growing bone and cartilage, these same tissues, when fully developed in the adult, are relatively insensitive and under therapeutic conditions, provided overdosage, trauma and infection are avoided, can be irradiated with impunity.

### *Radionecrosis of Bone*

The bony structures in the head and neck that may undergo radionecrosis are the mandible, the bones forming the upper jaw, the floor of the sphenoidal sinus and the temporal bone. Fortunately, although frequently irradiated, the hyoid bone and the vertebral column seem relatively immune to radionecrotic complications.

Osteoradionecrosis is usually associated with recurrent or persistent cancer, and its signs and symptoms have a common pattern. The onset is usually 6 to 18 months after radiation, the shorter period occurring in those cases in which the tumor has shown the least response and healing has been incomplete. The dominant clinical symptom is severe and persistent pain, at first localized to the affected bone but later radiating to neighbouring areas; fever, fetor, discharge, and ulceration with exposed necrotic bone detectable in the ulcer base complete the picture.

If necrosis affects a bone that is free of cancer, an expectant policy is usually rewarded by sequestration of the dead bone and healing. Occasionally, a sequestrectomy may be necessary. If, however, cancer is present, then a patient's survival will depend on whether or not radical surgery is possible.

From the earliest days of radiotherapy, the occurrence of radionecrosis with all its attendant problems has acted as a brake on the expansion of radiation as a treatment method for carcinoma of the head and neck. The radiotherapists have largely themselves to blame for this state of affairs, since many will not accept that radionecrosis is almost entirely avoidable and that the only occasion on which the risk of this complication should be deliberately accepted is when there is no alternative to radiotherapy available to the patient.

The concept that a necrosis rate, however small, is an acceptable part of the radiation treatment of early carcinoma, e.g., of the larynx, is to be condemned, since it merely reflects the sacrifice of the patient to technical expediency. Equally, the concept that, in an advanced case, it is better for a patient to survive with radionecrosis than to die of cancer is fallacious. It engenders a policy that, if pursued, can only result in patients having to undergo the slow miseries of ne-

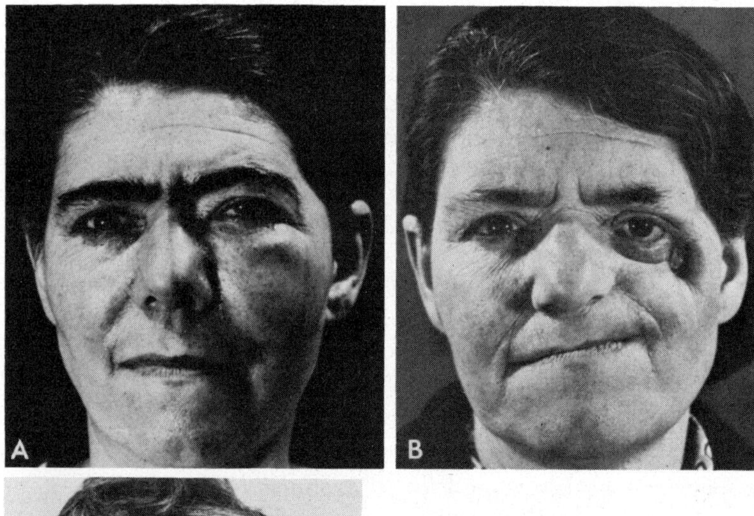


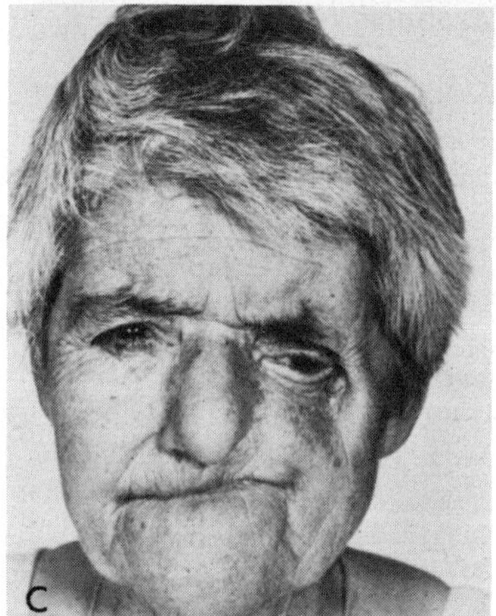


**Figure 23–3** Extensive carcinoma of the left antrum with malar bone invasion. *A,* Before treatment — June, 1948. *B,* After treatment — April, 1952 — showing the fistula following sequestration of the involved malar bone. *C,* Patient alive and well 30 years.

crosis, for which they must ultimately seek the help of the surgeon. The use of surgery as part of the initial treatment would achieve the same end result without the intervening necrotic stage.

The policy of prevention of radionecrosis of bone and cartilage is based on the acceptance, in principle, that once these tissues are involved by cancer, there will be diminished response to radiation and surgery will become necessary at some stage of treatment to remove all invaded tissues that cannot be safely eradicated by radiation. Because of the structural variations that exist in the bones forming the different regions of the head and neck, the precise manner of this association between radiation and surgery will vary accordingly.

### THE UPPER JAW

The tolerance to radiation varies with the bone structure. Thus, the mucoperiosteal bones of the maxilloethmoidal region, if invaded by neoplasm, can be sequestrated and discharged through the natural passages without any problem. The hard palate and alveolar ridge, if the seat of a malignant osteitis, can also be easily sequestrated without the associated complications of a major necrotic process. The only bone in the facial skeleton that occasions problems is the malar bone (Fig. 23–3).

The compact malar bone, if invaded by neoplasm and irradiated, will readily become the seat of a malignant osteitis, and, since the antrum is in these circumstances a closed cavity, sequestration can only take place through an external fistula. This undesirable event can be avoided by removing the invaded malar bone endorally prior to radiation. This removal is not meant to be a curative procedure but rather a "toilet" operation performed so as to make the preoperative course of irradiation as trouble-free as possible.

### THE LOWER JAW (FIGS. 23–4 AND 23–5)

The mandible is the most common bone in the head and neck to undergo radionecrosis. The reasons for this are as follows:

1. The compact bone is, by its structure, more vulnerable to radiation damage than other facial bones.
2. Because of its situation and relation to the many cancers occurring in the buccopharyngeal region and their metastatic nodes, it undergoes irradiation more frequently than any other facial bone.
3. The ease with which the mucous membrane of the alveolar ridges can be breached allows a pathway for infection; the presence of the teeth and their special radiation problems are also factors.

If the problems of mandibular radionecrosis are to be avoided, the patient with an invaded lower jaw should be treated by a

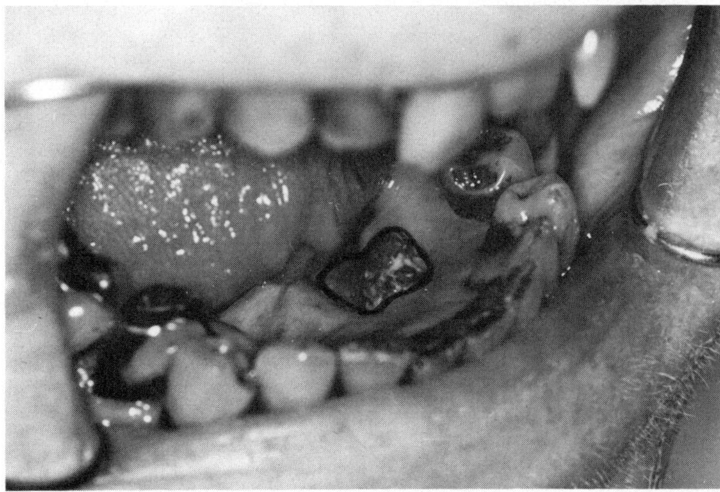

**Figure 23–4** Small area of radionecrosis of the mandible, sequestrating spontaneously. Patient initially had a carcinoma of the floor of the mouth treated by radioactive implant and subsequently developed a lymph node metastasis, treated by block dissection and postoperative radiotherapy.

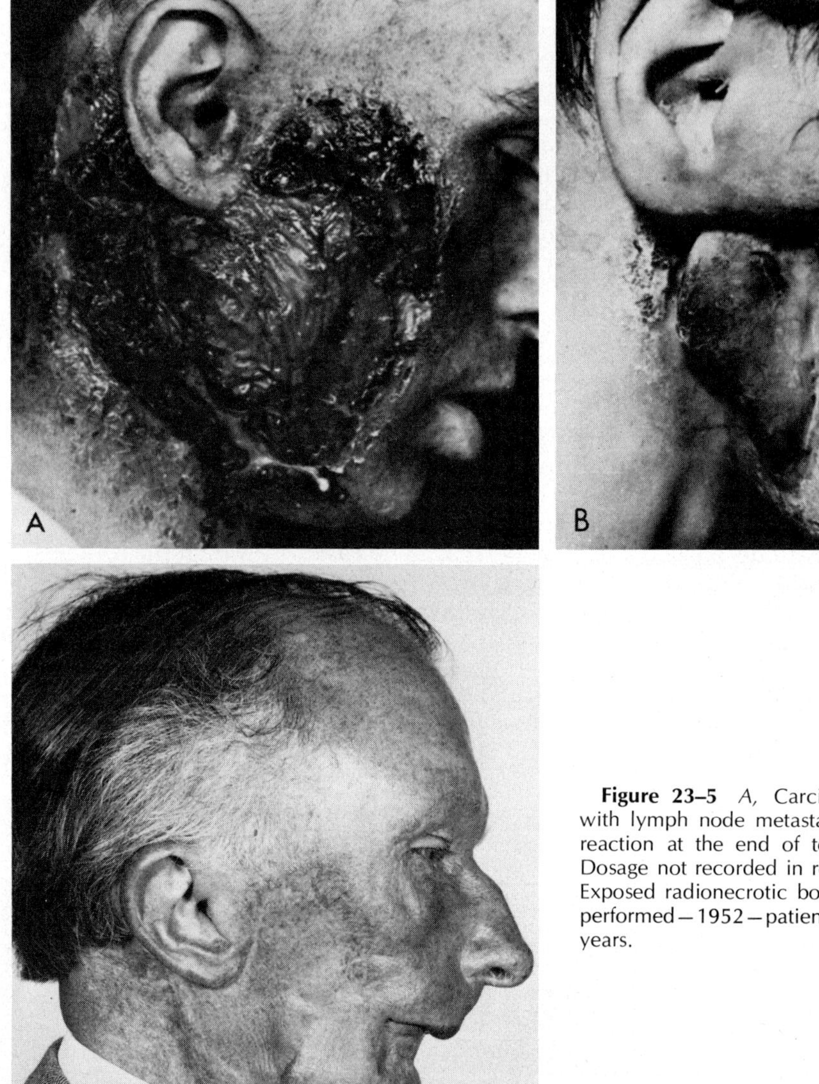


**Figure 23–5** *A,* Carcinoma of the tonsil with lymph node metastases. Extensive moist reaction at the end of teleradium treatment. Dosage not recorded in roentgens — 1938. *B,* Exposed radionecrotic bone — 1939. *C,* Graft performed—1952—patient alive and well 40 years.

combination of preoperative radiotherapy and surgery, so that the invaded bone is removed.

There are two occasions on which radiotherapy may yet achieve success even though mandibular bone invasion be present:

1. When there is superficial involvement of the alveolar ridge, a limited amount of cancellous bone can be sequestrated, with subsequent healing.

2. Paradoxically, if the whole thickness of the mandible (i.e., the alveolar ridge and the body of the mandible) is destroyed by neoplasm, radiation, by destroying the neoplasm, which has itself destroyed the bone, is followed by healing without sequestration, a pseudoarthrosis forming between the free ends of the bone.

### TEMPORAL BONE

The cancers occurring in the temporal bone that may be associated with a malignant osteitis or complicated by postradiation osteonecrosis are those involving the bony external meatus, the middle ear or the mastoid process.

The temporal bone itself is the densest and most compact bone in the base of the skull and is therefore not particularly tolerant of radiation even when normal. It is essential, therefore, in the presence of cancer to take steps to control sepsis and to establish drainage prior to embarking on radiation treatment. In order to achieve this aim, relieve the patient of the severe pain of a malignant osteitis and, at the same time, offer protection against the risks of postradiation osteonecrosis, a radical mastoidectomy is advised as a pretreatment toilet procedure. By this means, the extent of the disease can be assessed, dead bone can be removed and a freely draining inspection cavity can be provided. A full course of radiotherapy given after this procedure is usually uncomplicated, and in successful cases (30 percent of squamous cancers), the cancer is controlled and epithelialization of the cavity takes place. Development of an osteitis after radiotherapy usually denotes persistent or recurrent cancer and demands radical surgical treatment whenever possible.

### SPHENOIDAL SINUS

Primary carcinoma arising in the sphenoidal sinus or sphenoethmoidal region is not as rare as is generally thought, since these tumors are customarily misdiagnosed as being of nasopharyngeal origin because of their presenting signs and symptoms. Their separation is possible on clinical and radiological grounds, however.[6, 9] Apart from any clinical interest derived from their identification, these sphenoidal sinus tumors destroy the floor of the sinus by invading the vault of the nasopharynx, and if control of the cancer is achieved, sequestration of the bony sinus floor takes place. Severe occipitofrontal pain with postnasal discharge is the chief symptom, and ulceration of the nasopharyngeal vault is present, leading to a diagnosis of recurrent neoplasm. On direct examination under anesthesia, however, the exposed bone can be seen; biopsy from the ulcer edge is negative. Sequestration may occur spontaneously but usually minor surgical assistance is required.

## *Cartilage Necrosis*

Radionecrosis of cartilage occurs in various sites in the head and neck and, as with osteonecrosis, its importance differs with the site and nature of the cartilage affected.

As a general rule, the presence of a mesodermal supporting tissue, such as cartilage, or dense fibrous tissue adversely affects the tolerance to radiation of the organ or structure it supports. There are three supporting tissues found in the head and neck that are of importance to the radiotherapist:

1. The hyaline cartilage forming the thyroid and arytenoid cartilages.
2. The elastic fibrocartilage supporting the pinna, external nose and epiglottis.
3. The specialized condensations of fibrous tissue that form the pharyngeal aponeurosis and the tarsal plates of the eyelids.

In all cases, invasion of these tissues by cancer cells is accompanied by a diminished response to radiation and delay, or even total failure, to heal. By contrast, if these tissues are normal and uninvolved by cancer, they tolerate therapeutic doses of radiation well, provided infection is avoided.

### THE LARYNX AND ITS CARTILAGES

The patient with an early carcinoma of the larynx whose cartilages are not involved by cancer should not develop either perichondritis or necrosis after radiotherapy. Postradiation laryngeal edema may occur when either high doses have to be given or infection supervenes on an irradiated larynx. Its onset may be any time after the completion of radiation treatment. The symptoms of edema are vocal or respiratory and, if mild, usually settle with voice rest, antibiotics and steroids. A perichondritis is heralded by pain referred to the cartilage affected, with localized tenderness of the larynx and respiratory symptoms. Frank chondronecrosis is evidenced by severe pain, fever, fetor and respiratory obstruction; pieces of necrotic sequestrated cartilage may be expectorated.

When the cancer is controlled, the treatment of established perichondritis and chondronecrosis is expectant, although a tracheostomy is often essential. Special care is also necessary to maintain the nutrition of the patient and to avoid pulmonary complications. As with osteonecrosis, attention to irradiation technique will go far to eliminate edema and perichondritis; chondronecrosis can be avoided with surgery for those who are candidates for this complication because of the advanced stage of their disease.

The arytenoids are the laryngeal cartilages that cause the greatest problems, being made up largely of hyaline cartilage and functionally active in vocalization and swallowing. Their sequestration, if necrotic, is a long and burdensome process, and the patient is left with a stenotic, poorly functioning larynx and often with a permanent tracheostomy.

By contrast, the fibrocartilage of the suprahyoid epiglottis is, in humans, relatively functionless and readily sequestrates with-

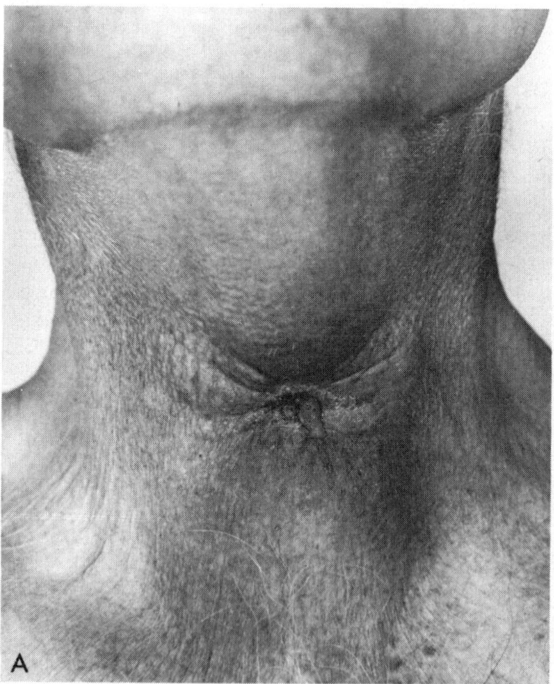


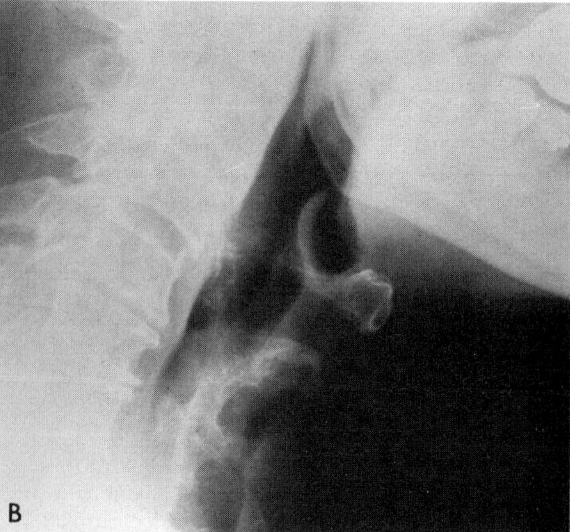


**Figure 23–6** *A,* Carcinoma of the right vocal cord treated in 1957. Dose: 6400 rads in 48 days — 1975. Further carcinoma of the left vocal cord, retreated by telecobalt therapy since patient refused laryngectomy. Dose: 6500 rads in 43 days. Necrosis of the Adam's apple — 1975. Patient remains well. *B,* X-ray of the damaged cartilage.

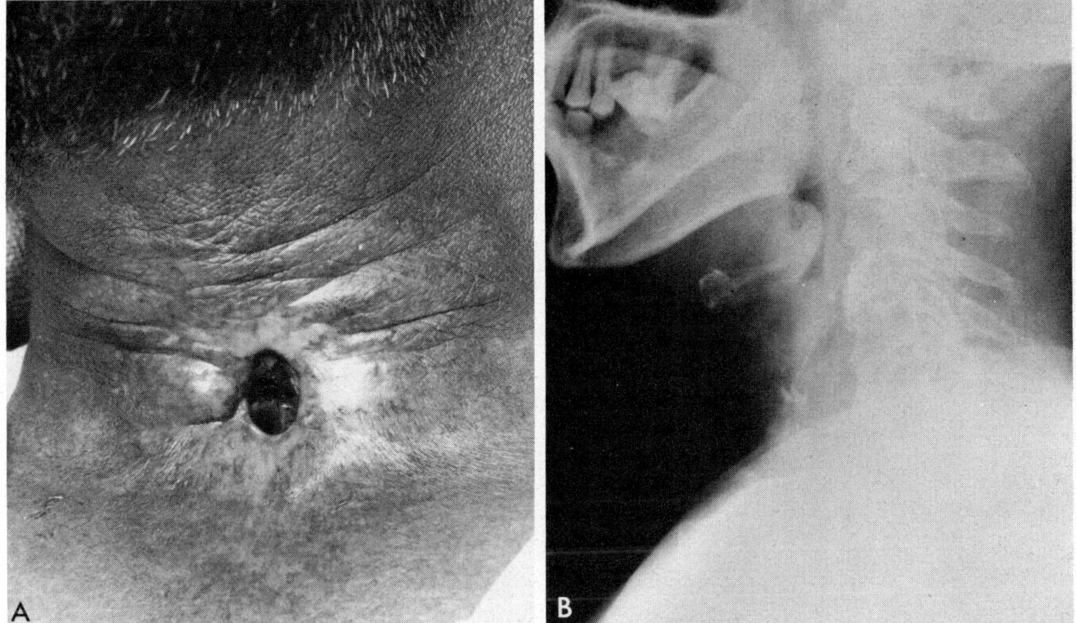


**Figure 23–7** *A,* Carcinoma of the subglottis treated by radiotherapy in 1973. Dose: 6800 rads in 47 days. Recurrence in upper trachea with right cervical lymph node metastasis and recurrent nerve paralysis in 1974, retreated by a combination of radiotherapy and chemotherapy since lesion was regarded as inoperable. Dose: 5500 rads in 42 days. Patient developed radionecrosis of the cricoid cartilage within six months. Patient remains well. *B,* X-ray showing necrosis of cartilage.

out much resultant disability. The suprahyoid epiglottis is in practice the one portion of the cartilaginous framework of the larynx that the radiotherapist can sequestrate with impunity.

The thyroid cartilage, which largely has a protective function, tends to undergo necrosis in the region of the Adam's apple, where sequestration is easy and closing the resulting fistula is not a major surgical problem (Figs. 23–6 and 23–7).

### THE FIBROCARTILAGE OF THE PINNA AND EXTERNAL NOSE

These cartilages, if uninvolved, should not become the seat of a chondritis. If, however, they are invaded by cancer, the diseased cartilage will sequestrate and healing will be slow and followed by deformity. Invasion of fibrocartilage by cancer is not a contraindication to radiotherapy (Fig. 23–8). It should be especially stressed that a normal pinna should not be removed as part of an operation for cancer of the external auditory canal or middle ear on the assumption that this step helps the radiotherapist should the patient require postoperative treatment. The normal cartilage of the pinna tolerates radiation well and does not require removal on these grounds.

### THE PHARYNGEAL APONEUROSIS

The posterior pharyngeal wall is a not uncommon site for cancer, and if the well-developed portions of the pharyngeal aponeurosis are invaded, particularly the pharyngobasilar fascia and the raphe on the posterior pharyngeal wall, then healing after radiotherapy may either be long-delayed or fail entirely. If there is simultaneous invasion of both the pharyngeal aponeurosis and the prevertebral fascia, then healing and cure by radiation are most unlikely.

### THE TARSAL PLATES

The structures behave in almost the same fashion as fibrocartilage in that healing is

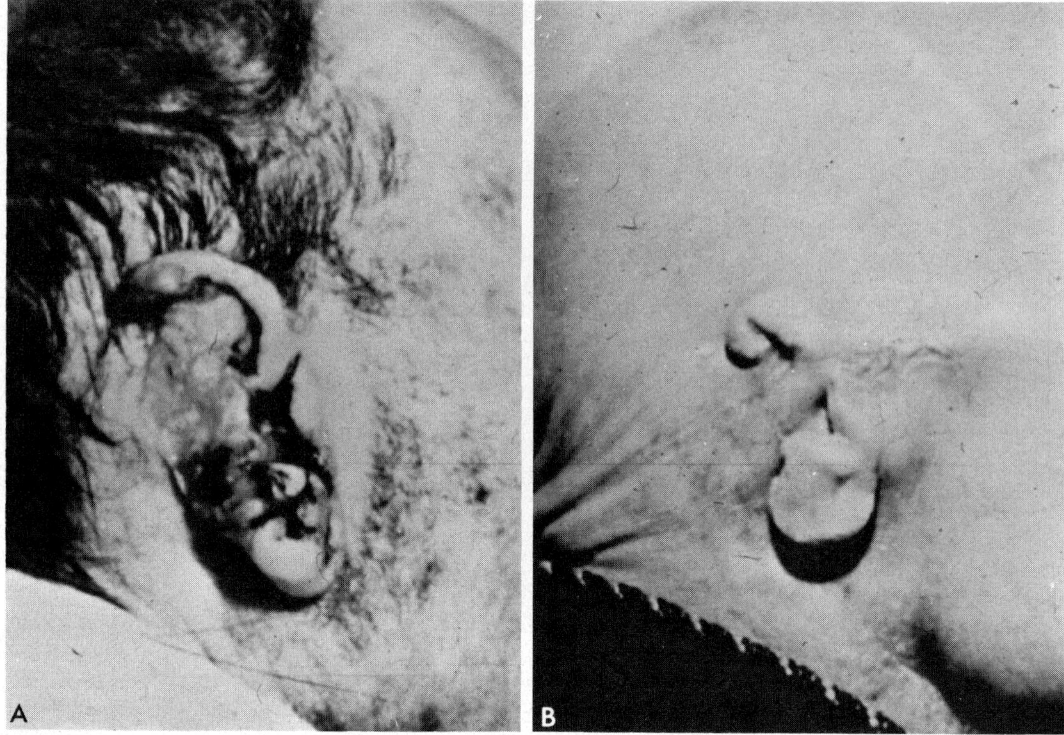

**Figure 23–8** Recurrent carcinoma of the pinna. *A,* Before radiation treatment. *B,* Afterward: healing has taken place without postirradiation perichondritis or necrosis.

followed by deformity, but since avascular cartilage is not present, there is no prior process of sequestration.

## EFFECTS OF RADIATION ON THE TEETH

A hypersensitivity of the teeth to extremes of temperature and sweet foods is noticed by many patients within months of the completion of radiation treatment. Dental caries, however, is the characteristic postradiation complication, the process following radiotherapy being similar to that occurring in the unirradiated mouth (Fig. 23–9). As a rule, the onset and progress of radiation caries is slow, appearing two to four years after treatment, and in moderately severe cases, with careful dentistry, the process may be kept in check for years. On the other hand, the rate of disruption may be so rapid that a complete dentition may be destroyed in a year or two.

The characteristic changes are (1) Decay on the labial surface of the neck of the teeth; (2) erosion, eventually resulting in amputation of the crown from the root; and (3) an increased rate of occlusal attrition.[14]

The dental changes occur first in the molar teeth, if they have been exposed to direct irradiation, but the incisor teeth outside the field of direct irradiation also suffer. It is rare to see one arcade or an isolated group of teeth alone affected. Since dental caries does not follow buccal cavity irradiation, if the salivary glands are excluded from the field of radiation (Fig. 23–10), the factors chiefly responsible for the carious process would seem to be the alteration in the character and quality of the saliva, although a possible effect on the vasculature of the teeth and jaws may also be significant. As a result of loss of taste and of dryness associated with the salivary changes, mastication becomes difficult and the patient adopts a fluid or semi-solid carbohydrate diet to maintain nourishment. Conditions of

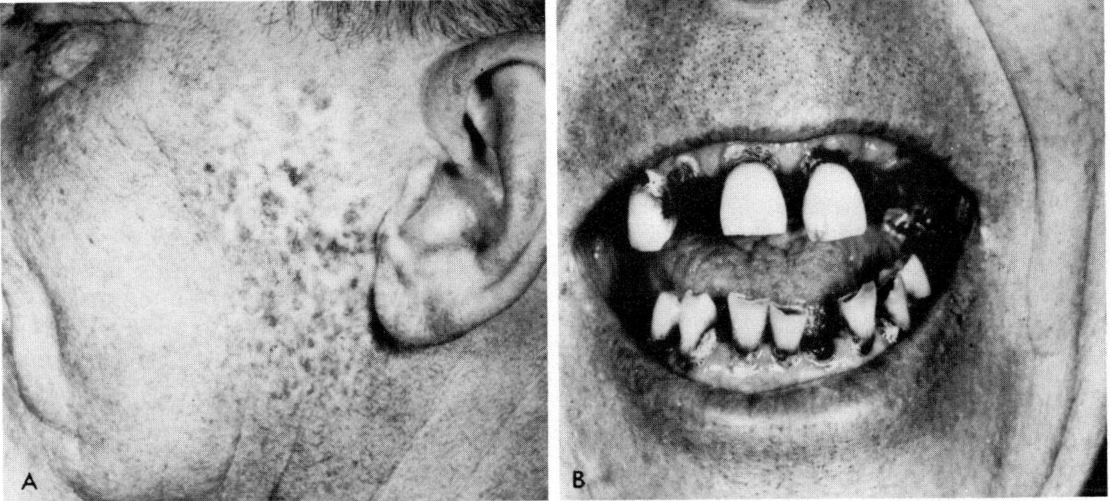

**Figure 23–9** *A*, Carcinoma of the soft palate showing extensive skin changes. *B*, Caries of teeth outside the radiation field. Patient developed carcinoma of the left external auditory canal 11 years later, possibly radiation-induced.

stagnation are thereby set up, with the result that food debris tends to cling around the teeth and sulci, and the carious process in both the irradiated and nonirradiated teeth is thus started.

The importance of postradiation dental changes lies not only in the undesirable dental signs and symptoms they produce but also in the risk of osteonecrosis of the irradiated jaw associated with their treatment.

One simple solution to the dental problems of patients undergoing irradiation for head and neck cancer would lie in wholesale extraction of all teeth. A procedure of this sort, although advocated at one time, is both brutal and unnecessary since it is possible that by proper care and management a pa-

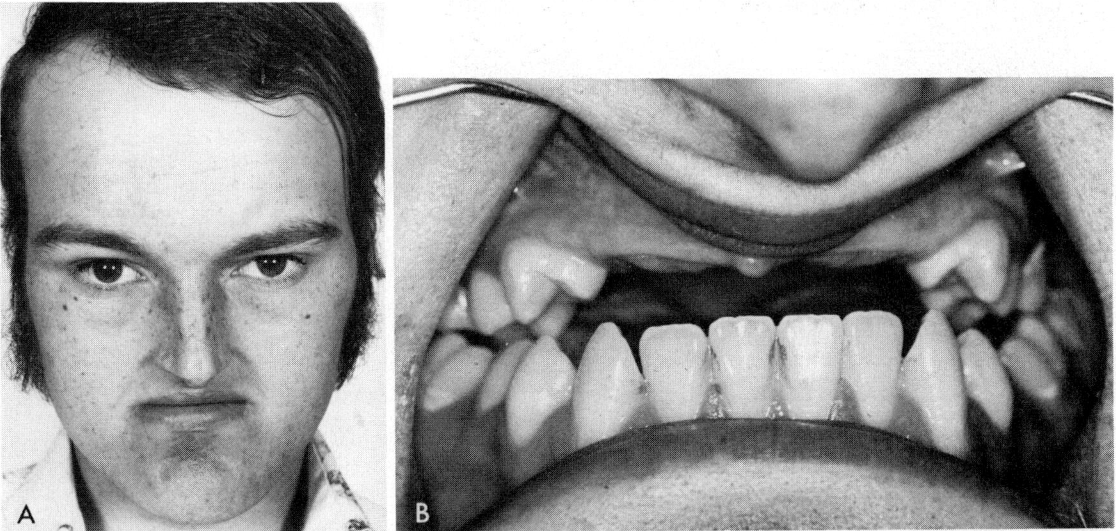

**Figure 23–10** *A*, Rhabdomyosarcoma of the nasal septum 16 years after treatment by orthovoltage x-rays. Dose: 6000 rads in 53 days. Patient now 20 years old. *B*, Teeth within radiation field undeveloped. Remaining teeth do not show caries since the salivary glands were not irradiated.

tient may retain sound teeth and avoid the postradiation caries and the risks of mandibular necrosis.

It is recommended that all carious and septic teeth be removed prior to radiation on the sound principle that treatment should not be given to a septic area without dealing with the sepsis first.

An attempt should be made to retain and conserve sound teeth except for teeth related to a buccal or lingual cancer that is going to be treated by a radioactive implant. Removal of teeth immediately adjacent to the neoplasm facilitates the radiotherapist's manipulations within the mouth and also adds to the patient's subsequent comfort, in that irritation of the edematous, irradiated area of the adjacent teeth is avoided. Extractions should be undertaken under antibiotic cover and radiation treatment should be delayed for seven days.

At one time, the author recommended the routine removal of the lower back molar teeth in those buccal cavity or pharyngeal cases in which this area came within the treatment field.[6] The reason for this recommendation was the high incidence of lower jaw necrosis, when removal of these particular teeth became necessary after radiotherapy. This pretreatment procedure has since been abandoned because of the delay necessary for healing prior to starting radiation. Moreover, the adverse effect of radiation on the healing process often resulted in failure of the sockets to heal and so becoming ever-present sources of pocketing and infection.

Postextraction osteitis or necrosis of the upper alveolus is most unusual, partly because there is much less tendency for food to pocket or stagnate in this region and partly because the bone of the upper alveolus is much more cancellous than the lower and there is therefore less risk of traumatic damage during dental extraction.

The risk of necrosis is greatest in the lower jaw after extraction of the back molar

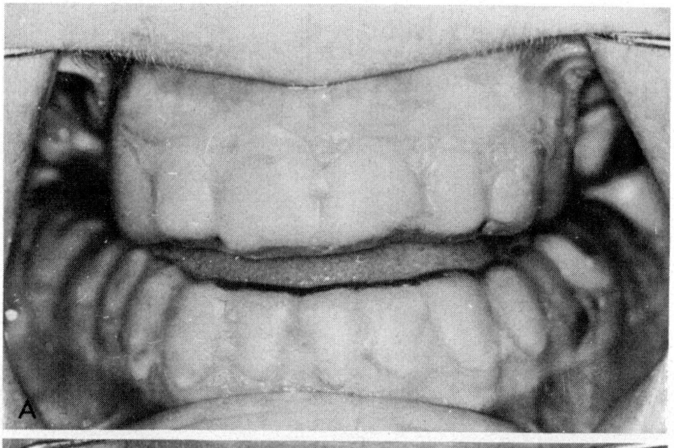


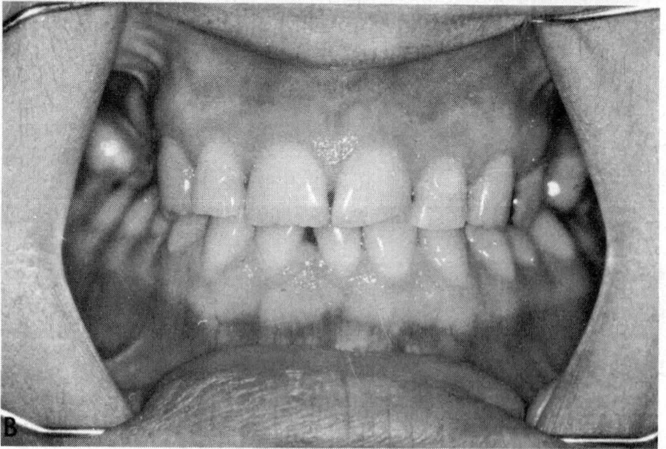


**Figure 23–11** *A,* Carcinoma of the nasopharynx. Acrylic splints in place. *B,* Splints removed one year later. No caries visible.

teeth. Necrosis may occur after extraction of lower teeth anterior to the premolars but is rarely so serious an event. Special caution is necessary if unerupted lower molars are present, since these should in all circumstances be left alone.

Apart from meticulous care in maintaining a clean mouth during and after treatment, the risk of dental caries can be reduced by the application of specially constructed acrylic splints that cover the teeth completely and are left in place for up to two years or until such time as some return of salivary secretion has taken place (Fig. 23–11). The rationale underlying the use of these protective splints is based on the observation that, in young patients, irradiated unerupted teeth show a much slower onset of caries when they later erupt into the dry mouth. It was therefore assumed that early and full coverage of the erupted teeth might achieve protection against caries by insulating them against the abnormal environment furnished by the postirradiated mouth. This assumption in practice seems to be justified.[3]

### *Effects on Developing Teeth*

Information concerning the effects of irradiation on the developing teeth in children is scarce, although the literature does contain accounts of the effects seen on the teeth of experimental animals.

Radiation will produce retardation of development of bone and teeth in children during the first few years of postnatal life. The defects most frequently seen in the permanent dentition of children whose teeth were irradiated during their developing phase are dwarfed teeth or failure of tooth development, incomplete root structure and premature eruption or calcification (Fig. 23–10).

## THE CENTRAL NERVOUS SYSTEM

The central and peripheral nervous systems are relatively tolerant to radiation, the latter especially so. In treating certain tumors of the head and neck it is impossible to avoid irradiating some part of the cerebral hemispheres, the brain stem or the cervical spinal cord. Chief among these particular tumors are those affecting the nasopharynx, upper jaw and temporal bone.

### *Cerebral Hemispheres*

Damage to the cerebral hemispheres is rare because, although part of the anterior and middle cranial fossae are irradiated when treating neoplasms of the paranasal sinuses and nasopharynx, it is largely the floor of these fossae that enters the field of radiation, and the volume of the brain tissue treated is, therefore, minimal. Nevertheless, ischemic necrosis of the temporal lobe can occur when treating nasopharyngeal cancer in elderly arteriosclerotic patients. Such an event occurs a year or two after treatment in a patient whose cancer is controlled, and the presenting symptoms are those of a brain tumor. The true diagnosis is usually made at or after operation. The posterior cranial fossa receives irradiation during the treatment of nasopharyngeal and middle ear tumors, and the brain stem lying in this region appears to be more sensitive to radiation than the cerebral hemispheres or cerebellum. Damage to the brain stem appears after a latent period of one to two years; there is an onset of ataxia, paresis of the limbs and a sixth nerve paralysis. The lesion may be unilateral, and the signs and symptoms become accordingly modified.

Radiation myelitis affecting the spinal cord is now well recognized and may occur after aggressive irradiation of oro- or hypopharyngeal tumors, particularly if associated with cervical lymph node metastases. After a variable latent period, which may be as short as six months, initial symptoms are numbness and tingling radiating from the neck to the arms and hands and made worse by flexion and extension. Lhermitte's sign is often present before any definite neurologic signs appear. There is an electric shock–like sensation radiating from the neck and back to the extremities on flexion of the neck.[17]

The symptoms present at the onset may disappear gradually or alternatively may progress and be accompanied by neurologic signs of progressive paresis and paralysis of the extremities ultimately associated with incontinence.

These disastrous nervous complications are permanent and without remedy, and most patients die shortly after their onset. It is difficult to assess the real risk of producing a radiation myelitis, since the patients at risk, particularly those with cervical lymph node metastases requiring high doses of radiation, are rarely successfully treated and die before any such damage becomes evident. Fortunately, prevention is not difficult and largely depends on avoiding or limiting the amount of central nervous tissue irradiated. The peripheral nerves are completely insensitive and require no special precautions if they enter the field of radiation. When the brain or brain stem has to be irradiated, the treatment fields can be reduced as the dose increases. Equally, toward the end of treatment, if dosage is going to be high and the irradiation of nervous tissue cannot be avoided, a change from high energy x-rays to electrons will reduce the risks. It is much easier to guard against damage to the cervical cord than to the brain stem, and the following measures help:

1. Reduction in field size, the use of electrons and the use of tangential fields help if high doses are to be given to residual nodes.

2. The key to safety in the neck, however, lies in recognizing the significant relationship the posterior triangle of the neck bears to the cervical spinal cord. The avoidance of heavy irradiation of the posterior triangles of the neck through parallel opposed fields will go far to eliminate radiation myelopathy of the cervical cord.

3. As a further guidance to safety, there is evidence to show that it is safe to deliver 4000 rads in four weeks to a 10 cm. segment of the spinal cord. If this guideline cannot be followed, the appropriate modifications of technique should be made.[11]

## THE SPECIAL SENSES

It is somewhat surprising that, although four special sense organs are related to the head and neck and are frequently irradiated, with the exception of the eyes, little is known concerning the mechanism whereby radiation exerts its effects or even the precise nature of these effects.

### *Taste*

The effects of radiation on taste and the underlying mechanism whereby gustatory changes are produced are ill understood. There is no doubt that patients undergoing radiation who reject food do so more on account of changes in taste than the discomfort of a radiation mucositis. The changes found presumably result from the direct effect of radiation on the taste buds, since the circumvallate papillae become red and prominent, giving an appearance not unlike a strawberry tongue even before a mucositis appears. There is no uniform pattern displayed by the changes, which seemingly vary from patient to patient. Generally speaking, however, bitter and acid taste is affected more than sweet and salt. Although there is no means of influencing these taste changes during treatment, a return to normal usually occurs within a year of completion of treatment.

The dryness experienced by patients is due to radiation damage to the mucous glands both of the lining epithelium of the mouth and pharynx and of the major and minor salivary glands. The latter may be affected by (1) partial duct obstruction following edema of the duct epithelium; (2) damage to the acini, resulting in alteration in the quantity and quality of the saliva secreted; (3) after healing, fibrous atrophy of the glands followed by permanent diminution of secretion owing to loss of gland substance.[12]

When glands produce a serous or mucous secretion, or both, it is the serous secretion that is most affected, leading to viscidity and acidity of the saliva with a reduction in quantity. The degree of postradiation dryness depends on the extent of the destruction of the secretory glands, which is rarely total and there is often therefore some belated return of secretion. When dryness is persistent and severe, however, it is surprising how patients develop their own ways of coping with this problem: many carry a bottle of water in their pockets; acid sweets sometimes help, as does artificial saliva (glycerine, 4 parts; simple syrup, 1 part; tincture of lemon 10 ml. to 2 l.); and when dryness wakes the patient at night, a small quantity of liquid paraffin is most useful.

Two important sequelae to the changes in the salivary secretions are: (1) a marked tendency to develop monilial infection (thrush), which can usually be prevented or controlled by attention to oral hygiene and the use of nystatin; and (2) dental caries, which has already been discussed.

### *Smell*

Least is known concerning the effect of radiotherapy on the sense of smell, since patients very rarely notice or complain of its loss. During radiotherapy, however, blockage of the nose by disease, reaction or crusts will result in impairment of smell, and after radiotherapy, stenosis, adhesions or excessive crusting in the nasal passages will have the same effect. That there should be some deleterious effect on the sense of smell should be expected, since olfactory stimuli are probably chemical in nature, and hence the surface of the olfactory mucous membrane must be kept moist so as to furnish the necessary solvent for these stimulating agents.

The olfactory glands of Bowman are the source of the secretion that serves this function, and since they are serous glands, they are readily damaged by radiation with resulting functional loss. The olfactory glands appear to have a function similar to that of the glands connected with the taste buds. Fortunately, the radiation perversions and disturbances occurring with the sense of taste are not encountered with the sense of smell, a fact that may be due to the relative unimportance of the latter sense in man.

### *Hearing*

The effects of therapeutic irradiation on the normal external auditory canal and tympanic membrane have received scant description in the literature, but the following changes may be observed:

1. The wax in the external canal thickens and dries.

2. The tympanic membrane becomes red and congested, particularly in the region of the handle of the malleus.

3. Edema may next occur and is more marked anteroinferiorly in the region of the junction of the bony and cartilaginous parts of the canal and where the canal overlies the temporomandibular joint. The edema in this region may be sufficiently marked to hide most of the drum from view.

4. Irradiation membrane may form along the floor of the external canal, but in the absence of ulceration within the canal, widespread membrane formation is rarely apparent. If, however, excessive irradiation is given, the canal becomes edematous, its walls are covered by membrane and the drum head is obscured. It is very rare to see irradiation membrane on the normal drum.

The vestibular apparatus appears to be relatively immune to radiation; only exceptionally are vestibular symptoms encountered. The patient who is already a sufferer from tinnitus or nerve deafness is uninfluenced for better or worse by irradiation. Under proper therapeutic conditions, nerve deafness induced by radiation in a previously normal ear must be almost unknown. This is to be expected in light of the known tolerance of nervous tissue to radiation and the fact that the nervous components of other special sense organs rarely suffer permanent or chronic injury from radiation. This is manifestly so in the case of the olfactory mucous membrane, the taste buds and retina.

Deafness of conduction type is commonly encountered and may be due to the following:

1. *Thick mucus* in the nasopharynx with constant downward drip into the lower pharynx may plague the patient for a long time after radiation treatment. The mucus may pocket in the lateral nasopharynx and block either temporarily or repeatedly the eustachian opening with consequent impaired hearing. In some cases of this kind, a serous effusion in the middle ear may also follow and subsequently become infected.

2. *Atresia of the eustachian orifice* may occur when there has been extensive neoplastic destruction of the eustachian orifice followed by healing. In these cases, fibrosis and narrowing of the orifice ensue. A rare cause of atresia is necrosis of the eustachian cartilage, characterized by severe earache and trismus. The exposed cartilage can usually be seen on examination, and in the absence of sepsis, no special treatment is required.

Healing usually takes place with resultant deformity of the eustachian orifice.

3. *Fibrosis* of the fascial space surrounding the levator muscle of velum palatini.

### *Sight*[7]

Radiation has an unfortunate reputation among ophthalmologists, who have never forgotten the disasters following its use in the early days of radiotherapy. A sound eye that is normal in position will tolerate radiation well, provided infection and trauma are avoided. The only complication that might occur in these circumstances is cataract formation, a risk that is acceptable. Since the treatment we recommend for upper jaw cancer[9] is a combination of radiotherapy and surgery, ocular problems inevitably arise when, as is the custom, the eye is retained during the preoperative radiation. In particular, the decision has to be made as to whether or not the eye should be sacrificed during the subsequent operation, especially if there is need for an extended maxillectomy.

The common so-called extended maxillectomy becomes necessary when there is simultaneous involvement of the maxilloethmoidal region and the orbitomalar region, if the lesion crosses the midline at the ethmoidal or palatal levels or there is gross involvement of the nasal fossa. Exenteration of the orbit should not be routinely performed as part of an extended operation on the jaw unless orbital disease with ocular displacement persists after a full course of irradiation.

## ENDOCRINE GLANDS

There are three endocrine glands that are often irradiated during the treatment of head and neck cancer.

These are the pituitary gland, which should always be included in the treatment field when irradiating nasopharyngeal neoplasms, and the thyroid and parathyroid glands, which are irradiated when treating laryngeal and hypopharyngeal cancer and metastatic cervical lymph node deposits.

It may be accepted that these endocrine glands, if normal at the beginning of treatment, will tolerate without significant change the necessary therapeutic doses of radiation that may be given to a neighboring neoplasm.

Occasional reports exist on the occurrence of hypothyroidism after external beam therapy and pituitary dwarfism in children suffering from nasopharyngeal cancer. There is, however, no recorded case of parathyroid damage following irradiation.

Although from a practical point of view it would seem that these particular endocrine glands are not especially vulnerable, it is clearly prudent for the radiotherapist to preserve them from irradiation when this can be achieved without risk of inadequately irradiating the primary lesion.

## RADIATION CARCINOGENESIS

The fact that ionizing radiation can give rise to malignant neoplasms has long been known. The precise magnitude of this risk to a patient undergoing radiotherapy is unknown but, on available evidence, must be so small as not to act as a contraindication to this form of treatment.

The radiation-induced cancers that are seen at the moment are largely a heritage from previous generations when there was a wide use of radiation in the treatment of many nonmalignant conditions for which specific remedies now exist.

Ringworm, acne, sycosis barbae, tuberculous cervical adenitis, hyperthyroidism and hypertrophy of the tonsils and the thymus gland were all at one time favorably influenced and treated by radiation, frequently and repeatedly. Unfortunately, the treatment techniques then prevailing depended on the use of low voltage x-rays and small doses being given over long periods of time. As a result, whatever improvement may have taken place in the disease being treated, permanent changes were inflicted on the normal skin and subcutaneous tissues, the mucosa and the salivary and thyroid glands. Most of the patients submitted to this form of radiation in this era were children or young adults, and a latent period of 10 to 20 years or more appears to be necessary before a malignant neoplasm manifests itself. Such neoplasms may affect the skin, pharynx, larynx and thyroid gland.

The occurrence of late radiation-induced carcinoma in patients who have already had therapeutic radiation for a previous malignant tumor is rare but is seen in patients who as children received treatment, usually for a malignant tumor in the neighborhood of the eye and orbit (Fig. 23–12).

In the case of adults suffering from the common epitheliomata of the head and neck region, the development of radiation-induced neoplasms is unlikely to be a serious hazard, since the age of the patient is usually such that the majority will die either of their disease or intercurrent causes long before the expiry of the long latent period the onset of this particular malignant process requires. With modern techniques of treatment, the gross tissue changes that seem to be a prerequisite to carcinogenesis are infrequently produced.

In the author's experience, covering the treatment of nearly 10,000 patients suffering from head and neck neoplasms over the past 40 years, there are two cases in which it is possible that the patients died of radiation-induced carcinoma. In one, a case of cancer of the soft palate, the patient developed carcinoma of the external auditory canal, which was just within the treatment fields 11 years after healing of the palate. In the second, a case of advanced cancer of the antrum, a carcinoma involving the base of skull appeared 29 years after treatment. There are two further observations that deserve attention.

1. The risk of radiation-induced cancer should not be invoked as a reason for denying young patients radiotherapy if the lesion is otherwise suitable for this treatment.

2. In the author's experience, radiation-induced cancer is amenable to successful treatment by radiation (Fig. 23–12). Although it is desirable to offer these patients primary surgical treatment, if this is impractical for any reason, radiotherapy, although technically often more difficult and hazardous, can usually be undertaken and may be successful because a radiation-induced neoplasm does not lose its radiosensitivity owing to its etiology. It would seem that these tumors are comparable in radiosensitivity to similar spontaneously occurring tumors of the same histology and involving the same site. In these circumstances, the radiotherapist's problems lie partly in destroying the tumor but above all in insuring that, once this is done, healing will take place in the abnormal radiation-damaged tumor bed.

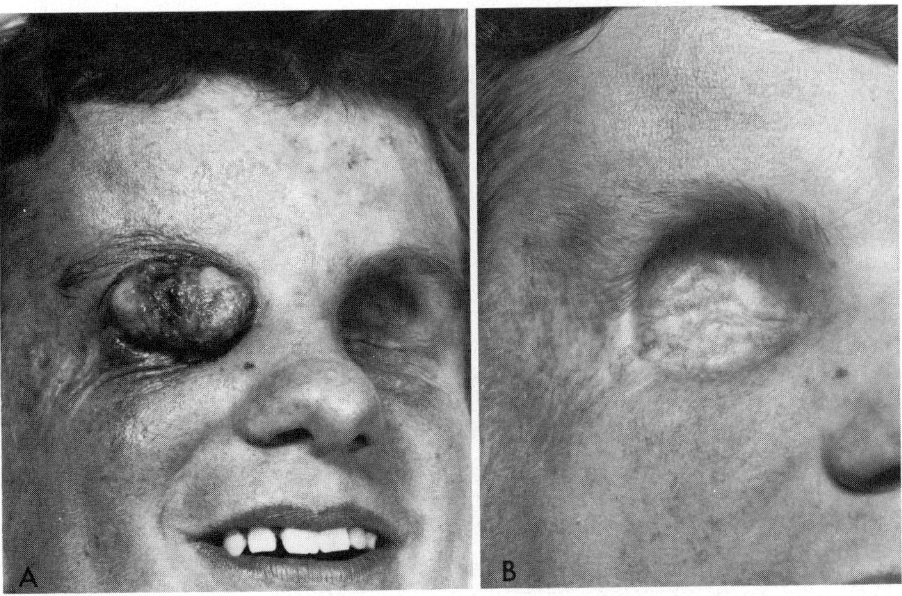


**Figure 23–12** *A,* Radiation-induced fibrosarcoma of lids 20 years after radiation treatment and enucleation of the eyes for bilateral retinoblastoma. *B,* After treatment: radium needle implant to right orbit. Dose: 3200 rads in 51 hours. Patient well 7 years later.

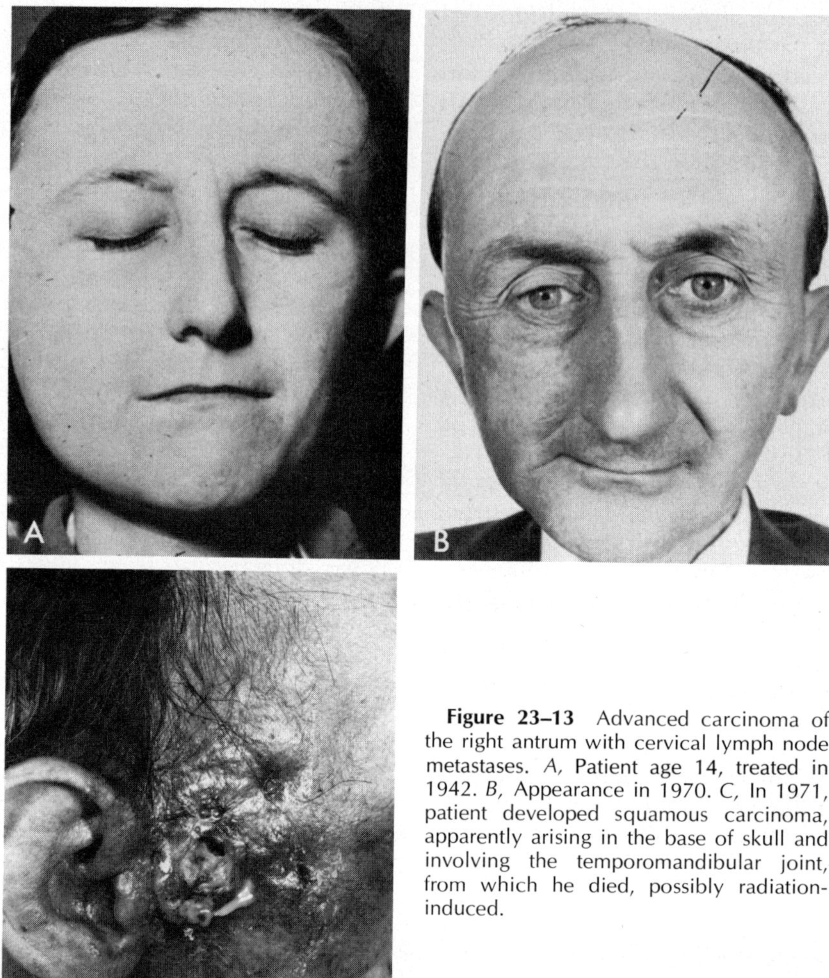


**Figure 23–13** Advanced carcinoma of the right antrum with cervical lymph node metastases. *A,* Patient age 14, treated in 1942. *B,* Appearance in 1970. *C,* In 1971, patient developed squamous carcinoma, apparently arising in the base of skull and involving the temporomandibular joint, from which he died, possibly radiation-induced.

To do this often means that reliance cannot be placed on external beam therapy; other more localized techniques, particularly those of radioactive implantation, may have to be employed.

## PREVENTION OF COMPLICATIONS

Observations have already been made suggesting ways in which some of the more serious radiation complications might be prevented. In general terms, most of these complications can be avoided or certainly reduced in frequency if a number of common sense rules are observed.

**Selection of cases.** In the same way as a surgeon refrains from operating if conditions are not reasonably favorable for success, so the radiotherapist should avoid using radiation indiscriminately. Whatever the emotional pressures brought to bear, some patients are better not treated by radiotherapy. In some cases, radiotherapy can be profitably used as an adjunct to surgery, particularly as a preoperative measure when cartilage or bone invasion or metastatic lymph nodes are present. The need for care in the retreatment of recurrent cases needs no emphasis.

**Technical factors.** The use of large fields, high doses and short treatment times will carry risks. During the course of irradiation treatment there should be a regular change of fields in conformity with the change in the tumor, and as doses are increased, so treatment times should be lengthened. A standard tumor dose does not exist, and therefore there is no justification for the routine use of rigid standard field arrangements and time-dose relationships.

**Control of reactions.** Although the use of high-energy radiation reduces the general and local reactions encountered, they cannot be entirely eliminated. Fortunately, radiation reactons can be put to use in the sense that their clinical interpretation furnishes some guide to treatment and moreover they can be controlled in degree by attention to dose and timing of treatments. In this way, the patient's discomforts can be minimized and late damaging effects can be avoided.

**Trauma and infection.** Dental extraction, badly fitting dentures and ill-advised biopsy, particularly from the larynx, may all open up pathways of infection of irradiated tissues, with resulting osteitis and chondritis, and should therefore be avoided. In the case of heavily irradiated skin, trauma and exposure to intense sunlight should be avoided.

## CERVICAL LYMPH NODE IRRADIATION

In the attempt to achieve both adequate irradiation of the cervical lymph nodes and at the same time avoid damage to normal structures, the following measures can be considered:

**Technique of limited risk.** Depending on the site of origin and histology of the primary tumor, it is permissible to omit certain lymph node stations from the field of irradiation. With squamous cancer limited to the upper or lower segments of the pharynx, the submaxillary and submental nodes can be excluded, and the lower cervical and upper cervical lymph nodes when the primary is in the upper and lower parts of the pharynx, respectively. Elective irradiation of the posterior triangle of the neck is mainly necessary for primary squamous cell carcinoma of the nasopharynx and malignant lymphomata arising from Waldeyer's ring.

**Selection of apparatus.** When using fields directed laterally to the neck, an electron beam has obvious advantages, particularly in helping to avoid irradiation of the spinal cord.

**Dosage.** When using large fields involving simultaneous irradiation of the head and neck, reassessment of technique is essential at the fourth week after a tumor dose of 4000 rads has been delivered.

When the spinal cord has been included in the field of radiation and received 4000 rads in four weeks, steps should be taken so as to avoid its further irradiation.

**Protective shielding.** In the attempt to avoid the unnecessary irradiation of adjacent normal tissue and above all to protect nearby organs or tissues that have important functions and may be vulnerable to irradiation, protective shielding may be employed.

At orthovoltage energies, protection can be achieved by placing some absorbing material, such as lead, directly over the part to be shielded. At high energies, the thickness of lead required to do this could not be supported by the patient. In these circumstances, an indirect method of shielding is used whereby the radiation field is first delineated by a light beam, and a lead absorber is then placed in the beam of irradiation so that the tissue requiring protection is brought within the shadow produced by the interposed absorbing material. This indirect method of shielding is of great value in protecting the eye and lacrimal gland during orbital irradiation and the anterior compartment of the neck and cervical spinal cord during cervical node irradiation, when a "split field" technique is used.

### Bibliography

1. Ackerman, L. V., and Del Regato, J. A.: Cancer: Diagnosis, Treatment and Prognosis. Rev. ed. St. Louis, The C. V. Mosby Company, 1970.
2. Catterall, M., Sutherland, S., and Bewley, D.: First results of a randomized clinical trial of fast neutrons compared with X or gamma rays in treatment of advanced tumors of the head and

neck. Report to the Medical Research Council. Br. Med. J., *2*:653–656, 1975.

3. Coffin, F.: The control of radiation caries. Br. J. Radiol., *46*:365–368, 1973.
4. Grise, J. W., Rubin, P., Ryplansky, A., et al.: Factors influencing response and recovery of grafted skin to ionizing irradiation; experimental observations. Am. J. Roentgenol., *83*:1087–1096, 1960.
5. Lawrence, J. H., and Tobias, C. A.: Heavy particles in therapy. *In* Wood, C., and Deeley, T. (eds.): Modern Trends in Radiotherapy. New York, Appleton-Century Crofts, 1967, p. 267.
6. Lederman, M.: Cancer of the Nasopharynx. Springfield, Illinois, Charles C Thomas, 1960.
7. Lederman, M.: Systems of Ophthalmology. *In* Duke-Elder, S. (ed.): Textbook of Ophthalmology. Vol. VII. St. Louis, The C. V. Mosby Company, 1962, pp. 764–797.
8. Lederman, M.: Malignant tumors of the ear. J. Laryngol., *79*:85–119, 1965.
9. Lederman, M., Busby, E. R., and Mould, R. F.: The treatment of tumors of the upper jaw. Br. J. Radiol., *42*:561–581, 1969.
10. Lederman, M.: Tumors of the upper jaw: Natural history and treatment. J. Laryngol., *84*:369–401, 1970.
11. Pallis, C. A., Louis, S., and Morgan, R. L.: Radiation myelopathy. Brain, *84*:460–479, 1961.
12. Rafla, S., and Rotman, M.: Introduction to Radiotherapy. St. Louis, The C. V. Mosby Company, 1974.
13. Reese, A.: Tumors of the Eye. 2nd ed. New York, Harper and Row, Publishers, 1963.
14. Rubin, P., and Casarett, G. W.: Clinical Radiation Pathology. Philadelphia, W. B. Saunders Company, 1968.
15. Stone, R. S., Lawrence, J. H., and Aebersold, P. C.: Preliminary report on use of fast neutrons in treatment of malignant disease. Radiology, *35*:322–327, 1940.
16. Stone, R. S.: Neutron therapy and specific ionization: Janeway memorial lecture. Am. J. Roentgenol., *59*:771–785, 1948.
17. Vaeth, J.: Radiation induced myelitis. *In* Buschke, F. (ed.): Progress in Radiation Therapy. Vol. 3. New York, Grune and Stratton, 1965, pp. 16–27.

# 24 COMPLICATIONS OF FACIAL TRAUMA

*Reed O. Dingman*
*Paul H. Izenberg*

Facial trauma complications frequently occur as a result of inadequate primary diagnosis and treatment. Numerous publications have covered this primary care; however, some important diagnostic features and initial treatment of facial fractures will be reviewed here. Only through adequate primary treatment can many of these secondary complications be avoided.

## ASSOCIATED INJURIES

Facial fractures, especially those resulting from high speed deceleration accidents, may be associated with multiple system injuries (Fig. 24–1). Recognition of these problems by the primary surgeon is important and frequently lifesaving.

### AIRWAY OBSTRUCTION

Respiratory insufficiency resulting from severe facial trauma calls for immediate assessment and prompt treatment. Frequently, such simple procedures as forward traction on the tongue and suctioning with removal of blood, tooth fragments and debris from the pharynx will save a life. If there is comminution of the mandible with loss of anterior tongue support, the base of the tongue may fall back on the posterior pharynx and obstruct the airway. Anterior traction on the tongue and fractured mandibular segment along with insertion of an oral or nasopharyngeal airway may suffice. If an airway cannot be established by these simpler methods, endotracheal intubation or emergency tracheostomy is necessary. In an unconscious patient, reflex maintenance of the airway frequently is difficult or impossible. In addition, although the conscious patient with facial fractures may initially be able to maintain his airway, with progressive fatigue or tissue edema the probability of needing intubation or tracheostomy increases. Endotracheal intubation is preferable to tracheostomy if the need for respiratory assistance appears to be of relatively short duration. Especially in children, tracheostomy should be avoided if possible because of the complications associated with decanulation and potential tracheal stenosis.

### ASPIRATION

Aspiration of blood, gastric contents and debris is not uncommon. McCoy and his associates (1966)[62] discuss aspiration as a frequently overlooked complication in facial fractures in children. Passage of a nasogastric tube to remove gastric contents and to relieve gastric dilation secondary to trauma should be routine. If anesthesia is to be given, use of a cuffed endotracheal tube and a cuffed tracheostomy tube may help prevent this. Once aspiration does occur, prompt treatment with vigorous suctioning, irrigation and fiberoptic bronchoscopy should be performed to avoid or lessen the subsequent bronchospasm, edema and pneumonia. Aspiration of solid materials (dentures, teeth, food and so on) should be

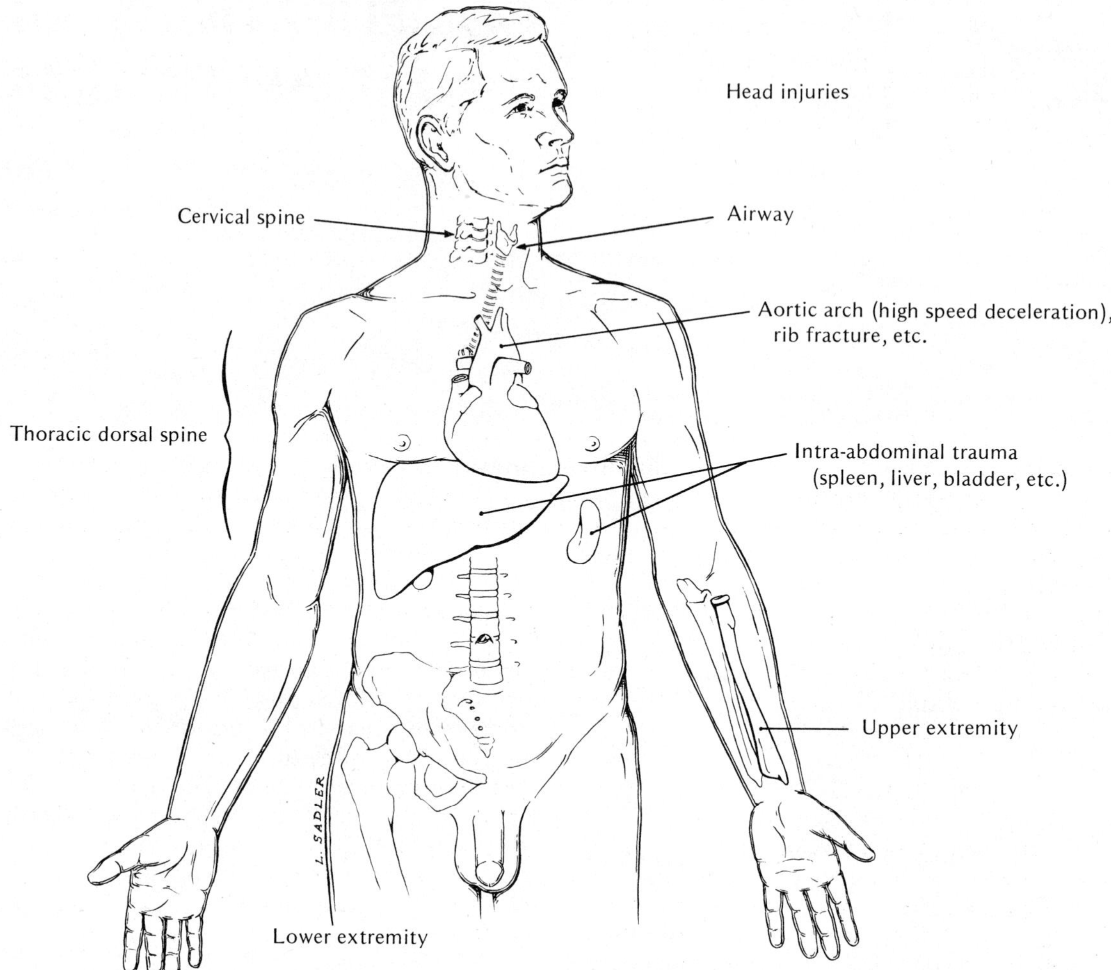


**Figure 24–1** Diagram depicting the multiple injuries frequently associated with facial fractures.

suspected if maintenance of an adequate upper airway does not improve the respiratory status. Chest x-ray may reveal the location of a foreign body, which should be removed if possible.

## CERVICAL SPINE INJURY

In the excitement of establishing an airway, controlling hemorrhage, doing a brief neurologic evaluation and checking facial injuries, a cervical spine injury may be overlooked. The consequence may be paraplegia, quadriplegia or death. Cervical spine fracture is not uncommon in association with facial fractures resulting from high speed injuries. On admission to the emergency room, the patient's head is immediately supported with sandbags to avoid unnecessary movement and to remind all emergency room personnel of the potential neck injury. The patient is evaluated for posterior neck pain or discomfort. The neck is carefully palpated but flexion is avoided. If emergency endotracheal intubation is needed, minimal head manipulation should be the rule. Grip strength, movement of all extremities and deep tendon reflexes can help establish the gross neurologic status of the patient. All patients with facial injuries secondary to deceleration accidents must have cervical spine films done as soon as possible while they are in the emergency room.

### OTHER INJURIES

The larynx is vulnerable to fracture. A laryngeal fracture should be suspected if subcutaneous emphysema or aphonia is present. Pneumomediastinum and pneumothorax may result also. If examination reveals a laryngeal fracture, tracheostomy is the immediate treatment. An unrecognized laryngeal fracture may be fatal.

Chest and abdominal injuries should be suspected, and the patient should be fully evaluated in this light. Aortic arch and tracheal tears related to deceleration injuries are seen occasionally.

### SOFT TISSUE INJURIES

A better understanding of individual soft tissue complications may be obtained if one quickly reviews the process of normal and abnormal healing of the soft tissues.

Soft tissue healing can be divided into three phases: (1) acute inflammatory, (2) cellular and (3) maturation. During these phases, the wound may heal normally with minimal granulation tissue and contracture, or abnormal delayed healing may occur with increased scar formation and resulting complications.[59, 66]

Epithelialization is a separate process, with mobilization of basal cells, migration, proliferation and differentiation of the migrated cells.

A clean surgical wound healing follows these phases, usually resulting in a nondistorting, well-healed wound. The healing of a traumatic wound frequently differs. If severe tissue damage is present, as with crush injuries, or if the wound is grossly contaminated with irritants or pathogenic bacteria, the healing process is delayed, with resulting increased scar formation and contracture deformities. This is felt to be due to the plugging of lymphatics, vascular stasis and anoxia resulting in local destructive inflammation. This can progress, especially with the presence of foreign bodies (dirt, grease, and so on), to a chronic inflammatory reaction and granuloma formation. This emphasizes the need for meticulous surgical technique, hemostasis, asepsis, adequate debridement and avoidance of strangulating sutures in order to permit normal wound healing and minimization of scar. Many of the poor results called complications could have been completely avoided if simple wound care principles had been adhered to.

The length of time from injury to repair is important. A clean laceration up to 24-hours-old on the face may be closed after adequate local preparation. A contaminated wound a few hours old or a human bite would should not be closed primarily. The results of delayed primary repair may be better than primary wound closure complicated by infection.

Local anesthesia may be difficult to attain in facial injury patients because of local tissue edema, but it is important to have a quiet, cooperative patient while evaluating, cleansing or closing a wound. Sensory and motor nerves should be evaluated prior to anesthetizing any wound.

The injury site is carefully debrided of only fully devascularized tissue. Surrounding soft tissue should be explored for foreign bodies (glass, tooth fragments, clothing fragments or road gravel). Irrigation with saline under moderate pressure (syringe, commercial irrigator) should be used. Prophylactic antibiotics are used in contaminated wounds.

A few factors that may lead to poor results are as follows: (1) a contused wound; (2) wounds crossing natural lines of skin tension; (3) wounds closed under tension; (4) fair skin, which predisposes to scars that remain red for longer periods; (5) skin elasticity — young skin tends to stretch and the scars widen, while older skin shows less of this; and (6) darker skin, which is predisposed to hyperpigmented scars.

### LACERATIONS

Proper repair of straight line uncomplicated lacerations has been well described.[39] The need for accurate, tension-free approximation of wound edges with slight eversion cannot be overstressed. Skin suture marks (scars) are related to tension and length of time the sutures are in place.[15] Sutures should be removed from the face in five to seven days. If there is need for longer wound support, "Steristrips" or paper tape may be used after suture removal. A running subcuticular suture frequently will assure accurate approximation of wound edges with no suture marks. If a wound is closed under slight tension, a running dermal suture is used for initial approximation, followed by a second, more superficial subcuticular running suture. Keeping the suture line clean and free of blood and serum crusts minimizes infection and allows better primary epithelialization. With multiple small parallel lacerations from windshield trauma, some of the skin bridges between lacerations may be excised prior to suturing. If areas heal irregularly, later dermabrasion may be useful in improving the appearance. Stellate lacerations frequently heal with a central pitting scar. Small irregular lacerations may be totally excised to give straight margins before primary closure.

The beveled laceration will usually slough some of the thin skin edge and re-epithelialization results in a wider, thicker scar. This may be avoided by cutting the skin edges perpendicularly, elminating the thin bevel, and closing the wound as a simple straight laceration. An avulsion flap or "trap-door" laceration, unless small enough to be excised primarily, will frequently heal with venous and lymphatic engorgement of the flap. This plus circular contracture of the scar results in a thick contracted mound of tissue with an obvious stepoff. Revision should be postponed until re-establishment of the lymphatic circulation and softening of the tissues (six months to one year). The technique of revision is well described (Fig. 24–2).[2, 41]

Full thickness skin loss may necessitate flaps or graft reconstruction and cannot be adequately discussed here. The defect should be primarily closed, if possible, or covered with skin grafts. In most cases, we attempt to get primary wound closure with a split or full thickness skin graft and correct any subsequent defect at a later time. Contracture of a split thickness skin graft may allow simple excision of the graft and direct closure after several months. Replantation of an avulsed segment of facial skin has been tried many times, sometimes with success. Usually, the replaced avulsed segment acts as a biologic dressing for a few days, but necrosis and local infection will eventually occur with loss of tissue. Replaced small (1.5 cm.) segments may survive as free grafts. Microvascular techniques now make replantation of large avulsed segments of tissue possible. Microsurgical replantation of an avulsed lip and nose[44] and a total scalp[57] have been reported.

If the full thickness loss is small, a pre- or postauricular full thickness skin replacement should be primarily considered, for example, at the nasal tip. This usually gives a better cosmetic result than a split thickness skin graft.

#### DERMA TATTOO

Blast and abrasion injuries to the face can result in severe derma tattoo. Once these particles are fixed in the tissues (approximately 12 hours), they are extremely difficult to remove primarily. The involved skin should be scrubbed with a stiff brush under local or general anesthesia. For deeper particles, immediate individual excision[34] appears to work well. If the foreign bodies are already fixed, formal dermabrasion is necessary. Unfortunately, late treatment is never as effective as removal of the pigment at the time of primary care.

### *Individual Facial Soft Tissue Injuries*

#### THE PINNA

The external ear, if managed properly, can recover from significant trauma. The blood supply to the ear is excellent, and vigorous debridement usually is not necessary. Most auricular tissue will survive even if attached by only a very small pedicle. All tissue should be reapproximated by careful suturing and supported by a wet cotton dressing packed carefully into contours of the ear anteriorly and posteriorly.

A subperichondrial hematoma must be aspirated or drained to avoid cartilaginous thickening and "cauliflower" ear deformity. If the injury is six weeks old, curetting the granulation tissue and scar may reproduce the normal contour. A tie-over bolster to hold the skin against the cartilage helps avoid recurrent hematoma. True "cauliflower" ears are difficult to recontour, although the ear may be significantly improved by surgery.

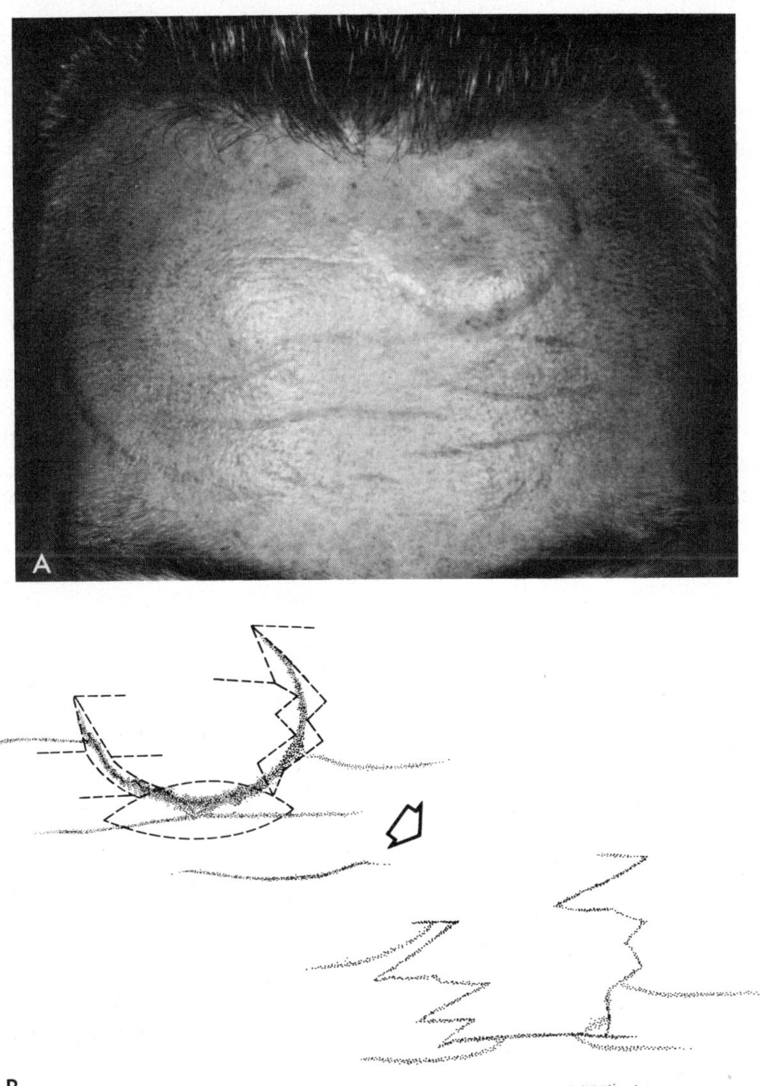

**Figure 24–2** *A,* A trapdoor scar deformity. *B,* Diagram of surgical treatment of trapdoor deformities. Partial simple excision in conjunction with multiple W and Z plasties.

**EYELIDS**

Reliance on primary care to avoid secondary complications is extremely important in eyelid injuries. Most authors agree that the best possibility of avoiding lid contractures and dysfunction is anatomic primary closure in three layers: (1) conjunctiva, tarsal plate, (2) muscle and (3) skin, with attention to exact approximation of the gray line. Before any soft tissue repair is attempted, thorough eye examination including visual acuity and corneal inspection is mandatory. If there is any question of direct ocular trauma or compromised vision, an ophthalmology consult should be obtained. Ocular complications of facial trauma will be discussed in the section on orbital fractures (p. 383). The eye may be protected during repair by a plastic corneal lens.

Secondary contracture of the upper lid can be tragic if desiccation of the cornea is persistent. Contracture may first be noted as a small upper lid notch and progress to gross ectropion. Opening the scar, recreating the original defect and proper repair may be all that is required. Local Z-plasties sometimes suffice if full thickness deficiency of eyelid skin is the problem. Full thickness skin from the opposite upper lid provides the most natural tissue for upper eyelid repair. If sufficient skin is not available, a thin split skin graft is useful. Full thickness skin from the pre- and postauricular areas placed on the mobile lid frequently results in a stiff, poorly functioning lid. Postauricular skin is adequate for lower lid reconstruction.[60]

Lid ptosis may result as a complication of a missed levator palpebral muscle or aponeurosis laceration. Although the levator is frequently difficult to find in the original injury, it is important to repair primarily if at all possible. Secondary repair is difficult and the results are inconsistent.[4] A wait of six months is recommended before a secondary repair procedure is attempted.

#### LACRIMAL APPARATUS

Damage to the lacrimal drainage system may be associated with an isolated soft tissue injury with nasal and naso-orbital bony trauma. The treatment principles and complications are similar.

If a disruption of the lacrimal drainage apparatus is suspected, primary repair should be attempted, since secondary repairs are fraught with difficulty and frequent failure. Repair of an individual canaliculus (upper or lower) is not absolutely necessary if one is sure that the uninvolved canaliculus is functioning. If repair is attempted, care to avoid damage to the functioning canaliculus is mandatory. Even with adequate primary treatment, stricture is still not uncommon and dilatation or surgery may be necessary. Medial canthal ligament injury should be looked for and be repaired primarily, as secondary repair is also difficult.

A stricture of the common canaliculus proximally may be resected and reanastomosis attempted. This complication usually will have to be treated by dacryocystorhinostomy. The success of this operation is 70 to 100 per cent, with few complications or reobstructions.

Destruction of the medial 3 to 4 mm. of both canaliculi or failure of the dacryocystorhinostomy may be treated with a conjunctivodacryocystorhinostomy.[45] These complications should be handled in conjunction with an oculoplastic surgeon. This procedure and others mentioned are described in detail in other publications.[4, 45, 87]

#### PAROTID DUCT

Lacerations of the parotid duct should be repaired at the time of initial injury if at all possible. Facial lacerations that cross the middle third of a line drawn from the tragus of the ear to the mid portion of the upper lip should be suspect. Saliva draining from the wound, significant swelling at the wound site and paralysis of muscles of the upper lip and nose (buccal branch of the seventh cranial nerve) may be associated findings. The duct should be cannulated and, if lacerated, repaired.

#### FACIAL NERVE

Laceration of the facial nerve and associated complications are not within the scope of this chapter. Needless to say, it is important to recognize this injury initially because it is now well known that primary repair yields the best functional results. The repair should be accomplished within 72 hours post injury if possible. Fine peripheral branches (those medial to a line dropped from the lateral canthus of the eye) need not be repaired, with usual return of function.

## COMPLICATIONS OF MANDIBULAR FRACTURES

The complications of mandibular fractures will be discussed as acute and late and in relation to the individual modes of treatment.

### *Acute Complications*

#### RESPIRATORY COMPLICATIONS

Respiratory complications of mandibular fractures are classified in two categories: (1) upper airway obstruction related to fracture of surgery and (2) aspiration.

A comminuted fracture of the mandible may be associated with significant bony and soft tissue displacement posteriorly secondary to muscle pull and loss of support to the floor of the mouth and the hyoid tissues. Posterior displacement may result in upper airway obstruction. If this occurs, immediate anterior support to the retroplaced segment of the mandible and soft tissues by traction on a large suture passed through the tongue may suffice. If this fails to establish adequate airway, an oropharyngeal or nasopharyngeal airway is placed. If the patient continues to remain obstructed, endotracheal intubation or tracheostomy should be done. Occasionally, parapharyngeal edema and interstitial hemorrhage will cause incomplete but dangerous airway obstruction, correctable by insertion of a nasopharyngeal tube, which also provides a passageway for sunctioning.

Early mandibular surgery may significantly increase existing soft tissue edema, resulting in obstructive symptoms not originally present post trauma.

When planning corrective operations that require postoperative intermaxillary fixation by interdental ligation, splints or other appliances, careful consideration of means to guarantee an adequate airway will prevent troublesome complications and even death of the patient. The methods used will vary with

1. the age of the patient
2. the severity of associated injuries
3. presence or absence of respiratory tract reflexes
4. suspected presence of intracranial injury
5. injury to air passage structures
6. duration of potential airway problems
7. presence of food in the upper GI tract

The following methods are useful in maintaining an airway and in aiding airway toilet in the injured, semicomatose or unconscious, aged or weakened postoperative patient:

1. Nasogastric suction to prevent aspiration of vomitus.
2. Maintain the endotracheal cuffed tube until the patient recovers respiratory reflexes.
3. Nasopharyngeal flexible airway tube if anticipated need is less than 24 hours.
4. Planned elective tracheostomy at the beginning or the termination of the operation. If a long, protracted postoperative course is anticipated, as in aged patients, those with multiple associated serious injuries, absent tracheal reflexes, fractures of the larynx and intracranial injuries with coma and others with potential airway problems, do not wait until the situation is emergent before doing a tracheostomy. Do it early!
5. Delay intermaxillary fixation until the patient recovers from the general anesthetic and reflexly is able to maintain his airway. Appliances may be placed under general anesthesia and the mouth left open until completely recovered from the general anesthesia. Fixation of jaws can be done as soon as the patient recovers or the next day, if necessary, under mild sedation.
6. Operate under local anesthesia if general anesthesia poses an airway problem. Adequate sedation and deep V and cervical block anesthesia with lidocaine (Xylocaine) will be adequate for most maxillofacial operations.
7. Suction at bedside with flexible catheters. Suction through the nose, mouth, endotracheal tube or tracheostomy tube will aid in airway toilet. House staff and other attendants should receive instructions regarding its use.
8. Vaporization of inspired air. Lungs need moisture to transport oxygen and $CO_2$. If inspired air does not pass over normal upper respiratory mucosa, it should be humidified, e.g., in retained endotracheal tubes and tracheotomy tubes.

Airway complications may occur after intermaxillary fixation in patients who ordinarily would be expected to have an uncomplicated course. These are rare situations. Nausea and vomiting following intermaxillary fixation is one of these possibilities. The story is perpetuated of the death of American and British troops with jaws wired together who drowned in their own vomitus while crossing the English Channel from France to England during World War I. Vilroy Blair, Robert Ivy and Varastaad Kazanjian, in personal communications, deny knowledge of these reports, and the files of the Surgeon General fail to substantiate the story.

Threatened vomiting might be relieved by nasogastric suction and, if imminent, by release of intermaxillary wire fixation with wire cutters kept with the patient in the postoperative period.

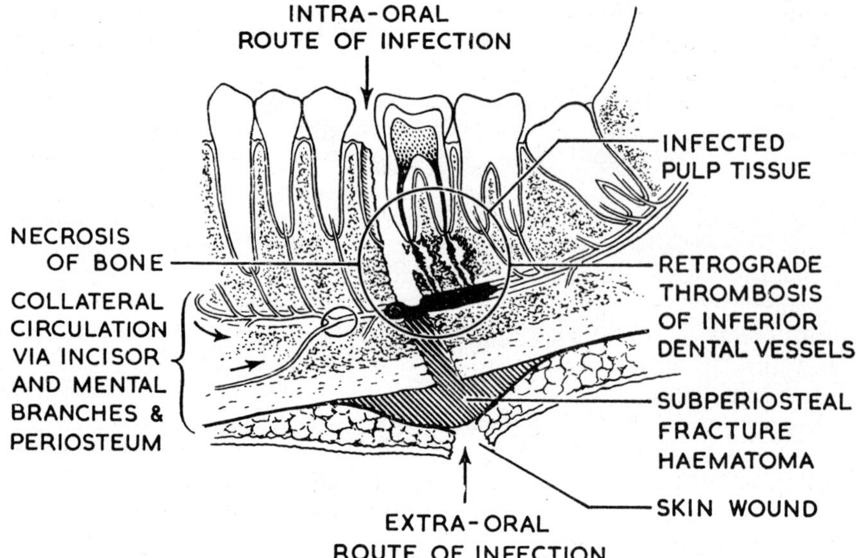


**Figure 24–3** The causes of infection in mandibular fractures. (From Rowe, N. L., and Killey, H. C.: Fractures of the Facial Skeleton. Baltimore, Williams and Wilkins Co., 1968.)

## HEMORRHAGE

Severe primary hemorrhage from mandibular fractures is uncommon except in gunshot wounds or severe avulsion injuries in which direct trauma to the facial, internal maxillary or external carotid vessels presents a more serious problem. Hemorrhage may result in aspiration and airway problems but is usually effectively controlled by pressure or direct ligation of the bleeding vessels. Local hematoma formation is common with mandibular fractures but usually is not significant enough to require drainage.

Late or delayed hemorrhage between the 4th and 12th days may occur after a gunshot wound as a result of clot disintegration or local infection. Bleeding may be from the facial, lingual or maxillary artery. Treatment consists of arresting the bleeding by packing the wound, direct ligation or external carotid ligation if necessary. Traumatic arteriovenous aneurysms occurring in areas of facial injury have been reported.[80] The treatment is surgical.

## INFECTION

The causes of infection are multiple (Fig. 24–3). Most fractures of the body of the mandible, even with slight displacement, are compound fractures and are initially contaminated through intraoral mucosal tears, from infected teeth in the fracture line or by compound external wounds.

Rarely are fractures of the ramus of the mandible infected at the initial injury except those compounded in the area of the ramus through facial lacerations or penetrating wounds, such as gunshot or shrapnel injuries.

Factors predisposing to infection of mandibular fracture site are:

Local

1. Poor oral hygiene, gingivitis, calculi, pyorrhea and local infection
2. Devitalized, infected or abscessed teeth in the area of the fracture
3. Hematoma in fracture area — ideal medium for infection
4. Delayed immobilization with moving open wounds
5. Lymphatic stasis due to direct injury
6. Edema and local tissue damage
7. Destruction of periosteum
8. Foreign bodies in wound: dirt, glass, wood, metal and so on
9. Devitalization and abscess of fractured teeth

General

1. Age
2. Malnutrition

3. Debilitating disease
4. Constitutional disease, i. e., diabetes, blood dyscrasia and so on

**PREVENTION AND AVOIDANCE OF INFECTION**

Infection is a serious complication because of increased morbidity, disability and such undesirable results as (1) delayed healing; (2) nonunion; (3) osteomyelitis; (4) loss of tooth and bone structure; (5) extension of infection from local site to adjacent areas, i.e., soft tissue, abscess of neck, floor of mouth and temporomandibular joint; and (6) prolonged hospitalization, disability and greater expense.

Some factors, such as age, constitutional diseases, lowered resistance and debilitating disease, are beyond the initial control of the surgeon. Other factors predisposing to infection may be controlled or measures may be instituted to reduce the incidence of complications. For example,

1. Correction of anemia or total blood volume by transfusion.

2. Early use of antibiotics. Streptococci and staphylococci are the usual offending organisms in mandibular wound infections. Well-controlled series of fractures managed with and without prophylactic antibiotics are not available. Since the antibiotic era began, however, we have noted a dramatic decrease in the incidence of infection at the fracture site, and rarely do we encounter osteomyelitis as a complication. Undoubtedly, other factors in wound management and general care of the patients influence the decreased incidence of these complications. But there seem to be no adverse effects to the use of prophylactic antibiotics. Broad-spectrum drugs should be used intensively, early. Later, if infection is a problem, wound culture and sensitivity may indicate use of more specific drugs.

3. Institute immediate oral hygiene program: (a) frequent mouthwash with weak solution of hydrogen peroxide and water (1:4); (b) removal of debris, devitalized tissue, nonusable loose bone and tooth structure; (c) dental prophylaxis to remove plaque, calculus and film from the teeth; (d) brush the teeth three times a day with soft brush; (e) mechanical water pulsating device (WaterPik)

4. Early immobilization of fractures by supportive head bandages early (A Barton bandage decreases movement, reduces pain and may prevent pumping action at the wound site.) and wiring of selected teeth. (One or two wires on each side between maxillary and mandibular teeth will give immobilization until definitive surgery can be done.)

5. Early definitive treatment. Fractures of the mandible are seldom acute surgical emergencies but should be treated as early as is consistent with the general condition of the patient. An early aggressive approach reduces complications and shortens the convalescent period. For example, if an injured patient arrives at the emergency room with an extensive facial laceration compounding a mandibular fracture and in satisfactory general condition for surgery, there is no better time at which to carry out definitive treatment. The wound can be debrided of loose bone and tooth fragments, foreign material, infected teeth and so on, and bone fragment wiring can be done immediately before closure of the soft tissue wound. In some instances, loss of segments of bone might be immediately replaced by bone grafts and local flaps used to provide tissue for wound closure (Fig. 24–4). Intermaxillary fixation, bone plates, intramedullary pins or external pin fixation are methods used to provide immobilization. Aggressive early surgery may reduce the possibility of wound infection, osteomyelitis, delayed union, malunion, nonunion, scar contracture and difficult secondary reconstructive procedures. Extensive wounds, or those in the presence of gross infection or contamination, should be drained to prevent hematoma or seroma, which provide ideal media for infection.

6. Teeth in the line of fracture. Teeth should be removed if they are loose and interfere with reduction of fragments, are devitalized and potentially a source of infection, are damaged beyond usefulness or may become devital and interfere with healing by becoming infected. Teeth should be retained if bony attachments are adequate for survival, the tooth is sound and important in maintaining fixation of fractured segments of bone (for example, a single molar on the proximal segment may prevent displacement if in contact with an

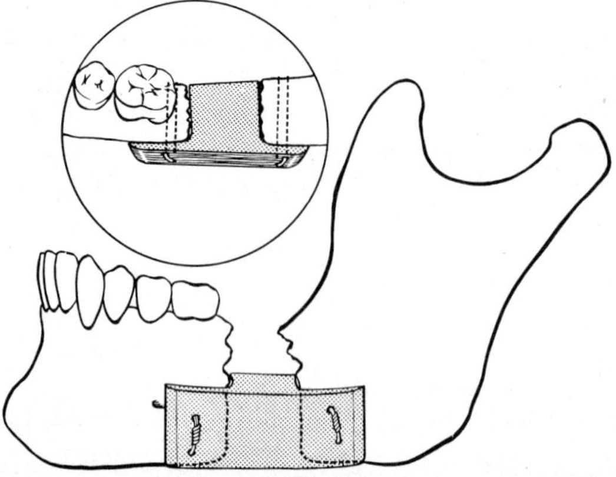

**Figure 24–4** Use of immediate iliac bone graft for stabilization of bone fragments in the case of traumatic bone loss. This method is applicable only if adequate soft tissue is available for covering the bone graft. (From Dingman, R. O., and Natvig, P.: Surgery of Facial Fractures. Philadelphia, W. B. Saunders Co., 1964.)

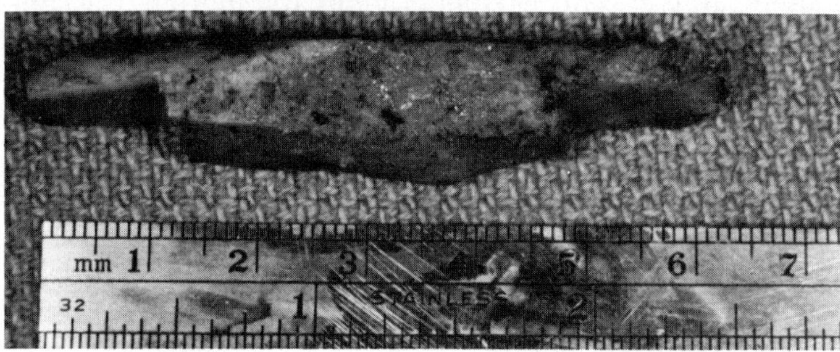


upper tooth) and its removal will add increased trauma, extend the severity of the wound and increase the possibility of infection (for example, a deeply impacted tooth in the line of fracture).

7. Bone fragments in the line of fracture usually will survive if they have an adequate periosteal attachment and should be preserved if they do not interfere with reduction. Free bone fragments should be retained and wired in a jigsaw pattern to the main fragments in cases of extensive damage. They often will survive as free grafts if the main segments are adequately immobilized and soft tissue coverage is adequate. Such wounds should be drained. Nonunion may be prevented in this manner.

8. Provide adequate drainage. If infection occurs before or after treatment, early drainage is imperative to prevent the spread of infection (Fig. 24–5). Drainage may be provided by removal of a loose or infected involved tooth in the line of fracture, incision through buccal sulcus mucosa to site of fracture with insertion of a drain, and submandibular incision for abscess drainage. Incision should be made in the direction of the skin folds and from 1 to 2 cm. below the mandibular border to avoid the ramus mandibularis and to minimize the scar. If a previously closed wound or scar is in the area of fluctuation, it may be opened for drainage and thus avoid an additional scar. Removal of foreign bodies, such as a tooth structure or devitalized bone fragments, should be accomplished. Do not make a direct attack on the bone ends at this time; you may spread infection. Interosseous wires, if implicated in the etiology of the infection, should be removed. If infection is due to other foreign material, the infection should clear with the wires still effectively supporting the fragments. Infections spreading to or localizing in the floor of the mouth usually are best drained through extraoral incision. Remember, to be effective, drainage of an abscess must be adequate. When infection is localized, antibiotic use is not a substitute for adequate drainage. Do not delay!

Osteitis is a limited inflammatory reaction involving bone. The bone may recover. Osteomyelitis is an extension of an acute infectious process extending into bone with necrosis, destruction and sequestration. Clinical differentiation between these two processes may be difficult. Osteomyelitis is usually associated with deep bone pain and extension of bony involvement even with adequate drainage. In the early stages, these processes are impossible to differentiate radiologically because in the early phase of normal physiologic repair there is a small degree of osteoporosis adjacent to the line of fracture.[73]

Ongoing osteomyelitis should be suspected if there is persistent pain after adequate immobilization and continued generous drainage at the fracture site. It may be several weeks before definite sequestra can be identified radiologically. Once osteomyelitis is diagnosed, adequacy of drainage and antibiotic coverage must be reassessed. Infectious osteomyelitis is best treated conservatively by correcting general deficiencies, generous drainage, antibiotics and careful removal of sequestra as they form. It is possible to have periodic sequestration involving most of the mandible over a prolonged period with total regeneration under conservative treatment.

## *Late Complications*

### DELAYED UNION, NONUNION AND MALUNION

There are multiple factors in the causes for delayed union, nonunion and malunion of mandibular fractures. Lack of adequate apposition of fragments, inadequate fragment immobilization, displacement of comminuted fracture fragments, aseptic necrosis of bone and soft tissue interposition are the major causes.

**Delayed union.** Mandibular fractures in the usual course of uncomplicated events and with adequate management heal with clinical stability within four to eight weeks. Healing may be protracted or delayed due to one or a combination of factors, including

1. Inadequate fixation with movement at the fracture site
2. Chronic infection at the line of fracture that finally resolves

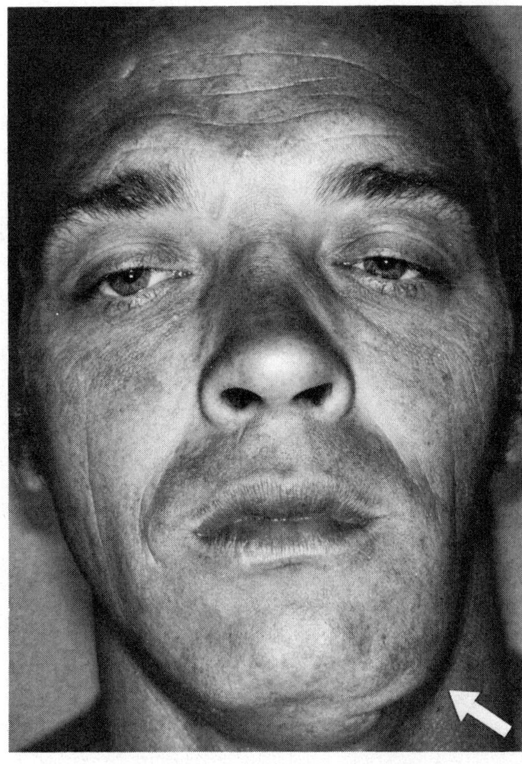

**Figure 24–5** Submandibular abscess complicating a fracture of the body of the mandible.

3. Presence of a foreign body at the fracture site, i.e., tooth root fragment, piece of devitalized bone, and so on
4. Inaccurate initial alignment of fragments
5. Separation of fragments
6. Advanced age
7. Debilitation, malnutrition, avitaminosis, and blood dyscrasia.

The eventual result is healing. If, upon removing fixation appliances at six to eight weeks, there is notable movement at the fracture site on bimanual manipulation or painful function with no unusual x-ray or clinical findings, the jaw should be immobilized for another period of eight to twelve weeks. Re-evaluation of all the above factors should be done and corrections made when feasible.

**Nonunion.** The usual causes of nonunion are

1. Inadequate approximation of fracture segments with lack of adequate contact between bone segments
2. Instability of fixation
3. Displacement and lack of alignment of comminuted bone segments
4. Aseptic necrosis of bone fragments
5. Soft tissue interposition between fragments
6. Osteomyelitis and bone absorption
7. Any of the constitutional, general or debilitating diseases.

Mathog[53] reported 2.4 per cent incidence of nonunion in 577 mandibular fractures over a five-year period. Eight of 14 cases of malunion were treated adequately with debridement, interosseous wiring and intermaxillary fixation; the remaining six required bone grafts because of significant defects. Because 50 per cent of these patients were edentulous, recommendations that additional means beyond splints and circumandibular wires should be seriously considered in the edentulous patient. Early incision and drainage with removal of tooth roots at the first sign of infection helps avoid osteomyelitis and subsequent nonunion.

Nonunion results in fibrous pseudoarthrosis at the fracture site with instability that, once formed, does not improve spontaneously.

Treatment of nonunion fractures. Some patients with minor disability do not wish or require treatment. Those with contour defects and malfunction because of the flail pseudoarthrosis and asymmetry wish to have treatment to facilitate dental reconstruction and to improve function and appearance. Surgery is the usual treatment, although dental appliances may be effective in some cases.

*Surgical Procedures*:

1. With minimal bone loss, exposure of the fracture site, removal of fibrous tissue, removal of eburnated bone ends and reapproximation of bone ends with interosseous wire fixation may result in union.
2. In cases with large bone defects, removal of fibrous tissue and scar, excision of eburnated bone from the ends of the fragments and iliac bone grafting usually produce an adequate reconstruction (Fig. 24–6). Iliac bone, cancellous block or chips are the best material for mandibular bone grafts in our hands. For small defects, grafts from adjacent mandible have been used. Methods of support and fixation after grafting vary with the individual problem. Fixation is from eight to twelve weeks.

The end result of treatment should be restoration of function and appearance.

The following brief discussion of bone healing as it pertains to the mandible is helpful in understanding its complications. At the moment of injury, disruption of the periosteum at the fracture site initiates reactivation of the osteogenic function of the inner periosteal layer. Hypertrophy of the osteoblasts not only takes place at the fracture site but also away from the site to assist in the formation of the callus. After resorption of necrotic bone, the osteoblasts from the endosteal surface of the bone, along with osteogenic cells derived from bone marrow, form a woven pattern of primary bone trabeculae. Fibroblasts also proliferate from the external surface of the periosteum and from the contiguous soft tissue. An inelastic fibrous investing layer forms around the entire fracture site. If the fracture segments are maintained in apposition, osseous union takes place without difficulty. If the fracture site is unstable, the fibroblastic layer is unable to invest the entire callus and advances between the masses of primary bone trabeculae before they fuse. Thus a fibroblastic barrier is formed that prevents bony union. If the fracture site is fixed in apposition at this time, as with a delayed repair, delayed and osseous union will occur. If the bony fragments remain unstable, pseudoarthrosis results with fibrocartilage formation and nonunion. Solid bone union therefore depends upon rigid immobilization in the early stages of healing.[73]

**Malunion.** Malunion of the mandibular fracture most frequently results from inadequate primary alignment or fixation. Malunion also is seen in cases in which primary repair was delayed by misdiagnosis or lack of treatment or when more serious injuries took precedence in treatment, also resulting in delay.

Multiple muscular contractile forces operate upon the mandible, with essentially four vectors of pull. The depressor-retractors pull the symphyseal area inferiorly and posteriorly. The elevators pull the angle superiorly. The protrusor (lateral pterygoid muscle) pulls the mandibular condyle anteriorly while the retractors (posterior fibers of temporalis, digastrics, geniohyoid and mylohyoid) pull the coronoid process posteriorly (Fig. 24–7). Depending on the direction of the fracture, these resultant forces may act to make a fracture either favorable or unfavorable in terms of stable bony apposition. Knowledge of this muscular pull is important in determining whether a fracture may be adequately immobilized using only interdental wiring or intermaxillary fixation as opposed to the need for direct interosseous wiring of the fracture site or other more rigid means of stabilization.

Malunion may present in a number of ways. A vertical malunion, such as those from condylar fractures or fractures of the mandibular rami, may present as open bite on the side opposite the injury. Malunion of fractures of the body and the angle of the mandible may present as a short mandibular arch on the involved side with malocclusion (crossbite, retrognathia). Obtaining normal post-treatment occlusion depends as much upon the type of primary fixation used as on proper initial alignment. If a patient has good dentition, the teeth should be aligned and fixed in functional occlusion. If abnormal dental occlusion is suspected to have existed prior to the fracture, preinjury photographs, dental casts (rarely available) and careful examination of the occlusal surfaces for wear facets may give clues to pretrauma occlusion. In cases of delayed primary reduction with firm callus formation, realignment of occlusion may be accomplished by slow intermaxillary traction with elastic bands passing from upper to lower arch bars. This traction frequently will bring the teeth and fragments into proper alignment.

If malunion does occur, the method of treatment will depend upon the cosmetic and functional severity. With an edentulous patient, frequently a change in dentures will suffice. If dentition is present and the occlusal abnormalities are minimal, they may be correctable by selective occlusal grinding or orthodontics. If the malunion only presents as a cosmetic deformity, improvement with augmentation onlay chin implants of autogenous bone or cartilage, irradiated cartilage or synthetic materials is adequate.

## *Other Complications*

### INFERIOR ALVEOLAR NERVE ANESTHESIA

Anesthesia in the distribution of the inferior alveolar nerve is a frequent sequella of mandibular fracture, especially in those involving the body proximal to the mental foramen. If the nerve is severed, recovery is related to a number of factors:[73]

1. The accurate reduction and approximation of the fragments
2. elimination of infection
3. adequate immobilization
4. no soft tissue obstructing the inferior dental canal

This will allow for regeneration of the nerve or release of compression if the nerve is still intact. In fractures with bone loss or requiring bond grafting, total anesthesia is frequently permanent. In some patients, anesthesia may be noted less after 12 to 18 months due to partial reinervation from surrounding sensory nerve branches. During surgery, if the nerve is accidentally severed, repair should be accomplished, if at all possible.

### TEETH

The most common complication of these fractures is devitalization of teeth with subsequent abscess and tooth loss. Traumatically devitalized teeth in the line of a fracture also represent a potential source of infection and should be removed. Chronic gingival disease and the loss of bony alveolar support may also result if the tooth is left in place. A

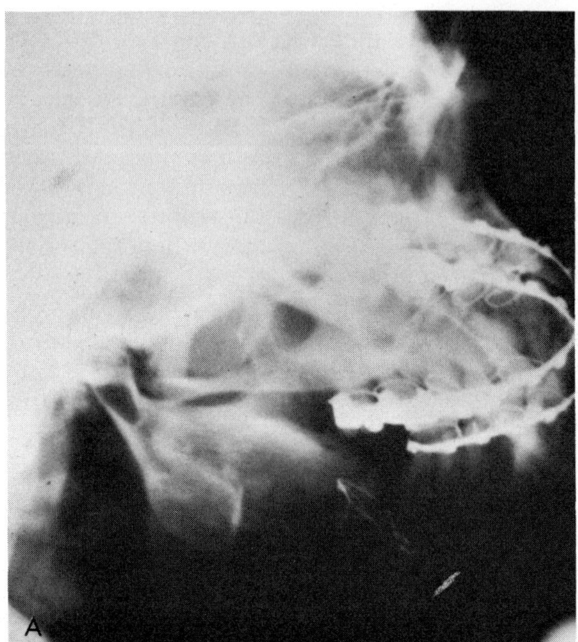


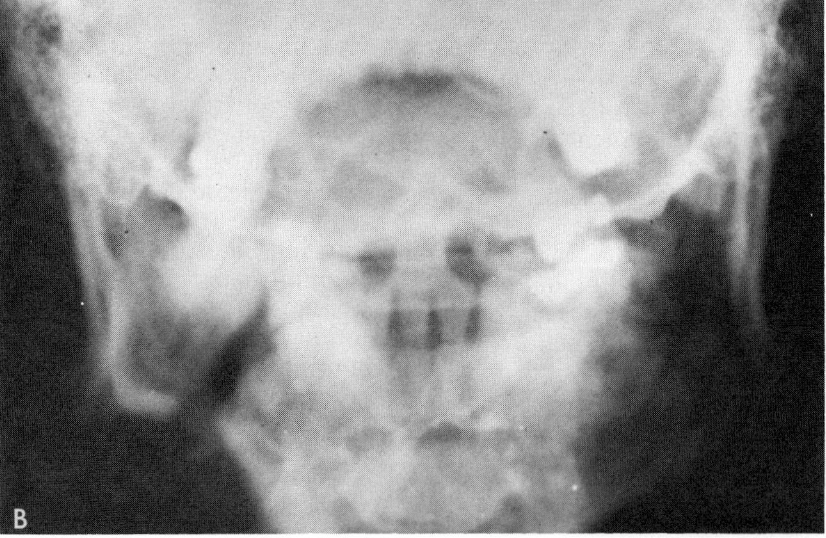


**Figure 24–6** *A* and *B*, X-rays showing bilateral mandibular fractures, healed on the right, nonunion on the left. This was treated by exposure of the fractured bone ends *(C)*, curetting the pseudocapsule, packing the defects with cancellous iliac bone graft *(D)* and interosseous wiring.

*(Figure 24–6 continued on opposite page.)*

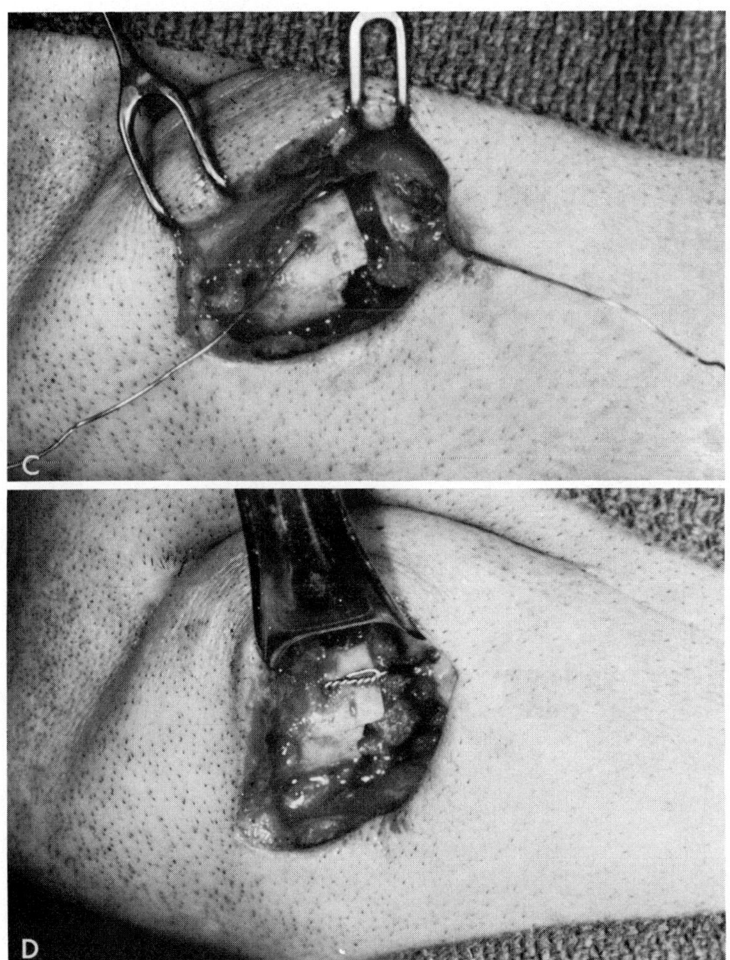


**Figure 24–6** *Continued.*

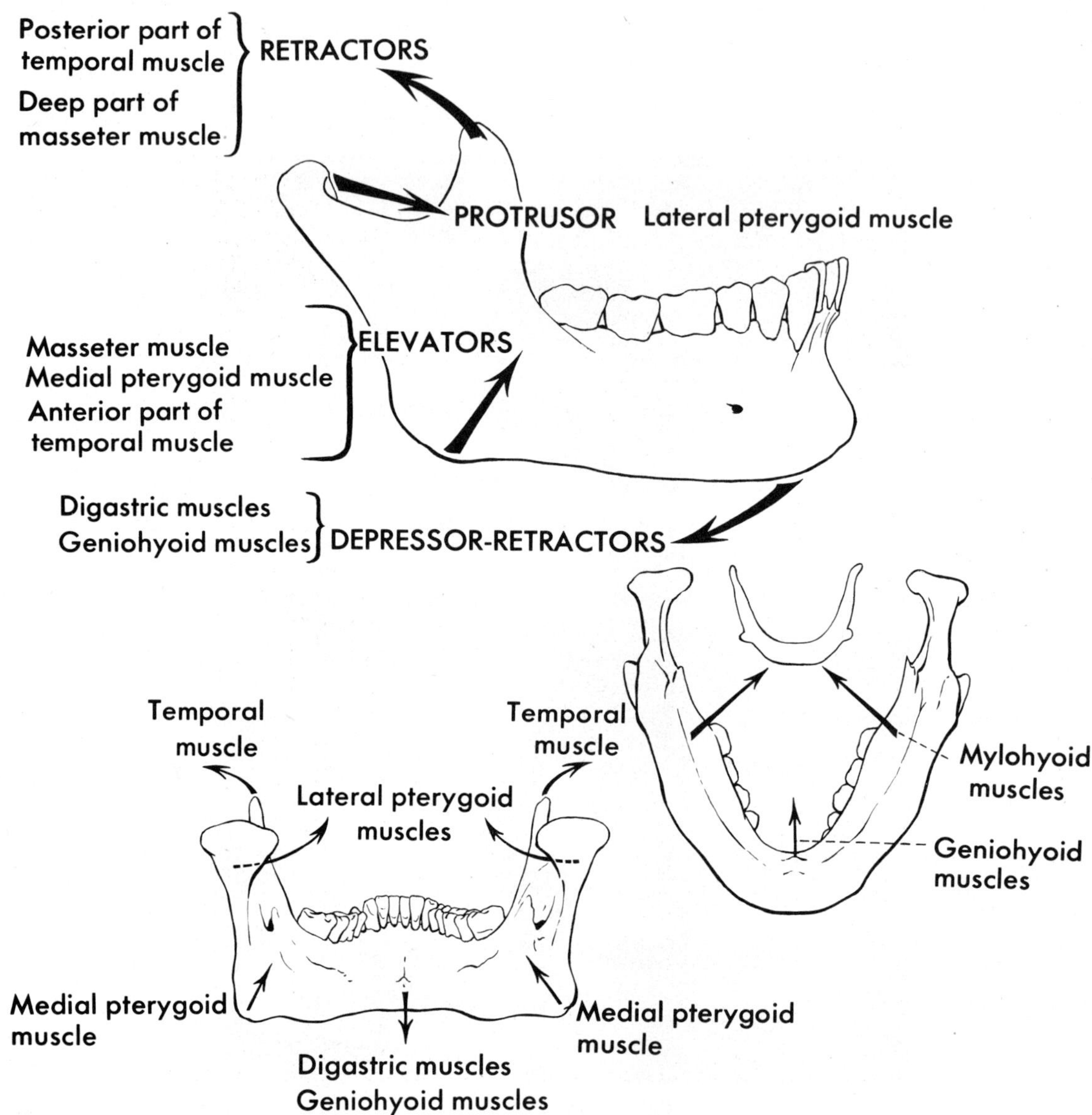


**Figure 24–7** Diagrammatic representation of the main directions of the composite forces of the mandibular muscles. (From Dingman, R. O., and Natvig, P.: Surgery of Facial Fractures. Philadelphia, W. B. Saunders Co., 1964.)

general rule is that a tooth with both crown and roots fractured, situated in the fracture line, should be extracted.[48] A questionable tooth, if possible, should be left out of the fixation device, because this may tend to further compromise the vascular supply. Partial tooth avulsion with attached alveolus should be reinserted properly and stabilized with direct simple wiring, circumferential wiring, cast, splint or arch bars.[49] Dental consultation should be obtained in all these cases.

### TRISMUS AND ANKYLOSIS

The great majority of condylar fractures can be managed successfully by either no treatment or a limited period of intermaxillary fixation. Late trismus may be due to scarring directly around the joint or in attached muscles. Some muscle shortening may be associated with intermaxillary fixation. Progressive mechanical oral dilatation or direct release of the scar contractures may relieve the trismus.

Internal derangement of the temporomandibular joint with resulting pain and joint dysfunction may be treated conservatively with local anesthesia, interarticular steroids and rest. If there is failure to respond to conservative measures with persistent chronic joint tenderness, crepitus or x-ray evidence of joint changes, surgery is indicated. This may vary from a simple meniscectomy to arthroplasty or complete replacement of the condylar head.

True bony ankylosis of the temporomandibular joint is probably due to intracapsular fracture and hemorrhage with articular surface destruction and fibrosis resulting in bony union between the articular head of the condyle and the glenoid fossa. Fibrous or bony ankylosis of the coronoid process of the mandible with the zygoma may also occur. Both of these are relatively rare. If the condylar head is fractured, movement as early as possible and as extensive as possible will decrease the chances of bony ankylosis. If ankylosis does occur, the treatment is surgical. X-rays and tomograms (two planes) will confirm the diagnosis. The treatment then consists of resection of the bony union with interposition of muscle, fascia,[19] dermal graft,[35] interposed Silastic[8] or other materials. One recent report showed fairly good results using full thickness skin interposition.[72] Bilateral sliding osteotomies or vertical osteotomies may be unnecessary for the treatment of associated mandibular growth deformities.

Treatment of ankylosis of the mandibular coronoid process to the zygomatic arch or maxilla may be treated through the intraoral approach with resection of the coronoid process.

### *Complications of Individual Modes of Treatment*

The indications and applications of individual types of mandibular fracture fixation are well described.[28, 46, 73, 75] There are problems associated with each device used.

**Interdental wiring.** Although the simplest method of fracture fixation, interdental wiring may allow the bone at the fracture to rotate because of the inability to counteract muscle pull. Melmed and Koonin (1975)[56] reported a relatively low incidence of complications with fractures treated in this manner. We rarely use this technique and feel that this type of fracture fixation should be used only in favorable simple fractures occurring in the body of the mandible, distal to the molar teeth. It may also be used as an adjunct to open reduction.

**Arch bars.** Arch bar fixation may result in similiar difficulty with rotation at the fracture site. The fracture must be distal to the molars to avoid this rotation. Careful limited use of the elastic traction is necessary to avoid the distractive forces of the elastics, possibly resulting in a malunion (Fig. 24–8). Intermaxillary wires should replace the elastics as soon as adequate reduction and stabilization are obtained. Intermaxillary fixation in the elderly may result in malnutrition; therefore, diet supplementation and vitamins should be recommended.

**Circumferential mandibular wires with splints.** In children, when interdental wiring and arch bars are impractical, this method may suffice, but care must be taken to avoid pulling the circumferential wires through the mandible. Fractures in the edentulous mandible have about twice the number of complications as those of the mandible with normal dentition.[31] In the edentulous patient with an undisplaced or

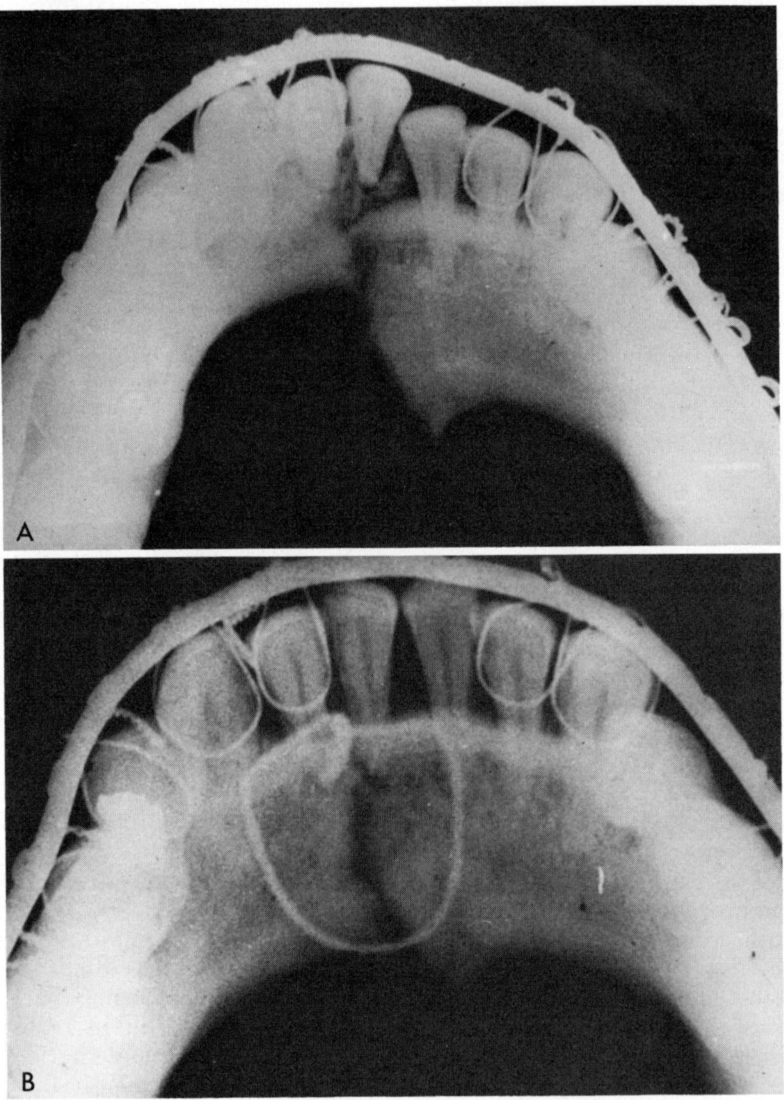


**Figure 24–8** *A,* Fracture of the symphyseal region of the mandible and displacement; the intraoral appliance failed to provide stabilization in the line of fracture. *B,* Stabilization of the fracture by open reduction and interosseous wire fixation. (From Dingman, R. O., and Natvig, P.: Surgery of Facial Fractures. Philadelphia, W. B. Saunders Co., 1964.)

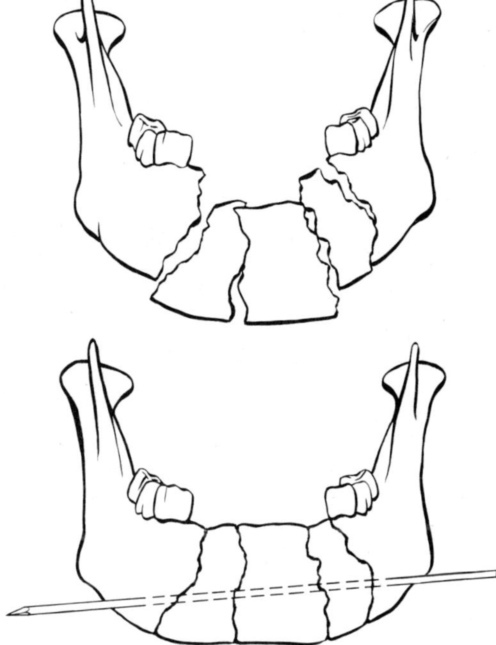

**Figure 24–9** Kirschner wire fixation of mandibular fractures. (From Dingman, R. O., and Natvig, P.: Surgery of Facial Fractures. Philadelphia, W. B. Saunders Co., 1964.)

slightly displaced fracture, splints with circumandibular wires may be sufficient. In the mandible with an unfavorable fracture line or comminution, however, transosseous wiring should also be accomplished in association with this type of splinting. Obwegeser (1973)[65] reports a series of cases in which the atrophic edentulous mandible was stabilized with onlay bone grafts over the fracture (rib, iliac crest and banked ribs). He states that this adds additional strength and speeds the bony healing while assisting in later prosthetic support.

**Kirschner wires.** The problem with this type of stabilization is that wires stabilize the fracture site but may not directly reduce or hold the fragments (Fig. 24–9). The potential exists for rotation around a single Kirschner wire. The use of K-wires is discouraged by Grabb (1972),[38] who describes a case in which a chronic infected K-wire tract had to be curetted to allow healing. Other authors also avoid K-wire fixation.[42]

**External mandibular fixation.** External fixation screws with acrylic connecting bars can give excellent bony stabilization and soft tissue support while allowing limited mandibular function. The appliance usually is well tolerated and is especially useful with significant bony loss, since it allows maintenance of normal muscular and soft tissue positioning until bone grafting is done. Complications of this method usually are associated with placement of the external mandibular screw.[46] The facial artery and facial vein must be avoided, and external screws should be placed below the inferior alveolar canal. If a hematoma exists near the fracture, the screws should be placed away from it to avoid infection. Soft tissues are protected from the drill when placing the screws to avoid local maceration or damage to the facial nerve. This may be accomplished by protecting the tissue with a nasal or metal ear speculum. Most importantly, the bony fragments must be in good apposition in the edentulous patient by use of a preoperatively applied intraoral splint. Since the bar is rigid, failure to impact the fragments with the initial fixation of the screws may result in nonunion or malunion. One must watch for skin ulcerations secondary to pressure from the screws and bar due to postoperative or traumatic edema.

## COMPLICATIONS OF MAXILLARY FRACTURES

Fractures of the maxilla are usually the result of a significant direct force to the midface against the instrument panel of a car.

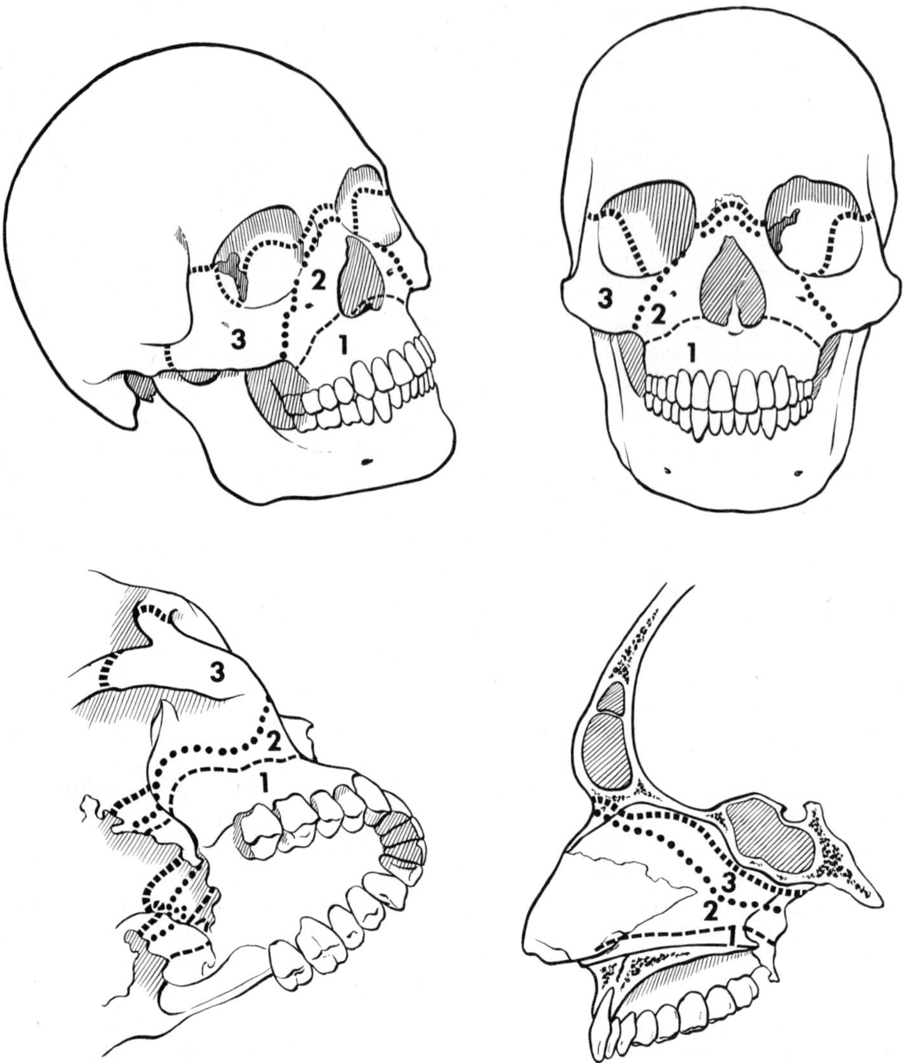


**Figure 24–10** Fractures of the maxilla. (1) LeFort I (transverse or Guérin fracture); (2) LeFort II (pyramided fracture); (3) LeFort III (craniofacial disjunction). (From Dingman, R. O., and Natvig, P.: Surgery of Facial Fractures. Philadelphia, W. B. Saunders Co., 1964.)

They may range from simple alveolar fractures to those involving multiple midfacial bones. Associated complications are discussed in the sections discussing individual facial bones.

Since LeFort's classic experimental study in 1901,[52] concise descriptions of the diagnosis and primary treatment of maxillary fractures have been published.[28, 46, 73, 74] Actual clinical fractures are infrequently along the classic lines of greatest structural weakness as demonstrated by LeFort (Fig. 24–10).

The transverse maxillary fracture, LeFort I, involves the maxilla above the teeth, and the fracture segment contains the alveolar process, portions of the maxillary sinus, the palate and the lower portion of the pterygoid process of the sphenoid bone.

The LeFort II, or pyramidal fracture, produces fractures of the nasal bones, frontal process of the maxilla, lacrimal bones, inferior rim of the orbit, floor of the orbit and near or through the zygomaticomaxillary suture. The fracture involves the lateral wall of the maxilla, the pterygoid plates and the pterygoid maxillary fossa.

LeFort III fracture, or craniofacial dysjunction, separates the facial bones from

| Subdivisional Involvement | Per Cent of Total |
|---|---|
| Zygomatic arch only | 16 |
| Zygomaticomaxillary compound | 66 |
| Orbit | 46 |
| Infraorbital margin | 45 |
| Floor | 41 |
| Lateral wall | 16 |
| Supraorbital margin and roof | 3 |
| Nasoethmoid pyramid | 6 |
| Upper jaw | 25 |
| Transverse separation | 13 |
| Midline | 4 |
| Alveolar segment | 7 |

**Figure 24–11** Individual facial bones involved in fractures of the middle one third of the facial skeleton. (From McCoy, F. J., Chandler, R. A., Magnan, C. G., et al.: Analysis of facial fractures and their complications. Plast. Reconstr. Surg., *29*:301, 1962.)

their cranial attachments. The fracture involves zygomaticofrontal, maxillofrontal and nasofrontal sutures, the orbital floors, the ethmoid sinus and the sphenoid bones.

Fractures of the middle third of the face tend to involve multiple bones. McCoy (1962)[63] tabulated the percentage of individual and multiple bones involved in midthird fractures (Fig. 24–11).

### *Acute Complications*

#### RESPIRATORY

As with mandibular fractures, aspiration in maxillary fractures should be watched for closely. A nasogastric tube can be lifesaving. Upper airway obstruction may also occur from progressive edema. Nasal obstruction is frequently related to associated nasal fractures. An oral airway placed along the buccal sulcus may temporarily suffice. For severe midface fractures or planned craniofacial surgery, a tracheostomy frequently is necessary. In children, tracheostomy should be avoided and, if possible, another method should be used.

#### HEMORRHAGE

Limited hemorrhage after maxillary fracture is common. This usually can be controlled by nasal cavity or nasopharyngeal packing.

#### INFECTION

Although infection following maxillary fracture is infrequent, patients are routinely placed on prophylactic antibiotics. Antral hematoma and stasis is a potential nidus for acute sinusitis.[73] Patients with chronic maxillary sinusitis may progress to acute purulent maxillary sinus infection. This may be secondary to a foreign body or free bone fragments in the sinus. If acute suppuration occurs, drainage is necessary. Progression of acute sinus trauma to chronic sinusitis was evaluated in a recent study of maxillary sinus after middle face fractures.[51] Using fiberoptic investigation of the sinuses, it was concluded that, in spite of chronic inflammatory mucosal changes in 35 per cent of post-midfacial fracture patients, all of them were asymptomatic. Primary revisional sinus surgery is not recommended for these patients.

#### NERVE DYSFUNCTION

McCoy (1962)[63] reports permanent cranial nerve dysfunction in 6 per cent of middle third facial fractures. Anosmia and ocular palsy are the presenting symptoms and are usually transient but on occasion may be permanent.[73] Superior orbital nerve syndrome presents as (1) ocular proptosis secondary to loss of extraocular muscle tone; (2) a fixed dilated pupil due to loss of parasympathetic innervation; (3) ptosis secondary to interruption of the tonus of Mueller's lid muscle;(4) ophthalmoplegia caused by involvement of cranial nerves III, IV and VI; and (5) sensory abnormality secondary to frontal and lacrimal nerve damage.

The infraorbital nerve may be involved in a high maxillary or pyramidal fracture. Occasionally, nerves VII, VIII and XII may be involved with cranial base fractures. Causalgia of cranial nerve V has been reported.

#### CSF RHINORRHEA

A maxillary fracture may be associated with a CSF leak secondary to a dural tear in the cribriform area. Rhinorrhea presents as clear nasal or pharyngeal drainage that initially may be mixed with blood and be difficult to identify. All patients with midface fractures who have a questionable cerebrospinal fluid leak are placed on prophylactic antibiotics. Leakage may not occur until a few days following trauma. Most leaks stop spontaneously, especially following fracture reduction and immobilization. Maxillary fractures should be reduced as soon as possible after neurosurgical clearance. Occasionally, the CSF leak persists. If it does not gradually diminish and stop in three weeks, neurosurgical intervention may be necessary. Meningitis has been reported months and years following facial trauma and long-term follow-up is necessary.

Other less common complications of midthird facial fractures include oronasal fistula and oral antral fistula following fractures involving the midline palate or alveolus of the maxilla. When present, repair of the fistula requires obliteration of the fistulous tract and closure by a local mucosal advancement or rotation flap. Other complications include traumatic diabetes insipidus and pneumomediastinum.[73, 83]

### *Late Complications*

#### NONUNION

Unlike mandibular fractures, nonunion of the maxilla is rare. In a case treated at our institution, a nonunion of a LeFort I fracture existed seven months after initial craniofacial suspension and intermaxillary fixation. He was treated with open reduction, K-wire fixation and iliac bone grafts, which resulted in stability and good occlusion (Fig. 24–12). The maxilla consists primarily of cancellous bone nourished by an extensive vascular network, which accounts for the infrequency of nonunion. Factors as described in nonunion of the mandible (infection, soft tissue interposition, poor bony apposition and foreign bodies) are much less apt to occur. The treatment of maxillary nonunion fracture is open reduction and bone graft with cancellous and cortical bone. This is followed by immobilization for eight to twelve weeks, or longer.

#### DELAYED UNION

If primary treatment of maxillary fractures is postponed due to concurrent life-threatening injuries, delayed union may result. The basic principles for treatment of delayed union are as follows:

1. Early reduction and fixation: From 10 to 14 days the fracture may be reduced by conventional means. In children, however, this rule may not apply, as the time for fracture healing in children is significantly reduced.

2. Up to six weeks, slow traction via suspension from a headcap, halo or extraskeletal traction usually will reduce the fracture and provide fixation.

3. Horizontal fractures up to four months old may also be corrected by traction. A rapid and satisfactory reduction may be accomplished by the method described by Dingman and Harding (1951)[27] (Fig. 24–13). In this method, a dental tray with dental compound is used to make a mold of the maxillary teeth. With the patient under general anesthesia, the tray is grasped and moved from side to side and up and down in an attempt to rupture the fibrous tissue attachments at the fracture site. This frequently will release the fracture and allow reduction and fixation.

#### MALUNION

Initial inadequate reduction and immobilization of a maxillary fracture frequently results in malunion. Avoidance of this complication depends upon careful primary reduction and suspension. The technique for suspension in LeFort I, II and III fractures has been adequately described.[28, 46] The following points are suggested to avoid malunion after suspension. The suspension wires must support but not decrease the vertical height of the midface by compression. If associated with a unilateral or bilateral fracture of the mandibular condyle, the maxilla should not be suspended from the zygomatic arch as it may heal in retrusion by shifting posteriorly with the unrestrained mandible.

When malunion occurs, significant facial deformity may result, including a dished out facies, irregular retromaxillism with Angle's Class III malocclusion, open anterior bite, nasal collapse, telecanthus and malar flattening (Fig. 24–14). The planning of any surgical approach to this problem includes cephalometric evaluation, anterior and lateral

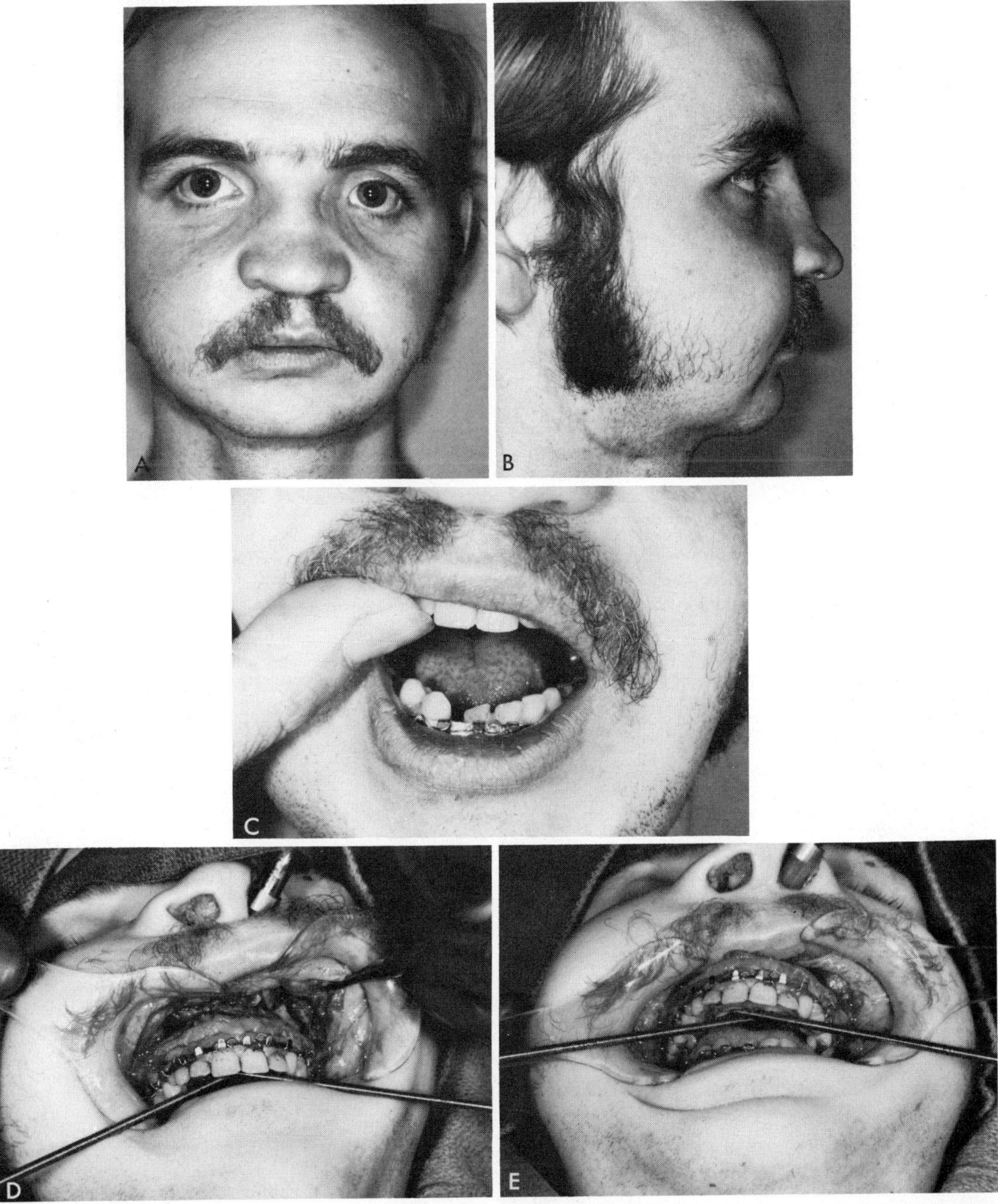


**Figure 24–12** 22-year-old white male involved in an auto accident. Initial fractures included: (1) fracture of the angle of the mandible, (2) LeFort II fracture on right, (3) LeFort III fracture on left, (4) nasal fracture and (5) LeFort I fracture bilaterally. Initial treatment included: 1. ORIF mandible, 2. ORIF left zygoma, 3. intermaxillary fixation and 4. bilateral craniofacial suspension from zygomatic processes of the frontal bones. Five months post accident he complained of a mobile maxilla when biting. (*A,B,C*). Clinically this was a nonunion of the LeFort I fracture. He was treated with an iliac bone graft and pin fixation of the palate to the zygoma bilaterally (*D* and *E*). One month later the maxilla was clinically solid and the fixation devices were removed after three and four months. He has done well since.

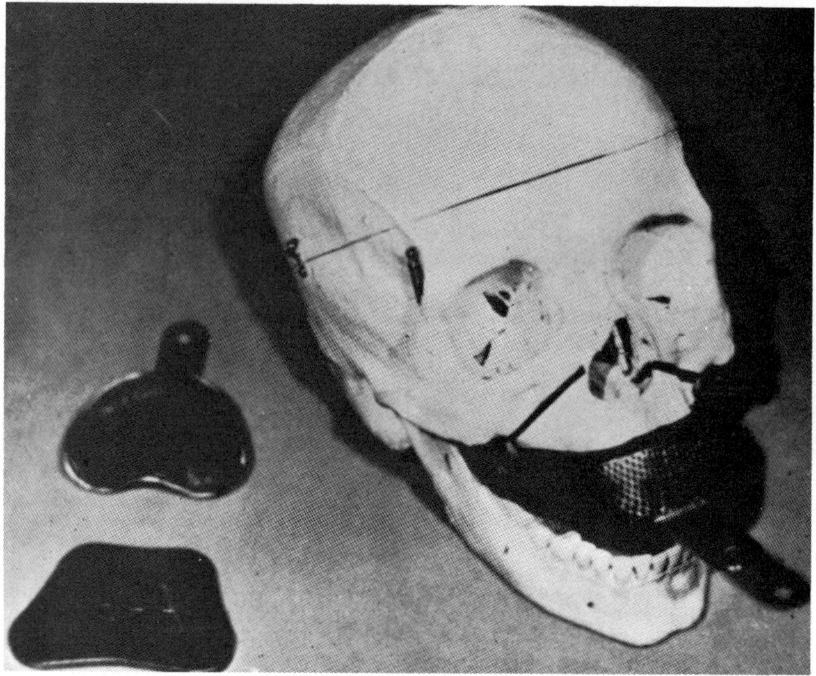

**Figure 24–13** Dental tray with dental compound used to break up the fracture site. (From Dingman, R. O., and Harding, R. L.: Treatment of malunion fractures of facial bones. Plast. Reconstr. Surg., *7*:505, 1951.)

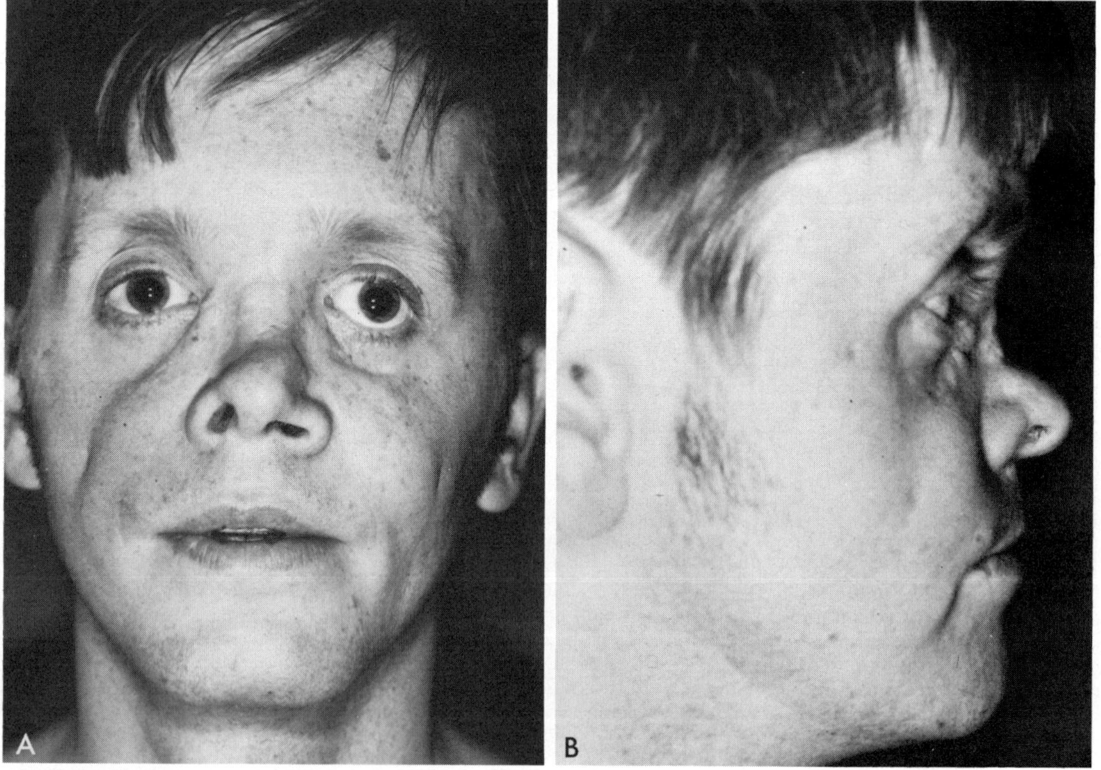


**Figure 24–14** Classic picture of a maxillary malunion with dished out facies, retromaxillism, nasal collapse, malar flattening and telecanthus.

tomograms, dental casts, photographs and orthodontic and dental planning.

Some late deformities may be treated by autogenous bone or cartilage onlay grafts with fairly good results. Others may be treated, as in malunion of a LeFort I fracture in the edentulous, by simply changing dentures. With advancement in craniofacial surgical techniques, the treatment of LeFort II and III maxillary malunion fractures by osteotomy and autogenous bone grafts is giving better results.

The LeFort I–controlled transverse maxillary osteotomy may be used for the retromaxillism due to malunion of a LeFort I fracture. This requires preoperative cephalometric evaluation with orthodontic planning and preoperative preparation of a plastic dental splint for intermaxillary fixation. The osteotomy is performed through the labial sulci bilaterally. If the fractured segment is severely retruded with comminution of the pterygoid plates, care must be taken in separating the maxillary segment to avoid injury to the greater palatine neurovascular bundle.[71] If postoperative fixation is unstable, external skeletal fixation as described by Georgiade (1966)[36] is necessary. Careful surgical planning and mucosal flap design may help avoid the complication of bony avascular necrosis with loss of tooth vitality, periodontal disease and relapse of the malunion. Splint pressure and vascular compromise are reduced with proper splint design. Strict postoperative oral hygiene must be emphasized as important to avoid infection.

The technique for LeFort II and III osteotomies was developed originally for the treatment of Crouzon's and Apert's disease and other craniofacial anomalies.[65, 82] Correction of major deformities may be accomplished quickly and accurately in this manner.[82] If the zygomatic bones are only slightly displaced and well consolidated, excluding them from the main block liberated by the osteotomies is recommended. The zygomas then support grafts for orbital floor reconstruction in prevention and treatment of enophthalmos. If the reduction is not possible or satisfactory cosmetically, primary consideration must be given to ocular function and proper occlusion. After the primary procedure, secondary operations such as rhinoplasty, septal reconstruction, medial and lateral canthoplasty and scar revisions may still be necessary. Avoidance of the dura mater at the cribriform plates because of potential adhesions associated with a fracture, of the lacrimal apparatus and of hemorrhage from the internal maxillary artery are pointed out as important by Tessier.

| | |
|---|---|
| Death | 2 (1.3%) |
| Infection | 9 |
| CSF Leaks | 5 |
| Bleeding | 13 |
| Ocular | 24 |
| Orbital | 16 |
| Bone Graft | 11 |
| Soft Tissue | 8 |
| Relapse of Midface | 6 |
| Other | 12 |

**Figure 24–15** Chart of complications associated with craniofacial surgery in a series of 141 patients (20 post-traumatic). (From Whitaker, L. A., Monroe, I. R., Jackson, I. T., et al.: Problems in craniofacial surgery. J. Maxillofac. Surg., *4*:135, 1976.)

A recent review of problems encountered with craniofacial surgery included a series of 141 cases (20 of which were post-traumatic) of which 60 per cent had no complications. The remaining complications are described (Fig. 24–15). Death occurred in 1.3 per cent of the cases. Infections may present as meningitis, subgaleal abscess and cellulitis and may result in loss of a bone graft. Five patients developed CSF leaks, all requiring corrective operations. One case of hematoma required drainage. No cases of blindness were seen in this series; however, four cases of VI nerve ophthalmoplegia were reported, three of which recovered spontaneously. Nasolacrimal obstruction in two cases was seen requiring operative correction.

Other complications included partial bone graft loss, small amounts of skin necrosis and occipital and sacral pressure sores. Pressure sores possibly can be avoided with careful intraoperative padding.

The tendency for relapse was minimal. Whittaker reported three cases of LeFort II and three cases of LeFort III osteotomies with relapse. Freihofer (1973)[31] reports three cases of relapse attributed to improperly immobilized bony segment. Additional operations after the facial bone osteotomy frequently include medial canthoplasty, dacryocystorhinostomy, rhinoplasty, septal reconstruction and onlay bony augmentation.

## COMPLICATIONS OF ZYGOMATIC FRACTURES

The zygoma, because of its structure and location, is the second most frequently fractured midfacial bone. Schultz (1970)[74] reported incidence of 15 per cent in 1031 facial fractures. The zygomatic arch and body are second only to the nasal bones in their inability to withstand direct trauma.[64] The fractured zygoma is subject to considerable displacement and forced rotation by strong muscle pulls. The immediately adjacent articulating bones most frequently involved are the frontal, sphenoid, temporal and maxillary bones. The zygoma also participates in the formation of the orbital floor, maxillary sinus, zygomatic arch and temporal fossa.

Edema and ecchymosis immediately following zygomatic injury may conceal the fracture and its deformity. The patient may be unaware of the fracture until resolution of the swelling when the deformity becomes obvious. When diplopia occurs as an initial symptom of orbital floor fracture or zygomatic displacement, the diagnosis is more easily made. Primary diagnosis and treatment of zygomatic fractures is discussed thoroughly by Dingman and Natvig (1964),[28] Rowe and Killey (1968)[73] and Kazanjian and Converse (1974).[46] Some classic physical signs of zygomatic fracture include (1) flattening of the malar eminence, (2) edema of the cheek and eyelids, (3) epistaxis (unilateral), (4) anesthesia in the infraorbital and zygomatic nerve distribution, (5) palpable step off deformity of the infraorbital rim, (6) diplopia and (7) trismus. Displacements of the zygomatic compound should be realigned, as even a small degree of abnormal bony contour may produce a conspicuous and prominent deformity after resolution of edema.

Complications appear to be directly related to the degree of zygomatic displacement and rotation and the subsequent treatment. Knight and North (1961)[50] classify zygomatic fractures into six groups:

| | |
|---|---|
| Group I | Undisplaced fractures — 6% |
| Group II | Zygomatic arch — 10% |
| Group III | Depression of zygomatic body without rotation — 33% |
| Group IV | Depression of zygomatic body with medial rotation — 11% |
| Group V | Depression of zygomatic body with lateral rotation — 22% |
| Group VI | Complex zygomatic fractures — 18% |

Most late complications involve rotated depressed zygomatic fractures and are related to inadequate fracture fixation.

### *Early Complications*

#### DIPLOPIA

Barkley (1958)[3] reports 10 per cent of patients with zygomaticomaxillary fractures suffering diplopia — 50 per cent transient and 50 per cent permanent. Knight and North saw the highest incidence of diplopia in Group IV fractures (depression with medial rotation), probably because of displacement of both orbital floor and the lateral orbital wall. The total incidence of diplopia in their series was 14.2 per cent (17 of 120). With loss of integrity of the lateral orbital wall there is depression of Lockwood's ligament and the lateral palpebral ligament. This also contributes to enophthalmos, and antimongoloid slant of the eye is frequently seen. Fragmentation of the orbital floor or infraorbital margin may also contribute to diplopia by mechanisms described in the section on orbital floor fractures. The reduction of a zygomatic fracture results in reconstitution of the lateral orbital wall and orbital floor with lateral suspensory support for the eye.

#### ACUTE TRISMUS

This may be the patient's primary complaint. Knight and North report 20.8 per cent of zygomatic fractures have associated trismus with the highest incidence in depressed zygomatic arch fractures. This may also occur more frequently in medially rotated body fractures. The lateral excursion of the mandible is restricted toward the affected side. Treatment is by elevation of the zygomatic arch depression or reduction of the body fracture.

### *Late Complications*

#### MALUNION

Late complications following zygomatic fractures are usually a result of inadequate primary reduction and fixation techniques.

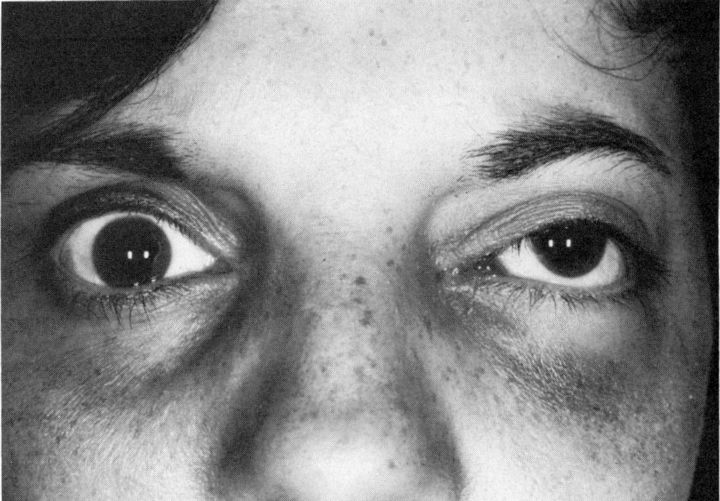

**Figure 24–16** Total blindness in left eye following open reduction of zygomatic fractures. A maxillary antrostomy with manipulation of the orbital floor was done. There was no evidence of bony fragments or fractures in the orbital floor posteriorly that may have directly injured the optic nerve.

Knight and North showed that all medially rotated fractures were unstable and 70 per cent of complex fractures were unstable. Malar fractures in children are frequently unstable. Dingman (1953)[20] reported that what appears to be adequate reduction using blind zygomatic elevation frequently is found to be inadequate on further exploration. Some depressed fractures of the zygoma-maxilla with herniation of the orbital contents through the orbital floor went unrecognized. We still feel that the majority of displaced fractures of the zygoma should be treated by open reduction and direct wire fixation. Our approach is through two incisions:(1) at the lateral aspect of the eyebrow (to avoid conspicuous scars) for exploration, reduction and, if necessary, wiring of the zygomaticofrontal suture and (2) through the skin at the junction of lid and cheek (parallel to the skin lines), a subciliary or transconjunctival incision. Through this approach, one may wire the zygomatic maxillary fracture line and explore the orbital floor. If necessary, the maxillary sinus may be packed through a Caldwell-Luc approach. A nasal antrostomy for pack removal permits closure of the incision.

### VISUAL CHANGES

Visual acuity changes, and blindness after reduction of zygomatic fractures have been reported.[37, 67] Three possible mechanisms are suggested: (1) hemorrhage and pressure within the optic nerve sheath, (2) direct injury to the nerve by bony spicule and (3) hemorrhage or thrombosis within the nerve itself. It was postulated that the most likely was hemorrhage within the nerve sheath. Early splitting of the intraorbital portion of the optic nerve sheath has been suggested as possibly beneficial in saving some of the patient's sight. Penn and Epstein reported severe intraorbital hemorrhage with rapid visual deterioration after reduction of a seven-day-old fracture. Immediate hematoma drainage of the lateral orbit was done with the gradual return of visual acuity. A case of blindness following blind Caldwell-Luc reduction of a zygomatic fracture was referred to our institution (Fig. 24–16).

In our experience, malunion is less frequent with open reduction and internal fixation than with blind reduction, antral packing alone or single interosseous wires at the zygomatic-frontal suture line. If stability of the fracture is not obtained by the described open reduction and internal fixation, zygomatic K-wire fixation (Fig. 24–17), external frontozygomatic pin fixation or craniozygomatic fixation with halo or plaster headcap may be used. The K-wire fixation has worked well for us in these difficult cases. The K-wire is removed in four to six weeks; however, if bone grafts are used, it is removed in eight to ten weeks.

Malunion of the zygoma frequently results in significant cosmetic deformity, with antimongoloid slant from inferior displacement of the lateral canthal ligament and loss of malar prominence. The ocular level is

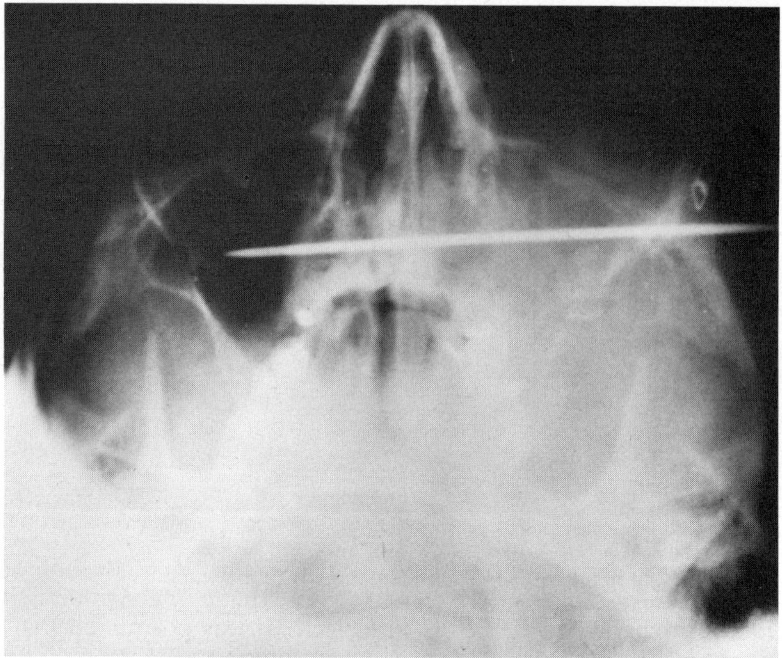

**Figure 24–17** K-wire fixation of an unstable zygomatic fracture.

frequently lowered, with disappearance of the supratarsal fold and associated pseudoptosis. Diplopia may or may not be present.

For correction of a zygomatic malunion, we feel osteotomy with repositioning of the zygoma gives a more satisfactory long-term result than onlay grafting with cartilage, bone or alloplastic material. In delayed union, open reduction and internal fixation can be done by usual methods up to six weeks after injury. It may be necessary to curette the callus and scar from the fracture lines and then elevate the zygoma by the preferred route.

If more than six weeks since injury has elapsed, more agressive treatment frequently is necessary to free the zygoma. We have corrected malunion of the zygoma from three months to six years after injury. This usually necessitates transverse osteotomy extending across the floor and upward through the lateral orbital wall. The AP osteotomy is through the rim at the fracture line. Care is used to avoid damage to the infraorbital nerve. The zygoma is realigned and fixed with #24 or #26 gauge wire. If necessary, soft tissues are freed from the bone for redraping. K-wire fixation from the osteotomized zygoma to the solid uninjured normal bone may be necessary. The K-wire is removed as an office procedure under local anesthesia six to eight weeks later.

For minimal residual defects after osteotomy, onlay grafting through intraoral or transcutaneous route may be of help.

## ANESTHESIA

Infraorbital nerve anesthesia with the initial zygomatic injury is common owing to contusion or impingement of the nerve at the fracture site. Anesthesia may last from six to twelve months. After eighteen months, surgical exploration of the nerve looking for entrapment is justified. A 10 per cent incidence of permanent anesthesia in this distribution has been reported.[1]

Direct injury also may be sustained by zygomaticofacial and zygomaticotemporal branches of the maxillary nerve. Careful instrumentation and bony realignment will avoid further nerve damage and aid in initial recovery.

Superior orbital fissure syndrome (ophthalmoplegia, ptosis, proptosis, fixed dilated pupil and sensory disturbance of the ophthalmic division of the trigeminal nerve) may occur in zygomatic fractures. This may lead to severe and intractable retro-orbital neuralgia. The treatment is expectant with no additional surgery warranted.

## COMPLICATIONS OF NASAL TRAUMA

Trauma to the cartilaginous and bony nasal framework is the most common facial injury excluding soft tissue trauma. Nasal injuries are frequently overlooked or inadequately treated, resulting in significant complications both functional and cosmetic. Even with the early recognition and proper primary treatment of nasal fractures, there is no assurance that airway obstruction or external nasal deviation will not occur.

Nasal fractures in children are difficult to detect and frequently overlooked. It may be assumed that a child with epistaxis following nasal injury has sustained a fracture. Careful evaluation, if necessary under general anesthesia, may reveal septal or bony fractures with displacement otherwise not evident. If fractures go untreated, severe nasal deformities, extremely difficult to correct, may become evident after puberty.

The interlocking stress forces in nasal septal cartilage as described by Fry (1966)[32] are present in the fetus, and deforming nasal trauma may occur during birth. The septum appears to play an important role in maxillary growth, and its destruction or absence has been shown to result in significant maxillary hypoplasia.[47] This further emphasizes the importance of properly examining and treating any child with suspected nasal fracture.

Nasal fractures may be associated with other injuries, such as damage to the nasolacrimal duct, perpendicular plate of the ethmoid, ethmoid sinuses, cribriform plate and orbital margins of the frontal bone. Comminution of the nasal bones with widening of the intercanthal distance is sometimes seen (telecanthus). Injury to the lacrimal sac may result in chronic dacryocystitis. These complications are discussed separately.

### Isolated Nasal Trauma

#### *Acute Complications*

##### HEMORRHAGE

Nasal hemorrhage of short duration from one or both nostrils is common after trauma resulting in nasal mucosa tears. Occasionally, intranasal packing, anterior or posterior, may be required for control.

##### SEPTAL HEMATOMA

Although not common, a subperichondrial hematoma from a septal fracture without a mucosal tear may accumulate unilaterally or bilaterally. If not drained, it may result in thickening, fibrosis and new septal cartilage formation with septal deviation, deformity and airway obstruction. If the hematoma is further complicated by infection, septal necrosis with perforation, cartilaginous collapse, loss of nasal support and saddle deformity can result. These are difficult problems to treat.

If a large hematoma occurs, it should be aspirated, and, if necessary, the inferior septal mucosa should be incised to establish drainage. The nose is gently packed. Prophylactic antibiotics are given. If infection occurs, drainage, culture and sensitivity and appropriate antibiotics are the treatments of choice. Subperichondrial and subperiosteal fibrosis with cartilage formation results in thickening of the septum up to 1 cm. or more. This usually will require submucosal septal cartilage contouring or submucous resection of the involved septum in order to obtain a satisfactory airway.

#### *Late Complications*

Even with careful primary treatment of trauma, external nasal deformity and airway obstruction frequently result. In some, deformity is due only to bony malunion; in others, only cartilaginous or bony septal deviation exists. A combination of the bony and cartilaginous deformity is most common, and both must be treated for good results (Fig. 24–18).

Edema, hematoma and ecchymosis may obscure the severity in an acute nasal fracture. Unless seen within an hour or two of the injury, when the fractures are more easily identified, we usually wait for four to seven days until the edema subsides before attempting reduction of the nasal bones. In children, consolidation of fractured bones is rapid, and after two weeks definitive repair may require osteotomy. In an adult, closed

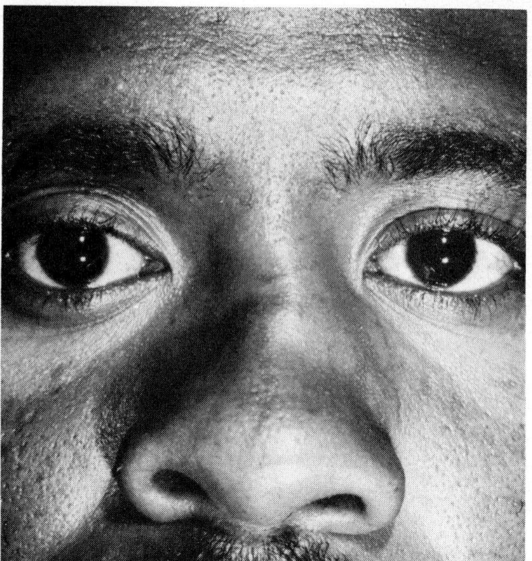

**Figure 24–18** An example of the bony and cartilaginous deformity commonly seen post nasal trauma.

reduction of nasal fractures may be attempted up to four weeks following trauma.

### SEPTAL DEFORMITY

Septal dislocation off the vomerine groove may be repositioned primarily. Fry (1967)[33] showed *in vivo* and *in vitro* that interlock stresses in human septal cartilages are present, and partial fracture of the septum releases only half of these stresses. This results in septal deviation away from the fracture at the point at which the cartilage distortion is most significant. Here, he recommends completing the fracture on the concave side, resulting in release of all the interlock stresses and allowing the septum to heal without deformity. We do not use this technique primarily.

As previously mentioned, external nasal deviation with malunion of the nasal bones and septal deformities can occur regardless of adequate primary treatment (Fig. 24–19). Septal fractures may occur independently of bone fractures, but nasal bone fractures without septal damage are infrequent. Careful planning of the repair is essential. A combined operation upon bony and septal structures is necessary to assure an adequate result. In some cases, corrective external rhinoplasty is impossible without septal reconstruction, and in other cases, the septum cannot be adequately repositioned to give a good airway without osteotomy of the bony malunion.

The techniques of septal reconstruction and rhinoplasty are discussed fully in many plastic surgical and otolaryngological texts and journals. The following are principles used by us for repair of nasal deformities.

At operation, repair of the septal deformity precedes the bony osteotomy to assure better airway correction and defers the traumatic and bloody part of the procedure (the osteotomy) until the end of the procedure. Septal deviation is corrected by a combination of resection of the obstructing cartilaginous and bony spurs, release of scar and interlocking cartilaginous stresses by scoring, resection of septal strips and morsalization. Retention of mucoperichondrial at-

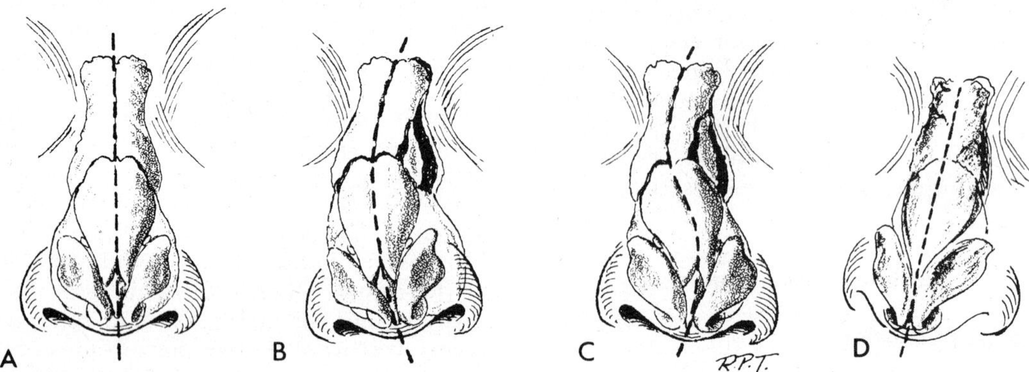


**Figure 24–19** Various types of nasal deviations. *A,* Straight nose. *B,* C curvature. *C,* S curvature. *D,* Total deviation to one side. (From Kazanjian, V. H., and Converse, J. M.: The Surgical Treatment of Facial Injuries. Baltimore, Williams and Wilkins Co., 1974.)

tachments to the septum on one side allows for both support and intact blood supply to the septal cartilage. The cartilaginous septum, if off the vomerine groove, is repositioned by resection of the inferior overlapping cartilaginous septum or by partial vomer osteotomy and repositioning. Frequently, it is necessary to correct overlap at the junction of the quadrangular cartilage and the perpendicular ethmoid plate. If the deviated caudal end of the septum has lost its attachment to the anterior nasal spine, it should be detached from the floor of the nose, scored or morsalized to relieve any stress, replaced on the vomer crest and sutured to the nasal spine. All except hopelessly deformed cartilage and bone should be salvaged, repositioned, and saved to preserve or improve nasal physiology. It is unnecessary to have an obviously straight septum to have a functional airway. Overzealous excision of septal tissues may result in distressing problems, such as septal perforation, retracted columella and recurrent nasal deformity.

When the septum is in the midline and abnormal spring has been released, the bony osteotomy is performed to realign the external bony malunion. Plastic intranasal septal splints are sometimes used to assist in initial septal support and maintenance of the septum in the midline.

A depression along the nasal dorsum immediately below the nasal bones may be due to loss or dislocation of the dorsal portion of the septal cartilage. This may be treated using eversion or sliding flaps of lateral nasal cartilage, with suturing of the released nasal cartilages beneath the skin in midline (Fig. 24–20). Defects of the lower cartilaginous dorsum may be corrected by rotating flaps of the cephalic edges of the lateral crus of the alar cartilages and suturing them to the periosteum of the nasal bones (Fig. 24–21). Techniques for obtaining or inserting cartilaginous or bony nasal grafts cannot be fully discussed here. If the deficiency cannot be reconstructed with local tissues, autogenous cartilage (Fig. 24–22) or iliac bone graft (Fig. 24–23) is used. Nasal tip support may require a single dorsal strut or one with a columella supporting strut attached to the anterior nasal spine. Wide contact of the graft to the nasal bones, stripped of periosteum, along with wire fixation to hold the graft in place usually insures a good result.

### SYNECHIA

Partial airway obstruction may be due to synechia between the turbinates and the septum. Treatment consists of local topical anesthesia, lysis of the synechia and interposition of plastic septal splints for one or two weeks to allow for complete epithelialization of the turbinate and septal mucosa.

## COMPLICATIONS OF ORBITAL FRACTURES

Schultz, in a study of 1031 facial fracture patients, showed that 12 per cent involved the orbital floor.[74] McCoy (1962)[63] reported a loss of integrity of the orbital floor in 41 per cent of zygomaticomaxillary injuries, proved by x-ray or exploration. Many orbital floor fractures associated with zygomatic fracture involve the infraorbital foramen and canal but are asymptomatic, requiring no orbital floor surgery, and heal without complications. The number of late complications following adequate primary treatment of orbital floor fractures is significantly less than in cases of delayed treatment.[13, 40] Therefore, an acute awareness of the mechanism of trauma, the signs and symptoms of orbital floor fractures and the proper primary treatment are essential.

Percentages vary but most series[13, 63, 74] indicate auto accidents, followed by human fist and household accidents as the most common causes of orbital fractures. The characteristics of the fractures vary, depending upon the mechanism of trauma. A blow directly to the globe, as with a fist or ball, tends to result in a "true" blow-out fracture with comminution and collapse of the orbital floor. If the mechanism is severe direct trauma to a periorbital bone, most often the zygoma, with posterior dislocation of the orbital rim and comminution of the orbital floor, the result is termed "impure" blow-out fracture.[46] These fractures frequently involve multiple bony structures, as shown in the following classification:[22]

A. Orbital rim fractures
   1. Zygomatic fracture
   2. Frontal bone fracture
   3. Maxillary fracture
B. Intraorbital fractures not involving the rim of the orbit, relatively uncommon ("true" blow-out)

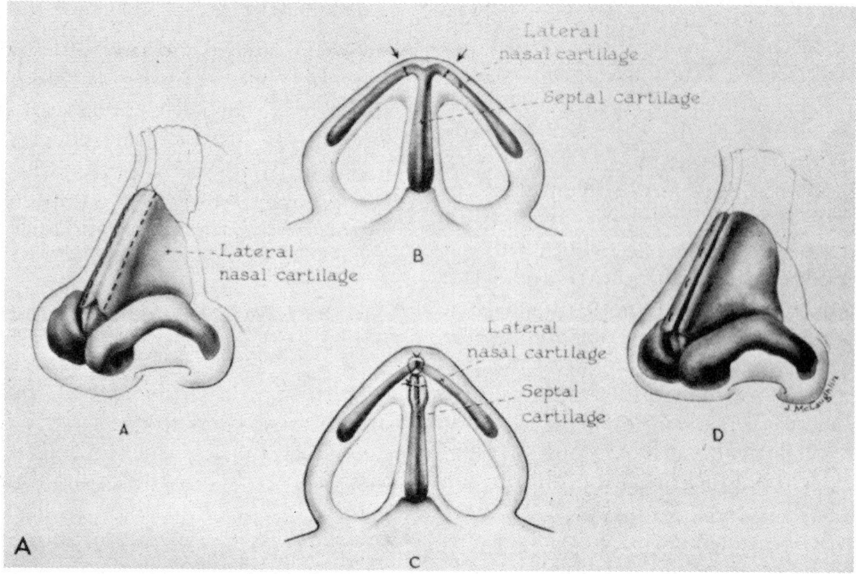


**Figure 24–20** *A,* Correction of minor depression of the upper cartilaginous vault. (From Dingman, R. O.: Correction of nasal deformities due to defects of the septum. Plast. Reconstr. Surg., *18*:241, 1956.)

(*Figure 24–20 continued on opposite page.*)

1. Blowout fractures involving the floor of the orbit through the thin bone of the maxilla
2. Medial orbital wall fractures through the lamina papyracea of the ethmoid
3. Combination of 1 and 2
4. Blow-out fracture of the orbital roof or the lateral orbital wall (rare)

C. Rim and infraorbital fractures combined, most common orbital fracture, occurs in cases of unusual and severe force, as auto accident or high velocity missile injury.

The function of the orbital cavity is to delicately suspend and adequately protect the orbital globes and their accessory structures. The bony rim surrounding the globe affords good protection of the globe, except in the lateral area where the rim is recessed 1.5 to 2 cm. behind the infraorbital and supraorbital plane. This allows protective vision through an arc of approximately 190 degrees but leaves the globe more vulnerable laterally. Of the bones of the orbit, the most frequently fractured is the zygoma. Because of its prominent position, it is vulnerable and displacement may be significant. The thin roof of the maxillary antrum in the orbital floor and the medial wall made up of the fragile lamina papyracea of the ethmoid offer little resistance to force. These thin, easily fractured bones provide a built-in protective mechanism, allowing fracture and rapid decompression of the orbital cavity, thereby decreasing the possibility of rupture of the globe. Discussion of the following complications applies to true blow-out fractures and to fractures involving the rim and the orbital floor.

### *Ocular Injuries*

The clinician must have an acute awareness of the potential for eye injuries in patients with facial fractures. Ocular injuries are frequently overlooked in patients with facial trauma.[43] Fortunately, most ocular injuries do not result in permanent damage. The more severe the fracture, the greater the likelihood of eye injury. Jabaley reports that 18.4 per cent of orbital fractures are complicated by ocular injuries. Others report 10 per cent of midface fractures with ocular complications.[58]

If ocular injury is suspected, visual acuity

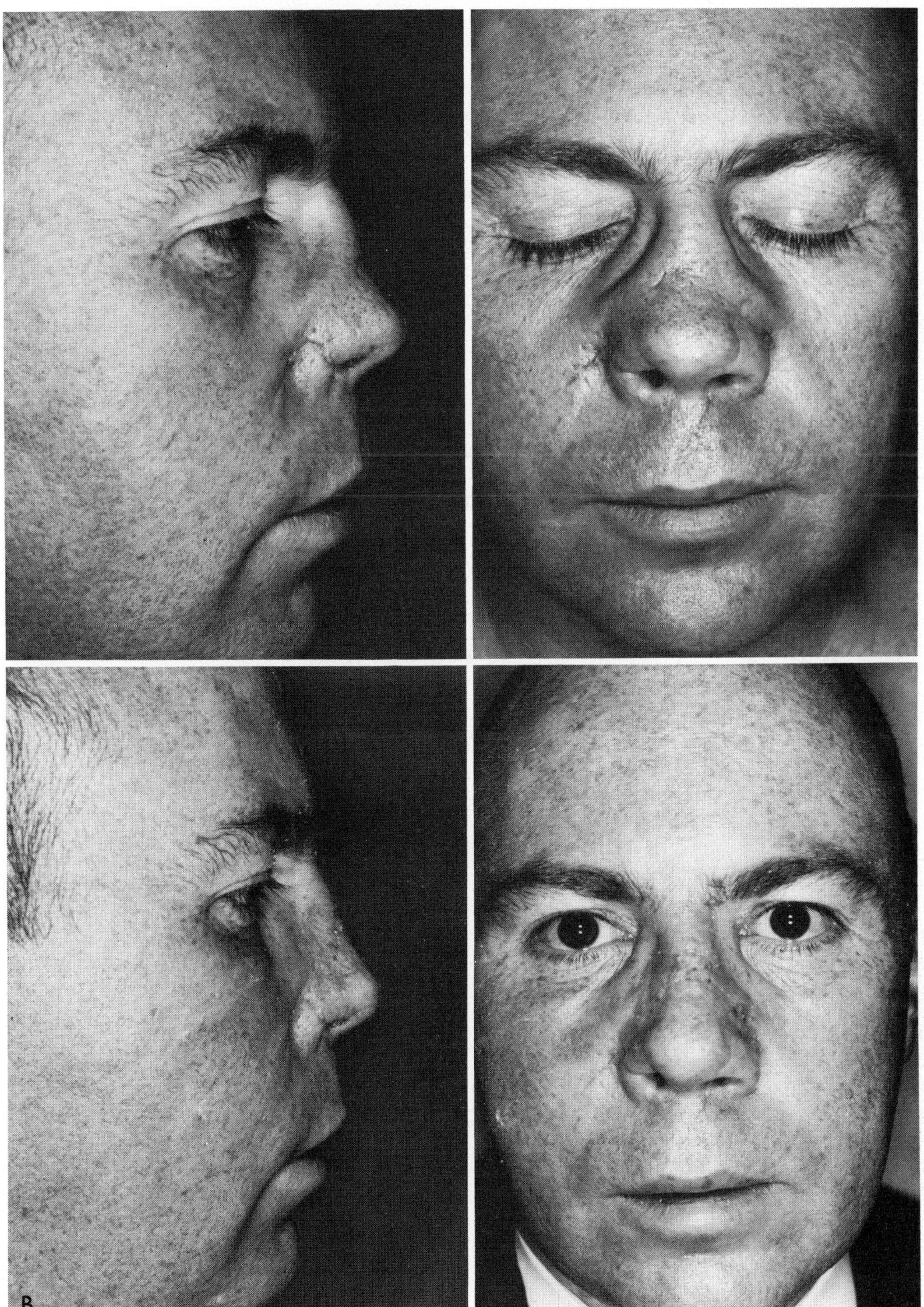


**Figure 24–20** *Continued. B,* Preoperative and postoperative photos of this technique in conjunction with nasal bone osteotomies.

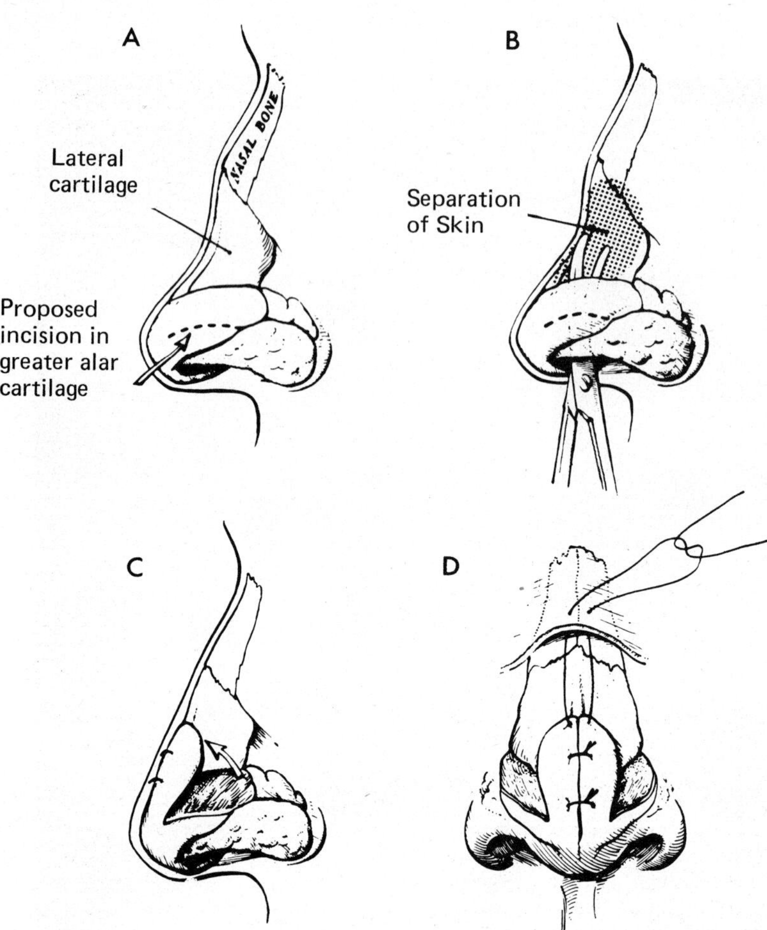


**Figure 24–21** Cephalic edges of the lateral crus of the alar cartilages to correct supratip depression. (From Dingman, R. O.: Correction of nasal deformities due to defects of the septum. Plast. Reconstr. Surg., *18*:241, 1956.)

examination should precede any treatment. If a wall or pocket chart is not available, use standard newsprint, which read at 13 inches represents near vision of 20/50.[58] If there is visual loss or if the patient is unconscious, the pupillary light reflex is sometimes helpful. The Marcus Gunn syndrome suggests a major injury to the eye and allows the examiner to locate the lesion somewhere between the optic chiasm and the retina. The eyes are examined with a direct light source. The light is moved back and forth between both eyes. If conduction in the optic nerve is diminished on the involved side because of injury, then the consensual response of that pupil will be greater than its response to direct light. This will give the appearance that the pupil on the injured side is dilating as light is brought from the uninvolved eye.

Significant eye pain, changes in gross vision and pupillary abnormalities may indicate direct ocular injury. The sclera and cornea should be examined for abrasions, lacerations or rupture. Blood in the anterior chamber (hyphema), lens subluxation and dislocation and iris disruption are among the types of damage to the anterior structures. Retinal injuries are most difficult to detect and require evaluation by an ophthalmologic consultant. Figure 24–24 shows ocular injuries frequently associated with orbital fractures.

If direct ocular injury is suspected, ophthalmologic consultation and treatment may help avoid permanent visual impairment.

McCoy (1962)[63] reported blindness in 0.6 per cent of 337 patients with fractures of the middle third of the face. There is a much higher incidence of permanent ocular impairment with direct trauma to the globe.

Intraoperative ocular injury may be

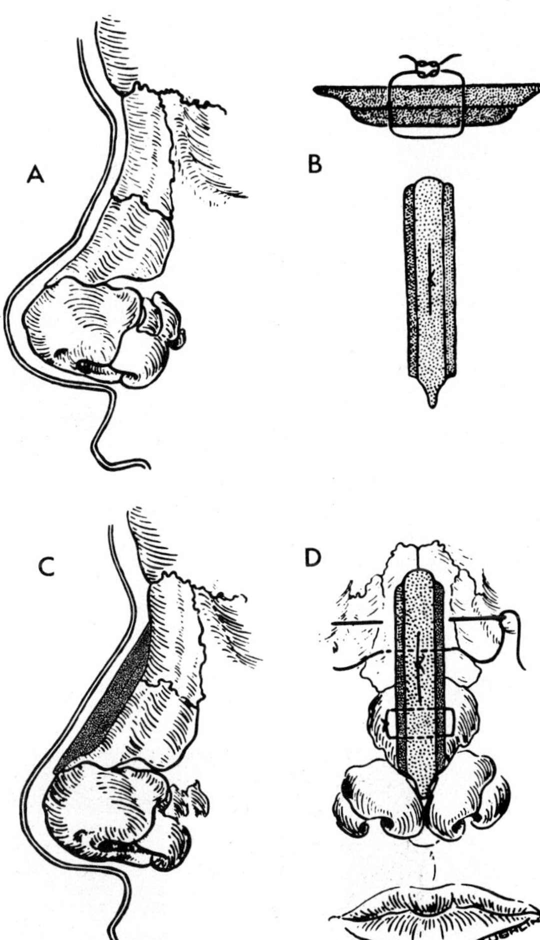


**Figure 24–22** Autogenous (septal) cartilage sutured together for correction of dorsal defect. (From Dingman, R. O.: Correction of nasal deformities due to defects of the septum. Plast. Reconstr. Surg., *18*:241, 1956.)

avoided by use of a large soft plastic corneal lens and protection of the globe with small malleable retractors while exploring the orbital floor. Cases of reduced visual acuity following surgery for treatment of zygomatic and maxillary fractures have been reported.[37, 38, 67] The mechanism for this appears to be pressure secondary to hemorrhage into the orbit. Grabb recommends placing lateral orbital drains when there is evidence of significant intraoperative bleeding within the orbit or any orbital proptosis.

The prevention of diplopia and enophthalmos, the most frequent sequelae of inadequately treated blow-out fracture, also may depend upon early diagnosis and treatment. Clinical examination and x-ray findings will usually give an accurate determination of an orbital floor fracture, the severity of which may not be determined without surgical exploration. Diplopia, or the symptom of double vision, may present immediately or be delayed. Diplopia alone is not diagnostic of orbital fracture, since intraorbital hematoma and edema may displace the globe or limit its movement. The patient may initially complain of diplopia or blurred vision, or examination may show extraocular muscle imbalance. Minimal degrees of diplopia may be documented by having the patient look at a white light source while covering one eye with a red lens. If minimal degrees of limitation of extraocular movement exist, the patient will see separate white and red images. Diplopia may not be evident, however, until a few days or longer post injury when tissue edema subsides or some muscle shortening begins.

Periorbital swelling and ecchymosis, palpable orbital rim defect and infraorbital nerve anesthesia are other signs of orbital

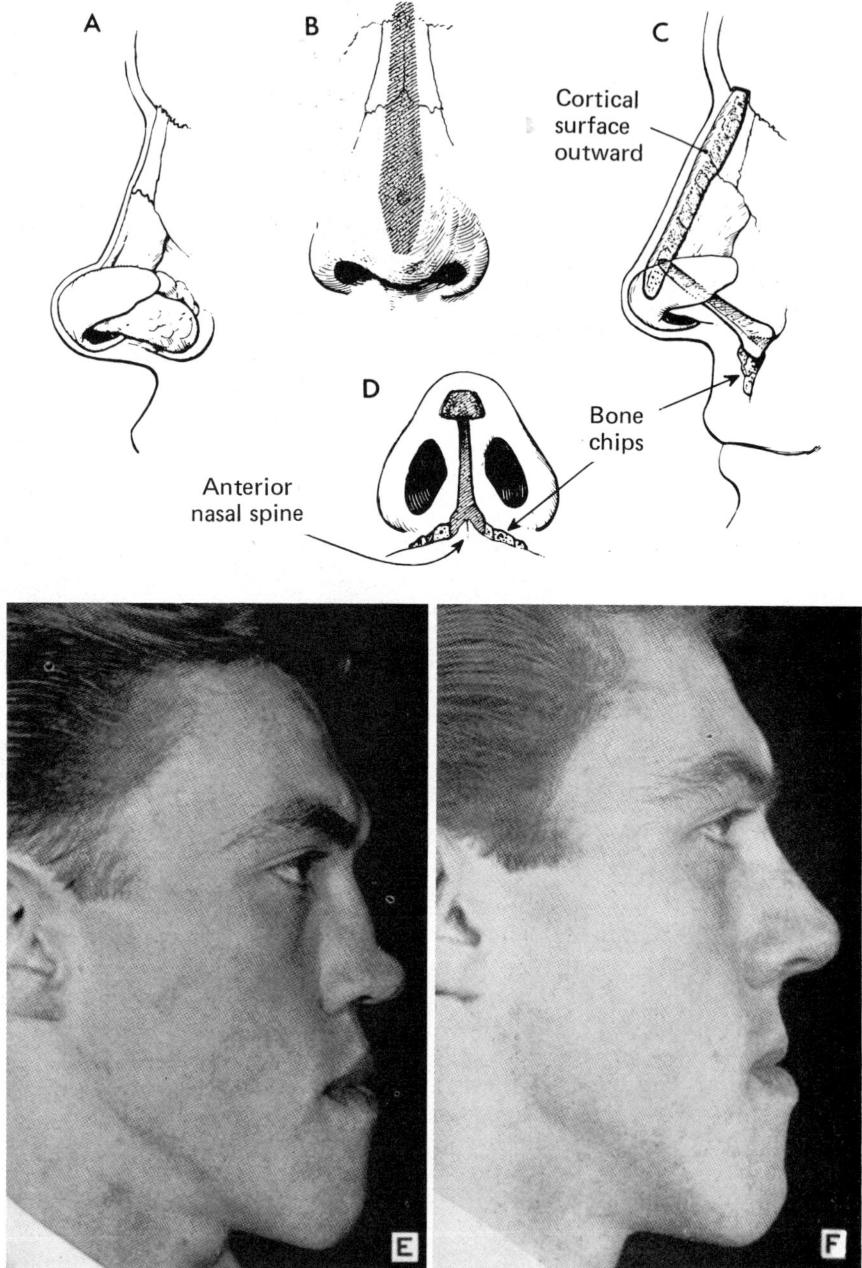


**Figure 24–23** Iliac bone graft (dorsal and collumellar strut). (From Dingman, R. O.: Correction of nasal deformities due to defects of the septum. Plast. Reconstr. Surg., *18*:241, 1956.)

| Structure | Structure Divisions | Injury |
|---|---|---|
| Integument of eye | Cornea | Abrasion, laceration |
| | Sclera | Laceration |
| Anterior structures | Anterior chamber | Hemorrhage |
| | Lens | Subluxation/dislocation, traumatic cataract |
| | Iris | Perforation (iridodialysis) |
| | Iris sphincter | Rupture |
| | Anterior chamber angle | Recession/contusion (absorption blockage) |
| | Ciliary body | Rupture |
| Posterior structures | Vitreous humor | Hemorrhage |
| | Retina | Edema, contusion, hematoma, detachment, hole |
| | Choroid | Hemorrhage, rupture |
| | Optic nerve | Contusion, hematoma, secondary atrophy |

**Figure 24–24** (Ocular structures and their injuries that may be associated with orbital fractures. (From Jabaley, M. E., Lerman, M., and Sanders, H. J.: Ocular injuries in orbital fractures. A review of 119 cases. Plast. Reconstr. Surg., *56*:410, 1975.)

floor fracture. X-ray examination may be helpful. Anteroposterior, lateral and Waters views are routine in orbital injuries but felt by some authors to be subject to a high rate of false positive findings.[14] We feel that these studies, in addition to orbital floor tomography, correlate well with surgical findings and should be an integral part of the preoperative evaluation.[14, 40] Tomograms frequently will show fragmentation of the orbital floor, depression of the fragments and prolapse of orbital soft tissues into the upper maxillary sinus.

An analysis of 300 orbital fractures[70] indicated 1.6 per cent incidence of medial wall blow-out. These may present with subcutaneous emphysema, epistaxis and crepitus over the side of the nasal bridge. Diplopia will usually be in lateral gaze. Tomography may show air in the orbit with lateral displacement of the globe.

The forced duction test for muscle entrapment is helpful in both the conscious and the unconscious patient. With the conjunctiva anesthetized, the sclera at the insertion of the inferior rectus muscle is grasped with a forceps and pulled forward. If there is no entrapment of the inferior rectus muscle in the orbital fracture site, the eye will rotate vertically with ease. This test assists in differentiating muscle entrapment from direct nerve or muscle damage (Fig. 24–25).

Causes of immediate diplopia are (1) direct injury to extraocular muscles, (2) muscle entrapment by the fracture fragments (medial, superior, lateral or inferior), (3) cranial nerve damage (III, IV, VI), (4) periorbital edema and (5) direct damage to the muscle attachments. Diplopia secondary to periorbital edema should resolve in a few days.

The objective of surgery is to elevate and reconstruct the bony floor of the orbit, thereby preventing irreversible incorporation of the suspensory (Lockwood's) ligament, extraocular muscles and sometimes the globe into the healed fracture. If on initial examination a blow-out fracture is certain and there is clinical enophthalmus, ptosis of the globe, diplopia, restricted vertical movement of the globe and supratarsal depression, early surgery is recommended by most authors. If in doubt, a wait of 7 to 10 days may be advisable, since the clinical symptoms and signs may become more indicative if a blow-out fracture is present. If the initial findings are related to edema only, symptoms will usually resolve. Waiting too long, however, may result in increased complications later. Converse (1967) reports difficulty with treatment after 21 days because of early malunion, established diplopia, and enophthalmos.

Three approaches or combination approaches have been advocated for exploration of the orbital floor.

### ANTRAL APPROACH

The Caldwell-Luc maxillary antrostomy and antral packing for blow-out fracture continues to be popular. In a study[48] of 56 patients with orbital floor fracture treated

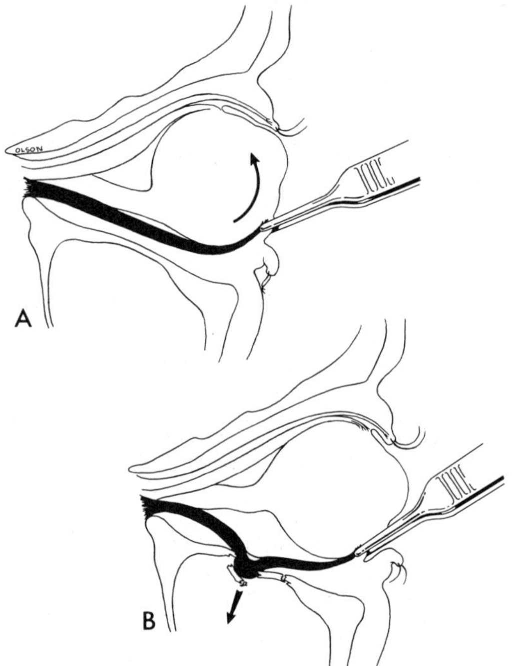


**Figure 24–25** Forced duction test to examine for muscle entrapment associated with "blow out" of orbit. *A*, Negative exam. *B*, Positive exam with entrapment.

with maxillary antrostomy and packing, 30 of these patients had complications, including diplopia, enophthalmos, trigeminal neuralgia and iridocyclitis. Others also reject this method in all cases because the blind packing may potentially push bone spicules into the optic nerve or globe and result in blindness.[63]

We feel that the Caldwell-Luc antrostomy has many shortcomings. The blind treatment of a blow-out fracture does not permit accurate fragment control and maintenance of orbital floor elevation. Trapped muscle or infraorbital fat may not be fully released and bone spicules may be displaced into the orbit with resulting nerve or globe injury. If used, it should be in combination with adequate infraorbital exposure to provide accurate bone reduction.

We have seen two patients with unilateral postoperative blindness and one with bilateral blindness following transantral orbital floor reduction. Others have been reported. We know of none following the direct orbital approach to the orbital floor for blow-out fracture treatment.

#### DIRECT ORBITAL APPROACH

Access may be obtained through any of three acceptable incisions:

1. Through the skin, 2 to 3 mm. below the lash line. The subciliary incision extends from lateral to the punctum to the lateral canthus. Skin and orbicular muscle are separated from the orbital septum to the infraorbital rim. An incision is made through the periosteum at the rim, and subperiosteal dissection is used to expose the orbital floor. Access may be limited with this exposure, and transient (three to six months) mild ectropion has been noted in 25 per cent of a small series in our clinic. The scar is negligible.
2. Skin incision at junction of lid and cheek skin. This gives easy exposure of orbital rim where periosteum is incised and subperiosteal dissection is carried to the orbital floor. Wide exploration is possible, but the scar may be slightly noticeable.
3. The conjunctival approach for orbital floor fractures is a "spin off" of Tessier's technique for orbital floor approach in craniofacial surgery.[84] The incision is made transversely in the depth of the lower conjunctival cul-de-sac; dissection is made anterior to the orbital septum to the orbital rim where the periosteum is incised. Subperiosteal dissection gives exposure of orbital floor. If wider exposure is necessary, the conjunctival incision is extended into a lateral canthotomy. The cornea must be protected. The exposure is excellent, and the scar is well hidden.

In all these approaches, the surgeon should avoid cutting through the orbital septum above the orbital rim since herniation of orbital fat occurs and is difficult to control intraoperatively. This may not be preventable if the orbital septum or periosteum is already torn. The globe should be elevated with great care with malleable ribbon retractors to avoid iatrogenic complications.

After the periosteum is incised at the rim and carefully elevated, the orbital floor is fully explored. If a blow-out fracture is present, the herniated contents (periorbital fat, muscles and globe) are carefully elevated out of the defect. If Lockwood's suspensory ligament is intact, herniation will be minimal. With careful evaluation of the comminuted bony fragments, the maxillary sinus mucosa may be left intact, reducing the possibility of infection or bone necrosis. The orbital floor defect should be restored to continuity. We prefer irradiated homograft cartilage,[24] since it is inexpensive, easily cut to size and in our hands has few complications. Fresh autogenous costal cartilage grafts, iliac bone, anterior maxillary sinus wall, perpendicular plate of the ethmoid and septal cartilage have been used successfully. Converse[46] prefers split rib grafts in children and iliac grafts for wide defects. Synthetic materials are now popular, especially for small and noncontaminated fractures. These include Teflon, Silastic, Supramed and collagen sheets. With these materials, secondary operations (hip or chest) are unnecessary. A recent study[72] reports good results with denatured porcine collagen (Gelfilm) as the choice for small blow-outs. It is nonallergenic and noninflammatory and appears to discourage adhesions. Metal screen and mesh are undesirable materials for orbital floor reconstruction.

Implants should be placed subperiosteally and should not protrude beyond the infraorbital rim, since extrusion may occur. The potential for infection exists, especially if the sinus is open and infected. Patients with blow-out fractures should receive prophylactic antibiotics to reduce the potential for orbital cellulitis and sepsis, a serious complication. Antibiotics should be continued for 7 to 10 days after orbital reconstruction with implants.

Medial wall blow-out fractures with entrapment are managed in a similar manner. Great care must be exercised while dissecting posteromedially in the region of the optic nerve and the inferior orbital fissure.

The primary objective of this surgery is to restore fully the ocular rotary movements with restoration of the orbital floor. This can be checked interoperatively again, using the forced duction test. Relief of actual or potential enophthalmos is also important, but function comes first.

Close observation is important postoperatively. Orbital pain, absent pupillary reflex or decreased visual acuity may be signs of impaired retinal circulation, requiring immediate removal of the orbital floor implant.

### PERSISTENT OCULAR ROTARY IMBALANCES

Late persistent muscle dysfunction may be secondary to direct cranial nerve damage, ocular muscle damage, displacement of muscles on the globe or late adhesions.[29] Function of the eye is altered in the field of action of the specific muscle involved. The forced duction test will assist in differential diagnosis. Muscle dysfunction in the absence of fracture usually subsides in a short time. After initial surgery for blow-out fracture, muscle imbalance may persist for two or three months. Muscle surgery should be deferred for this period. Limited treatment includes patching (partial or complete occlusion) and prisms. Muscle shortening or lengthening is considered if the other measures do not correct the problem.

### ENOPHTHALMOS

Post-traumatic enophthalmos is not fully understood. Even with standard techniques, including adequate and early exploration with repair of orbital floor fractures, this occurs. If seen immediately post injury, enophthalmos is usually a certain sign of significant orbital floor fracture requiring exploration and treatment. Pseudoptosis and deepening of the supratarsal fold are noted secondary to loss of globe support. Diplopia also frequently occurs with acute enophthalmos. With blow-out fracture, the periorbital fat herniates, decreasing the volume of the intraorbital contents and allowing the globe to recede. Even with adequate repair of the floor defect, fat necrosis probably due to trauma pressure and inflammation decreases intraorbital volume. Muscles, nerves and fascia may shorten with delayed repair, entrapment or fibrosis. Minimal enophthalmos, even 2 to 3 mm., is significantly disfiguring and functionally disabling.

Acute enophthalmos may be corrected by replacement of the periorbital fat and muscles into the orbit and orbital floor implant, thus restoring the normal volume of orbital contents. Late enophthalmos is usually uncorrectable. Converse uses the forward traction test to determine if surgery will improve this condition. If traction with sutures placed on the medial and lateral rectus insertions does not produce forward movement of the globe, enophthalmos will not improve with infraorbital implant. Preoperatively, specific orbital measurements from multiple x-ray views may help determine anatomic orbital changes. Surgical repair consists of placing implants (bone, cartilage or Silastic) over the orbital floor, lateral wall and medial wall behind the lacrimal sac. A movement of 6 mm. has been reported, using Silastic sponge.[77] Grabb (1972)[38] reports three cases treated with irradiated cartilage graft. One patient was improved slightly, but two were failures. The use of Silastic bead placement in nonseeing eyes has also been reported.[78] Pseudoptosis may be worse after implant. Augmentation of the infraorbital rim in patients with enophthalmos should be avoided, since it may produce an optical illusion of increased deformity.

Orbital roof fractures are uncommon. They may involve the supraorbital rim, be linear or be associated with comminution of the frontal bone. The rim fractures may result in permanent diplopia and ptosis if not treated. Open reduction and wire fixation is necessary. Frontal bone fracture, including the orbital roof, also should be managed by open reduction and wire fixation of fragments. Bone fragments should be used when possible in reconstruction. The linear roof fracture may have associated diplopia secondary to hematoma, which usually resolves in two to three weeks.[7] Persistent ptosis with comminuted roof fractures may be secondary to herniation of the frontal lobe. These must be surgically treated. Large defects are approached intracranially with rib or iliac bone graft to the roof to separate the periorbita from the dura. Dural defects should be repaired. Smaller defects have been treated via the intraorbital approach.[14] Reconstruction of the orbital roof using methylmerthacrylate prostheses has also been reported.[55]

Other complications of orbital fractures include (1) damage to the lacrimal system with epiphora and dacryocystitis, subsequently requiring nasolacrimal surgery; (2) infraorbital nerve damage with anesthesia; (3) ptosis secondary to levator palpebral muscle trans-section or paresis; and (4) bony rim defects.

Orbital bone injuries may be complex and serious and associated with injured globe and adnexa. The results of treatment may frequently be less than normal restoration of contour and function. It therefore seems prudent for the maxillofacial surgeon to work closely with his colleagues in ophthalmology and neurosurgery to give the patient the greatest opportunity for restoration of normal function and appearance.

## NASO-ORBITAL INJURIES

Trauma to the naso-orbital area can lead to severe cosmetic and functional deformity. Avoidance depends greatly on early primary diagnosis, accurate fracture reduction and treatment of soft tissue injuries. Studies[79] have shown that the nasal area is the weakest of the facial skeleton. The nasal-interorbital space contains thin, fragile bony structures —nasal bones, ethmoid cells, and lamina papyracea, superior and middle turbinates and the perpendicular plate of the ethmoid. A direct force, depending on its intensity and vector, may shatter and displace these structures. Less violent forces, as from a fist, may cause fracture with displacement of large segments of bone and minimal soft tissue damage. High speed forces, as in a facial smash from automobile accidents or missiles, cause more severe soft tissue damage, extensive comminution, displacement and injury to the adjacent tissues. Frequent findings in these cases include posterior and lateral displacement of the nasal bones, fractures of the septum, lacrimal system injuries, widening of the interorbital space with encroachment on the orbital cavities and their contents and paranasal sinus damage.

The normal medial palpebral ligament divides into two heads, the deep head of the pretarsal muscles inserting on the posterior lacrimal crest and the superficial anterior segment inserting on the anterior lacrimal crest. Between these insertions lies the lacrimal sac. Interorbital fractures usually involve the lacrimal bones and frequently result in lateral displacement of the attachments of the medial palpebral ligament. This occurs by either laceration of the ligaments or, more commonly, comminution of the bony ligamentous attachments. Displacement of the ligaments with loss of support permits lateral and downward pull by the orbicular muscles, resulting in an increase in the intercanthal distance (telecanthus), blunting of the canthal angle and epicanthal folds. The horizontal dimension of the palpebral fissure is frequently shortened.

X-ray examination as described by Dingman and Natvig (1964)[28] will assist in the diagnosis. Naso-orbital injury may be associated with blow-out fracture, cribriform plate fracture with CSF leak, extraocular muscle trauma, frontal sinus fractures, cranial nerve damage and ocular injuries. As with other injuries of this magnitude of the head and neck, the patient should be fully evaluated for cervical spine injuries.

A CSF leak frequently will cease spontaneously in two to four weeks. Antibiotic coverage is used in all naso-orbital injuries because of this potential leak and possible subsequent meningitis. If the leak persists, exploration of the anterior cranial fossa may be indicated.

Epiphora may result from injury to the lacrimal apparatus, disturbance of normal lacrimal pump mechanism or injuries of the punctum. Lacrimogram may be helpful in assessing the patency of the lacrimal system.

Orbital emphysema from ethmoid sinus fracture may be detected on x-ray.

Primary repair of naso-orbital fractures should be done as early as the patient will tolerate surgery. Fractures are easier to manage primarily, and results are better if treated early. Open wounds may give excellent access to the fracture site, permitting reduction and fixation under direct vision. In closed fractures, judiciously placed incisions will provide access and give an opportunity to replace and fix fragments before hematoma, fibrosis and malunion occur. If associated with cranial and orbital injuries, naso-orbital fractures may be treated concurrently with intracranial or orbital exposure in cooperation with the neurosurgical consultants. Close cooperative team effort usually gives the best results with fewer complications.

Reduction and fixation of facial bone fractures and other necessary repairs should be accomplished primarily, if possible, because of greater difficulty encountered after the structures are fixed in malposition by scar. Bony fractures should be carefully reduced (Fig. 24–26). If comminuted, it may be necessary to fix the fractures with fine wire splints, wire pins, intranasal packs or extraskeletal appliances. Early repair of the nasolacrimal system injuries is recommended. Laceration and separation of the palpebral ligaments are treated by replacement and fixation with transosseous wires, as described by Converse and Smith (1966).[12]

### LATE COMPLICATIONS

A. External nasal deformity
   1. Saddle nose
   2. Twisted nose
   3. Deviation
   4. Shortened nose
   5. Retraction of the columella
B. Intranasal problems
   1. Obstruction
   2. Synechia
   3. Septal perforation
C. Telecanthus
D. Increased interorbital distance
E. Lacrimal system problems
   1. Epiphora
   2. Dacryocystitis
F. Cerebral abscess — may occur many months or years after injury if dural leak is persistent

After the early golden opportunity for repair has passed, a wait of several months after injury is advisable before reconstruction to allow resolution of edema and maturation of scar.

### LATE SURGERY

The objective of any surgical repair is to restore bony contour, establish nasolacrimal duct drainage, correct the telecanthus by re-establishing normal medial palpebral ligament insertion, establish a functional airway and restore normal appearance of the face. Converse and Smith emphasize attempting these repairs during the same operative session (1966),[12] and we favor an early aggressive approach whenever possible and safe for the patient.[19]

Incisions for the repairs may be combined with the correction of traumatic epicanthal folds. Mustarde's rectangular flap operation

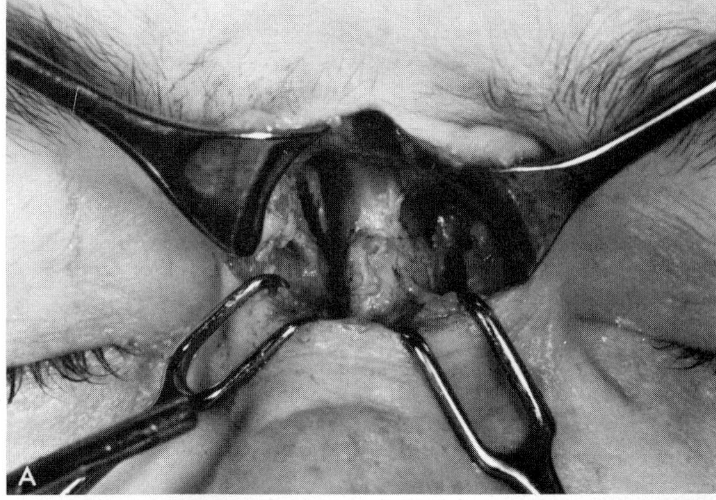


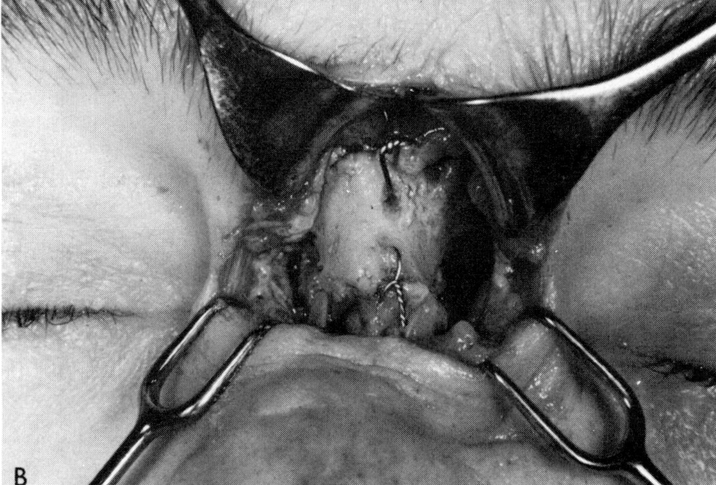


**Figure 24–26** Interosseous wiring of a relatively recent malunion of a naso-orbital fracture.

(Fig. 24–27) (1959)[61] or the double opposing Z-plasties as described by Converse and Smith (1966)[12] (Fig. 24–28) are most frequently used. These incisions permit adequate subperiosteal dissection of the nasal bones and medial orbit. If the fracture is relatively recent, realignment and wiring of the fracture fragments sometimes is possible. If late, the nasal dorsum is usually wide and thick due to bony overlap and osteogenesis and must be contoured by osteotomies, high speed drill contouring or bone grafts. Subperiosteal dissection is used to avoid damage to the scarred lacrimal sac, which is difficult to identify. Probing the canaliculus or staining of the lacrimal system by irrigation with dilute methylene blue dye may assist in identification. Care must be used since dye leakage staining the surrounding tissues will make dissection more difficult. Dacryocystorhinostomy may be necessary to correct epiphora if the nasolacrimal duct or lower lacrimal sac has been destroyed. If destruction of the common canaliculus has occurred, conjunctivorhinostomy, as described by Jones (1976),[45] may be indicated.

The scarred medial palpebral ligament is identified. If the ligament is lacerated, location may be difficult, but if it is still attached to a piece of avulsed lacrimal bone, it may be easier to find. When the ligament is difficult to mobilize medially, Converse suggests that the septum orbitali be detached subperiosteally and incised at its insertion along the medial half of the upper and lower orbital rims. A lateral canthotomy may be necessary to get relaxation.[26] After the ligament has

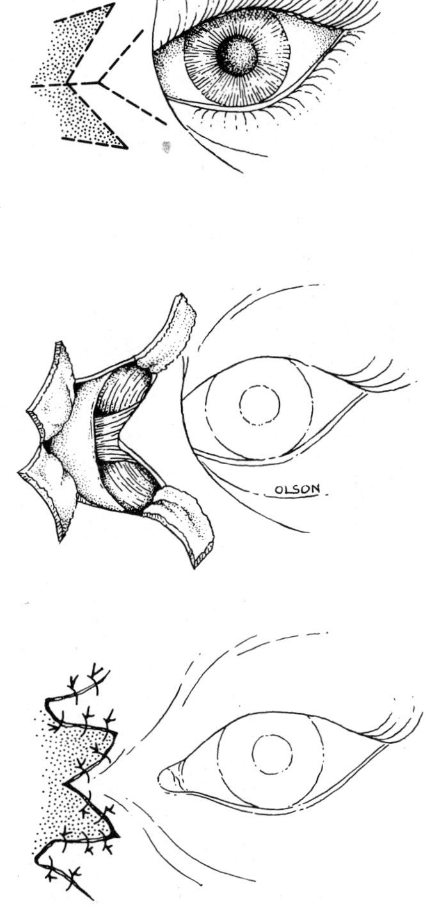


**Figure 24–28** Mustardé's rectangular flap technique for correction of an epicanthal fold.

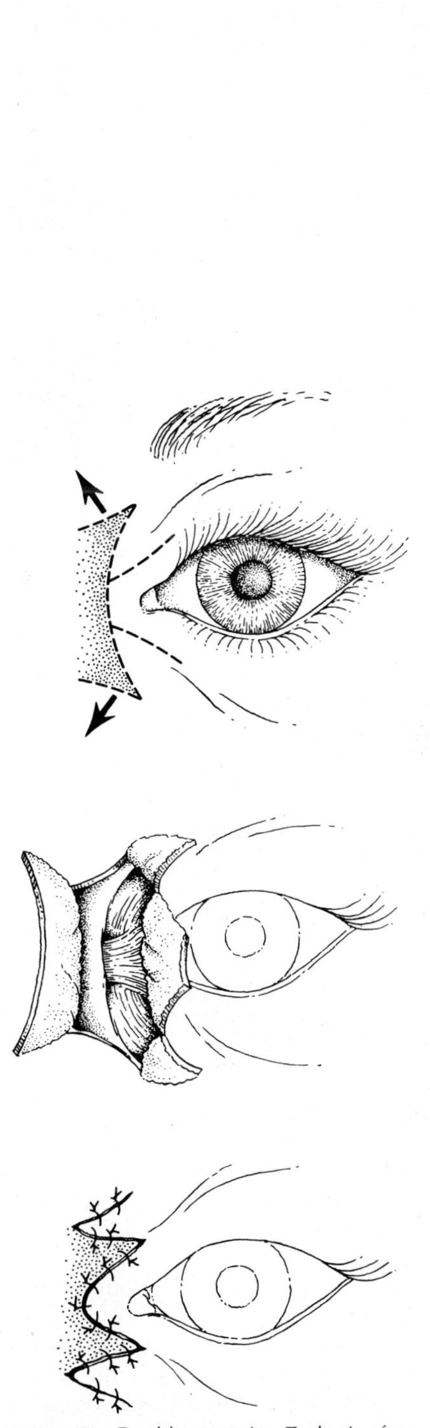

**Figure 24–27** Double opposing Z-plasties for correction of an epicanthal fold (arrows represent pull obliterating fold). (Adapted from Converse, J. M., and Smith, B.: Naso-orbital fractures and traumatic deformities of the medial canthus. Plast. Reconstr. Surg., 38:147, 1966.)

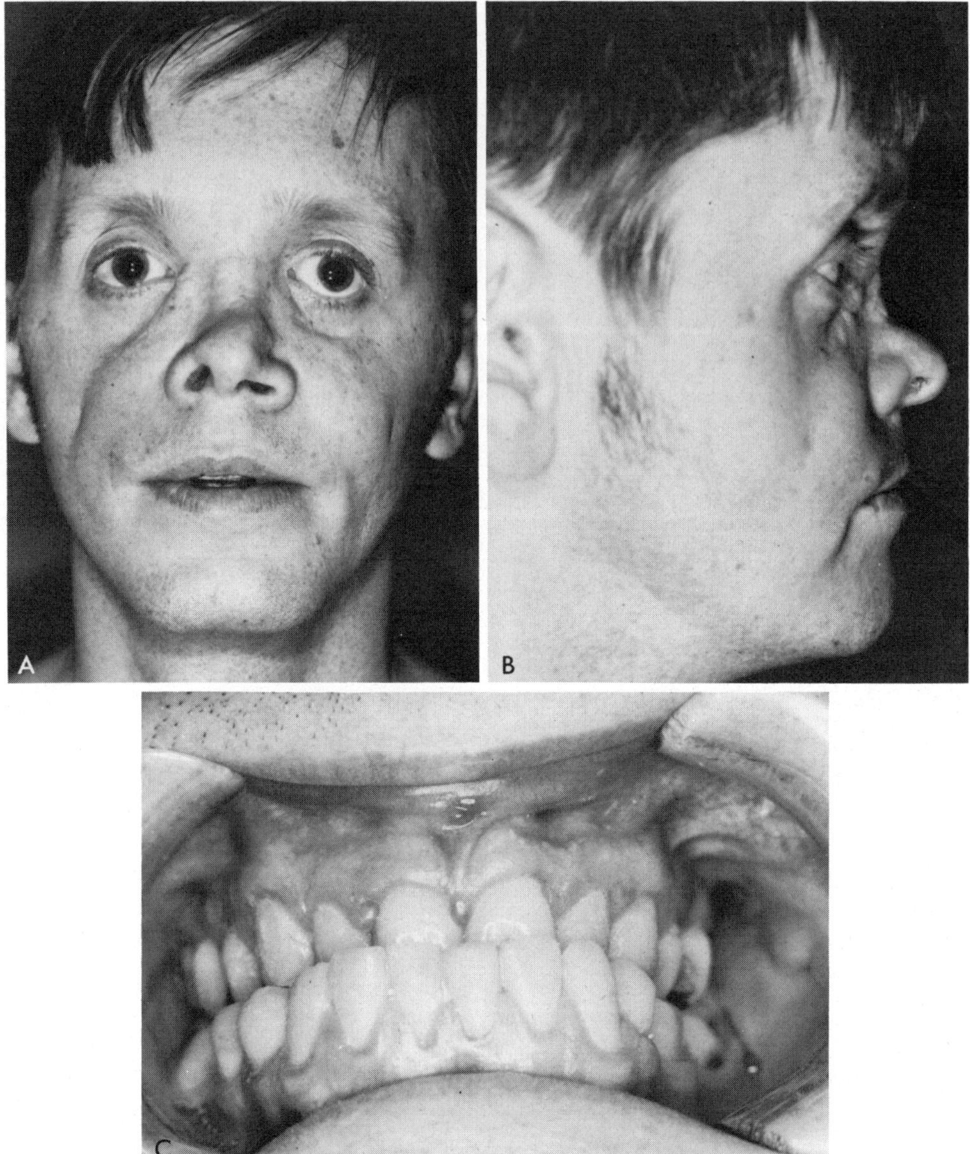

(*Figure 24–29 Legend and illustrations continued on opposite page.*)

been freed, it should be reattached to the medial orbital wall just posterior and superior to the lacrimal fossa with transosseous wires. Additional transosseous wires are tied over acrylic splints for 10 to 14 days to hold the skin against the bony structures. Late follow-up surgery may include bone grafts to the nasal dorsum and septal reconstruction.

## MULTIPLE FACIAL BONE FRACTURES

Avoidance of complications in injuries involving multiple facial bones lies in the full determination of the extent of the injury and meticulous repair. The complications associated with individual soft tissue or bone trauma have been discussed. Multiple facial bone fractures with or without severe soft tissue damage are not uncommon, especially in high-speed automobile accidents. Although the incidence of facial smash injuries has decreased since the advent of the 55 m.p.h. speed limit, the principles of treatment have not changed.

Facial fractures are not surgical emergencies except when contributing to airway obstruction or threatened exsanguination.

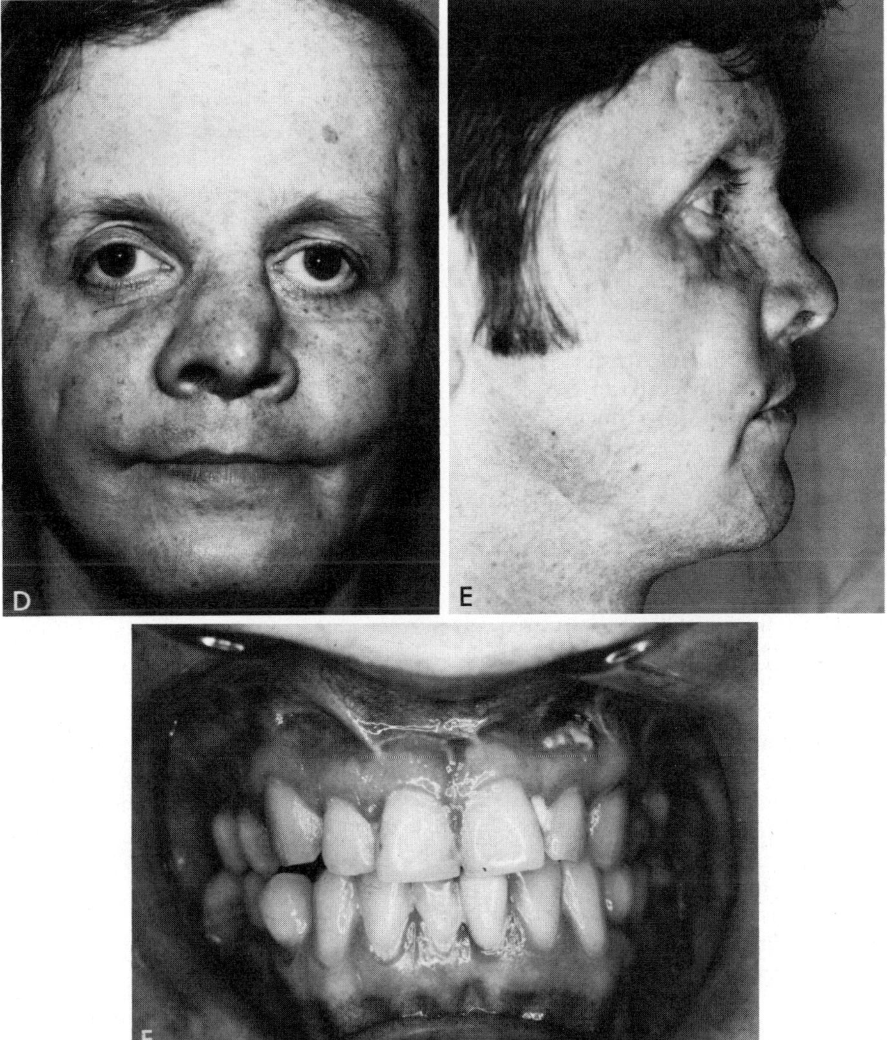


**Figure 24–29** *Continued. A,* Severe facial fractures with multiple deformities. *B,* Postoperative multiple reconstructive procedures, as described in the text.

Work-up of the severely injured patient, including cervical spine, thoracic, abdomen and central nervous system is indicated. The initial findings of panfacial fractures may be masked by edema and hematoma. Careful physical and x-ray evaluation can, however, demonstrate the extent of injury. If conditions warrant, aggressive early surgical exploration and fracture reduction is optimal. Frequently severe edema obscures the picture, but if the patient is stable, operative correction within the first six hours after injury is ideal and may decrease the necessity for later secondary surgical procedures.

The objective management of severe facial injuries is to restore the patient to normal, or as nearly normal as possible from the standpoint of function and appearance, in the shortest time possible consistent with good care.

The principles of fracture management include reduction of the fracture, fixation during the process of healing and prevention of infection.

Successful management of multiple facial fractures requires an orderly approach to reduction and fixation. When multiple bones are fractured and displaced, points of reference are sometimes difficult to establish. If the mandible is not involved, the maxillary segment may be oriented in relationship to the mandible through tooth or denture relationships and the fractured midface segments may be arranged in perspective and fixed by appropriate measures in position for optimum healing.

If the mandible is broken in one or several areas, reconstruction of it by open methods is first done, and the maxilla and midfacial bones are fixed to the mandible to establish occlusion. The maxillary mandibular complex is then forced upward into anatomic position, where it is fixed with appropriate wires, splints, pins or appliances to the immediately intact suprastructure, i.e., to the frontal bone, zygomatic bone, nasal process of the frontal bone, pyriform margin of the maxilla, nasal spine or other solid structures. Surgical approach by elective transcoronal, lateral brow, lower lid, conjunctival, intraoral, submandibular and preauricular incisions may be necessary to obtain access to the areas of bone fracture.

To minimize complications, the surgeon, on the basis of his clinical, x-ray and laboratory findings, should develop a surgical plan of approach individualized for each patient. Although neither definitive nor all-inclusive, the following sequential steps are suggested for the development of the surgical plan:

1. Establish an airway system that will permit administration of anesthesia and guarantee postoperative airway patency.
2. Tracheostomy should be used if deemed necessary.
3. Local anesthesia with sedation should be used if practical. For prolonged procedures use general anesthesia.
4. Explore open wounds for presence of underlying fractures.
5. Reduce and fix the fractures through open wounds and, if necessary, surgically extend lacerations to provide exposure or make new incisions for adequate exposure.
6. Conservative debridement is advisable. Save all useful bone and soft tissue.
7. Wire bone fragments together with fine wire.
8. Use local bone for immediate grafts if indicated. If necessary, use rib or iliac bone grafts for large bone defects.
9. Cover exposed bone or bone grafts with local soft tissues. Skin or mucosa provide adequate drainage.
10. Use drains in grossly contaminated wounds or where seroma or hematoma may occur.
11. Provide positive fixation of bone fragments in anatomic position.
12. Close wounds carefully.
13. Give broad-spectrum antibiotic coverage.
14. Provide detailed complete postoperative supportive measures.

The basic principle is to establish fixation of loose fragments to stable bone. In some cases, if adequate skin coverage is present, primary iliac bone grafts provide reconstruction and stability and avoid later deformity.

The soft tissue and bony complications, contour defect, malunion and so on are approached individually with emphasis on both function and appearance as secondary procedures (Fig. 24–29).

## Bibliography


1. Altonen, M., Hohonen, A., and Dickhoff, K.: The treatment of zygomatic fractures: Internal wiring — antral packing — reposition without fixation. J. Maxillofac. Surg., *4*:107, 1976.
2. Ausin, A.: The "trap door" scar deformity. Clin. Plast. Surg., *4*:255, 1977.
3. Barclay, T. L.: Diplopia in association with fractures involving the zygomatic bone. Br. J. Plast. Surg., *11*:147, 1958.
4. Beard, C.: Ptosis. St. Louis, C. V. Mosby Co., 1976.
5. Beyer, C., and Smith, B.: Naso-orbital fractures: Complications and treatment. Ophthalmologica, *163*:418, 1971.
6. Blevins, C., and Gores, R. T.: Fractures of the mandibular condyloid process: Results of conservative treatment in 140 patients. J. Oral Surg., *19*:392, 1961.
7. Bloem, J. J., Meulen, J. C., and Ramselar, J. M.: Orbital roof fracture. Mod. Probl. Ophthalmol., *14*:510, 1975.
8. Bromberg, E. B., Sorg, I. C., and Radlaver, C. P.: Surgical treatment of massive bony ankylosis of the temporomandibular joint. Plast. Reconstr. Surg., *43*:66, 1969.
9. Brown, J. B., Fryer, M. P., and McDowell, F.: Internal wire fixation for fractures of upper jaw, orbit, zygoma, and severe facial crushes. Plast. Reconstr. Surg., *9*:276, 1952.
10. Chalmers, J.: Lyons Club members: Fractures involving the mandibular condyle: A post treatment survey of 120 cases. J. Oral Surg., *5*:45, 1947.
11. Converse, J. M., and Smith, B.: Canthoplasty and dacryocystorhinostomy in malunited fractures of the medial wall of the orbit. Am. J. Ophthalmol., *35*:1103, 1952.

12. Converse, J. M., and Smith, B.: Naso-orbital fractures and traumatic deformities of the medial canthus. Plast. Reconstr. Surg., *38*:147, 1966.
13. Converse, J. M., Smith, B., Obear, M., et al.: Orbital blowout fractures: A ten-year survey. Plast. Reconstruc. Surg., *39*:20, 1967.
14. Converse, J. M., Smith, B., and Wood-Smith, D.: Deformities of the midface from malunited fractures. Clin. Plast. Surg., *2*:107, 1975.
15. Crikelair, G. F.: Skin suture marks. Am. J. Surg., *96*:631, 1958.
16. Crikelair, G., Rein, J., Potter, G., et al.: A critical look at the "blowout" fracture. Plast. Reconstr. Surg., *49*:326, 1972.
17. DeFries, H. O., and Marble, H. B.: Reconstruction of the mandible: Use of homograft combined with autogenous bone and marrow. Arch. Otol., *93*:426, 1973.
18. Dingman, R. O.: Correction of nasal deformities due to defects of the septum. Plast. Reconstr. Surg., *18*:241, 1956.
19. Dingman, R. O.: Ankylosis of the temporomandibular joint. Am. J. Orthod., *32*:120, 1946.
20. Dingman, R. O.: Symposium: malunited fractures of the zygoma: repair of the deformity. Trans. Am. Acad. Ophthal. Otolaryngol., *57*:889, 1953.
21. Dingman, R. O.: Introduction to orbital fractures. *In* Tessier, P., et al. (eds.): Symposium on Plastic Surgery in the Orbital Region. St. Louis, C. V. Mosby Co., 1976, p. 63.
22. Dingman, R. O.: Surgical correction of deformities secondary to rhinoplasty. *In* Symposium on Corrective Rhinoplasty. St. Louis, C. V. Mosby Co., 1976.
23. Dingman, R. O., and Converse, J. M.: The clinical management of facial injuries and fractures of the facial bones. *In* Converse, J. M. (ed.): Reconstructive Plastic Surgery. Philadelphia, W. B. Saunders Co., 1977, p. 599.
24. Dingman, R. O., and Grabb, W. C.: Cartilage homografts preserved by irradiation. Plast. Reconstr. Surg., *28*:562, 1961.
25. Dingman, R. O., and Grabb, W. C.: Reconstruction of both mandibular condyles with metatarsal bone grafts. Plast. Reconstr. Surg., *34*:411, 1964.
26. Dingman, R. O., Grabb, W. C., and O'Neal, R. M.: Managment of injuries of the naso-orbital complex. Arch. Surg., *98*:566, 1969.
27. Dingman, R. O., and Harding, R. L.: Treatment of malunion fractures of facial bones. Plast. Reconstr. Surg., 7:505, 1951.
28. Dingman, R. O., and Natvig, P.: Surgery of Facial Fractures. Philadelphia, W. B. Saunders Co., 1964.
29. Dunlap, E. A.: Management of persistent oculorotary imbalances in orbital fractures. *In* Troutman, R. C., Converse, J. M., and Smith, B. (eds.): Plastic and Reconstructive Surgery of the Eye and Adnexa. Philadelphia, F. A. Davis (Butterworth), 1962.
30. Freihofer, H. P.: Results after midface osteotomies. J. Maxillofac. Surg., *1*:30, 1975.
31. Freihofer, H. P., and Sailer, H. F.: Experiences with intraoral transosseous wiring of mandibular fractures. J. Maxillofac. Surg., *1*:248, 1973.
32. Fry, H.: Interlocked stress in human nasal septal cartilage. Br. J. Plast. Surg., *19*:276, 1966.
33. Fry, H.: The importance of the septal cartilage in nasal trauma. Br. J. Plast. Surg., *20*:392, 1967.
34. Furnas, D. W., and Somers, G.: Microsurgery in the prevention of traumatic tattoos. Plast. Reconstr. Surg., *58*:631, 1976.
35. Georgiade, N.: The surgical correction of temporomandibular joint dysfunction by means of autogenous dermal grafts. Plast. Reconstr. Surg., *30*:68, 1962.
36. Georgiade, N., and Nash, T., Jr.: An external cranial fixation apparatus for severe maxillofacial injuries. Plast. Reconstr. Surg., *38*:142–146, 1966.
37. Gordon, S., and Macrae, H.: Monocular blindness as a complication of the treatment of malar fracture. Plast. Reconstr. Surg., *6*:228, 1950.
38. Grabb, W. C., and Berner, C. F.: Treatment of facial fractures. *In* Goldwyn, R. M. (ed): The Unfavorable Result in Plastic Surgery. Boston, Little, Brown and Co., 1972.
39. Grabb, W. C., and Smith, J. W.: Plastic Surgery: A Concise Guide to Clinical Practice. Boston, Little, Brown and Co., 1973.
40. Hakelius, L., and Ponten, B.: Results of immediate and delayed surgical treatment of facial fractures with diplopia. J. Maxillofac. Surg., *1*:150, 1973.
41. Hinderer, U. T.: Prevention of unsatisfactory scarring. Clin. Plast. Surg., *4*:199, 1977.
42. Irby, W.: Facial Trauma and Concomitant Problems. St. Louis, C. V. Mosby Co., 1974.
43. Jabaley, M. E., Lerman, M., and Sanders, H. J.: Ocular injuries in orbital fractures. A review of 119 cases. Plast. Reconstr. Surg., *5*:410, 1975.
44. James, N.: Survival of a large replanted segment of upper lip and nose. Plast. Reconstr. Surg., *58*:623, 1976.
45. Jones, L. T.: Surgery of the lacriminal sac. *In* Tessier, P., et al. (eds): Symposium on Plastic Surgery in the Orbital Region. St. Louis, C. V. Mosby Co., 1976, pp. 129–135.
46. Kazanjian, V. H., and Converse, J. M.: The Surgical Treatment of Facial Injuries. Baltimore, Williams and Wilkins Company, 1974.
47. Kemble, J. V.: Importance of nasal septum in facial development. J. Laryngol. Otol., *87*:4, 1973.
48. Kingsbury, B. C.: Alveolar fractures. J. Oral Surg., *27*:530, 1969.
49. Knapp, N., Whitaker, L., and Graham, W.: Evaluation of maxillary antrostomy in the treatment of fractures of the middle one-third of the face. J. Trauma, *13*:884, 1973.
50. Knight, J. S., and North, J. F.: The classification of malar fractures: An analysis of displacement as a guide to treatment. Br. J. Plast. Surg., *13*:325, 1961.
51. Kreidler, J. F., and Koch, H.: Endoscopic findings of maxillary sinus after middle face fractures. J. Maxillofac. Surg., *3*:10, 1975.

52. LeFort, R. (trans. by Dr. Paul Tessier): Experimental study of fractures of the upper jaw. Part III. Plast. Reconstr. Surg., *30*:6, 1963.
53. Mathog, R., and Boies, L.: Nonunion of mandible. Laryngology, *86*:908, 1976.
54. Mathog, R., and Rosenberg, Z.: Complications in the treatment of facial fractures. Otolaryngol. Clin. North Am., *9*:533, 1976.
55. Mayer, R., Brihaye, J., Brihaye-vanGeartruyden, M., et al.: Reconstruction of the orbital roof by acrylic prosthesis. Mod. Probl. Ophthalmol., *14*:506, 1975.
56. Melmed, E., and Koonin, A. J.: Fractures of the mandible: Review of 909 cases. Plast. Reconstr. Surg., *56*:323, 1975.
57. Miller, G., Anstee, E. J., and Snell, J. A.: Successful replantation of an avulsed scalp by microvascular anastomosis. Plast. Reconstr. Surg., *58*:133, 1976.
58. Miller, G., and Tenzel, R.: Ocular complications of midface fractures. Plast. Reconstr. Surg., *39*:37, 1967.
59. Montandon, D., D'Andrian, G., and Gabbiani, G.: The mechanism of wound contracture and epithelialization. Clin. Plast. Surg., *4*:325, 1977.
60. Mustardé, J. C.: Repair and Reconstruction in the Orbital Region. Baltimore, Williams and Wilkins Co., 1966.
61. Mustardé, J. C.: The treatment of ptosis and epicanthal folds. Br. J. Plast. Surg., *12*:252, 1959.
62. McCoy, F., Chandler, R. A., and Crow, M.: Facial fractures in children. Plast. Reconstr. Surg., *37*:209, 1966.
63. McCoy, F. J., Chandler, R. A., Magnan, C. G., et al.: Analysis of facial fractures and their complications. Plast. Reconstr. Surg., *29*:301, 1962.
64. Nahum, A.: The biomechanics of maxillofacial trauma. Clin. Plast. Surg., *2*:63, 1975.
65. Obwegeser, H. L., and Sailer, H. F.: Another way of treating fractures of the atrophic edentulous mandible. J. Maxillofac. Surg., *1*:213, 1973.
66. Peacock, E. E., Jr., and VanWinkle, W., Jr.: Wound Repair. Philadelphia, W. B. Saunders Co., 1976.
67. Penn, J., and Epstein, E.: Complications following late manipulation of impacted fracture of the malar bone. Plast. Reconstr. Surg., *6*:65, 1953.
68. Pirsig, W., and Lebmann, I.: The influence of trauma on the growing septal cartilage. Rhinology, *13*:39, 1975.
69. Popescu, V., and Vasiliu, D.: Treatment of temporomandibular ankylosis with particular reference to the interposition of full-thickness skin autotransplant. J. Maxillofac. Surg., *5*:3, 1977.
70. Prasad, S.: Blowout fracture of the medial wall of the orbit. Mod. Probl. Ophthal., *14*:493, 1975.
71. Rabuzzi, D.: Revision surgery of malaligned midface fractures. Otolaryngol. Clin. North Am., *7*:112, 1974.
72. Raz, S.: Gelfilm and blowout fractures. J. Laryngol. Otol., *90*:699, 1976.
73. Rowe, N. L., and Killey, H. C.: Fractures of the Facial Skeleton. Baltimore, Williams and Wilkins Co., 1968.
74. Schultz, R. C.: Facial Injuries. Chicago, Yearbook Medical Publishers, 1970.
75. Schultz, R. C.: Facial injuries from auto accidents: A study of 400 consecutive cases. Plast. Reconstr. Surg., *40*:415, 1967.
76. Skoog, T.: Plastic Surgery, New Methods and Refinements. Philadelphia, W. B. Saunders Co., 1974, p. 253.
77. Stallings, J. D., Pakiam, A. I., and Cory, C. C.: The late treatment of enophthalmos: A case report. Br. J. Plast. Surg., *1*:57, 1973.
78. Smith, B., Obear, M., and Leone, C. R.: The correction of enophthalmos associated with anophthalmos by glass bead implantation. Am. J. Ophthalmol., *64*:1088, 1967.
79. Swearington, J. J.: Tolerance of Human Face to Impact. Swearingen, J. J.: Tolerance of human face to crash impact. Office of Aviation Medicine, F.A.A. Civil Aeromedical Research Institute, Oklahoma City, July, 1965.
80. Taylor, D. V.: Traumatic aneurysm and facial palsy as complications of a mandibular fracture. Br. J. Oral Surg., *4*:202, 1967.
81. Tessier, P.: The conjunctival approach to the orbital floor and maxilla in congenital malformation and trauma. J. Maxillofac. Surg., *1*:3, 1973.
82. Tessier, P.: Total osteotomy of the middle third of the face for faciostenosis or for sequelae of LeFort III fractures. Plast. Reconstr. Surg., *48*:533, 1971.
83. Tofield, J.: Pneumomediastinum following fractures of the maxillary antrum. Br. J. Plast. Surg., *30*:179, 1977.
84. Van Winkle, W., Jr.: Wound Contraction. Surg. Obstet. Gynecol., *125*:131, 1967.
85. Walker, R. O.: Maxillofacial injuries. Br. J. Plast. Surg., *56*:726, 1969.
86. Whitaker, L. A., Monroe, I. R., Jackson, I. T., et al.: Problems in craniofacial surgery. J. Maxillofac. Surg., *4*:131, 1976.
87. Wobig, J. L.: Lacerations of the lacrimal excretory system. *In* Tessier, P., et al. (eds.): Symposium on Plastic Surgery in the Orbital Region. St. Louis, C. V. Mosby Co., 1976, pp. 50–54.

# 25 COMPLICATIONS OF AESTHETIC FACIAL SURGERY

*Thomas D. Rees*
*Daniel C. Baker*

The present widespread demand for aesthetic surgery as well as for improvements in results and safety of procedures has done much to dispel the older misguided attitudes about "cosmetic surgery." In no other field of surgery is there such a constant demand for perfection. Particularly in aesthetic facial surgery, miniscule deformities resulting from surgical error or complication can be seen by everyone.

The surgeon who commits himself to performing cosmetic surgery must face the challenges and mysteries of that most delicate of all human perceptions — the self-image. The doctor-patient relationship between the cosmetic patient and surgeon is more in the nature of that which exists between psychiatrist and patient.[3] Although there is extensive literature on the psychology of the cosmetic patient, there is no definitive evaluation technique that can anticipate or prevent all postoperative emotional problems.

To avoid complications, there is no substitute for thorough personal interviewing and consultation prior to surgery. The motivations of the patient must be analyzed along with his expectations from the surgery. If the decision is made to operate, the indications, limitations and complications of the procedure should be explained to the patient and so recorded on his chart. In his desire to have aesthetic surgery, a patient not infrequently denies the unpleasant possibility of a postoperative complication or represses being told of the realistic result.[53]

Complications of cosmetic facial surgery may be of minor or major degree and may or may not affect the final result. Some patients will refuse to accept anything short of perfection and will always be dissatisfied. The cosmetic surgeon, on the other hand, aims for perfection — "to surpass the normal," as Gilles said. In so doing, he is often highly critical of his work and may not be pleased with a result that is entirely satisfactory to the patient. Complications and unfavorable results are unavoidable with any operation, but the fact that cosmetic surgery is performed on physiologically normal patients makes any complication or untoward result all the more critical.

The following discussion of complications of aesthetic facial surgery deals with the most common procedures: rhinoplasty, blepharoplasty, rhytidectomy, otoplasty and augmentation mentoplasty. Emphasis is on the avoidance, recognition and treatment of postoperative complications. Discussion of surgical techniques has been purposefully kept to a minimum. Most of these procedures are performed under local anesthesia for which the intraoperative complications could constitute a chapter in itself. Therefore, any surgeon who uses local anesthetic agents supplemented by intravenous narcosis must be thoroughly familiar with the allergic manifestations, and toxic doses of these agents as well as with cardiopulmonary resuscitation.

## COMPLICATIONS OF RHINOPLASTY

### *General Considerations*

Unquestionably, rhinoplasty is technically the most difficult of all operations in plastic surgery; part of this difficulty is that the operation must be conceptualized as a three-dimensional technique requiring essentially a blind approach. This is further compounded by the difficulty in prediction of the final result; many factors combine to produce this result, such as the surgeon's skill, anatomic variations in the skin and subcutaneous tissues and cartilages of the nose, healing idiosyncrasy of the patient and complications. The final result of rhinoplasty is evident only after months or years, during which time the nose changes continuously. The concept of a long-term gradual metamorphosis is extremely important for the surgeon to grasp, since a common cause of failure, the overoperated nose, occurs because of steadfast determination at the operating table to achieve a result that fits a preconceived vision without real appreciation of the long-term effects of the healing process.

There are few articles in the literature concerned with a statistical analysis of complications and unsatisfactory results in cosmetic rhinoplasties. Klaubunde and Falces[12] surveyed 300 rhinoplasties; 42 patients, or 14 per cent, expressed dissatisfaction with the result of the primary procedure. The authors stated that approximately 10 per cent may have needed one or more secondary procedures. Most authors feel that this figure is too high and agree that the experienced surgeon should not exceed a 5 to 10 per cent secondary operation rate.[3, 20] Each surgeon's personal incidence will decrease as his skill and experience increase. Although it is not possible to be absolutely accurate in predicting the result of rhinoplasty because of the many variables encountered, certain complications from a primary rhinoplasty are avoidable. Many can be minimized.

In no other cosmetic operation is the preoperative evaluation and patient selection more crucial to minimizing complications. Much has been written about the neuroses and psychoses of the rhinoplasty patient, and a careful evaluation of the patient's motivations and self-image is essential. The surgeon must determine whether the patient is emotionally suited to the operation and to what degree the nose can be improved in contour. A poor decision at this time can result in the ultimate failure of the operation, even though a technically successful contour has been achieved. Age is an important consideration, for the patient of 40 years or older presents an entirely different set of problems than the teenager. Bones become more brittle, skin is inelastic, cartilage is calcified and vessels are fragile with advancing age, increasing the possibility of complications.

Anatomic factors that may influence the result of rhinoplasty are the thickness of the nasal bones, the presence or absence of the nasion and the thickness and position of the septum.[3] Deviations of the cartilaginous septum pose the most difficult and challenging problem. Despite all surgical maneuvers, the attainment of a completely straight dorsum may not be possible, and some curvature or external deviation of the nose may still be present immediately postoperatively or become apparent only after several weeks or months.[7, 8] Evaluating the tip preoperatively and predicting with any degree of accuracy the postoperative result requires considerable experience. The most difficult tips to correct are in those patients with thick oily skin and a marked excess of subcutaneous fatty tissue. This extremely thick, inelastic skin with large pores does not conform well to the new, smaller cartilaginous and bony framework. Blemishes, scars, pigmentation and uncorrectable asymmetries should be pointed out to the patient preoperatively; otherwise, these faults might be wrongly attributed to the surgery.

A thorough physical examination including anterior and posterior rhinoscopy is important to evaluate septal abnormalities and nasal obstruction. If a structural abnormality such as deviated septum warrants correction, and the patient also has findings of allergic or vasomotor rhinitis, he should be told that the operation will improve but not cure his nasal obstruction. The attitude "when in doubt, do a submucous resection" is fraught with error, for many pre-and postoperative nasal obstruction problems are physiologic rather than structural and can be treated with patience and medical care.[4]

It is simply not possible to do a standard operative procedure on every patient and obtain satisfactory results. The surgeon must appreciate the anatomic limitations and problems, and he should command at least three or four basic surgical approaches in order to adequately treat the individual nasal plastic problem. Even the most experienced and expert of surgeons must accept the necessity of secondary operation in a certain percentage of rhinoplasty patients. The most common deformities requiring secondary surgery are minor irregularities of the dorsum, such as depressions or elevation of the septal dorsum or upper lateral cartilages; asymmetry of the nostrils or tip; and malposition of the bones. Secondary surgery should not be performed before six months or a year, since low-grade edema can persist for long periods of time. Secondary surgery before edema is resolved only aggravates the vicious cycle of edema→resolution→scar tissue.

### *Early Postoperative Complications*

#### HEMORRHAGE

The most common troublesome complication of rhinoplasty is hemorrhage or epistaxis, which can occur any time from immediately after surgery to several weeks later. Usually, bleeding occurs during the first 48 hours or at 10 to 14 days postoperatively. Excluding blood dyscrasias, which should have been detected preoperatively, bleeding that occurs during the first 48 hours is particularly apt to come from the raw edge of the anterior septal mucosal incision.[3] If septoplasty or submucous resection has been performed in conjunction with rhinoplasty, the chances of bleeding are increased considerably. The second period during which epistaxis is most common is from the 10th to the 14th postoperative day, when the eschars along the incisions separate. When vigorous bleeding occurs, the intranasal packing must be removed; the nasal cavity is suctioned free of clots; and, using a nasal speculum under good lighting, an attempt should be made to locate the exact bleeding point. The nose may be gently repacked with epinephrine-soaked cotton pledgets, which usually control the bleeding. It is then wise to insert a pack of oxidized cellulose (Oxycel) or similar material that forms a natural clot and may be teased out several days after the bleeding ceases. If hemorrhage is severe and the bleeding site cannot be located, the nose must be packed with a nonadherent or greased gauze extending as far posteriorly as possible and exerting pressure against the splint or cast. Posterior bleeding must be controlled with nasopharyngeal packs as well as anterior packing. For persistent bleeding, the patient may require hospitalization and sedation. Uncontrolled epistaxis from the posterior septum can occur as the result of radical septal surgery, particularly in the older patient prone to hypertension. Trans-sinus ligation of the internal maxillary artery may rarely become necessary in such patients. Postoperatively, patients must be admonished not to blow, pick, touch or insert applicators into the nose.

#### HEMATOMA

Uncontrolled hemorrhage may result in hematoma that could cause displacement of the alar cartilage or distortion of the nasal tip with eventual thickening and excessive scar tissue. Septal hematomas, if not properly evacuated, may later cause nasal obstruction and lead to septal perforation. Prompt treatment of hemorrhage and careful inspection of the septum following submucous resection will minimize these complications.

Hematomas under the dorsal skin flaps can occur immediately if the dorsal splint is not accurately applied, or even several days following surgery if the skin flap is elevated from the underlying framework during removal of the cast or taping.

#### INFECTION

An infection following rhinoplasty is surprisingly rare, even though one of the most potentially contaminated areas in the body is transgressed. Klabunde and Falces[12] reported five infections in 300 cases (1.6 per cent), although this seems high. Flowers and

Anderson,[9] in reviewing 1000 rhinoplasties, found eight (0.8 per cent) instances of localized infection somewhere along the course of the lateral osteotomy. Even before the advent of antibiotics, infections following rhinoplasty were infrequent. When an infection does occur, it is usually found in a hematoma site or in areas surrounding retained bone dust or loose bony fragments.[20] To prevent this, bone dust, spicules and clots should be removed from the osteotomy site and nasal dorsum by a curette, frequently called a "nasal sweeper." Fortunately, the majority of potentially invasive organisms of the nose are controlled by antibiotics which most surgeons use prophylactically. It is best to postpone surgery on patients with active pustules or infection around the nose. Localized abscesses can occur at the transfixion incision in the columella, the tip (between the undermined domes of the alar cartilages) and the base of the prefrontal process of the maxilla along the lateral osteotomy. These should be treated with incision and drainage, local heat applications and broad-spectrum antibiotics pending culture results, when the appropriate antibiotic should be given. The offending organism is most often *Staphylococcus aureus*. A most dreaded but rare complication is septic cavernous sinus thrombosis, which if undiagnosed can lead to brain abscess and death. It must be treated vigorously with massive doses of broad-spectrum antibiotics.

## PERIOSTITIS

Along fracture lines in the nasal bones, periostitis can begin as a low-grade infection and smolder for weeks or months. This is most apt to occur when the saw osteotomy technique is used and sawdust or debris is left behind. The presenting symptoms are swelling and pain and later erythema. When recognized, vigorous broad-spectrum antibiotics should be given. Inadvertent or purposeful comminution of the nasal bones can very rarely result in a sequestrum that becomes the site of a localized osteomyelitis. Intensive antibiotic therapy may control the infection; however, removal of the sequestrum may be required if conservative therapy fails.

## EDEMA AND ECCHYMOSIS

This is a universal occurrence following rhinoplasty, although there is a tremendous variation among individuals as to the extent and the amount of time required for swelling, edema and ecchymosis to subside. Swelling[6] of the tip in a patient with thick, sebaceous skin may take many months to resolve. For most patients, it takes six to 12 months before all swelling has cleared and the final result can be seen. It is not unusual, however, for patients to have residual swelling for up to two years postoperatively. Gentle support and reassurance by the surgeon are necessary to bolster the patient. Ecchymosis usually subsides promptly in two to four weeks after surgery. There are some patients in whom dark circles remain beneath the eyes — presumably blood breakdown products — for many months, even up to a year or more, however. The cause is unknown, but it usually occurs in patients of Mediterranean heritage, especially Italians. Except in those patients with a family predisposition to darkly pigmented eyelid skin, this condition is never permanent. A tendency to increased pigmentation of the lower eyelid skin should be looked at before surgery, and the patient should be advised of the possibility of prolonged "black eyes." There is no effective treatment to hasten the absorption of blood pigments.

## SKIN PROBLEMS

Minor skin complications include tape reaction, skin pustules and the formation of telangiectases. Tape reactions have been minimized by the use of paper tape, but they may still occur in highly sensitive individuals. Allergic reactions are treated with topical steroid creams and systemic antihistamines. Pustules should be expressed as they occur, and a drying desquamating soap is prescribed. Patients with a diathesis toward capillary telangiectasis will sometimes develop these small spider lesions after rhinoplasty. They may be treated by electrodesiccation using an epilating needle that is passed under magnification into the lumen of the vessel. Several treatments may be required.

Skin necrosis over the dorsum resulting from excessive pressure from the splint or tape or from circulatory problems can occur but is very rare. The best treatment is a conservative "watch and wait" attitude. An eschar will form that eventually separates as healing progresses beneath. The final scar may require excision or even full thickness skin grafting. If a full thickness slough of dorsal skin is evident, with the danger that the nasal bones and cartilage will become exposed, the slough can be excised and the defect covered with a local flap.

Necrosis of the tip skin can result from excessive dissection of the tip and undue surgical trauma. This represents a surgical disaster, and little can be done either at the time of the slough or subsequently to obtain an acceptable result. Such patients become nasal cripples and often begin an odyssey from surgeon to surgeon to obtain help.

#### INJURY TO LACRIMAL APPARATUS

Because of the proximity of the lacrimal apparatus to the lateral osteotomy site during rhinoplasty, lacrimal sac injury is not an uncommon occurrence, as reported by Flowers and Anderson.[9] They demonstrated first anatomically in cadavers and then clinically in patients undergoing rhinoplasty that significant disruption of the lacrimal sac occurred during osteotomy; 21 of 27 patients showed lacrimal obstruction on one or both sides on the second postoperative day. At two weeks postoperatively, however, only one patient had obstruction, which cleared at three months. They concluded that postoperative obstruction of the lacrimal apparatus was functional, of short duration and without sequelae. Although there is no report in the literature of permanent damage to the lacrimal apparatus, it could conceivably happen with a careless osteotomy or technical error. A study of the skull confirms the difficulty of injuring the nasolacrimal duct during the operation because of its well protected location below the maxillary rim.

#### SEPTAL PERFORATIONS

Septal perforations are less common today than several decades ago because of the infrequency of radical septal resection for septal deviation. The use of antibiotics for adequate early treatment of nasal infection has also reduced the complication of septal perforation. The main causes are an improperly executed submucous resection and unrecognized septal hematoma. Small anterior septal perforations may cause a disturbing whistling noise with respiration. Treatment is by use of local or buccal mucosal flaps if the patient is symptomatic.

### *Late Postoperative Complications*

#### NASAL OBSTRUCTION

After rhinoplasty, postoperative nasal obstructive symptoms are common. Almost all patients experience partial nasal obstruction from transient edema of the mucosa, coagulated blood or crusting along the incision lines. This type of obstruction usually resolves spontaneously in several weeks without treatment.

Patients with allergic disorders or vasomotor rhinitis may have an exacerbation of nasal obstruction postoperatively. In a review of 1000 consecutive rhinoplasties, Beekhuis[5] found approximately 10 per cent of patients developed a persistent enlargement of the inferior turbinates postoperatively, causing an obstructive vasomotor type of rhinitis. The obstruction usually began at the time of surgery and would persist for several months if left untreated. The use of intranasal, intramucosal injections of long-acting corticosteroids as described by Baker and Strauss[4] is the treatment of choice for these patients and will alleviate the majority of symptoms.

#### ALTERED SENSE OF SMELL AND ANOSMIA

The olfactory area is located high in each nasal cavity far from the operative field of rhinoplasty, and interference with the sense of smell should be an unusual complication. Champion,[6] however, questioned 200 patients who underwent rhinoplasty and found that 10 per cent had temporary anosmia lasting 6 to 18 months, and one patient had permanent anosmia. He did not perform olfaction tests on these patients. Goldwyn and Shore,[11] however, further studied this problem using olfactory testing on patients undergoing rhinoplasty or submu-

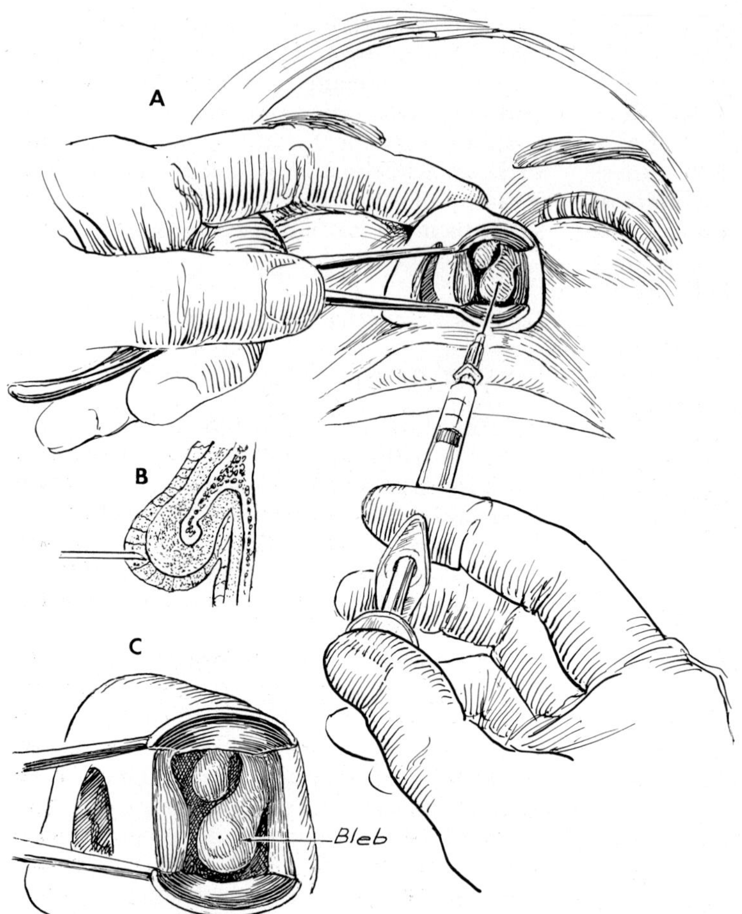


**Figure 25–1** The proper technique of injection of the inferior turbinate. *A,* A 25 gauge needle is inserted intramucosally. A very small dose suffices. (Before injection vasoconstrictors should be used to shrink the membranes.) *B,* Only the bevel of the needle is inserted intramucosally in the anterior tip of the inferior turbinate. *C,* 0.3 ml. of steroid is injected forming a bleb (similar to a PPD test). (From Baker, D. C., and Strauss, R. B.: The physiologic treatment of nasal obstruction. Clin. Plast. Surg., *4*:121, 1977.)

cous resection or a combination of the two. They found that at two weeks after surgery 80 per cent of patients had normal sense of smell, and at two months postoperatively no patients complained of anosmia or demonstrated it on testing. They concluded that submucous resection and rhinoplasty rarely produce permanent anosmia. Postoperative bleeding and edema can cause temporary anosmia lasting a few weeks. Nevertheless, a careful preoperative history questioning for anosmia could prevent a postoperative complaint.

## CALLUS FORMATION

Occasionally, bony callus can form at the site of bony hump removal or along lateral osteotomy sites. This is usually the result of an exaggerated response to bone dust, periosteal tags or blood clots that were not carefully removed at surgery.[20] This can result in a residual bony dorsal hump or, sometimes, irregularities along the lateral osteotomy site that appear several months after surgery. Treatment requires rasping of irregularities or repeat osteotomy.

## UNFAVORABLE RESULTS AND SECONDARY RHINOPLASTY

It has already been emphasized that adequate time for healing and softening of the tissues should be allowed before undertaking revision. Secondary rhinoplasties pose some of the most difficult problems in plastic surgery.[10, 15, 16, 17, 18] If the deformity is severe and particularly if scarring of the soft tissue exists, there may be little or nothing that can be accomplished by a secondary procedure. Certain patients should be ad-

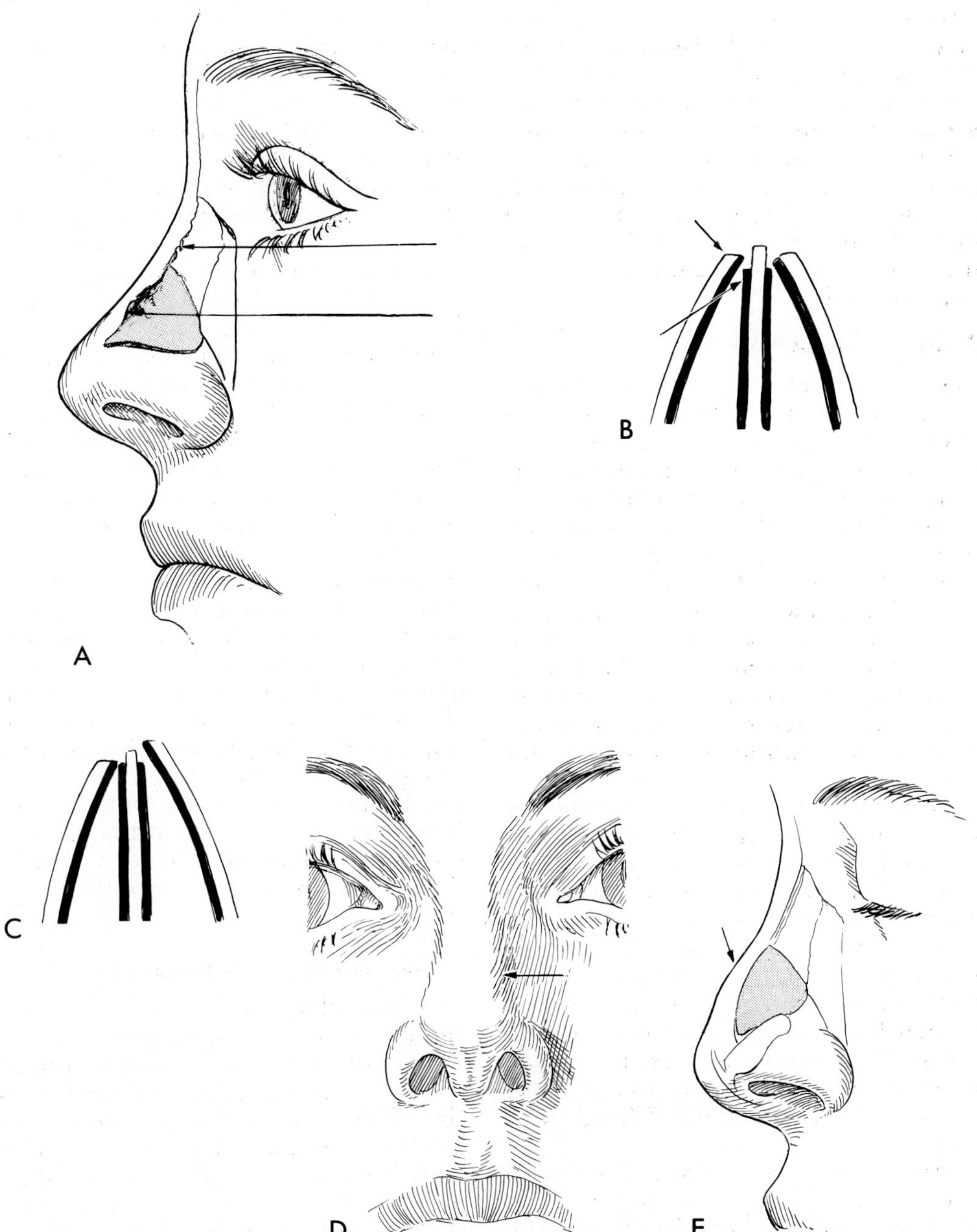


**Figure 25–2** *A,* An irregular bony dorsum with excess protrusion of the upper lateral cartilages. No intervention is necessary in a patient whose irregularity is palpable but not visible. *B,* Ideal postoperative relations of cartilage and mucosa. *C,* An irregular upper lateral cartilage border. *D,* Fullness of the supratip area that may result from excessive upper lateral cartilage. *E,* In the thin-skinned patient, a supratip hump may be more noticeable. (From Rees, T. D., and Wood-Smith, D.: Rhinoplasty. *In* Rees, T. D., and Wood-Smith, D. [eds.]: Cosmetic Facial Surgery. Philadelphia, W. B. Saunders Company, 1973.)

vised against further surgery because of a psychologic problem or insurmountable anatomic deformity. The subject of secondary rhinoplasty is too extensive to permit a detailed discussion of all the causes of secondary deformities and their correction, but the most common will be mentioned.

Secondary deformities following rhinoplasty are classified into those involving (1) the bony framework; (2) the cartilaginous framework, including the tip; (3) the soft tissues; (4) the tip alone; (5) the nostrils, vestibulum and columella; and (6) any combination of these.[3]

### The Bony Framework

Residual Hump and Palpable Irregularities. Insufficient resection of the hump during rhinoplasty may leave a secondary hump, requiring further removal. Palpable irregularities may follow comminution of the nasal bones. If these irregularities are visible, they may be rasped or chiseled away; if not visible, no further surgery is indicated, and the patient should be reassured.

Incomplete lateral osteotomy and incomplete fracture at the junction of the nasal and frontal bones are common postrhinoplasty problems. Refracture with comminution on the bony complex is necessary for correction.

External Deviation. Asymmetry or external deviation of the bony framework, commonly due to deviation of the bony septum, may have been caused by incomplete fracture or failure to perform an adequate medial osteotomy on one side. The correction requres surgical comminution of the nasal bones or fracture of the ethmoid plate and nasal bones at the nasofrontal suture and straightening of the septum. Percutaneous puncture with a 2 mm. osteotome is sometimes useful in accomplishing these fractures.

Postoperative Widening. Postoperative widening of the bony framework is usually the result of a high deviation of the septum that may have been unrecognized at the primary operation. Although difficult to correct, this problem can sometimes be solved by fracture and repositioning of the bony septum. Narrowing of the nasal bones, particularly at the nasofrontal angle, may have been prevented by incomplete osteotomy of the frontal process of the maxilla with a "greenstick" fracture. Marked thickness of the bone also may have prevented narrowing at the radix, and resection of a medial triangle or web of bone with osteotome or bone forceps may be necessary to allow room for medial displacement at infraction.[3]

"Stair-step" Deformities. Stair-step deformities have resulted from the lateral osteotomy having been placed too high on the frontal process of the maxilla. The lateral osteotomy should be located in the depths of the nasomaxillary groove and should pass through the nasofrontal process of the maxilla. "Stair-stepping" can be corrected by comminuting the frontal process with a 2 mm. osteotome or by rasping of the high bony ridge.

Saddle Nose. A saddle nose may have been caused by excessive bony hump removal or by the fractured nasal bones dropping into the pyriform aperture. The latter can often be avoided by never completely stripping the periosteum from the nasal bones, using the soft tissues to support the fractured bones. Later, should the surgeon recognize that he has removed an excessive amount of bony hump at operation, he should trim the bone free of mucous membrane and cartilage and replace the sculpted hump primarily. Correction of saddle nose deformities is best done with autogenous bone or cartilage grafts, since alloplastic materials are frequently extruded after insertion into scarred soft tissue of the nasal dorsum.

### The Cartilaginous Framework

It is possible that an external deviation of the nose may become apparent after rhinoplasty when none was visible before with a C- or S-shaped deviation of the dorsal border of the septal cartilage. These deformities are often difficult to correct, and complete freeing of the septum along the vomer groove combined with multiple incisions in the deviated cartilage may be necessary for straightening. Techniques to correct such deviations have recently been reviewed by Converse[7] and Dingman and Natvig.[8]

As a general rule, it is preferable to remove cartilage only when necessary to obtain an airway. Radical submucous resection of the septal cartilage, ethmoid plate and vomer is not advised during any rhinoplasty

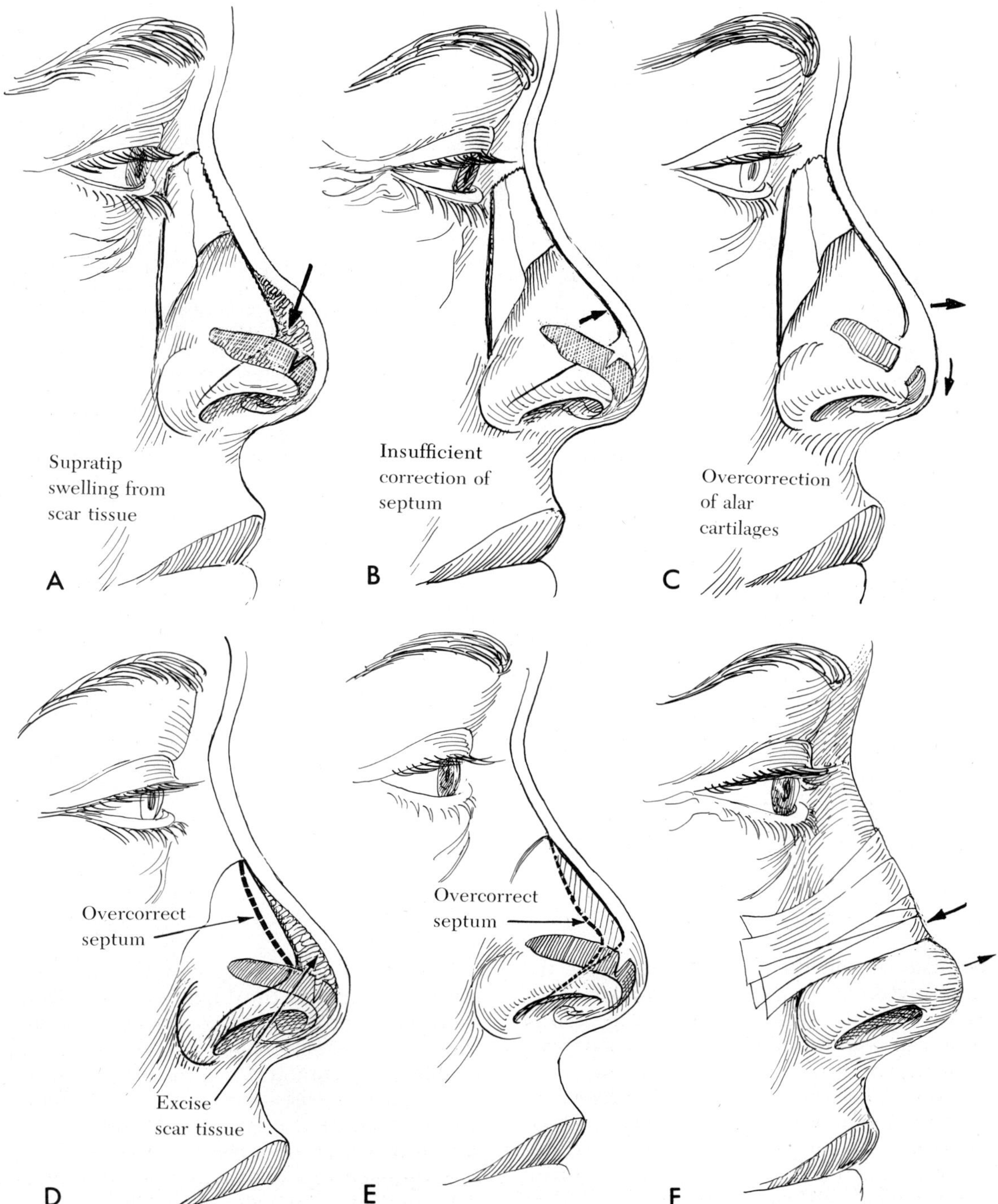


**Figure 25–3** Supratip swelling, commonly called "polly tip" or "ram's tip," is perhaps the most common reason for a secondary nasal plastic operation. It is usually the result of scar tissue formation in the dorsal dead space secondary to granulation tissue (*A*), inadequate reduction of the dorsal septal border (*B*), or excessive resection of the alar domes (*C*). The first two problems are usually correctable by a secondary procedure (*D* and *E*) and fixation of the soft tissues to the nasal framework. However, when too much alar cartilage has been removed, correction is almost impossible. (From Rees, T. D., Krupp, S., and Wood-Smith, D.: Plast. Reconstr. Surg. *46*:332, 1970. Reproduced with permission.)

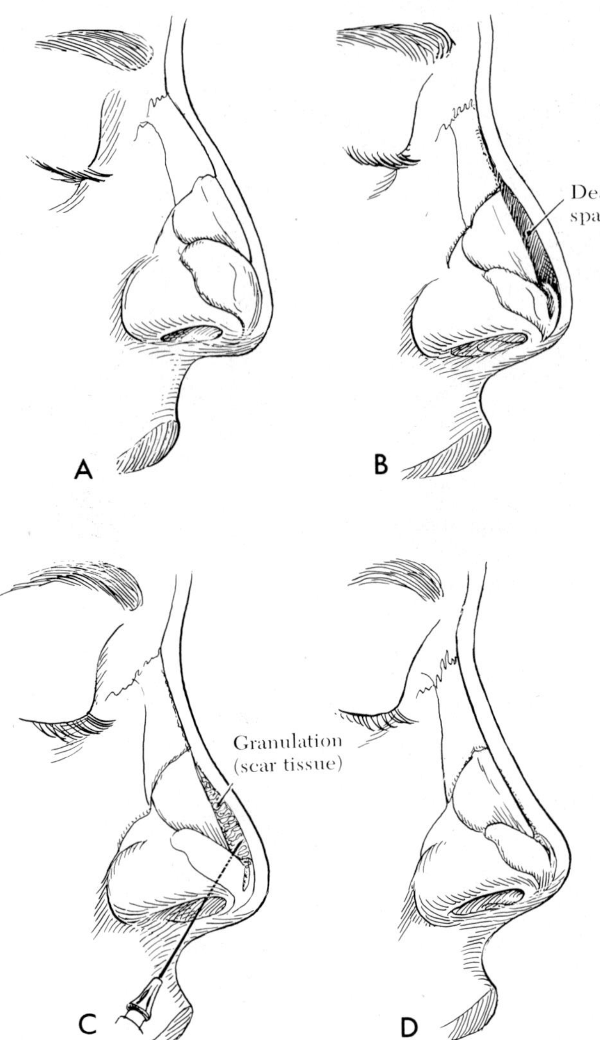


**Figure 25–4** Intralesional injections of steroid compounds have proved helpful in hastening resolution of granulation tissue causing supratip swelling. *A,* The preoperative anatomy. *B,* Potential dead space between skin and cartilage created by the operation. Dressings help to eliminate this space. *C,* Granulation tissue in the dead space. Injection of triamcinolone directly into this tissue at weekly intervals for two or three weeks, usually in a dose of 5 mg. per injection, will help to eliminate this tissue. *D,* The result after dissolution of the granulation tissue. (From Rees, T. D., and Wood-Smith, D.: Rhinoplasty. *In* Rees, T. D., and Wood-Smith, D. [eds.]: Cosmetic Facial Surgery. Philadelphia, W. B. Saunders Company, 1973.)

because of the danger of collapse of the nasal pyramid into the pyriform aperture. When radical resection appears indicated, it is best to plan it as a secondary procedure.

SUPRATIP SWELLING. This is the most common deformity requiring secondary rhinoplasty and is usually referred to as "parrot beak" or "polly tip." This can result from (1) insufficient lowering of the dorsal septum, (2) insufficient removal of the dorsal borders of the upper lateral cartilages, (3) insufficient trimming of the septal mucosa, (4) excessive resection of the alar cartilage domes, (5) inherent thickness of the skin and subcutaneous tissue and (6) a short columella.

Correction of supratip elevation may require lowering of the high septal dorsum, excision of scar tissue and resection of the upper lateral cartilages. When supratip swelling is secondary to granulation tissue, edema may persist for many months, sometimes years. If the surgeon becomes convinced that postoperative supratip convexity is not related to a high septal dorsum but is the result of dead space, granulation tissue and intermittent edema, good results may be obtained by subcutaneous injections of small doses of steroids, as described by Rees.[19]

Uneven trimming of the septum or upper lateral cartilages along their dorsal borders causes palpable or visible irregularities that may require secondary trimming. Excessive removal of the upper lateral cartilages may leave oblique grooves on either side of the nasal dorsum, which is almost impossible to correct.

## The Nasal Tip

Asymmetry, Sharp Points and Pinching. These are common deformities of the tip following rhinoplasty and are the result of injudicious carving of the alar cartilages along with, in the case of pinching, excision of excess vestibular lining. Correction of irregularities of the alar cartilages requires secondary trimming of the offending cartilage remnants.

Boxed Tip. The boxed tip may require total resection of the alar domes. This is usually safer in the secondary operation because of the added support given to the soft tissues by the cicatrix from the first operation. When the skin is very thin, however, resection of the alar cartilage must be conservative and accurate, with emphasis on shaping while maintaining cartilaginous support. Patients with thick skin or subcutaneous tissue can afford loss of most or all of the lateral crura of the alar cartilage without nostril collapse.

"Drooping" Tip. The drooping tip occurs if the upper lateral and alar cartilages have not been trimmed or sutured in suitable relationship to the shortened caudal margin of the septum. The tip also tends to plunge downward if excessive hump has been removed or if the nose has been shortened without tilting the tip. In older patients, loss of skin contractility may contribute to the drooped tip. Correction may require shortening the upper lateral cartilages or approximating them to the alar cartilages. Fixation of the medial crura of the alar cartilages to the caudal septal border is frequently needed. If the alar cartilages naturally plunge downward at the domes, it may be necessary to resect the domes and to reposition the medial and lateral crura in a new relationship.

Bifid Tip. Bifidity of the tip requires suturing together of the alar domes or their remnants, a technique that is often more easily described than done. Often, breaking up of the interdome fibroareolar tissue will produce sufficient scar tissue contraction to correct the problem.

Finally, many secondary deformities of the nasal tip cannot be corrected by surgery or would even be further damaged by revision and the problem exacerbated. The inexperienced surgeon is often tempted to take on these problem patients when really he should advise them against further surgery.

**Vestibular Scarring.** Cicatricial stenosis, synechiae or retraction of the nostrils has usually been the end result of secondary healing of raw surfaces left when lining was sacrificed. Replacement or reconstruction of missing soft tissue may require skin grafts, Z-plasty, local flaps and composite and cartilage grafts. When complete vestibular collapse is present, support can be provided only by a prosthetic insert that provides an airway at the critical junction of the nasal cartilages and septum.

**Nostril Irregularities and Flaring.** Irregularities or thickening of the nostrils that are accentuated after rhinoplasty can be improved by selective resection of the nostril rims by various methods described.[16, 18, 20] The scars are not infrequently prominent, however, and caution is advised before undertaking these corrections. Flaring of the nostrils may be accentuated following rhinoplasty when the tip has been recessed, and an alar base resection may be required for correction.

**Hanging Columella.** A hanging columella, a convexity or roundness of the caudal margin of the medial crura of the alar cartilages, may first become significant after rhinoplasty. This can be corrected by marginal incisions in the columella and trimming of the rounded cartilage and, sometimes, the lining.

**Retraction of the Columella.** This may result from excessive removal of the inferior or caudal margin of the septum, and sometimes from resection of the membranous septum or medial crura. Correction of this deformity is difficult, often impossible. For minor deformities, a septal cartilage implant may be effective if sufficient lateral crus or alar cartilage is present. A retracted columella can be improved by Millard's alar turnover flap;[14] however, rarely is there sufficient cartilage remaining after rhinoplasty. A composite graft can also be used in place

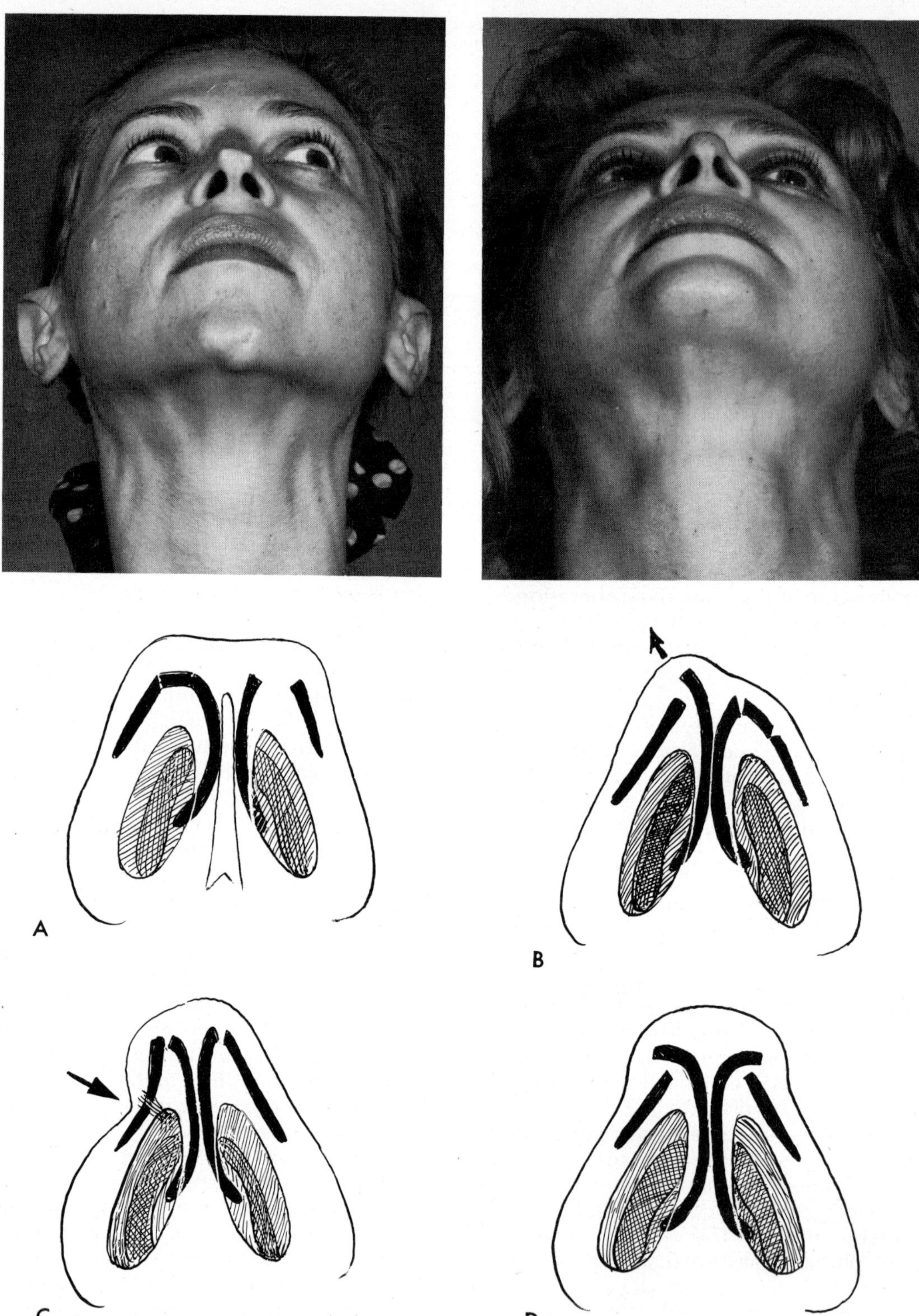


**Figure 25–5** The asymmetric nasal tip and some of its common causes. *A,* Unequal excision of alar dome cartilage, with weakening of the dome support on the (patient's) left. *B,* Disruption of the continuity of the lateral crus of the alar cartilage, with projection of a portion of the cartilage expressing itself as a palpable skin irregularity. *C,* Damage to the skin overlying the lateral crus of the alar cartilage, resulting in dimpling. *D,* Breaking of the continuity of the lateral crura and failure to adequately resect their medial portions results in a so-called boxed tip. (From Rees, T. D., and Wood-Smith, D.: Rhinoplasty. *In* Rees, T. D., and Wood-Smith, D. [eds.]: Cosmetic Facial Surgery. Philadelphia, W. B. Saunders Company, 1973.)

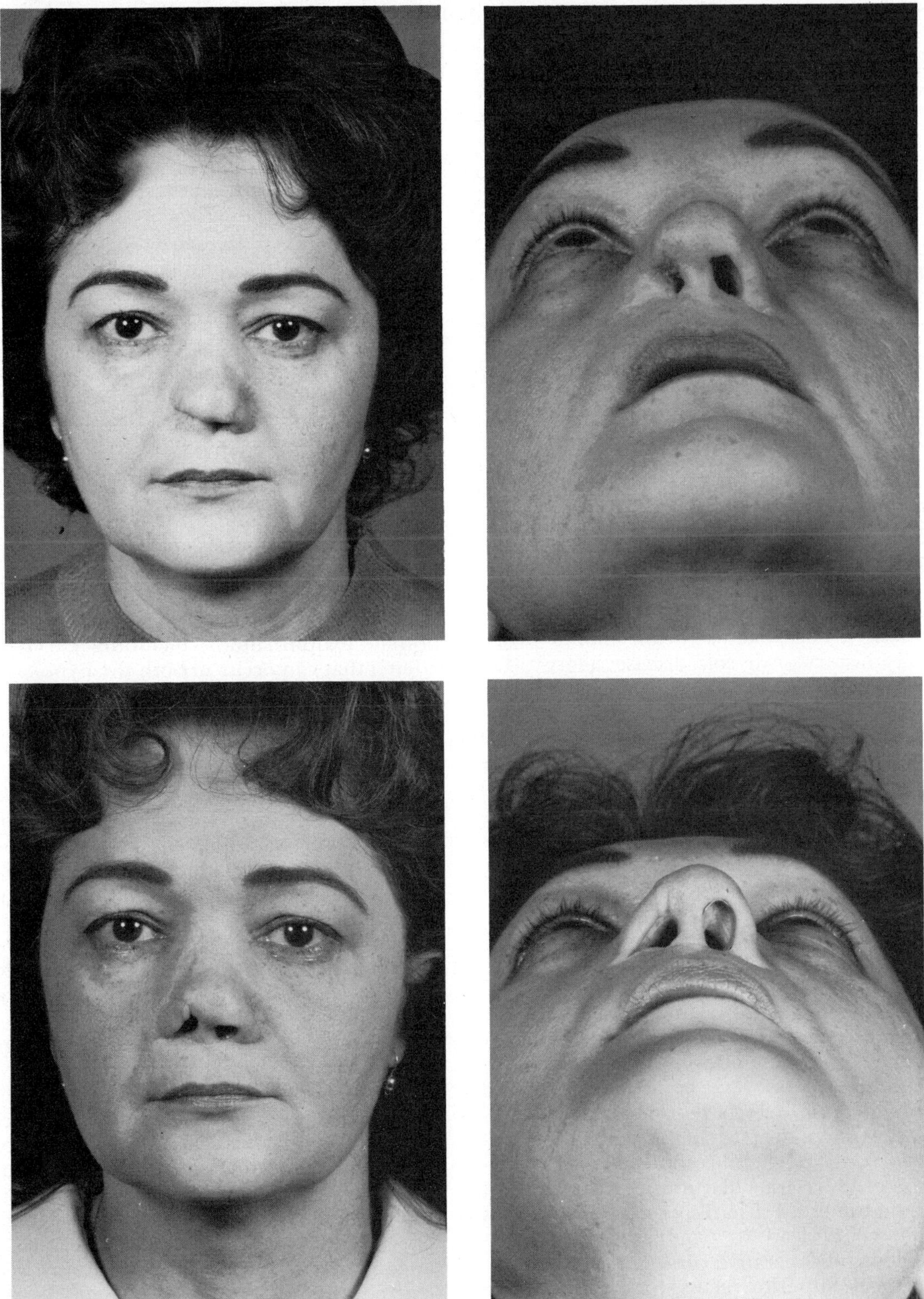

**Figure 25–6** A mutilated nose, the result of many inexpert procedures done in rapid order. The right nostril was almost completely blocked, and loss of cartilage support on the left resulted in a flaplike action during inspiration. Postoperative views were taken after a chondrocutaneous composite graft to the right nostril; also illustrated is the use of a continuously worn acrylic shell prosthesis in the left nostril to prevent collapse. (From Rees, T. D., and Wood-Smith, D.: Rhinoplasty. *In* Rees, T. D., and Wood-Smith, D. [eds.]: Cosmetic Facial Surgery. Philadelphia, W. B. Saunders Company, 1973.)

of the missing membranous septum in severe retraction. Bone and alloplastic implants are generally disappointing because of insufficient soft tissue coverage.

## COMPLICATIONS OF BLEPHAROPLASTY

### *General Considerations*

Complications of aesthetic blepharoplasty are best treated by prevention, which begins long before surgery, at the time of the first consultation. Since many of these complications result from aggravation of a pre-existing condition, an adequate general and ophthalmologic history followed by an ophthalmologic examination will bring into focus any pre-existing eye problems. History should include specific questioning about any major ocular disease, such as glaucoma, detached retina, cataract as well as corneal abrasions, epiphora and "dry-eye syndrome." The systems review should probe for a history of thyroid disease, allergy, diabetes and cardiovascular disease, since these conditions in particular may affect the eyes and adnexa. Examination of the eye should include its adnexal structures, the bony orbit, the extraocular muscles, a visual acuity test and an ophthalmoscopic examination for lenticular opacities or obvious retinal pathology.

### *Specific Considerations*

A miniature portable Snellen's chart is convenient to test acuity, and each eye should be tested separately. A patient may be unaware of amblyopia, poor vision or blindness in one eye before surgery, and should these defects become apparent following blepharoplasty, the surgeon could incorrectly be held responsible. Examination of the extraocular muscles is important to determine if a paresis or paralysis exists that could lead to troublesome, or even serious postoperative consequences. Paralysis of the superior rectus, for example, with an absent Bell's phenomenon, could promote desiccation leading to ulceration of the cornea, since temporary lagophthalmos after blepharoplasty is not uncommon. Although spasm of Müller's muscle is normal in some individuals, on the other hand, it can herald early thyrotoxicosis or expanding intraorbital lesions long before other symptoms occur.

A sign of levator spasm is a staring look caused by scleral "show" above the limbus of the cornea. Spasm may or may not be associated with exophthalmos. Such eye signs can precede the symptomatology of hyperthyroidism and even the changes in protein-bound iodine fractions by many months. A slight bulging of the globes, so-called normal exophthalmos or proptosis, occurs in some individuals without thyroid disease or ocular pathology. It can be a family trait that is genetically inherited. Asymmetry is also common. Unilateral exophthalmos may suggest occult orbital lesions. Investigations of the orbit by tomography may be indicated if suspicion of a space-filling lesion or bony deformity exists.

Thyroid disease can produce localized signs of the eye and orbital regions in addition to exophthalmos, including excessive edema that can occur in both the hypo- and hyperthyroid states.

Intermittent eyelid edema in women is often related to cyclic hormone influence. Many females are prone to collect periorbital edema in the immediate premenstrual days of their cycle. Fluid retention is common with interruptions of the normal hormonal balances at menopause. Periorbital edema related to hormonal influence can often be identified by history. The patient should be informed that swelling of the eyelids will continue even after a successful blepharoplasty with removal of redundant fat and skin.

Allergy may manifest not only as allergic dermatitis of the eyelid skin but also as recurrent episodes of intensive periorbital edema. An unusual but typical localized edema can occur over the malar eminences, just below the bony infraorbital rims and not involving the eyelid skin itself. This small saclike area of edema is usually intermittent and may eventually result in subcutaneous fibrosis. It is typical, and once recognized, never forgotten. It may be the source of misunderstanding between patient and surgeon unless identified preoperatively, since it is unlikely to be ablated by blepharoplasty. The patient should be so advised. It is helpful to positively point out this localized area of edema formation on the preoperative photographs.

Minor, or subclinical, forms of the so-called "dry-eye syndrome" are more prevalent than commonly believed.[27, 40, 42] When fully developed, the syndrome is known as keratoconjunctivitis sicca or Sjögren's syndrome. It can result in blindness from corneal opacities. Diminution in tear production occurs normally with advancing age. It also may be hereditary or as a consequence of certain systemic diseases such as thyrotoxicosis. A history of recurrent bouts of irritation of the eyes with burning and itching often combined with a slight protrusion of the globe (exophthalmos) is suggestive. A Schirmer's test is then advisable preoperatively to determine the amount of tear production. A small strip of absorbent paper is inserted into the inferior fornix. Tear production is measured in millimeters over a given time period. A Schirmer's test seems unnecessary in every potential blepharoplasty patient but can suggest the diagnosis when positive. A deficiency of lysozyme in the tears is also pathognomonic, although this test is more difficult than a simple Schirmer's. The dry-eye syndrome can be complicated and exacerbated by lid surgery because of normal wound contracture with the slight lagophthalmos and ectropion that frequently occur during the healing period. Patients with slight exophthalmos, a drooped lower lid and "scleral show" before surgery are particularly prone to these mechanical forces of wound healing that can aggravate the symptoms. Patients with such contours should be carefully questioned about irritative eye symptomatology.

Cosmetic blepharoplasty is not necessarily precluded because of diminished tear production, but extreme caution in the surgical approach should be exercised. Skin and fat excision must be conservative. If the surgeon and patient elect to proceed with the surgery, a two-stage procedure seems advisable, operating on the upper lids first, followed a few weeks later by the lower lids. Levator fixation of the upper lids in such patients is probably unwise. Some surgeons have also advocated a partial resection of a prominent lacrimal gland if present at the time of blepharoplasty. Because diminution in tear production occurs normally with advancing age, the aesthetic improvement gained by this procedure does not seem to warrant the possible medicolegal consequences of a postoperative "dry-eye syndrome."

Complications following blepharoplasty occur most often in the immediate postoperative period. They may be mild or severe, temporary or persistent, and may or may not require definitive surgical correction. Since most of these complications are the result of surgical trauma or the aggravation of a pre-existing condition, it is of utmost importance to reduce operative trauma to an absolute minimum, as well as to perform an accurate preoperative history and physical examination.

## *Minor Complications*

### WOUND SEPARATION

Separation of the wound immediately after suture removal is not unknown after blepharoplasty. It usually occcurs along the lateral segment of the incision in the superior eyelids lateral to the outer canthus. Should dehiscence occur it can be promptly resutured or brought together and splinted with sterile paper tape strips (steri-strips).

### INFECTION

Significant infection of blepharoplasty wounds is exceedingly uncommon, undoubtedly because of the rich and abundant blood supply to the area. Most surgeons do not employ prophylactic antibiotic therapy for blepharoplasty since infection is so uncommon. Should infection occur, however, prompt treatment with an appropriate antibiotic along with warm compresses is indicated. Superficial pustules will occur, in particular at the medial exit of the subcuticular suture of the upper eyelid, if the sutures are left in place more than four to five days. The exudate should be gently expressed and usually causes no further problem.

Chronic blepharitis of a nonspecific nature has been seen following blepharoplasty, but it is so rare as to lead one to the conclusion that its occurrence may be coincidental. Obvious deformities of the lids such as ectropion or lagophthalmos can obviously lead to blepharitis. Treatment by a competent ophthalmologist is recommended. Recurrent chalazions or styes have also been seen following blepharoplasty but are usually considered coincidental since there is frequently a history of prior occurrence.[3]

#### EPIPHORA

Epiphora — excessive tearing from the eyes — is common during the first 48 hours after surgery and may persist for longer periods. It is usually caused by the immediate postoperative reaction, such as edema of the skin, distortion of the canaliculus or tear-drainage mechanism or distortion of the lid margins. Often with subsidence of the wound reaction, the epiphora usually disappears. Rarely, intermittent epiphora, occurring nocturnally or with sudden changes of weather, can persist for several weeks or months. Permanent epiphora may occur but is extremely rare. It is most likely related to stenosis of the canaliculus or lacrimal sac resulting from injury at the time of surgery, from aggravation of a preoperative condition or from obstruction by concretions or mucous plugs. Probing of the lacrimal system should be performed by experienced hands, since injury to the thin walls of the ducts or sacs can occur, which could further aggravate the condition.

If injury to the lacrimal apparatus does occur at surgery and is recognized at that time, immediate repair should be done. To minimize injury, it is wise not to extend the incision of the lower eyelid into the extreme medial corner of the lid, particularly in the skin-muscle flap technique.

#### CORNEAL INJURY

Injury to the cornea is best prevented rather than treated after it occurs. Abrasive gauze sponges should be replaced with atraumatic absorbable synthetic sponges. A protective corneal shield is favored by many surgeons during the operation; however, a corneal lens shield can itself cause an abrasion if inserted improperly. It is important to prevent desiccation of the cornea during surgery, since drying can result in abrasion that can progress to ulceration because of the avascularity of the cornea. Frequent irrigations with sterile saline during the operation is therefore a good practice, particularly during suturing when the lids are apt to be open and the cornea exposed. At the conclusion of the procedure, a bland lubricating ointment should be liberally applied to the incisions and the conjunctival sac to protect the cornea during the first few hours following surgery until muscular closure is re-established.

Thorough irrigation of the conjunctival sac at the end of the procedure helps remove foreign matter, such as bits and pieces of suture and so forth. Foreign material can cause corneal abrasion, a most uncomfortable, even painful, condition.

Pain in the eye after surgery is a warning signal that requires investigation. Corneal injury such as abrasion must be ruled out. The cornea and conjunctival sac can be stained with fluorescein or rose bengal dye. Minute abrasions are sometimes only detected with a slit-lamp. One is available in most hospitals. If a corneal abrasion is found, the eye should be treated with appropriate topical medication and put at rest with an occlusive dressing until healing has occurred.

### *Dermatologic Complications*

#### TELANGIECTASIS

Small pre-existing telangiectases of the eyelid skin are likely to be intensified in size and numbers after surgery, particularly along the margins of the upper eyelids below the incision. Patients with such lesions should be advised of this possibility. Application of camouflaging cosmetics is the best treatment since telangiectases are not likely to improve.

#### SCARRING

Hypertrophic scarring of eyelid wounds is unusual but can occur, particularly in fair-skinned individuals. True keloids in the eyelid skin have not been reported and probably do not occur. Scar hypertrophy is most common along the medial portion of the incision near the epicanthus. The treatment of hypertrophic scarring is watchful waiting. The surgeon should not be in a hurry to perform Z-plasties, V-Y plasties or other maneuvers, since these may only complicate and prolong the scar resolution. Intralesional injections of minute doses of steroids may accelerate resolution of the hypertrophy.

Improvement almost always occurs with the passage of time, however.

### PIGMENTATION

Increased pigmentation of the skin should be noted prior to surgery since it is unlikely that the operation will improve the problem and may aggravate it. Sometimes, reducing the convex lid contour caused by bulging periorbital fat and redundant eyelid skin apparently improves dark pigmentation by flattening highlights. Prolonged postoperative ecchymosis can result in dark discoloration of the eyelids, sometimes for many months following surgery. This problem is, fortunately, uncommon and usually self-curing. Observation is the proper method of treatment. The discoloration disappears even after one to one and one-half years, except in rare individuals in whom it can apparently persist for life.

Superficial pigmentation of the eyelid skin can often be improved or eliminated by deep chemical peel, which can be done six to eight weeks after blepharoplasty. It can enhance the result of blepharoplasty not only by reducing superficial pigmentation but also by removing many of the remaining fine rhytides that cannot be safely removed at operation.

### INCLUSION CYSTS

The eyelid skin is very thin and rich in epithelial cells. Postoperative milia inclusion cysts are common after surgery, since epithelial debris may become trapped in the wound. Milia are easily evacuated through a stab wound made with a small hypodermic needle or a #11 blade. Larger inclusion cysts require excision. Epithelial tunnels will result if sutures are left in the eyelid skin for longer than four or five days. The epithelium grows rapidly along the suture tract and lines it to form a tunnel. It is therefore important to remove all interrupted sutures in the eyelid skin within 48 hours after surgery, leaving for another two or three days only subcuticular sutures and those in the lateral skin of the orbital region where epithelial tunnels are not likely to occur. If tunnels form, they are treated by exteriorization. A fine scissors blade is inserted into the tunnel and the covering epithelium snipped away.[22]

### POSTOPERATIVE WRINKLING

It is not uncommon for patients to complain of the appearance of small wrinkles of the eyelid skin after cosmetic blepharoplasty, particularly when the main problem to begin with was redundant fat. This is often a real observation rather than imagined and may be the result of reducing the ballooning effect on the skin caused by the bulging redundant periorbital fat. When the maximum amount of skin as well as fat has been resected in such an individual, a chemical abrasion may substantially improve such wrinkles.

### HEMATOMA

Hematomas can occur anywhere in the blepharoplasty wound. Retrobulbar hematoma occurs deep to the orbital septum and will be discussed subsequently.

Localized subcutaneous or submuscular hematomas following surgery often are not recognized until after much of the immediate swelling and ecchymosis have subsided. Such localized hematomas become liquefied in approximately 7 to 9 days after the surgery. They should be *thoroughly* evacuated. It is rare that aspiration of hematomas is completely effective; therefore, it is best to reopen the blepharoplasty incision adjacent to the hematoma or make a separate stab wound over it with a #11 blade. The clot should be painstakingly and thoroughly evacuated. Every effort should be made to completely evacuate the hematoma during its liquid stage. Any residual clot will contribute to the formation of a firm organizing scar that may persist for many months and be a source of annoyance to the patient. Such persistent scar nodules are best treated with injections of very dilute and small doses of intralesional steroids. Caution is advised in the use of steroids since there is considerable individual variation in response to steroid injections. Significant subcutaneous atrophy can occur in some patients. Rarely, more than 2 mg. of triamcinolone or related compounds are required at any one injection. It is wise to space the injections at least two to three weeks apart so that the effect can be measured and a cumulative effect avoided.

An acute hematoma discovered immediately following surgery is better left undisturbed until liquefaction occurs. Early clots

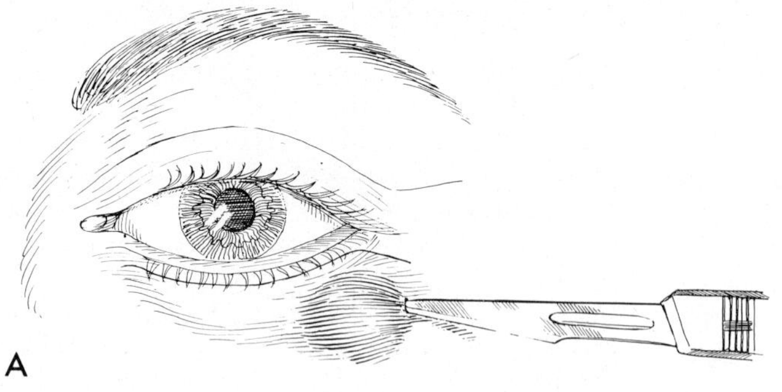


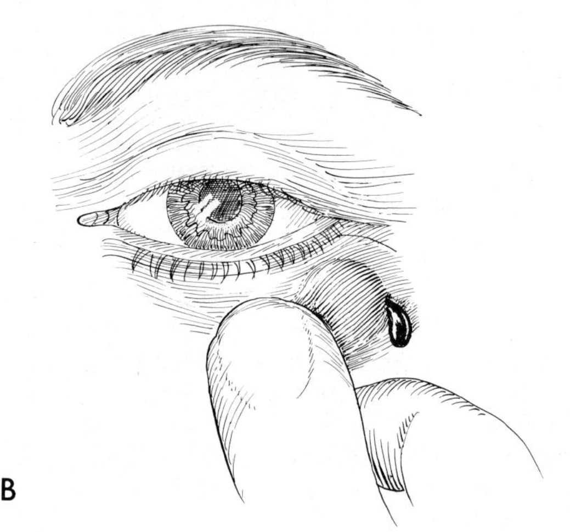


**Figure 25–7** If a small, localized hematoma of the eyelid develops postoperatively (*A*), it should be removed at about eight days by making a stab wound with a No. 11 blade and pressing out the contents with the thumb (*B*). (From Rees, T. D.: Blepharoplasty. *In* Rees, T. D., and Wood-Smith, D. [eds.]: Cosmetic Facial Surgery. Philadelphia, W. B. Saunders Company, 1973.)

are poorly defined, adherent to surrounding muscle and difficult to evacuate.

## ASYMMETRY

Almost everyone has some degree of asymmetry of the eyes, adnexae and orbits. Asymmetry is significant in many patients. When camouflaged with redundant skin or periorbital fat, asymmetry may not be obvious to the patient until after aesthetic blepharoplasty.[37] It is astonishing how few people are aware of asymmetry in their face. It is good practice to point out such differences preoperatively. Asymmetry may be related to unilateral ptosis. Plication of the levator expansion or fixation to the tarsal plate on one or both sides may then correct or improve the asymmetry in such patients.[41] Often asymmetry can be improved if not completely corrected by varying the soft tissue resection from side to side during surgery.

## LAGOPHTHALMOS

Lagophthalmos — the inability to completely close the eyes — is a common complaint during the immediate postoperative period. This can result in drying of the cornea and general desiccation and irritation of the conjunctiva and lid margins. A bland eye ointment to be applied at night should be prescribed for patients with this problem. The use of methylcellulose or other protective solution eye drops on retiring and during the daytime also provides protection until the condition has corrected itself. Occasionally, temporary lagophthalmos will continue for several weeks or months.

Lagophthalmos may result from excision of too much skin from the upper eyelids. Careful preincision marking of the upper lids will help avoid this mistake. The upper lid should not remain open more than 3 mm. at the end of the procedure. If the skin shortage causing lagophthalmos is severe, a serious situation exists, for the cornea is no longer covered and protected by the upper lid. This results in desiccation, exposure keratitis and eventual ulceration of the anterior chamber, with possible perforation — a set of circumstances frequently seen following thermal burns of the eyelids. This severe degree of what is really ectropion of the upper lid requires emergency consideration with release of the lid and immediate skin grafting. Such a problem is exceedingly rare in cosmetic blepharoplasty.

#### LOSS OF EYELASHES

Spontaneous loss of eyelashes, although rare, has been known to occur. The process is usually reversible, however, and the lashes grow in again. "Trimming" the lashes should be avoided, and they are especially susceptible during the subciliary incision in the lower eyelid. They can usually be retracted by an assistant with a cotton tip applicator.

### *Major Complications*

#### PTOSIS

Pseudoptosis from wound edema and reaction may be present in the early postoperative period. This, however, rapidly improves with resolution of the wound edema.

Persistent ptosis suggests injury to the levator expansion. Injury to the medial portion of the levator expansion can occur when the orbital septum is opened to remove redundant fat from the upper lid or the transverse fat on the outer surface of the levator just behind the orbital septum and the orbicularis. Furthermore, because the medial fibrofat extends deeply back into the orbit, the dissecting scissors can detach a portion of the medial levator unless proper caution is exercised. If the levator is injured, surgical repair is indicated.

Disparate resection of soft tissue or imbalance in the level of levator fixation can also result in "relative" ptosis. Unquestionably, levator fixation into the dermis or tarsus, as advocated by Sheen[41] and others, is a useful procedure in selected patients; however, great care should be exercised to suture the levator at exactly the same level on either side to prevent asymmetric ptosis, although such disparity usually corrects itself with time in such cases.

#### EXTRAOCULAR MUSCLE IMBALANCE

The inferior rectus muscle occupies a position straddling the medial and middle fat compartments of the lower eyelid. Because of its relatively superficial position and its anatomic location, it can be damaged during the course of blepharoplasty when these two fat compartments are decompressed. The muscle can be injured when the stumps of the excised fat are cauterized. It can also be traumatized by instrumental dissection in the area. Partial injuries usually heal without residual deformity shortly following the operation. Accidental complete resection of the muscle during the course of blepharoplasty is recognized by persistent postoperative diplopia readily identified by ophthalmologic and visual field examination. Temporary palsy of the muscle is usually restored within six weeks. If damage to the muscle is proved and persists beyond this time, a resection of the inferior rectus muscle and simple repair of the severed ends should be performed. In rare cases, if the deviation is severe enough, resection with a recession of the superior rectus muscle may be required to restore extraocular muscle balance.

Very rarely, the superior oblique muscle can be inadvertently severed at the tendon. In this situation, the superior oblique muscle should be freed from all scars in the area and a fat flap should be mobilized within the orbit and placed anterior to the tendon to prevent the recurrence of adhesions to the old scar.

#### RETROBULBAR HEMATOMA

This is a feared and spectacular complication of blepharoplasty. Blood collects in the deep tissues throughout the soft tissues of the orbit behind the orbital septum. Puncture of a small vessel during deep injection of the fat pockets is the usual cause.[34] It is therefore best to delay deep injections of local anesthetic into the fat pockets until immediately before making an incision into the orbital septum. Bleeding from open vessels of the fat pedicle stumps can also cause retrobulbar hematoma, but much less commonly than punctured vessels. The offending bleeder in a fat pedicle can often be identified and coagulated, whereas in the retrobulbar hematoma caused by deep needle injection, the exact point of bleeding is rarely identifiable.

The signs of retrobulbar hematoma are unmistakable.[29] The eye becomes stony hard and proptotic; the lids are forced back from the globe and the eye protrudes further and further. The treatment during operation consists of opening the orbital septum extensively and exploring the deeper orbit insofar as safe and practical.[38] As stated previously, it is rare that the offending bleeding point is found. The blood is not locally collected as it is in localized hematoma but is infiltrated throughout the fat and soft tissues, making effective drainage difficult or impossible. It is probably just as wise to continue the operation as to stop. It seems reasonable to assume that decompression of the orbital contents by opening the orbital septum widely would help. Likewise, the remote possibility of identifying the bleeding point is enhanced.

When retrobulbar hematoma is apparent, the intraocular pressure should be measured with a tonometer. A moderate elevation of pressure is not unusual and may persist for several hours. A temporary tarsorrhaphy suture through the eyelids may be helpful as a postoperative measure to protect the cornea if the proptosis is not too severe. Pressure dressings are not recommended since further pressure on the globe and central retinal vessels seems inadvisable. The postoperative treatment of retrobulbar hematoma consists primarily of observation, cold compresses, the use of diuretics to reduce the extracellular fluid volume and medical reduction of the blood pressure when elevated. The consultation and advice of a qualified ophthalmologist should be sought. Paracentesis of the anterior chamber of the eye has been suggested to decompress the elevated intraocular pressure,[33] but such treatment is controversial. Until the rationale is established by further investigation, the technique must be considered inadvisable in most cases, unless strongly suggested by a qualified ophthalmologist who is familiar with the problem. In the senior author's experience with five instances of retrobulbar hematoma, paracentesis was performed in none and a prompt recovery was experienced in all. A recent clinical report by Huang, Horowitz, and Lewis[32] of ten cases of retrobulbar hematoma from trauma or elective surgery resulted in no permanent visual disturbances. In their series, temporary elevation of the intraocular pressure readings was common. Anterior chamber paracentesis was not performed despite elevated pressures.

Retrobulbar hematoma, so frightening at onset, most often subsides dramatically within 12 to 24 hours following surgery. Although blindness has been attributed to retrobulbar hematoma, a direct cause and effect relationship has not been established. The mechanism is thought to be pressure on the central retinal vessels. Fry[26] injected large volumes of blood into the posterior orbit in monkeys, and although he produced temporary interference with vision, permanent blindness did not occur with this technique in any animal. Similar experiments in rabbits by DeMere, Wood, and Austin[23] as well as by Huang, Horowitz, and Lewis[32] failed to produce permanent blindness in these animals. Retrobulbar hematoma is well known to those eye surgeons who administer large numbers of local anesthetics by deep orbital injections. According to Duke-Elder,[24] retrobulbar hematoma rarely causes permanent blindness, and he reported only two instances in 2750 cases of retrobulbar hemorrhage. The general consensus is that it is more frightening than threatening, however, and the patient should be carefully followed until complete resolution has occurred.

### BLINDNESS

Blindness is the most feared complication, yet knowledge of the relationship of this tragic complication to the blepharoplasty operation is scant. Existing documentation seems too flimsy to draw definite conclusions. A national survey conducted by DeMere, Wood, and Austin[23] of plastic and ophthalmic surgeons found 40 cases of unilateral blindness after 98,514 eyelid operations (0.04 per cent incidence). The etiologic cause of the loss of vision could not be established, and there was no correlation with the type of anesthesia or the use of dressings. Most significant is the finding that adequate eye examinations were recorded preoperatively by only 15 per cent of plastic surgeons, 46 per cent of ear, nose and throat surgeons and 90 per cent of ophthalmic surgeons. It seems probable that progressive and unrelieved pressure from retrobulbar hematomas could result in blindness by choking the ophthalmic vessels. Such an end result must be exceedingly rare, however, since retrobulbar hematoma from all causes occurs with sufficient frequency to identify a causal relationship to blindness that is rarely reported in association with blepharoplasty or retrobulbar hematoma.

Idiopathic optic atrophy has been reported as a cause of blindness following blepharoplasty[30] but could well have been incidental to the surgery. It seems reasonable to assume that many cases of blindness following blepharoplasty have not been reported. It would be an important contribution if all such patients were documented. Preoperative binocular ophthalmologic evaluation of the patient is obviously important from a legal point of view, in the event such a serious problem as blindness should be discovered in the postoperative period.

A review of seven cases of blindness following blepharoplasty was reported by Moser, DiPirro, and McCoy.[35] In the group, they found three cases reportedly due to retrobulbar optic neuritis and one due to an optic nerve injury, which was unproved. They speculated that such changes were likely the result of fascicular changes from unrecognized central nervous system disease, such as multiple sclerosis or toxic amblyopia. Thrombosis of the retinal artery and vein was reported as the cause of two cases of blindness. The final conclusion of these investigators was that no causal relationship could be established. Hueston and Heinze[33] reported on a 37-year-old patient who, following an uneventful blepharoplasty, developed severe orbital ecchymosis and swelling and a rise in the intraocular tension that led to blindness. This patient apparently had a retrobulbar hematoma and was noted to have a general interstitial extravasation of blood. They could not determine a discrete orbital hematoma, which is not unusual since retrobulbar hematomas are not usually so circumscribed. A cessation of blood circulation in the retina and optic disc was noted. They performed paracentesis of the anterior chamber, and their patient made a complete recovery. This experience led to their primary recommendation, which was careful observation of patients following surgery.

## ENOPHTHALMOS

Enophthalmos following blepharoplasty can often be anticipated and therefore avoided by careful preoperative examination. Patients with "deep set" eyes or prominent infraorbital bony margins present an ideal anatomic predisposition for developing enophthalmos following removal of redundant periorbital fat. Great care should be exercised in such patients to remove a minimal amount of fat. If the surgeon suspects that he has removed too much fat during surgery, an appropriate amount of fat can be reinserted through the rent in the orbital septum to fill out the defect. When fat is replaced, the orbital septum should be sutured to retain the graft. It is unknown whether the fat survives as a free fat graft or simply fills in the contour from fibrous organization of the transplant.

Once established, there is no effective therapy for the cadaverous appearance of enophthalmos. Dermis-fat grafts performed subsequently are not successful. The use of prosthetic substances or liquid silicone injections in the periorbital tissues in the absence of blindness is considered unwise under most circumstances.

Careful reduction of the prominent bony orbital margins with an air-driven polishing bur might well be effective in some cases, but has not as yet been reported.

## KERATOCONJUNCTIVITIS SICCA ("DRY-EYE SYNDROME")

Should the dry-eye syndrome develop after aesthetic blepharoplasty, protracted conservative treatment must be anticipated.[43] Protection and lubrication of the cornea is the only treatment. Such treatment is important at night when lagophthalmos and corneal drying from exposure are likely to result from loss of the normal air seal of the lids. Bland protective agents such as Lacri-Lube or Duralube and a complete air seal of the lids may be required at night for weeks or months until the lids seal naturally again during sleep. An artificial lid seal eye dressing is commercially available or can be fashioned by applying thin plastic sheeting, such as saran wrap, over the eye and sealing it to the skin with Vaseline. During the day, frequent application of "artificial tears" may be required to maintain corneal lubrication. Several such compounds are commercially available. Valium may be helpful, since the combination of sleep loss and constant irritation of the eyes can extract a heavy emotional toll. Improvement may be slow in forthcoming. Many months may pass before significant improvement occurs. Ophthalmologic consultation should be obtained when the problem is first recognized and subsequently to follow the progress of treatment. Full-blown keratoconjunctivitis sicca is a serious and debilitating disease that can lead to xerophthalmia with multiple small filamentous ulcers of the cornea. Cicatricial replacement of the cornea and blindness can eventually result if the disease is untreated.[27, 40, 42]

## ECTROPION

A minor, temporary postoperative "scleral show" may occur no matter how conservatively the blepharoplasty was carried out. In some patients, such mild ectropion may be temporary, lasting several weeks or months; in other patients it may be permanent.[25] It sometimes can be anticipated before surgery if one takes note of unusual bulging of the globe, a relative shortness of soft tissue or excessive pseudoherniation of orbital fat.

Minimal postoperative ectropion or "scleral show" is often caused by the removal of fat in patients who have excessive periorbital fat with a marked convex curve of the lids. In such patients, it is extremely important to recontour the skin flap so that it fills all contours of the dissected muscle beneath.

The immediate problem of ectropion is usually the result of chemosis and generalized wound edema and reaction. Such ectropion is not the result of excessive tissue resection but of normal wound reaction. Severe chemosis can be rapidly resolved by the local application of topical steroids, often within a few hours.

Another cause of temporary pull-down of the lower lid in the immediate postblepharoplasty period is a temporary paresis of the orbicular muscle of the eye that results from surgical interference with terminal branches of the facial nerve and from wound edema and reaction within the muscle itself. Such muscle paresis is ordinarily short-lived and clears up promptly following resolution of the acute wound reaction or following reinnervation of the muscle from undamaged nerve filament.

Cicatricial ectropion is the result of excessive removal of skin or muscle or of damage to the orbital septum. If the surgeon suspects that he has removed too much skin at surgery, it should be replaced immediately as a free whole-thickness graft.[39] Usually such small grafts survive entirely and are difficult to identify in several months' time. The technique of skin excision of the lower eyelids is particularly important to prevent ectropion. Several useful "tricks" are available to aid the surgeon in excising the proper and safe amount of skin. Downward pressure on the eyeball will elevate the lid[36, 39] and opening the mouth widely stretches the lower lid downward and is useful with local anesthesia. The lid margins should be free and the resected fat stumps should be tucked beneath the orbital septum to prevent adherence to this structure. Another technique to increase the safety of skin excision is to carefully drape the skin in a cephalic direction and then make one or two vertical cuts with small scissors down to the line of proposed skin excision. The redraped skin is then excised exactly along the incision line with very fine scissors.

Cicatricial ectropion results from contracture resulting from excessive skin or soft tissue resection.[21] Observation for a period of several months, during which time wound reaction subsides and scar tissue resolves and softens, is the best first choice. When the wound stabilizes, the defect is surgically re-created and resurfaced with full thickness skin grafts. Occasionally, full thickness skin grafts are required if excessive scarring is present or the defect is very large. The deficiency is always larger than anticipated; therefore, the graft should not be measured or cut before the wound is made. Some degree of contraction of all skin grafts must be anticipated, and some residual "scleral show" will probably result

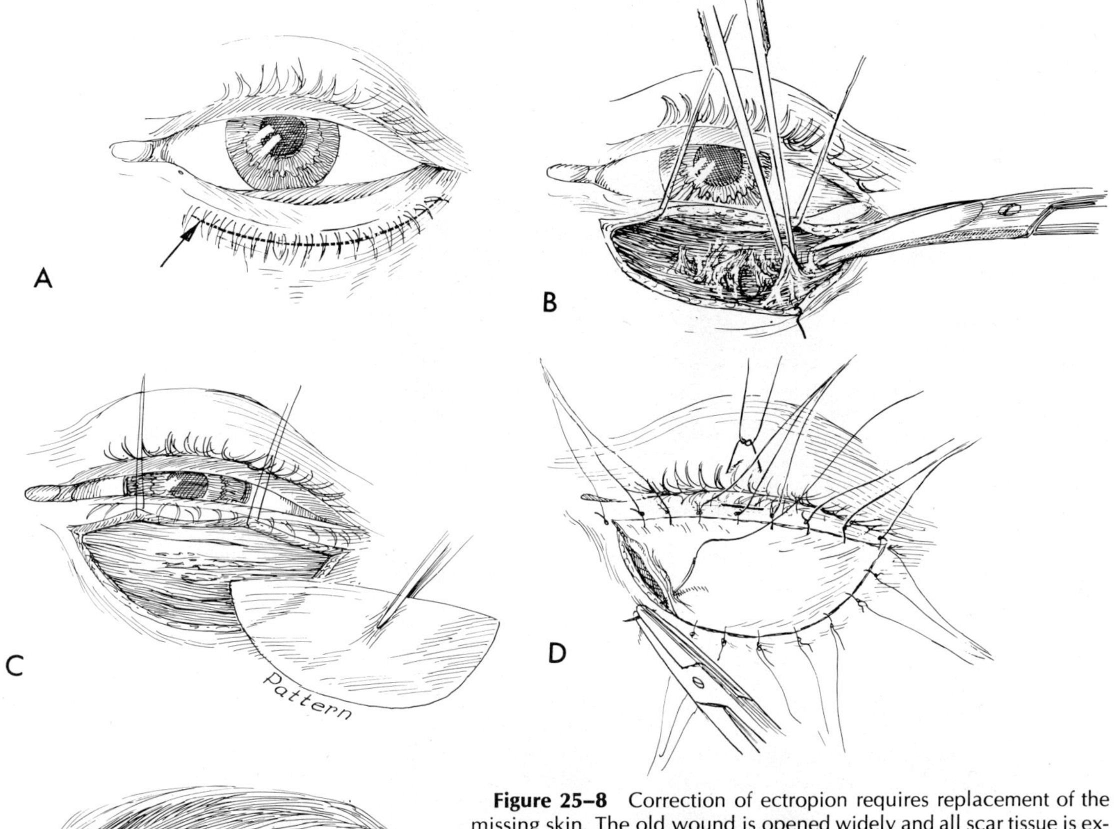


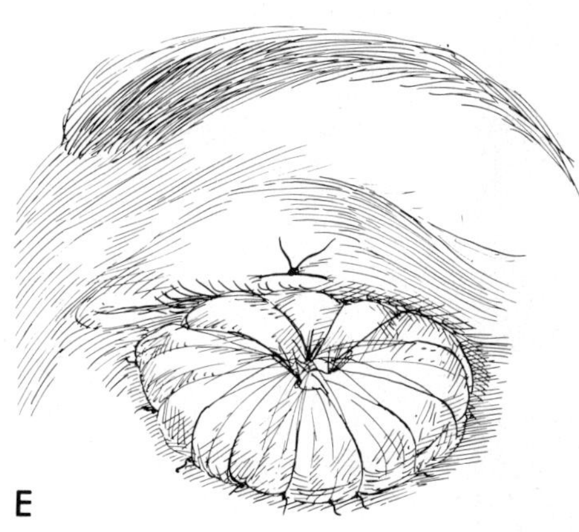


**Figure 25–8** Correction of ectropion requires replacement of the missing skin. The old wound is opened widely and all scar tissue is excised (*A, B*). The wound edges should not be undermined, because dead spaces beneath the skin can be the site of fluid accumulation or hematoma formation, which mitigates against graft survival. A pattern of the defect is then constructed with a thin sheet of plastic (*C*), and a full-thickness skin graft of the exact size is cut from the upper lid—provided a sufficient amount of skin is available. The graft is trimmed of all subcutaneous fat and sutured into place (*D*). A tie-over dressing is left in place for seven to ten days (*E*). The lids are closed during this period with a temporary tarsorrhaphy suture. A certain amount of contraction of the graft must be expected in the few weeks following surgery, but this is minimal with full-thickness grafts. If there is not enough skin on the upper lid to provide a graft of proper size, the graft should come from the retroauricular region, or, as a last resort, the supraclavicular area. The scar that results will probably be unsightly in this area, especially in a woman. (From Rees, T. D.: Blepharoplasty. *In* Rees, T. D., and Wood-Smith, D. [eds.]: Cosmetic Facial Surgery. Philadelphia, W. B. Saunders Company, 1973.)

even after the most successful reconstruction.

Redundancy of the lower lid with its tarsal plate is common in older patients (senile ectropion). A full thickness wedge V-excision lateral to the corneal limbus and repair of the defect should accompany aesthetic skin corrections. Patients with a tendency to senile ectropion should have a wedge resection at the time of blepharoplasty to prevent eversion of the lid margin. The technique is simple. Repair is accomplished by an accurate approximation of the tarsal plate with fine interrupted sutures or a Mustardé pullout suture. Careful line-up of the lid margin is crucial to success. Marked redundancy of herniated fat or skin can easily mask early senile ectropion or loss

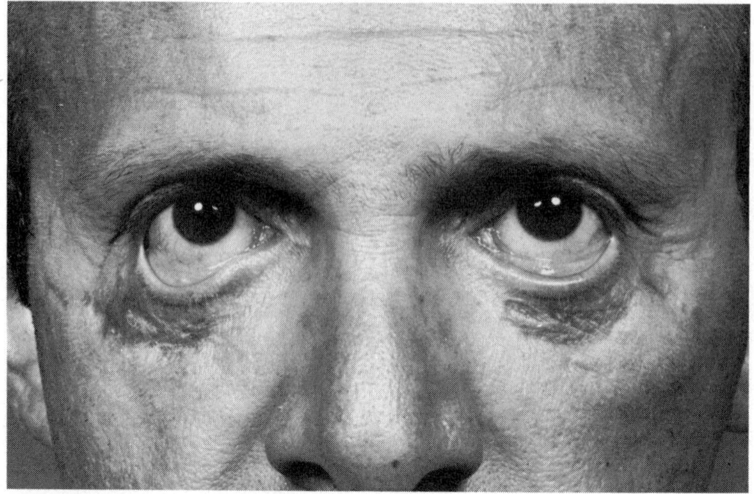

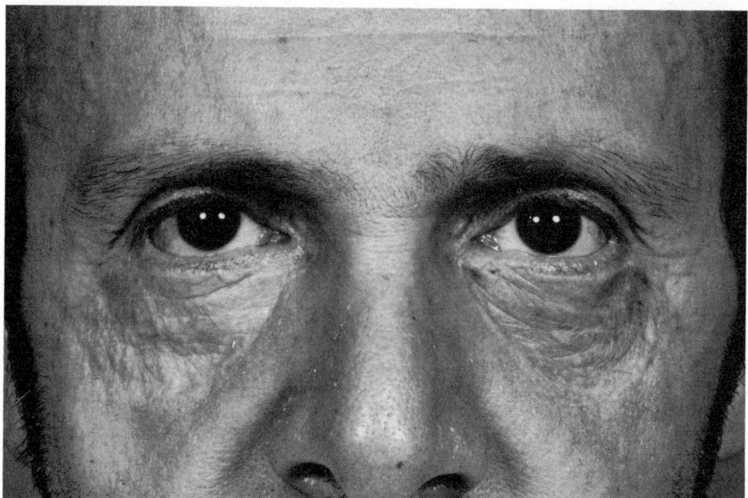

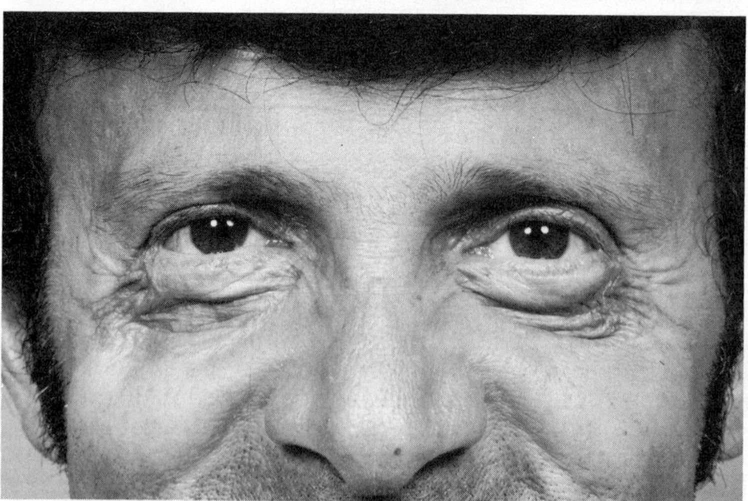

**Figure 25–9** Severe ectropion can result from excessive skin removal and poor timing of operations aimed at correcting the initial problem, as shown in this patient. Several attempts had already been made to correct bilateral ectropion that resulted from cosmetic blepharoplasty performed by another surgeon. Each of these procedures consisted of split-thickness skin grafting, and they were performed within several weeks of each other, during the period of maximum wound reaction and scar contracture. The final result consisted not only of severe ectropion but also of extensive scarring of surrounding skin and underlying muscle. The patient was not able to close his eyes.

The postoperative photographs of this patient demonstrate correction of the ectropion, but the large skin grafts are permanent cosmetic defects that cannot be eradicated. (From Rees, T. D.: Blepharoplasty. *In* Rees, T. D., and Wood-Smith, D. [eds.]: Cosmetic Facial Surgery. Philadelphia, W.B. Saunders Company, 1973.)

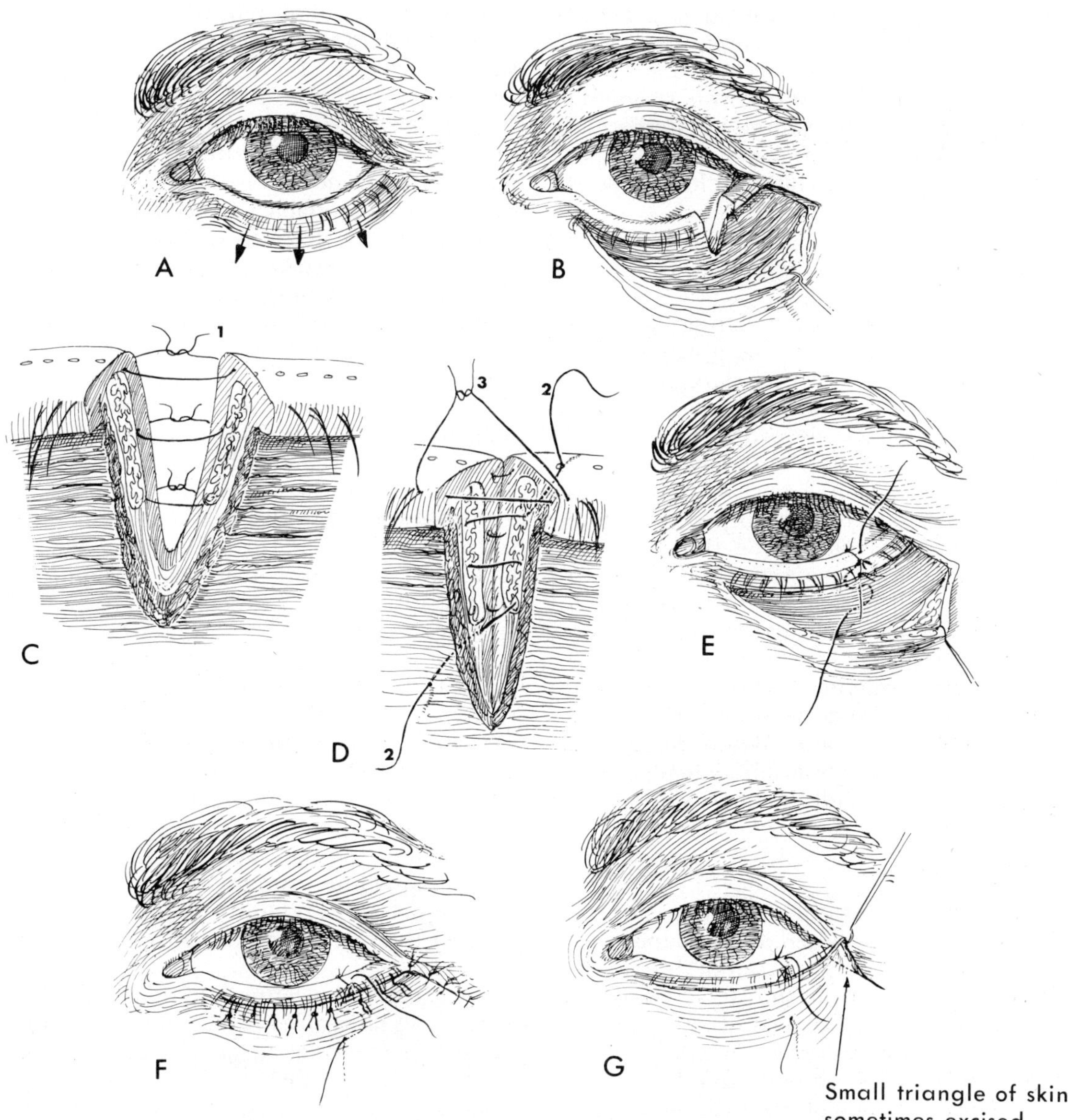


**Figure 25–10** In patients with atonicity of the lower lid, which can be familial in origin or the result of senile changes, the tendency toward ectropion can be aggravated by blepharoplasty. This is particularly true in males for some unknown reason. If ectropion develops after cosmetic blepharoplasty, and atonicity seems the primary cause (*A*), correction can be achieved by incising along the old blepharoplasty incision, undermining the skin flap, excising a suitably sized full-thickness wedge lateral to the limbus *(B)*, and repairing the defect according to Mustardé's technique, with layer closure and a pull-out as shown in *C, D, E, F,* and *G.* (From Rees, T. D.: Blepharoplasty. *In* Rees, T. D., and Wood-Smith, D. [eds.]: Cosmetic Facial Surgery. Philadelphia, W. B. Saunders Company, 1973.)

of lid tone. A slight drooping of the lateral third of the lids, the "hound dog look," should alert the surgeon.

The diagnosis is confirmed by testing the lower lid redundancy. The lid is grasped between thumb and forefinger and stretched. Excess tissue or loss of tone is readily apparent by comparison to young lids that are tight. One should not hesitate to perform a V-excision routinely in older patients in which a redundancy of lower eyelid is present.

## SKIN SLOUGH

It seems remarkable that skin slough does not occur more often after complete undermining of the lower eyelid skin, since this maneuver results in what is almost a full thickness skin graft; nevertheless, skin necrosis is exceedingly rare. Incipient or suspected slough should be treated conservatively, similar to a frost bite injury, since the extent of tissue viability beneath the eschar is unknown until it has separated. A situation that would initially seem to require a skin graft is usually salvaged. Complete epithelial healing usually occurs beneath the eschar. The surgeon should not be in a hurry to debride such wounds, and a conservative policy is best. When healing is complete, any remaining skin deficiency can be repaired with a full thickness skin graft.

## GLAUCOMA

Although there is only one report in the literature of acute closed-angle glaucoma[28] occurring as a complication of blepharoplasty, plastic surgeons must be aware of this risk, especially because of the marked female preponderance for acute closed-angle glaucoma. A preoperative history of migraine-like attacks, blurred vision or halos around lights should arouse suspicion, and an ophthalmologic consultation is recommended. Although the incidence of acute closed-angle glaucoma in a normal population has been reported as 0.09 per cent,[31] a blepharoplasty may precipitate the onset. A postoperative patient complaining of pain, blurred vision, corneal edema and a dilated pupil warrants an immediate ophthalmologic opinion.

### *Secondary Blepharoplasty and Undercorrection*

Secondary blepharoplasty is one of the most challenging and hazardous operations in the field of cosmetic surgery. It even ranks ahead of secondary rhinoplasty in technical difficulties and pitfalls awaiting the unwary surgeon. Such surgery should be undertaken only if, after careful assessment, the surgeon is certain that he can achieve a reasonable correction without creating further deformity. It is particularly perilous to undertake correction of minor secondary deformities, for, unfortunately, minor degrees of improvement are not always appreciated by the patient.

The most common deformities requiring secondary surgery after a primary blepharoplasty are (1) bulging of the medial fat pockets of the upper eyelids; (2) recurrence of a skin fold of the upper eyelid; (3) ptosis of the brow, often with a marked lateral skin fold; (4) residual herniated fat pockets of the lower eyelids, usually medial and middle and less often lateral; (5) elevated, irregular or uneven scars or scar contractures such as webbing near the lateral canthus; (6) varying degrees of ectropion because of excessive resection of the skin of the lower lids; (7) inability to close the upper lids with corneal exposure; (8) excessive skin of the lower lids because of inadequate excision at the primary operation; (9) excessive pigmentation of the skin; and (10) the appearance of many fine wrinkles not visible before the original surgery and thought to be the result of the release of skin tension after fat removal.

The cause and treatment of many of these deformities have already been described. Of prime importance in surgery is the fact that there is rarely sufficient skin to spare at a secondary operation, particularly on the lower lids. This is of utmost importance when planning a secondary operation. Occasionally, undercorrection at the time of primary blepharoplasty may be improved by a second operation. If the defect consists of a remnant bulge from a fat pocket, a stab wound immediately into the area with excision of the fat suffices. As a general rule, a secondary operation should not be carried out before six months have elapsed to allow for edema to subside and healing and softening of the scar tissue.

## COMPLICATIONS OF RHYTIDECTOMY

### *General Considerations*

Although the face lift operation has been practiced for at least seventy years, the demand for this type of surgery has risen sharply over the past decade. With safer anesthesia and improved techniques, the extent of the face lift operation has become more radical. That is, the amount of skin undermining is more extensive, reaching well down into the neck and toward the corners of the mouth. In general many of the complications following rhytidectomy occur in direct proportion to the extensiveness of undermining and in indirect proportion to the success of hemostasis.[49] Peterson[60] compared extensive and limited undermining in face lift patients and found that extensive undermining permitted the excision of only 15 per cent more skin by weight. Eighty per cent of the complications occurred in sides that had extensive undermining, and there was little discernible difference between the cosmetic result obtained by extensive undermining compared to limited undermining in patients with comparable facial types.

Although the recent introduction and popularization of the subplatysmal dissection and platysmal muscle flap surgery[55] has enhanced the result of some rhytidectomies, there may be a higher risk of serious complications. The wise surgeon will remember that his goal is improvement rather than "cure," and heroic surgical indulgence followed by complications only makes for an unsatisfactory aesthetic result and an unhappy patient.

As in rhinoplasty and blepharoplasty, the preoperative evaluation is of paramount importance in minimizing the possibility of postoperative complications. Those considerations that should be stressed in the preoperative evaluation are the patient's (1) attitude, psychologic state and anticipated improvement from surgery; (2) obesity, weight loss or gain that would affect the result; (3) skin texture, senile changes or atrophy; (4) bony framework of the face, mandibular retrusion, microgenia or retrognathia or the mandibular-cervical angle; (5) hairstyle, hair thickness and position of the sideburns, in the male; (6) previous scars, hypertrophied scars or keloid diathesis; and (7) facial asymmetry, which should be pointed out to the patient preoperatively.

Perhaps the most important part of the preoperative consultation is an explanation to the patient of the "realistic" expectations of the surgery, the duration of results as well as the possible postoperative complications. In spite of this detailed discussion by the surgeon, many patients exhibit an inability to retain or comprehend, as recently demonstrated by Goin, Burgoyne, and Goin.[53] For this reason, the surgeon must document what the patient has been told and be prepared to handle any negative postoperative responses. Considering the highly emotional aspects of face lift surgery, it is not surprising to find a high incidence of "niggling" complaints in the immediate postoperative period.[66]

No matter how completely the limitations and realities of the surgery are explained, the patient still dreams of regaining youth and may be motivated by magical hopes and expectations. This is not to say that the majority of patients undergoing rhytidectomy are not eventually pleased with the results. For the most part they are satisfied, and this satisfaction usually increases as the months pass after the operation. A continuous calm, reassuring attitude on the part of the surgeon and his staff often results in the transformation of what appeared at first to be a dissatisfied patient into a satisfied one.

### *Minor Postoperative Complications*

#### INFECTION

Primary or secondary infection following the face lift operation is extremely rare in spite of the presence of hair surrounding the wound. Undoubtedly the superb blood supply to the face is a factor in keeping the reported incidence of infection to less than 1 per cent.[45, 71] Prophylactic shampoo and face wash the night before and day of surgery is advised, and many surgeons use prophylactic antibiotics, although there is no

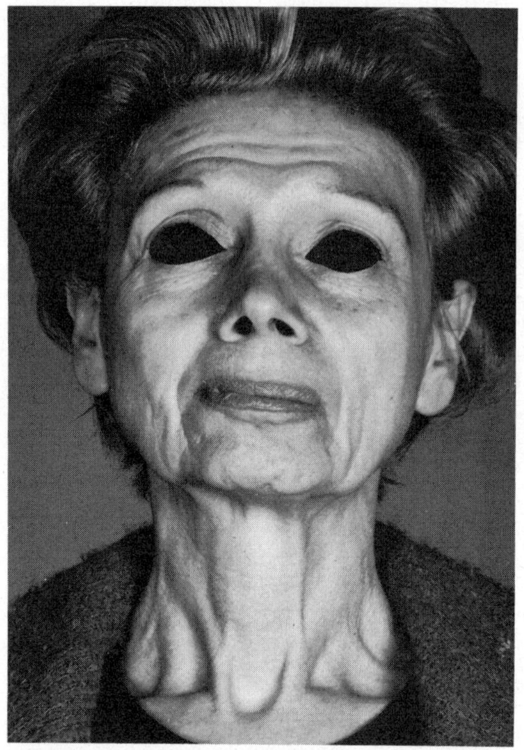

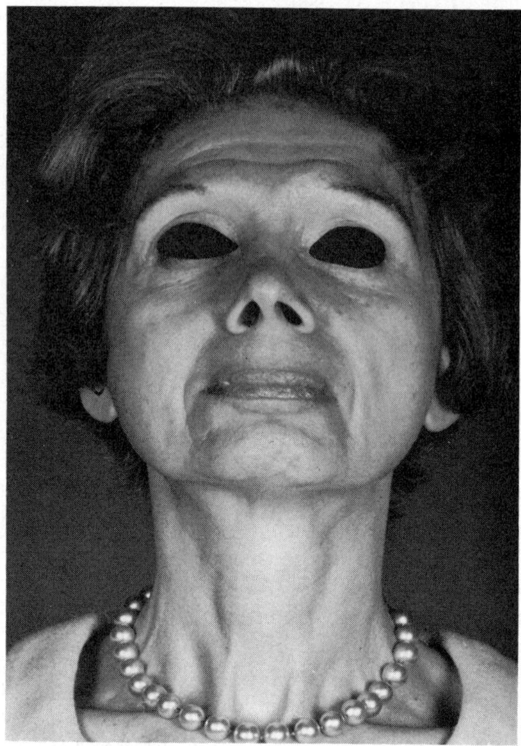

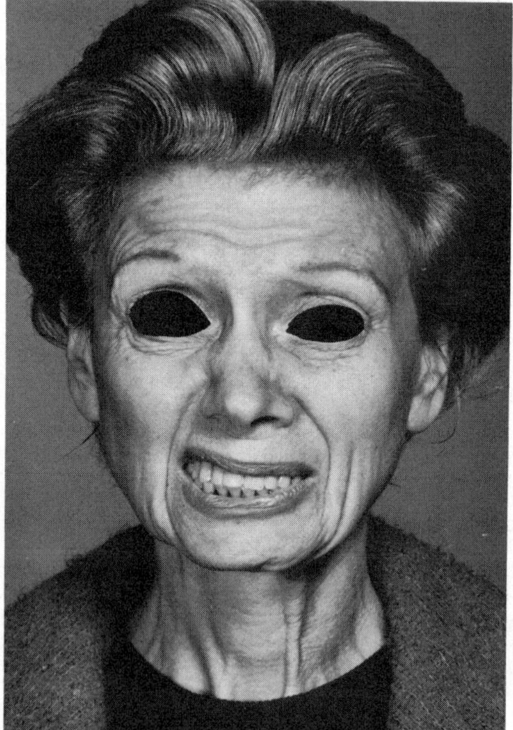

**Figure 25–11** Preoperative examination of every patient who is a candidate for facial plastic surgery should include a careful inspection of the facial musculature for evidence of unilateral weakness or paralysis. If such a condition can be shown to exist preoperatively, it cannot later be ascribed to the surgery performed. This patient exhibited a left partial hemiparesis, the residual of an old Bell's palsy, that was hardly noticeable except with extreme animation. The same principle applies to facial asymmetry, which can be accentuated by surgery. Minor degrees of asymmetry or even paralysis can be missed in the initial examination unless the patient is instructed to display marked facial animation. Such minor deformities must obviously be pointed out to the patient before surgery in order to avoid postoperative repercussions. (From Rees, T. D.: Face lift. *In* Rees, T. D., and Wood-Smith, D. [eds.]: Cosmetic Facial Surgery. Philadelphia, W. B. Saunders Company, 1973.)

evidence to support their efficacy. Minor localized infections can occur around sutures or hair follicles, and these are easily treated by suture removal and evacuation. Suppurative infections beneath the flaps usually occur in the presence of hematoma, and the treatment is suture removal, adequate drainage, local heat and specific antibiotics. Acute chondritis has been known to occur when postauricular sutures have been placed through the perichondrium and cartilage. Prompt therapy must be instituted to minimize cartilage destruction. (See treatment of chondritis following otoplasty.)

#### SMALL HEMATOMAS

Hematomas are by far the most significant and troublesome complication following rhytidectomy.[65] The most common are small localized collections of from 2 to 30 cc. with a reported incidence of about 15 per cent.[3] Very small hematomas are absorbed spontaneously within a few weeks and usually leave no sequelae. Often a discrete collection may not be detected until the edema subsides after a few days, when it will present as an area of firmness, ecchymosis or skin surface irregularity. Between the 7th and 14th days, these small hematomas liquefy, and at this time, every effort should be made to evacuate or aspirate them with a 15- or 16-gauge needle. If a small hematoma is located near a suture line, several sutures may be removed and the clot "milked out." If it is located some distance from the nearest suture line, it is sometimes possible to place a small stab incision in a natural skin crease overlying the hematoma and express it. After the 14th day, the clot becomes firm, and a puckering or minor contour deformity of the skin over the site may eventually occur that could take several months to resolve. Intralesional injections of small doses of steroids during the organizational phase of clot formation may help to minimize this deformity. Care must be taken to employ minute doses of steroid or subcutaneous atrophy will occur at the site of injection.

#### EXTENSIVE ECCHYMOSIS AND PIGMENTATION

Some localized ecchymosis is usually seen following a face lift operation, and this resolves in one to two weeks. Occasionally, a patient will develop extensive ecchymosis down to the lower aspect of the sternum that requires many weeks or months to resolve. Patients with thin, transparent skin and hypopigmentation are prone to severe ecchymosis, as are those patients with a preoperative history of unusual bruising. Although resolution of ecchymosis is usually complete, patients with darker complexions may have a residual brown pigmentation and should be forewarned of this possibility.

Telangiectasia may also be exacerbated following rhytidectomy, and a permanent reddish discoloration of the neck and cheeks may appear. Patients with small telangiectasias should be advised prior to surgery that new lesions may appear. The most appropriate treatment is with cosmetics; larger lesions can be electrocoagulated.

#### EDEMA

Edema following rhytidectomy normally subsides by the second postoperative week and is secondary to venous stasis. Persistent edema lasting more than three weeks is unusual and is presumably related to lymphatic stasis. Postoperative edema can be minimized by gentle tissue handling especially by avoiding undue pulling, pinching and squeezing of the skin flaps. Most edema eventually subsides with no residual. In patients with chronic postoperative swelling, other causes should be ruled out, such as allergy or kidney disease. Diuretics are not recommended to "hasten" the normal healing process.

### *Local Disfigurements*

#### EAR DEFORMITIES

With most rhytidectomy incisions, the pinna is circumscribed 75 per cent or more, and if excessive tension is applied to it in closing the wound, the ear may become dislocated or twisted on its axis. The most common type of ear deformity is the "pixie ear" that results from adherence of the lobe to the skin of the cheek. When trimming the pre- and postauricular skin flap, it is essential to obtain an exact fit of the lobe without tension if this deformity is to be avoided. In addition, the first suture of the postauricular flap should never be hung on the fascia of the ear lobe, but tension and fixation should be at the peak of the postauricular incision through the mastoid fascia. Preauricular incisions carried behind the tragus to minimize visible scars may result in distortion of the tragus and an unnatural look following normal wound contracture. A preauricular incision placed in a normal skin crease usually heals with minimal visibility and avoids the possibility of tragal deformity. A significant ear deformity may require a complete readjustment of the wound as a secondary procedure.

### "DOG EAR"

Despite all precautions taken at the time of surgery, a small "dog ear" may persist in the temporal region or nape of the neck. These usually resolve spontaneously within several months but can be quite annoying to the patient. If necessary, excision and correction can be carried out as a minor office procedure.

### SUBMENTAL DEPRESSION

When submental fat is removed, it is important to leave a small adipose layer attached to the skin in order to prevent adherence of the skin to the underlying strap muscles. Removal of all fat may result in adhesions, with fixation of skin to muscle causing unsightly contour irregularities that are emphasized during swallowing or motion of the neck. Small "dog ears" usually remain at the ends of the submental incision and must be carefully trimmed or unsightly bumps will remain. Suturing the wound from lateral to medial also helps eliminate this deformity. Excessive excision of fat and skin, particularly in patients with microgenia or mandibular retrusion, can result in webbing in the vertical dimension of the neck.

### WOUND SEPARATION

Wound dehiscence is usually secondary to trauma or excessive tension on the wound edges. Although some surgeons prefer to use buried dermis sutures to reduce the tension on the skin sutures, these are unnecessary if the redraping and fixation of the skin flaps has been properly done. There should be no tension on the preauricular and postauricular incisions. The preauricular incision is generally closed with #6–0 nylon, and these sutures are removed on the fifth postoperative day to prevent suture marks. Nylon of #4–0 is used to close the temporal scalp and mastoid skin, which supports the most tension, and these sutures are removed on the 10th to 12th postoperative days. Should wound dehiscence occur, Steri-Strips should be used for reapproximation or the wound should be resutured.

### SCARS AND KELOIDS

Hypertrophied scars and keloids following rhytidectomy are actually quite unusual. Scar hypertrophy is exceedingly rare in the preauricular region and is usually found in the postauricular area, where the greatest tension exists. Incisions closed under tension in the temporal and nape of the neck areas may result in wide or hypertrophied scars that are more obvious if there is an associated hair loss. The best prevention is wound closure without tension. Hypertrophic scars must be treated with patience, time and, occasionally, small doses of intralesional steroids.[54] Only after maturation should re-excision be considered. Keloids in face lift scars are rare but do occur and are more common in patients with darkly pigmented skin. Intralesional steroid injections should be tried first, and only if necessary, excision followed by steroid injections and radiation may be used.

### HAIR LOSS

Hair loss may result from superficial undermining with injury to the hair follicle, excessive tension or interference with blood supply to the hair follicles. MacGregor and Greenberg[57] reported a 2.8 per cent incidence of hair loss in the temporal region. Fortunately, temporary hair loss is more common than permanent loss, and patients with healthy hair and scalp usually have regrowth of hair in several months. An obvious hair loss may be noticed in the postauricular scalp as a "stair-step" if the hair line has not been accurately approximated. Male patients should be told preoperatively that the hairless preauricular area will be nar-

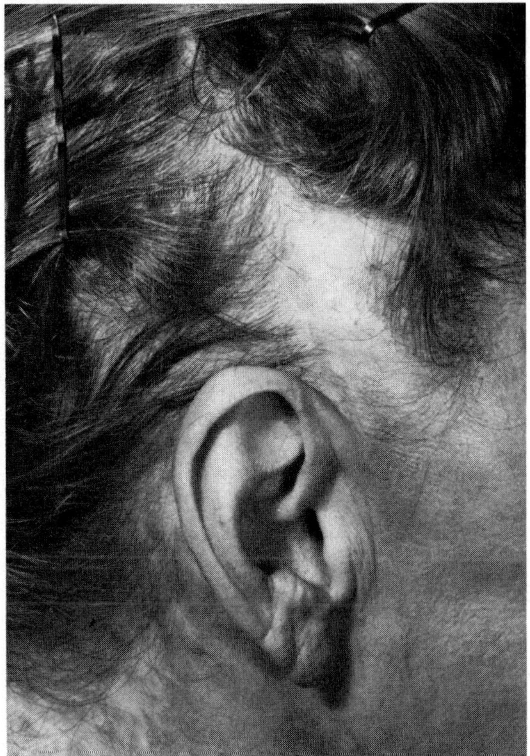

**Figure 25–12** Example of temporal alopecia probably secondary to excessive tension with resulting ischemia and loss of hair follicles. Too superficial undermining can also result in death to the hair follicles.

rowed and the beard pattern will change, possibly necessitating shaving behind the ear. When hair loss appears unusually extensive, a dermatologic consultation should be requested.[67]

#### SENSORY NERVE INJURY AND PARESTHESIAS

Temporary numbness and paresthesias over the earlobes and cheeks is quite common during the early postoperative period. This is usually the result of transection of the small sensory nerves, and full sensation generally returns in several weeks to months. Permanent injury to the great auricular nerve is uncommon but may occur if dissection is too deep over the upper third of the sternocleidomastoid muscle. If this injury is recognized at surgery, the nerve should be appropriately repaired to avoid a permanent anesthesia of the lower portion of the ear. Patients with anesthesia of the ear lobe should be cautioned about wearing compressive jewelry and the possibility of frostbite.

#### PAIN

Significant postoperative pain is unusual, and its occurrence, particularly if unilateral, should arouse suspicion of hematoma, which warrants investigation. Patients who have had plication of the platysma or the platysma flap not infrequently will complain of discomfort and tightness in the neck for the first few days or weeks postoperatively. Calm reassurance that this is normal will alleviate anxiety. Intractable, chronic pain is rare, and Conway[50] suggested that injury to branches of the cervical sensory nerves as they emerge from the posterior border of the sternocleidomastoid muscle might be a cause. Most pain invariably subsides within six months, and regional sensory nerve blocks or muscle relaxants, such as diazepam, may provide some relief.

### *Major Complications*

#### LARGE HEMATOMAS

As already stated, hematomas are by far the most frequent and troublesome complication following rhytidectomy. The treatment of small hematomas, which are the most common, has been discussed. Large, expanding hematomas that cause pain, swelling and ecchymosis demand immediate attention and should be evacuated as an emergency procedure. These usually occur within the first 24 hours after operation, although hematomas can occur as late as 10 days to two weeks postoperatively. Massive hematoma is almost always heralded by sudden and acute discomfort usually followed by unilateral swelling and ecchymosis. Since most patients have minimal discomfort after a face lift operation, excessive pain warrants an examination and removal of the dressing if there is any doubt. Failure or delay to evacuate a large hematoma may lead to venous engorgement and circulatory compromise of the flap with eventual necrosis. When a hematoma is identified, the sutures should be removed at the bedside and the

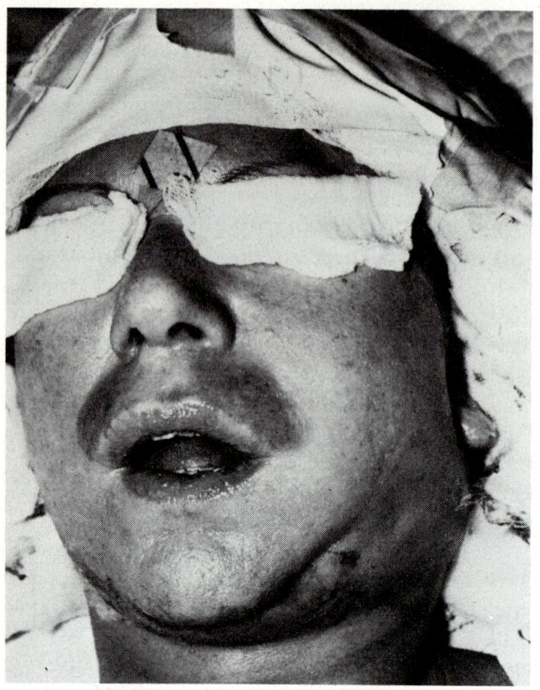

**Figure 25–13** Expanding hematoma of the left postauricular, parotid, and submental areas that was associated with pain, restlessness, and acute swelling of the left side of the face. Immediate evacuation will minimize complications resulting from large hematomas.

clots evacuated immediately to relieve tension on the skin flaps. The patient is then returned to the operating room where, under good lighting and anesthesia, the remainder of the hematoma is removed and bleeding stopped. Following successful treatment of a hematoma, there is generally more ecchymosis and prolonged edema, but the final result is not compromised.

The incidence of large hematomas that require surgical evacuation varies with individual series, but a compilation of the major series in the world literature is summarized in Table 25–1. In 8430 reported face lifts, the overall average incidence of large hematomas is 3.7 per cent. Few of these reports are analyzed by sex, but the actual literature indicates about 5 per cent of all rhytidec-

**TABLE 25–1** HEMATOMAS FOLLOWING RHYTIDECTOMY (Male and Female)

| Authors | Year | Number of Cases | Large Hematomas | Percentage |
|---|---|---|---|---|
| Serson-Neto | 1964 | 170 | 2 | 1.2 |
| Conway | 1970 | 325 | 21 | 6.6 |
| MacGregor and Greenberg | 1971 | 524 | 42 | 8.0 |
| McDowell | 1972 | 105 | 3 | 2.9 |
| Stark | 1972 | 100 | 3 | 3.0 |
| Webster | 1972 | 221 | 2 | 0.9 |
| Pitanguy, Ramos and Garcia | 1972 | 1600 | 89 | 5.5 |
| Morgan | 1973 | 40 | 1 | 2.5 |
| Rees, Lee and Coburn | 1973 | 806 | 23 | 2.9 |
| Barker* | 1974 | 163 | 2 | 1.3 |
| Black | 1976 | 1804 | 48 | 2.7 |
| Baker, Gordon and Mesienko | 1977 | 1500 | 46 | 3.0 |
| Stark | 1977 | 500 | 13 | 2.6 |
| Leist, Masson and Erich | 1977 | 180 | 6 | 3.3 |
| Straith, Raju and Hipps | 1977 | 500 | 8 | 1.6 |
| TOTALS | | 8538 | 309 | 3.5 |

*Barker, D. E.: Prevention of bleeding following rhytidectomy. Plast. Reconstr. Surg., *54*:651, 1974.

**TABLE 25–2** HEMATOMAS FOLLOWING RHYTIDECTOMY IN MALES

| Authors | Year | Number of Cases | Males | Large Hematomas | Per Cent | Small Hematomas | Per Cent |
|---|---|---|---|---|---|---|---|
| Pitanguy et al. | 1973 | 52 | 52 | 4 | 7.7 | 2 | 3.3 |
| Baker et al. | 1977 | 137 | 137 | 12 | 8.7 | 14 | 10.2 |

tomies are performed on males. Only two reports[44, 62] have specifically evaluated complications in male patients, and the incidence of large hematomas in these series was 7.7 per cent and 8.7 per cent (Table 25–2). These findings substantiate the general agreement among plastic surgeons that males have more bleeding at the time of surgery as well as a higher incidence of postoperative hematomas. Baker and his colleagues[44] suggested that this may be related to the increased blood supply to the beard, although this concept has not been proved.

There are numerous reports in the literature[44, 46, 57, 65, 66, 72] analyzing the causes of hematoma, and the majority of these reports concentrate on the operative period and intraoperative techniques. In general, the more extensive the undermining, the greater chances for a postoperative hematoma. Even the most meticulous hemostasis, various drainage methods, dressings or no dressings and immobilization have been tried and failed to prevent hematoma formation, however. Extensive evaluations for coagulation defects in hematoma patients are almost always normal. General anesthesia or hypotensive anesthesia does not prevent or reduce the incidence of hematoma as demonstrated by Rees, Lee and Coburn.[66]

The most recent and significant studies have evaluated postoperative hypertension as an etiological factor after rhytidectomy. Berner, Morain and Noe[46] studied pre- and postoperative blood pressures on 202 patients who had face lifts. They found that during the first two hours postoperatively blood pressure recordings were similar to the preoperative levels. During the succeeding three hours, however, most patients demonstrated blood pressures well in excess of their preoperative level. The authors pointed out that this was the period during which preoperative and intraoperative medications lose their effectiveness and the adrenergic response to pain and anxiety becomes manifest. They advocated the use of chlorpromazine in the early postoperative period to reduce "reactive hypertension" and this is a logical choice, for this drug has tranquilizing, antiemetic and antihypertensive effects. The recommended regimen is intramuscular injection of 25 mg. chlorpromazine one hour prior to completion of the operation, followed by a repetition of this dose at three hours postoperatively and four-hour intervals thereafter, when and if the systolic blood pressure exceeds 150 mm. Hg. Chlorpromazine is not recommended if no preoperative systolic pressure has exceeded 140 mm. Hg and if there are no hypertensive peaks postoperatively. More recently, Straith, Raju and Hipps[72] evaluated 500 consecutive face lifts and found that the incidence of hematoma correlated with the admission blood pressure; when the pressure was above 150/100 mm. Hg on admission, hematoma occurred 2.6 times more frequently than in normotensive patients.

The other important factor in minimizing bleeding and hematoma is the avoidance of aspirin and aspirin-containing compounds for two weeks prior to surgery and one week postoperatively. Aspirin is known to inhibit the adherence of platelets, and as little as 10 grains a day can act to prevent normal aggregation of platelets and predispose to postoperative bleeding. This effect persists for the entire lifetime of the platelet, which is about 10 days, and therefore all aspirin and aspirin-containing compounds should be discontinued, as mentioned previously.

### MOTOR NERVE INJURIES

The most commonly injured motor nerve is the facial, and this is exceedingly rare because the nerve is well protected by the parotid gland over the main trunk and the superficial fascia distally. The anatomy of this nerve and its common variations have been extensively reviewed,[51, 52, 63, 69] and the danger points during rhytidectomy have been emphasized: (1) over the mandibular body at the point the facial artery crosses the mandibular branch and the nerve becomes superficial; (2) over the malar eminence, where the frontal branch is superficial as it passes over the zygoma; and (3) at the midpoint of the patch of temporal skin between the outer canthus of the eye and the superior auricular angle. Extensive dissection in these regions should be avoided, especially in thin persons with atrophic skin and subcutaneous tissue, where the vulnerability of the nerve is obviously increased. The facial nerve will not be endangered if the plane of dissection is maintained at a superficial level. Dissecting as far anteriorly as the corner of the mouth or the nasolabial fold is not recommended, as the nerve branches are very superficial at this level and can be easily injured, resulting in partial or complete paralysis. Although nerve regeneration usually occurs at this level, in some instances it is accompanied by dissociated muscle fasciculations resulting in an annoying involuntary twitching.[3]

The various causes of facial nerve paralysis following rhytidectomy have been reviewed[48, 49] and include (1) transient paresis from local anesthetic solution, (2) stretching the nerve during blunt dissection, (3) pinching the nerve with forceps, (4) heat injury during electrodesiccation, (5) compression of the nerve by a plication suture, (6) partial or complete transection, (7) inflammation and infection, (8) coincidental Bell's palsy or other neurologic pathology and (9) distorted anatomy from subcutaneous fibrosis in secondary or tertiary face lifts.

Those nerve branches most frequently injured are the frontal, buccal and marginal mandibular. Fortunately, permanent paralysis is rare, and full function generally returns within weeks to months. Therefore, unless it is obvious that during the operation a branch has been transected, the treatment is expectant, with the justified hope that there will be little deficit. If it is recognized that a nerve has been cut during surgery, the best chance for full return of movement is microsurgical approximation of the cut ends. If there is permanent paralysis after one and one-half to two years with no evidence of return of function by electrical testing, lysis of the contralateral branch will re-create symmetry of the forehead or mouth.[49]

MacGregor and Greenberg[57] reported injury to the spinal accessory nerve following face lift, with the resultant loss of motion of the trapezius muscle and a "winged scapula." This is the only known report in the literature and probably resulted from too deep dissection along the posterior border of the sternocleidomastoid muscle, where the spinal accessory nerve exits. Dissection must remain supeficial to the sternocleidomastoid fascia, taking care not to expose muscle fibers.

### SKIN SLOUGH AND NECROSIS

The incidence of skin sloughs has been reported between 1.1 per cent[45] and 3.0 per cent.[57] This is one of the most feared complications of face lifting and results from a diminished blood supply to the flap. This vascular compromise can be caused by several factors: (1) most commonly, from delayed recognition of a hematoma; (2) too superficial dissection of the flap; (3) excessive trauma to the flap from retractors or "raking" the scissors; (4) excessive tension from too much pulling or tightening of the skin; (5) excessive pressure from tight dressings; (6) excessive undermining; (7) impaired circulation from previous scars, e.g., thyroidectomy; and (8) infection.

Skin necrosis and slough are first recognized by the typical pallor caused by arteriolar compromise or a bluish tinge due to venous congestion.[64] This is usually noted when the dressing is removed and occurs most over the mastoid area, where the skin flap is thinnest, the tension is greatest and the blood supply is farthest from the tip of the flap. Fortunately, these sloughs are rarely extensive, and the resulting scar is behind the ear, where it can be easily hidden by appropriate hair styling. All sloughs should be treated expectantly and conservatively and often heal with minimal scarring if the area involved is small. An eschar eventually develops where full thickness loss has occurred, and healing takes place by second intention. Patients understandably require much reassurance during the healing period, which may be several weeks or months. Superficial slough may resemble a

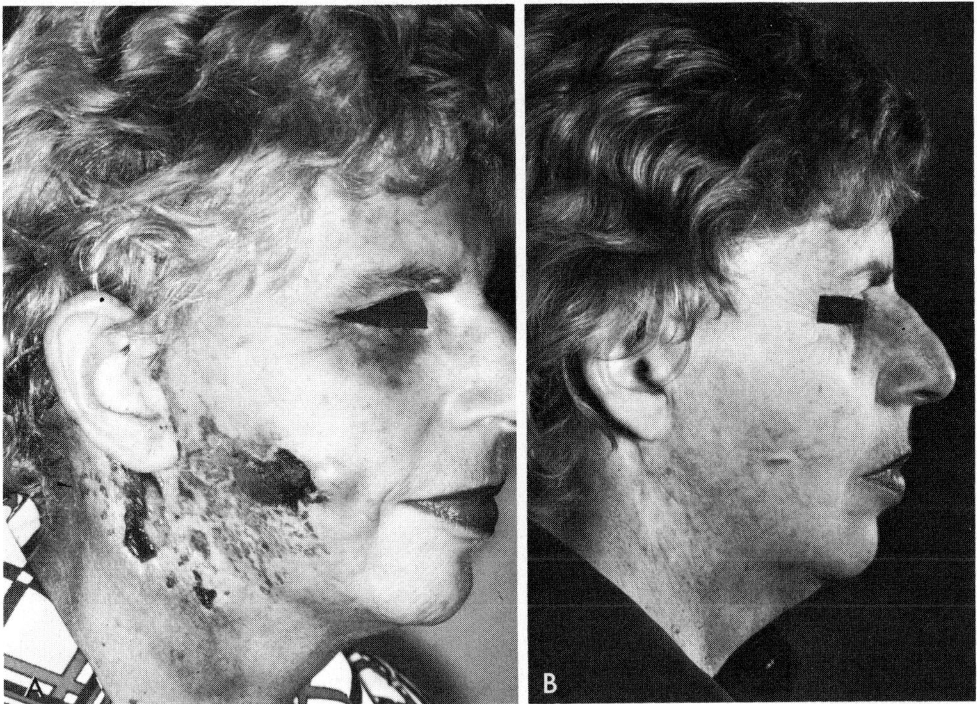


**Figure 25–14** *A,* Appearance of deep skin slough of the midcheek, postauricular area, and neck 2 weeks following rhytidectomy. Superficial "peeling" of the skin surrounds the areas of deeper slough. There is a small hematoma beneath and just anterior to the eschar on the cheek (note the small bulge). *B,* Six months postoperatively the scars are smaller than the original defects. Future scar revisions may be considered. (From Rees, T. D., and Aston, S. J.: Complications of rhytidectomy. Clin. Plast. Surg., *5*:109, 1978.)

second-degree burn and develop blistering and desquamation. Healing is generally satisfactory, but there may be residual pigmentation, coarseness or superficial scarring of the skin. Small doses of steroids injected into a hypertrophied scar may be of some help.

Major full thickness skin sloughs rarely occur and usually are secondary to a massive hematoma that has been neglected. In such cases, the resulting scar may be unsightly and require excision and repair or, rarely, skin grafting if the area is excessively large. The best treatment of skin slough is prevention, which requires gentle handling of tissue and meticulous hemostasis.

### *Causes of Failure and Secondary Rhytidectomy*

Causes of failure and unfavorable results of the face lift operation generally result from poor patient selection, improper surgical technique or changes in the patient's physiology. Physical factors in the face and neck can prevent a satisfactory result. These factors include a short, thick neck; an unfavorably low position of the hyoid bone in relation to the mandible; an overweight patient; badly sun-damaged skin; and unaesthetic angles and contours of the facial bones. Poor surgical technique with too much or too little undermining, improper rotation of the flaps and uneven tensions can cause facial imbalance and distortion or a quick postoperative relaxation. Any changes in the patient's general health that would promote premature degeneration of the skin could accelerate postoperative relaxation. These factors include weight fluctuations, hormonal imbalance, severe emotional upsets, excess alcoholic intake and certain systemic diseases.

It is not possible to predict with any reliable accuracy just when a secondary face lift operation will be required by an individual patient. Most patients should simply be told that the result is not permanent because the aging process continues; a second operation can be done when and if it becomes necessary or desirable for them, usually somewhere within 5 to 10 years. In general, younger patients obtain a more satisfactory and durable result than older patients with degenerative skin changes who have their first rhytidectomy in their 60's or 70's.

The first indications of relaxation usually occur at the cervicomental angle under the chin and along the jaw line. The timing of the second operation depends on the subjective feelings of the patient and the objective findings of the surgeon.[66] The secondary operation is almost invariably easier to perform than the first. Pre-excision is not recommended in secondary rhytidectomy, for despite extensive undermining of the skin, usually only a small amount of tissue can be resected in secondary operations.[64] The improvement from secondary rhytidectomy is more often the result of redistribution of the skin and whatever physical changes occur from undermining rather than from actual excision of excess skin. Repeated face lift operations at too frequent intervals can result in the skin losing its natural elastic properties, and the face assumes an unnatural appearance or "mask look."

## COMPLICATIONS OF OTOPLASTY

### *General Considerations*

Numerous operative methods exist for the correction of prominent ears that have produced acceptable results, and the technique chosen will be influenced by each surgeon's training and experience. It is often said that correction of prominent ears is easy, but actually, it is difficult to obtain a perfect result. The protruding or lop ear deformity is frequently associated with a psychologic disturbance for both the child and his parents, or even for the adult patient. Consequently, any improvement is gladly accepted by most patients, the majority of whom are pleased, although the surgeon may be unhappy with the final result. There are few reports[74, 78] in the literature discussing complications, which are surprisingly low. A recent 20-year retrospective review by Baker and Converse[74] of 292 patients (570 ears) who had undergone corrective otoplasties by a "tubing technique"[75] yielded the following most common complications:

| | | |
|---|---|---|
| Infection | 7 ears | (1.2%) |
| Chondritis | 4 ears | (0.7%) |
| Hematoma | 5 ears | (0.8%) |
| Hypertrophic scars | 4 ears | (0.7%) |
| Keloids | 1 Black | (11%) |
| | 12 Caucasian ears | (2.1%) |
| Telephone deformity | 9 patients | (3.0%) |
| Recurrence | 15 ears | (2.6%) |

### *Early Postoperative Complications*

#### HEMATOMA

Hematoma is the most immediate postoperative complication, although the incidence is less than 2 per cent. When a patient complains of persistent and excessive pain, particularly if unilateral and during the immediate 24 to 48 hours postoperatively, the dressing should be removed immediately and the ears inspected. A tense and bluish swelling in the retroauricular space confirms a hematoma, which requires vigorous treatment with evacuation of clot and coagulation of all bleeding points; this is best carried out in the operating room under sterile conditions with good anesthesia and lighting. Following wound closure, a pressure dressing is carefully reapplied and large doses of broad-spectrum antibiotics are continued.

#### INFECTION

Infection usually occurs early in the postoperative phase, on or about the fourth or fifth postoperative day, and is frequently a sequel to an undetected or inadequately treated hematoma. The initial symptom is usually excessive pain on the third or fourth postoperative day, and the signs include fever, erythema and swelling followed by purulent drainage. Sutures should be opened to provide adequate drainage, and necrotic debris should be irrigated from the wound after appropriate culture and sensitivity studies have been instituted. A localized cellulitis can sometimes be treated at home with broad-spectrum oral antibiotics and warm compresses. Patients with fulminant infections should be hospitalized and placed on intravenous antibiotics, and all buried nonabsorbable sutures should be removed. Small Silastic catheters through which a continuous slow drip of antibiotic solution can be administered can be placed in the wound.

Fortunately, infections following otoplasty are rare, perhaps because of the vigorous blood supply to this area. The following prophylactic measures are recommended, however: Careful shampoo and face wash with germicidal soap the evening before and morning of surgery; antibiotics begun prior to surgery; hair never shaved but carefully draped out of the field with a standard head drape, and a self-sticking (3M*) plastic drape with a central opening large enough for the ear is used to maintain sterility.

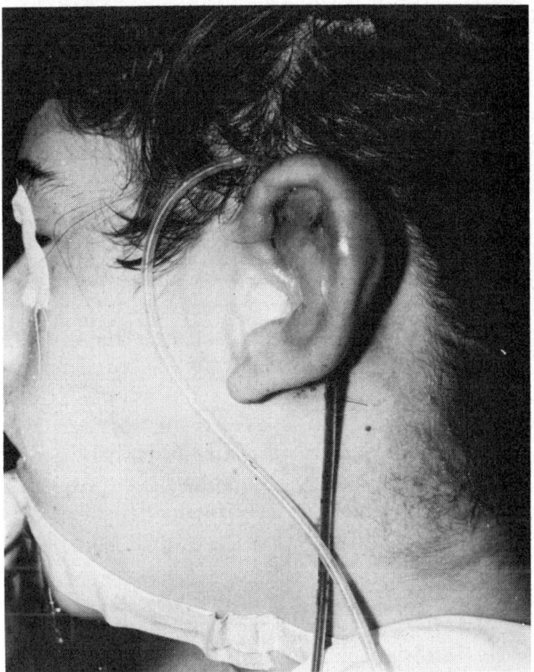

**Figure 25–16** Continuous catheter irrigation with broad spectrum antibiotics will minimize cartilage necrosis and help control infection in acute chondritis.

### CHONDRITIS

Chondritis, the sequela of infection, is the most dreaded complication following otoplasty. Although this is a common occurrence in the burned ear, only rarely does a frank chondritis with necrosis of the cartilage follow otoplasty. The characteristic clinical picture of suppurative chondritis has been described by Dowling, Foley and Moncrief:[76] Pain of increasing severity and often refractory to narcotics is the first and most prominent symptom; the ear is red, swollen, hot and exquisitely tender; marked edema causes an increase in the auriculocephalic angle with protrusion of the ear and loss of correction.

Usually, systemic antibiotics do not significantly alter the course when frank suppurative chondritis is present. Continuous antibiotic irrigation through small catheters can be helpful, but usually wide exposure and removal of all involved cartilage is necessary. Unfortunately, it is difficult to differentiate healthy from infected cartilage on the operating table, since there is no sharp demarcation between necrotic and viable cartilage. Persistent tenderness and induration are signs of recurrent chondritis, and repeated debridement is necessary. Disappearance of pain is the best indication of effective therapy.[83] When the entire ear is infected, almost total chondrectomy may be necessary. The end result of chondritis with cartilage loss may be a severe deformity that may seem to mimic a microtic ear. Recon-

*Minnesota Mining and Manufacturing

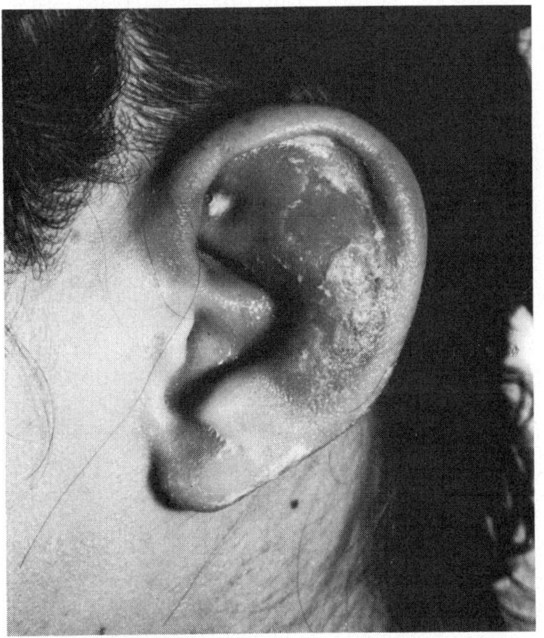

**Figure 25–15** Acute swelling, tenderness, and erythema associated with chondritis.

struction should not be considered for at least a year.

#### PAIN

Pain has already been mentioned as one of the initial signs of hematoma, infection and chondritis. If severe pain occurs postoperatively, particularly if unilateral and requiring narcotics for relief, the surgeon should be suspicious of a complication and remove the dressing to inspect the ear. A tight or shifted dressing may be causing excessive pressure on the ear, which could lead to avascular necrosis. Skin necrosis has not been reported but could certainly occur with excessive pressure, folding or twisting of the repaired ear. A simple dressing adjustment could prevent a major complication.

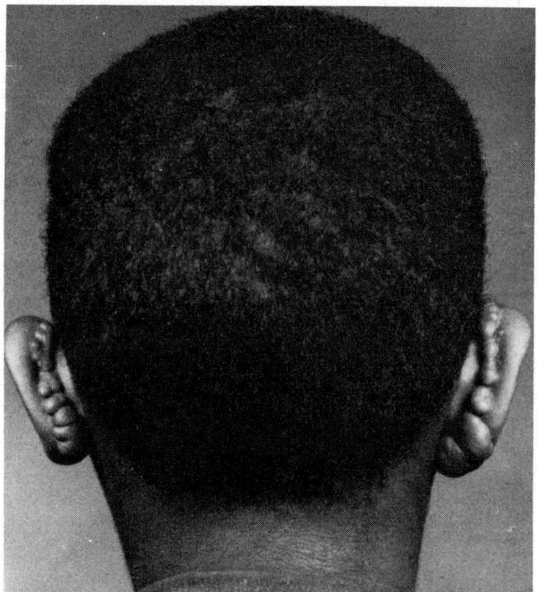

**Figure 25–17** Example of postauricular keloid formation in Negro patient following otoplasty. Successfully treated by steroid injections.

### *Late Postoperative Complications*

#### HYPESTHESIA

Patients not infrequently will complain of sensory deficit for varying periods of time, and this is usually secondary to trauma to the greater auricular nerve. The treatment is reassurance, for in several months to a year sensation usually returns. Paresthesias, neuromas and permanent sensory deficits are rare and have not been reported. Extreme care must be taken to avoid injury to the greater auricular nerve on the mastoid fascia when dissecting for exposure to obtain conchal reduction and setback.

#### HYPERTROPHIC SCARS AND KELOIDS

Fortunately, most otoplasty techniques utilize incisions in the postauricular skin, and hypertrophic scars are infrequent (0.7 per cent, Baker and Converse)[74] and unobtrusive in this area. They are more common in patients with deeply pigmented skin, and in those cases in which a large postauricular skin excision has been performed and closed under tension. It is therefore best to limit the skin excision to only the redundant skin after set-back, thus avoiding tension on the closure and minimizing the chances of scar formation. If a slight redundancy of skin remains after repair, it usually shrinks over several weeks to conform to the underlying cartilage. The normal scar maturation period must be kept in mind before considering revision, and it may take more than a year for some scars to mature sufficiently.

Keloids are always a risk, particularly in the darkly pigmented patient. The incidence reported by Baker and Converse[74] was 11 per cent in Negro and 2.1 per cent in Caucasian patients. In the early stages of hypertrophic scar and keloid formation, intralesional injections of triamcinolone acetonide (Kenalog 40 mg. per cc.) are repeated monthly until regression occurs and then tapered before terminating treatment.[54] Occasionally with unresponsive keloids, surgical excision must be combined with intralesional steroids and radiation, although the use of the latter in this area is fraught with the danger of chondritis and should be avoided.[3]

#### NARROWING OF EXTERNAL AUDITORY CANAL

Narrowing of the external auditory meatus can occur when a large concha is set back by employing sutures (Furnas technique)[77] that are incorrectly placed or under excessive tension. Care must be taken not to shift the conchal cartilage anteriorly but rather to put it posteriorly and inward. Excision of the excess concha will avoid this complication. Although the concha usually tends to spring out after several weeks, relieving the narrowing of the canal, it might be necessary to cut the concha-mastoid sutures and replace the ear in a more favorable position should a permanent partial stenosis be observed.[83]

#### SUTURE EXTRUSION AND BOWSTRINGING

Occasionally, the buried mattress sutures used in the Mustardé technique[80, 81] may become visible or outlined beneath the postauricular skin. This complication usually occurs when the ear cartilage is thick and the sutures are under a great amount of tension or if excess postauricular skin has been removed. No treatment is necessary unless sutures are extruded. This complication can occur months to years following otoplasty and usually results from excessive tension or sutures placed too superficially into the cartilage that tear out. The only treatment is to remove the extruded suture, which usually has no effect on the position of the ear in the late postoperative period. In general, when the antihelical deformity is severe and the cartilage is thick, a technique that breaks the spring of the cartilage by cutting or scratching will minimize the tension on sutures and avoid the problems of extrusion and bowstringing.

### *Unfavorable Results*

Unfavorable results may occur anytime following surgery and include inadequate correction, recurrence, contour distortions or asymmetric correction, which may require secondary operation. Caution is advised in undertaking correction of minor deformities, some of which can be very difficult to correct.

#### RECURRENCE OF DEFORMITY

Although there are few statistical analyses of various techniques of otoplasty, recurrence of the deformity is probably the most common unfavorable result and usually occurs unilaterally. Despite the fact that some experienced surgeons may obtain consistently good results with one technique, there are certain deformities that would seem to have a higher incidence of recurrence with the suture methods of Mustardé[80, 81] and Furnas.[77] These deformities include marked unfurling of the antihelix and excess concha with thick cartilage. These ears require a breaking of the cartilaginous spring by one of the cutting or scratching methods[84] as well as by excision of the excess concha. Cartilaginous incisions must be through the cartilage up to but not including the perichondrium over the anterolateral aspect of the auricular cartilage. If the anterior surface of the cartilage is scored by the Stenstrom technique, the use of some nonabsorbable sutures on the posterior surface helps to maintain the desired shape and position. If the Mustardé technique is used, an adequate number of sutures must be placed through full thickness cartilage with a "healthy bite" to avoid pulling through of the sutures. Nonabsorbable sutures, such as clear nylon or white dacron, are recommended. Finally, lack of patient cooperation with discontinuation of the dressing or accidental trauma might cause a disruption of sutures. Postoperatively, a headband or stockinette should be worn at night for three to four weeks. Should a recurrence warrant secondary correction, several months should elapse to allow for complete healing and disappearance of induration before revision.

#### TELEPHONE DEFORMITY

The telephone deformity is so named because the middle third of the ear is set against the side of the head while the root of the helix and lobule remain protruding. Strict attention must be given to the position of the upper and lower thirds of the pinna to avoid this deformity, especially in the large ear with a wide scapha. This deformity will result from insufficient removal of cartilage and skin in the superior and inferior thirds or from excessive removal of conchal cartilage in the central third. Correction is particularly unpleasant, since it requires a "plastering" of the ear to the side of the patient's head. When the root of the helix remains protruding, several sutures may be placed between the cartilage of the helix and the temporal fascia to close the angle

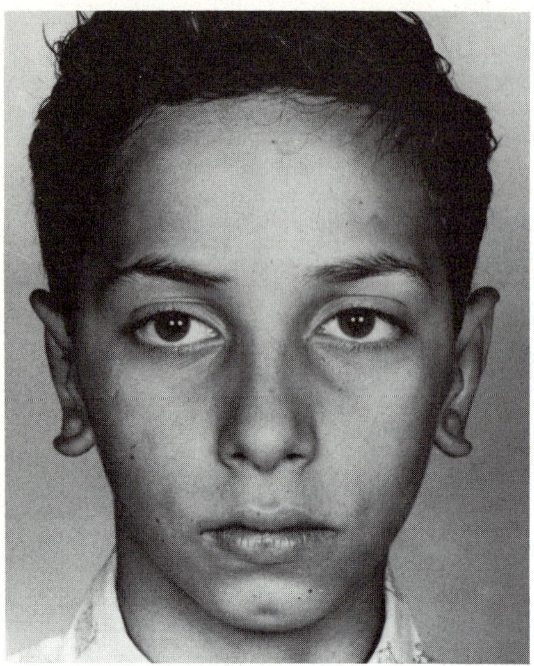

**Figure 25–18** Typical telephone deformity following otoplasty.

between the helix and scalp.[79] For the protruding lobule, a variety of skin excisions and Z-plasties have been recommended.[83, 85]

### EXCESSIVE SET-BACK

Fortunately patients rarely complain if the ears are "plastered" against the head, but it can be disturbing to the surgeon. According to Spira and his coworkers,[82] the average distance between the helical rim and the mastoid area in the "normal" ear is slightly less than 2 cm., and the helix is lateral to the antihelix. Avoiding excessive removal of conchal cartilage or obliteration of the postauricular sulcus by excessive resection of skin will minimize this deformity.

## COMPLICATIONS OF AUGMENTATION MENTOPLASTY

### *General Considerations*

The chin, nose and forehead are the three important balancing masses that form the aesthetic profile of the face. An understanding of the normal physical balance of these facial structures and a careful evaluation of the dental occlusion is necessary prior to undertaking chin augmentation. A severe malocclusion or marked microgenia might best be treated by one of the various osteotomies. The majority of patients with small or recessive chins can be corrected or improved by augmentation mentoplasty. Approximately 15 per cent of patients seeking rhinoplasty will benefit from chin augmentation, but approximately 75 per cent of these patients will be unaware of this "weakness" of the chin.[89, 90] In such instances, it behooves the surgeon to point out that augmentation mentoplasty may be as important to the final aesthetic result as the nasal plastic operation. In general, it is usually unwise for the surgeon to suggest an operation to correct a defect of which the patient is unaware. Chin augmentation is an exception to this rule.

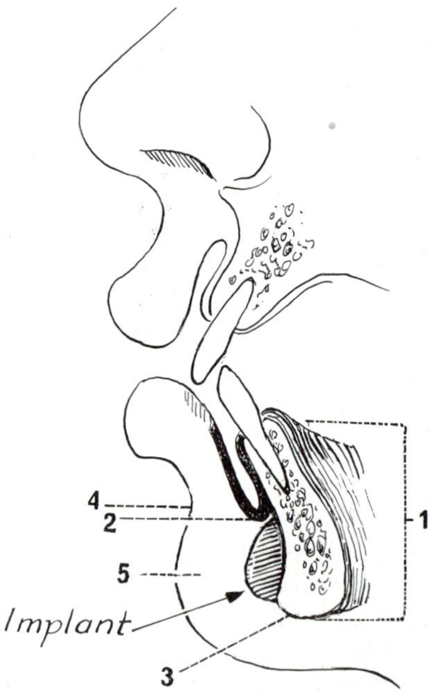


**Figure 25–19** The normal anatomy of the mandible and the adjacent soft tissues plays an important role in determining the success or failure of chin implants. Anatomical factors include (1) vertical height of the mandible at the symphysis; (2) depth of the gingivolabial sulcus; (3) configuration of the lower mandibular rim at the symphysis; (4) development of the labiomental groove; and (5) the amount of soft tissue over the chin. (From Rees, T. D., Horowitz, S. L., and Coburn, R. J.: Mentoplasty, prognathism, and cheiloplasty. *In* Rees, T. D., and Wood-Smith, D. [eds.]: Cosmetic Facial Surgery. Philadelphia, W. B. Saunders Company, 1973.)

Profile photographs can graphically demonstrate the point, and oriented lateral x-rays (cephalograms) provide further substantiation.

Whether it is advisable to perform rhinoplasty first, followed by mentoplasty, or the reverse depends upon the type and severity of the deformities of the nose and chin. Usually both procedures are done at the same operative session. If the chin is markedly retruded, however, it is advisable to augment this structure first, since the change in profile may be helpful in planning the nasal reduction. Not infrequently, patients are seen who have had simultaneous rhinoplasties and chin augmentation in which too much was removed from the nose and too much added to the chin. This overcorrection of both structures can result in a facial disharmony that is as unbecoming as the original condition.

### THE CHOICE OF IMPLANT

Prior to silicone implant materials, chin augmentation was accomplished usually with homologous or autogenous cartilage or bone grafts. Autogenous grafts required a second surgical wound to the rib cage or ileum, however, which was sometimes more troublesome to the patient than the operation on the chin. Furthermore, it was found that autogenous bone grafts to the chin had a marked tendency to resorb because of the strong forces placed on the grafts by constant mobility and the pressure of soft tissues and facial musculature. Cartilage grafts particularly, whether autogenous or homologous, tended to absorb or warp.[1] A second or third operation on the chin was not uncommon. Most foreign implants were criticized because of their unnatural consistency and tendency to extrude. With the development of the silicone rubber compounds, augmentation mentoplasty became simplified. During the past decade the use of such implants has become almost universally accepted. Proponents of bone and cartilage grafts have abandoned these more complicated techniques for the use of alloplasts in simple chin augmentation.

Silicone rubber (Silastic) is available in several degrees of firmness, as a fine-celled sponge or as a liquid. Prefabricated, commercially available implants are preferred. These implants need not impose a specific size upon the surgeon, since they can be trimmed at the operative table with scissors or scalpel to whatever dimension and shape desired. The preformed implants reduce operating time and do not impose the nuisance of sculpting an implant from raw blocks. Soft, gel-filled implants are also available but cannot be altered, and clinical experience with this type is limited.

Close-celled silicone sponge provides excellent results but has the disadvantage that the final result cannot be assessed for months because of pressure on the implant by the natural fibrous capsule with subsequent contraction of the sponge. If used, the sponge should be slightly oversized to allow for shrinkage following contraction of the scar capsule and compression of the sponge.

### INSERTION ROUTE

Chin implants can be inserted using the intraoral approach via the inferior gingivolabial sulcus or the external approach through an incision in the natural horizontal submental skin crease. The intraoral approach is simple, leaves no external scar and has a surprisingly low incidence of complications. Since Converse[86] demonstrated the safety and feasibility of introducing autogenous bone grafts through intraoral incision, this approach has been widely used for autogenous as well as synthetic implants. Certain factors militate against optimal results from the intraoral approach, however. A short mandibular body (micrognathia) associated with a shallow labial sulcus may cause the implant to be placed high if inserted intraorally. This results in loss of the natural lip-chin crease (labiomental fold). In addition, the implant is an annoying mass in the labial sulcus that the patient is able to feel with his tongue.

A short mandible and a shallow sulcus usually require the implant to be placed through the external submental incision. This approach permits the surgeon to elevate the periosteum only as high as required for the implant, thereby preserving the integrity of the sulcus and placing the implant at a lower level or even along the inferior mandibular margin, if so desired. The resulting scar is unnoticeable. Large implants

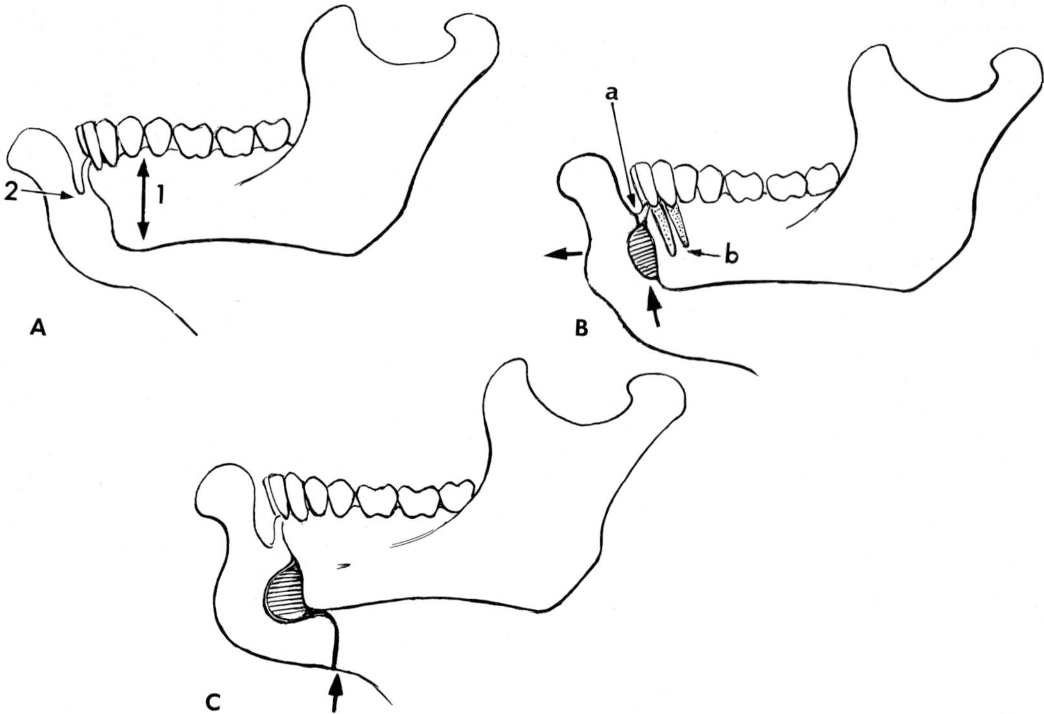


**Figure 25–20** Augmentation mentoplasty is difficult in the presence of certain anatomical variations of the lower jaw, such as decreased vertical height at the symphysis (1 in *A*) and shallowness of the gingivolabial sulcus (2 in *A*). An implant placed too high (as shown in *B*) would elevate the sulcus (*a*), creating an uncomfortable bulge and an unnatural chin shape (arrows). Horizontal osteotomy is also difficult in such patients because the roots of the teeth may extend into the customary plane of section (*b*). The proper placement of an implant in such a circumstance is shown in C. The pocket should not be dissected as high as the gingivolabial sulcus. The implant must be placed on the exact tip of the chin and not permitted to slip down. A two-layer soft tissue closure helps to maintain this position. (From Rees, T. D., Horowitz, S. L., and Coburn, R. J.: Mentoplasty, prognathism, and cheiloplasty. *In* Rees, T. D., and Wood-Smith, D. [eds.]: Cosmetic Facial Surgery. Philadelphia, W. B. Saunders Company, 1973.)

are best inserted from an incision in the submental crease so as to prevent excessive tension on the intraoral suture line that might lead to wound breakdown and extrusion. Accurate positioning of large implants is also facilitated by the external approach.

Implants may be placed directly on cortical bone or overlying the periosteum, and this makes little difference in the final result.[3] They should not be placed in a subcutaneous or intramuscular pocket where they can be readily palpated, however. The periosteum can be elevated and an implant placed beneath it on the bone, but only rarely is it possible to close the periosteum over the implant. The submental wound should be closed in two layers. The deep closure brings the muscles together and is helpful in fixing the implant and protects the skin incision from dehiscence. The danger of extrusion is thus minimized.

## INFECTION

The incidence of infection is very low and is rarely a problem with the intraoral or the submental approach and usually results from a hematoma. Preoperative attention to dental hygiene is an important preventative measure; teeth should be cleaned and caries repaired to minimize oral flora; antibiotic coverage is started in full therapeutic doses prior to surgery and continued for 10 days postoperatively. Should an infection occur, the implant (foreign body) should be removed and the tissues allowed to heal and soften for several months before attempting reimplantation. If infection has occurred via the intraoral approach, consideration should be given to the submental approach for the secondary procedure. When the intraoral approach is used, only a liquid diet is permitted for three days postoperatively until the wound is sealed. A Water Pik is helpful in maintaining oral hygiene in the postoperative period.

### HEMATOMA

Hematoma is an infrequent complication, but the occurrence of a large hematoma requires opening the wound and controlling the bleeding. Intraoperative hemostasis should be obtained prior to inserting the implant. This can usually be accomplished by packing the wound with an adrenalin-soaked sponge (well wrung out, 1:1000 concentration) and pressure. Cautery is used for larger bleeders. The pocket should be made only large enough to accommodate the implant, and a postoperative compression dressing is recommended, utilizing Elastoplast strips placed into the labiomental fold and beneath the chin, which also aids immobilization.

### ASYMMETRY — MALPOSITION

Sometimes the formation of a small hematoma will cause asymmetry of the chin for several months, but this usually subsides in time. Actual displacement or malposition, of course, must be corrected by adjusting the size and shape of the pocket. The implant must be placed exactly in the midline, and this can be confirmed by marking the midline of the chin with ink and notching the midline of the upper border of the implant and aligning them.

### VISUAL PROJECTIONS

The cause of this is usually inadequately formed pocket, improperly carved implant or too large, too long or too thick an implant. One end of the implant may show through the skin if the pocket in this area is too superficial. Patients not infrequently may also have some slight asymmetry of the mandible, and the surgeon must appreciate this preoperatively and carve the implant to contour the deformity.

### OVERCORRECTION — EXCESS CHIN PROMINENCE

One must allow at least six months for the postoperative edema or a small hematoma to resolve. This may be the cause of a temporary overcorrection. If the implant is too large, it must be removed and reduced. Most Silastic sponge implants can change in size. Initially, sponges fill with serum or fluid, causing swelling of the chin. As the fibrous capsule forms around the implant, the sponge contracts slowly, so that the chin size diminishes. The degree of change is usually not significant and should not contraindicate the use of the fine-celled sponge. Often, when an implant is removed, the residual pocket and scar tissue may preserve enough augmentation to please the patient. As has been mentioned, when simultaneous chin augmentation and rhinoplasty are performed, it is often advisable to do the mentoplasty first, since the change in profile will help in planning the nasal reduction and minimize the danger of overcorrection of both structures.

### EXTRUSION

Extrusion can occur with any implant, although perhaps not for many months or years after surgery. The best prophylaxis against this complication is adequately sized pockets and careful anatomic placement of the implant. Nevertheless, even the most carefully placed implant can shift in position and present itself as a pressure point, either within the mouth or externally at the chin. If the implant becomes extruded, it can be replaced. Implants must be placed into pockets of exact size over the anterior surface of the mandible. The pocket should be made so that the implant rides along the border of the mandible but does not extend higher than the natural labiomental sulcus. Meticulous layered closure is important in preventing extrusion.

According to Friedland, Coccaro and Converse,[87] exposure of an implant is likely to occur in cases of severe or even moderately severe retrusion of the mental symphysis because of the following reasons: (1) the implant necessary to correct the deformity is too large; (2) there is not sufficient laxity of the soft tissues to maintain coverage over such a large implant; or (3) in the presence of severe mandibular retrusion, hyperfunction of the chin muscles is necessary to obtain lip seal and may cause displacement or increase the soft tissue pressure over the implant. Therefore, in severely micrognathic patients, serious consideration must be given to osteotomies of the mandible to correct the deformity.

### NERVE INJURY

Temporary hypoesthesia or anesthesia of the chin and lower lip can occur if the mental nerves are excessively stretched, accidentally cauterized or otherwise traumatized. Numbness is usually transient but may persist for several weeks or even months. If the nerve is cut or irreversibly injured at the time of surgery, permanent anesthesia results. Protection of the nerve and its branches during surgery is of prime importance. If the mental nerve is cut during surgery, it should be repaired prior to closure.

### BONE ABSORPTION

Erosion of bone by onlay implants was reported by Robinson and Shuken.[91, 92] Recently Friedland, Coccaro and Converse[87] performed a cephalometric analysis on 85 randomly selected patients who had chin augmentation with silicone rubber prostheses. Some bone absorption was noted in over 50 per cent of the cases studied, and most of the patients studied showed 13 to 27 per cent absorption of the total thickness of the mandibular symphysis. Mandibular flattening beneath the implant was noted as early as two months postoperatively. The bone responds to the pressure of the implant by osteolytic activity. The position of the implant is the most important factor in bone absorption. The absorption was less when the implant was placed over the lower part of the mandible (pogonion or menton), where the bone is cortical and hard, as opposed to higher on the mandible (suprapogonion), where the bone is alveolar and cancellous. Placement of an implant on alveolar bone, overlying the roots of teeth, could cause root absorption and premature loss of teeth.[91, 92] If an implant should penetrate a softer tooth-bearing portion of the mandible, the implant should be removed to prevent damage to the apices of the teeth.

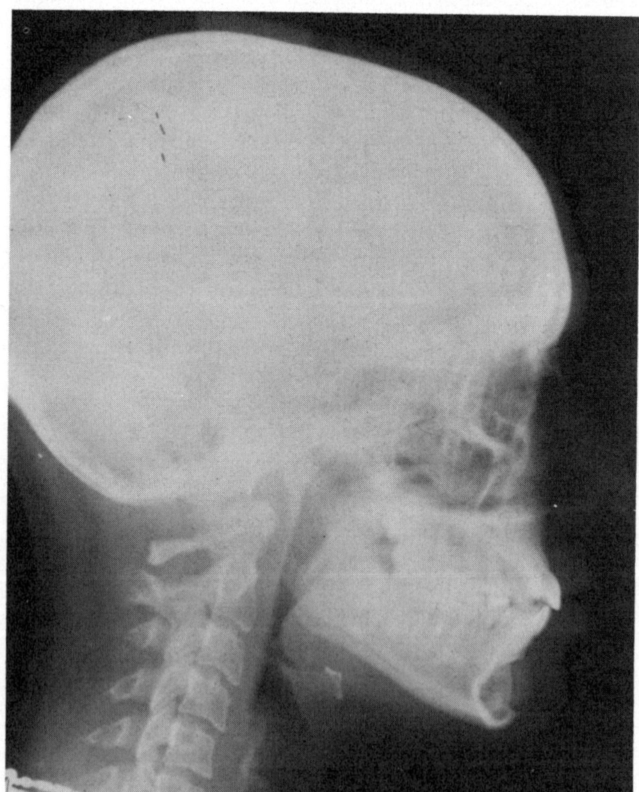

**Figure 25–21** Mandibular absorption six months following augmentation mentoplasty with silastic prosthesis.

When an implant is placed over the hard bone of the mental symphysis, absorption is minimal, the implant settles into the bone and becomes encapsulated and no further absorption occurs. Such erosion does not appear to represent a significant contraindication for implants, since apparently it is self-limiting and not reason for removal of the implant. As yet, it is uncertain whether the new, softer, gel-filled implants will cause less absorption or the placement of an implant supraperiosteally influences absorption. Despite this apparently adverse radiologic finding under silicone chin implants, the relative absence of morbidity and the high level of patient satisfaction with this operation (almost 100 per cent) dictates its continued use and acceptance.[88]

## Bibliography


### General References

1. Converse, J. M.: Reconstructive Plastic Surgery. Philadelphia, W. B. Saunders Company, 1977.
2. Goldwyn, R. M.: The Unfavorable Result in Plastic Surgery: Avoidance and Treatment. Boston, Little, Brown and Company, 1972.
3. Rees, T. D., and Wood-Smith, D.: Cosmetic Facial Surgery. Philadelphia, W. B. Saunders Company, 1973.

### Complications of Rhinoplasty

4. Baker, D. C., and Strauss, R. B.: The physiologic treatment of nasal obstruction. Clin. Plast. Surg., *4*:121, 1977.
5. Beekhuis, G. J.: Nasal obstruction after rhinoplasty; etiology and techniques for correction. Laryngoscope, *86*:540, 1976.
6. Champion, R.: Anosmia associated with corrective rhinoplasty. Br. J. Plast. Surg., *19*:182, 1966.
7. Converse, J. M.: The deviated nose. *In* Millard, D. R. (ed.): Symposium on Corrective Rhinoplasty. St. Louis, The C. V. Mosby Company, 1976.
8. Dingman, R. O., and Natvig, P.: The deviated nose. Clin. Plast. Surg., *4*:145, 1977.
9. Flowers, R. S., and Anderson, R.: Injury to the lacrimal apparatus during rhinoplasty. Plast. Reconstr. Surg., *42*:577, 1968.
10. Goldman, I. B.: Rhinoplasty: Its surgical complications and how to avoid them. J. Int. Coll. Surg., *13*:285, 1950.
11. Goldwyn, R. M., and Shore, S.: The effects of submucous resection and rhinoplasty on the sense of smell. Plast. Reconstr. Surg., *41*:427, 1968.
12. Klabunde, E. H., and Falces, E.: Incidence of complications in cosmetic rhinoplasties. Plast. Reconstr. Surg., *34*:192, 1964.
13. Lewis, M. L.: Prevention and correction of cicatricial intranasal adesions in rhinoplastic surgery. Arch. Otolaryngol., *60*:215, 1954.
14. Millard, D. R.: The triad of columella deformities. Plast. Reconstr. Surg., *31*:370, 1963.
15. Millard, D. R.: Secondary corrective rhinoplasty. Plast. Reconstr. Surg., *44*:545, 1969.
16. Millard, D. R.: Secondary rhinoplasty surgery. *In* Millard, D. R. (ed.): Symposium on Corrective Rhinoplasty. St. Louis, The C. V. Mosby Company, 1976.
17. O'Connor, G. B., and McGregor, M. W.: Secondary rhinoplasties; their cause and prevention. Plast. Reconstr. Surg., *15*:404, 1955.
18. Rees, T. D., Krupp, S., and Wood-Smith, D.: Secondary rhinoplasty. Plast. Reconstr. Surg., *46*:322, 1970.
19. Rees, T. D.: An aid in the treatment of supratip swelling after rhinoplasty. Laryngoscope, *81*:308, 1971.
20. Rogers, B. O.: Rhinoplasty. *In* Goldwyn, R. M. (ed.): The Unfavorable Result in Plastic Surgery. Boston, Little, Brown and Company, 1972.

### Complications of Blepharoplasty

21. Castanares, S.: Eyelid plasty. *In* Goldwyn, R. M. (ed.): The Unfavorable Result in Plastic Surgery: Avoidance and Treatment. Boston, Little, Brown and Company, 1972.
22. Converse, J. M.: Clinical note: Treatment of epithelized suture tracts of the eyelid by marsupialization. Plast. Reconstr. Surg., *38*:576, 1966.
23. DeMere, M., Wood, T., and Austin, W.: Eye complications with blepharoplasty or other eyelid surgery. Plast. Reconstr. Surg., *53*:634, 1974.
24. Duke-Elder, S.: Systems of Ophthalmology. St. Louis, The C. V. Mosby Company, 1972.
25. Edgerton, M. T.: Causes and prevention of lower lid ectropion following blepharoplasty. Plast. Reconstr. Surg., *49*:367, 1972.
26. Fry, J. H.: Reversible visual loss after proptosis from retrobulbar hemorrhage. Plast. Reconstr. Surg., *44*:480, 1969.
27. Graham, W. P., Messner, K. H., and Miller, S. H.: Keratoconjunctivitis sicca symptoms appearing after blepharoplasty. Plast. Reconstr. Surg., *57*:57, 1976.
28. Green, M. F., and Kadri, S. W. M.: Acute closed-angle glaucoma, a complication of blepharoplasty: Report of a case. Br. J. Plast. Surg., *27*:25, 1974.
29. Hartley, J. H., Lester, J. C., and Schatten, W. E.: Acute retrobulbar hemorrhage during elective blepharoplasty. Plast. Reconstr. Surg., *52*:8, 1973.
30. Hartman, E., Morax, P. V., and Vergez, A.: Complications visuelles graves de la chirurgie des poches palpebrales. Ann. Ocul. (Paris), *195*:142, 1962.
31. Hollows, F. C., and Graham, A. P.: Intraocular pressure, glaucoma and glaucoma suspects in a defined population. Br. J. Ophthalmol., *50*:570, 1966.
32. Huang, T. T., Horowitz, B., and Lewis, S. T.:

Retrobulbar hemorrhage. Plast. Reconstr. Surg., *59*:39, 1977.

33. Hueston, J. T., and Heinze, J. B.: Successful early relief of blindness occurring after blepharoplasty. Plast. Reconstr. Surg., *53*:588, 1972.
34. Kraushar, M. F., Seelenfreund, M. H., and Frelich, D. B.: Closure of the central artery following retrobulbar injection. Trans. Am. Acad. Ophthalmol. Otolaryngol., *78*:65, 1974.
35. Moser, M. H., DiPirro, E., and McCoy, F. J.: Sudden blindness following blepharoplasty. Plast. Reconstr. Surg., *51*:364, 1973.
36. Rees, T. D.: Technical aids in blepharoplasty. Plast. Reconstr. Surg., *41*:497, 1968.
37. Rees, T. D., and Guy, C. L.: Patient selection and techniques in blepharoplasty. Surg. Clin. North Am., *51*:353, 1971.
38. Rees, T. D.: Complications following blepharoplasty. *In* Symposium on Plastic Surgery in the Orbital Region, St. Louis, The C. V. Mosby Company, 1976.
39. Rees, T. D.: Correction of ectropion resulting from blepharoplasty. Plast. Reconstr. Surg., *50*:1, 1972.
40. Rees, T. D.: The "dry eye" complication after blepharoplasty. Plast. Reconstr. Surg., *56*:375, 1975.
41. Sheen, J. H.: Supratarsal fixation in upper blepharoplasty. Plast Reconstr. Surg., *54*:425, 1974.
42. Swartz, R. M., Schultz, R. C., and Seaton, J. R.: "Dry eye" following blepharoplasty. Plast. Reconstr. Surg., *54*:644, 1975.
43. Tenzel, R. R.: Cosmetic Blepharoplasty. *In* Soll, D. B. (ed.): Management of Complications in Ophthalmic Plastic Surgery. Birmingham, Alabama, Aescalapium Publishing Co., 1976.

### Complications of Rhytidectomy

44. Baker, D. C., Aston, S. J., Guy, C. L., et al.: The male rhytidectomy. Plast. Reconstr. Surg., *60*:514, 1977.
45. Baker, T. J., Gordon, H. L., and Mesienko, P.: Rhytidectomy. Plast. Reconstr. Surg., *59*:24, 1977.
46. Berner, R. E., Morian, W. D., and Noe, J. M.: Postoperative hypertension as an etiologic factor in hematoma after rhytidectomy. Plast. Reconstr. Surg., *57*:314, 1976.
47. Black, M. J. M.: Personal communication, 1976.
48. Castanares, S.: Facial nerve paralysis coincident with, or subsequent to, rhytidectomy. Plast. Reconstr. Surg., *54*:637, 1974.
49. Conley, J.: Face Lift Operation. Springfield, Ill., Charles C Thomas, 1968.
50. Conway, H.: Factors underlying prolonged pain following rhytidectomy. Transactions 4th Int. Congr. Plast. Surg., Amsterdam, Excerpta Medica Foundation, 1969.
51. DeCastro-Correia, P., and Zani, R.: Surgical anatomy of the facial nerve, as related to ancillary operations in rhytidoplasty. Plast. Reconstr. Surg., *52*:549, 1973.
52. Dingman, R. O., and Grabb, W. C.: Surgical anatomy of the mandibular ramus of the facial nerve based on the dissection of 100 facial halves. Plast. Reconstr. Surg., *29*:266, 1962.
53. Goin, M. K., Burgoyne, R. W., and Goin, J. M.: Face lift operation; the patient's secret motivations and reactions to "informed consent." Plast. Reconstr. Surg., *58*:273, 1976.
54. Griffith, H.: The treatment of keloids with triamcinolone acetonide. Plast. Reconstr. Surg., *38*:202, 1966.
55. Guerrero-Santos, J., Espaillat, L., and Morales, F.: Muscular lift in cervical rhytidoplasty. Plast. Reconstr. Surg., *54*:127, 1974.
56. Leist, F., Masson, J., and Erich, J. B.: A review of 324 rhytidectomies, emphasizing complications and patient dissatisfaction. Plast. Reconstr. Surg., *59*:525, 1977.
57. MacGregor, M. W., and Greenberg, R. L.: Rhytidectomy. *In* Goldwyn, R. M. (ed.): The Unfavorable Result in Plastic Surgery. Boston, Little, Brown and Company, 1972.
58. McDowell, A. J.: Effective practical steps to avoid complications in face lifting. Plast. Reconstr. Surg., *50*:563, 1972.
59. Morgan, B. L.: The aftercare of rhytidectomies with the no dressing technique. Plast. Reconstr. Surg., *51*:576, 1973.
60. Peterson, R. A.: Face lift — a personal concept. Presented at the meeting of the American Society for Aesthetic Plastic Surgery, Los Angeles, California, March, 1977.
61. Pitanguy, I., Ramos, H., and Garcia, L.: Filosofia, tecnica e complicões das ritidestomias através de observaçao e analise de 2600 casos pessoais consecutivos. Rev. Bras. de Cirurgia, *62*:277, 1972.
62. Pitanguy, I., Pinto, A. R., Garcia, L. C., et al.: Ritodoplastia em homens. Rev. Bras. de Cirurgia, *63*:209, 1973.
63. Pitanguy, I., and Ramos, A. S.: The frontal branch of the facial nerve; the importance of its variations in face lifting. Plast. Reconstr. Surg., *38*:352, 1966.
64. Rees, T. D.: Rhytidectomy: some observations on variations in technique. *In* Masters, F. W., and Lewis, J. R. (eds.): Symposium on Aesthetic Surgery of the Face, Eyelid, and Breast. St. Louis, The C. V. Mosby Company, 1972, p. 37.
65. Rees, T. D., and Aston, S. J.: Complications of rhytidectomy. Clin. Plast. Surg., *5*:109, 1978.
66. Rees, T. D., Lee, Y. C., and Coburn, R. J.: Expanding hematoma after rhytidectomy. Plast. Reconstr. Surg., *51*:149, 1973.
67. Rees, T. D.: Face Lift. *In* Rees, T. D., and Wood-Smith, D. (eds.): Cosmetic Facial Surgery. Philadelphia, W. B. Saunders Company, 1973.
68. Serson-Neto, D.: Rhytidoplasties: study of 170 consecutive cases. J. Internat. Coll. Surg., *42*:208, 1964.
69. Smith, J. W.: The aesthetic anatomy of the facial nerve. *In* Masters, F. W., and Lewis, J. R. (eds.): Symposium on Aesthetic Surgery of the Face, Eyelid, and Breast. St. Louis, The C. V. Mosby Company, 1972, p. 37.
70. Stark, R. B.: Follow-up clinic on deliberate hypo-

tension for blepharoplasty and rhytidectomy. Plast. Reconstr. Surg., *49*:453, 1972.

71. Stark, R. B.: A rhytidectomy series. Plast. Reconstr. Surg., *59*:373, 1977.
72. Straith, R. E., Raju, D., and Hipps, C.: The study of hematomas in 500 consecutive face lifts. Plast. Reconstr. Surg., *59*:694, 1977.
73. Webster, G. V.: The ischemic face lift. Plast. Reconstr. Surg., *50*:560, 1972.

### Complications of Otoplasty

74. Baker, D. C., and Converse, J. M.: Otoplasty: a 20 year retrospective. Aesthetic Plastic Surgery *2*:36, 1979.
75. Converse, J. M., Nigro, A., Wilson, F. A., et al.: A technique for surgical correction of lop ears. Plast. Reconstr. Surg., *15*:411, 1955.
76. Dowling, J. A., Foley, F. D., and Moncrief, J. A.: Chondritis in the burned ear. Plast. Reconstr. Surg., *42*:115, 1968.
77. Furnas, D. W.: Correction of prominent ears by conchal mastoid sutures. Plast. Reconstr. Surg., *24*:189, 1968.
78. Goode, R. L., Proffitt, S. D., and Rafaty, F. M.: Complications of otoplasty. Arch. Otolaryngol., *91*:352, 1970.
79. Hatch, M. D.: Common problems of otoplasty. J. Int. Coll. Surg., *30*:171, 1958.
80. Mustardé, J. C.: The correction of prominent ears using simple mattress sutures. Br. J. Plast. Surg., *16*:170, 1963.
81. Mustardé, J. C.: The treatment of prominent ears by buried mattress sutures: A ten year survey. Plast. Reconstr. Surg., *39*:382–386, 1967.
82. Spira, M., McCrea, R., Gerow, F. J., et al.: Correction of the principal deformities causing protruding ears. Plast. Reconstr. Surg., *44*:150, 1969.
83. Spira, M.: Reduction Otoplasty. *In* Goldwyn, R. M. (ed.): The Unfavorable Result in Plastic Surgery. Boston, Little, Brown and Company, 1972.
84. Stenstrom, S. J.: A "natural" technique for correction of congenitally prominent ears. Plast. Reconstr. Surg., *32*:509, 1963.
85. Wood-Smith, D., and Converse, J. M.: The lop ear deformity. Surg. Clin. North Am., *51*:417, 1971.

### Complications of Augmentation Mentoplasty

86. Converse, J. M.: Restoration of facial contour by bone grafts introduced through the oral cavity. Plast. Reconstr. Surg., *6*:295, 1950.
87. Friedland, J. A., Coccaro, P. J., and Converse, J. M.: Retrospective cephalometric analysis of mandibular bone absorption under silicone rubber chin implants. Plast. Reconstr. Surg., *57*:144, 1976.
88. Jobe, R., Iverson, R., and Vistnes, L.: Bone deformation beneath alloplastic implants. Plast. Reconstr. Surg., *51*:169, 1973. Discussions by Rees, T. D., and Spira, M.: Plast. Reconstr. Surg., *51*:174, 1973.
89. Millard, D. R.: Chin implants. Plast. Reconstr. Surg., *13*:70, 1954.
90. Millard, D. R.: Augmentation mentoplasty. Surg. Clin. North Am., *51*:333, 1971.
91. Robinson, M., and Shuken, R.: Bone resorption under plastic chin implants. J. Oral Surg., *27*:116, 1969.
92. Robinson, M.: Bone resorption under plastic chin implants. Follow-up of a preliminary report. Arch. Otol., *95*:30, 1972.

# SKIN FLAP AND SKIN GRAFT COMPLICATIONS

# 26

## Skin Flap Complications

*John J. Conley*

### INTRODUCTION

The skin flap has assumed such an important role in surgery of the head and neck that serious complications that affect its viability will lead to increased morbidity and additional operations, may diminish the quality of the result and will downgrade the prognosis. Its uses permit the immediate resurfacing of extensive skin and mucous membrane deficiencies in the neck and pharynx, protect the carotid artery system, establish a foundation for future reconstruction, replace heavily irradiated skin, protect the brain and subarachnoid space from external contamination, support vital structures and assist in the restoration of physiology. It is obvious that no single flap can accomplish all of these purposes, and it is therefore necessary to have available an assortment of potential flaps in various areas of the head and neck and their adjacent territories. These flaps are positioned on the scalp, face, cervical area, upper chest and upper back.

There has been considerable investigation of the advantages of delaying a flap for the purposes of increasing its blood supply, and thus its viability. These experiments have been carried out primarily on the skin of pigs, rabbits and rats and are reported in detail by Grabb and Myers (1975).[17] They state that this improved vascularity appears in three days, reaches a maximum in 8 to 10 days and then falls off after three months. McFarlane and his coworkers (1965)[24] and later Milton (1972)[25] and then Reinisch and Myers (1974)[34] reported that delayed flaps were less tolerant of ischemia than fresh flaps. It is obvious that not all of the physiologic principles applying to flap transfer have as yet been revealed. It is, however, accepted empirically by many surgeons that raising and delaying the transfer of a flap will enhance its viability. In the preparation of certain flaps, under certain conditions and in different regions of the body, this empiricism has merit.[8, 9, 10, 24, 25, 26, 27] The circumstances that dictate the need for the use of a regional flap and the rich arterial and cutaneous vascular connections in the area of the head and neck permit these particular flaps to be transferred without delay with few exceptions. Some of these exceptions consist of severe alterations from normalcy, such as inanition, certain types of malnutrition, organic disease, metabolic dysfunction, arteriosclerosis, advanced age and irradiation fibrosis. Other specific exceptions pertain to undue stress on the standard flap as a result of attempts to gain extra length, prefabrication, splitting or infolding or perforating the flap. In head and neck surgery, the delay often

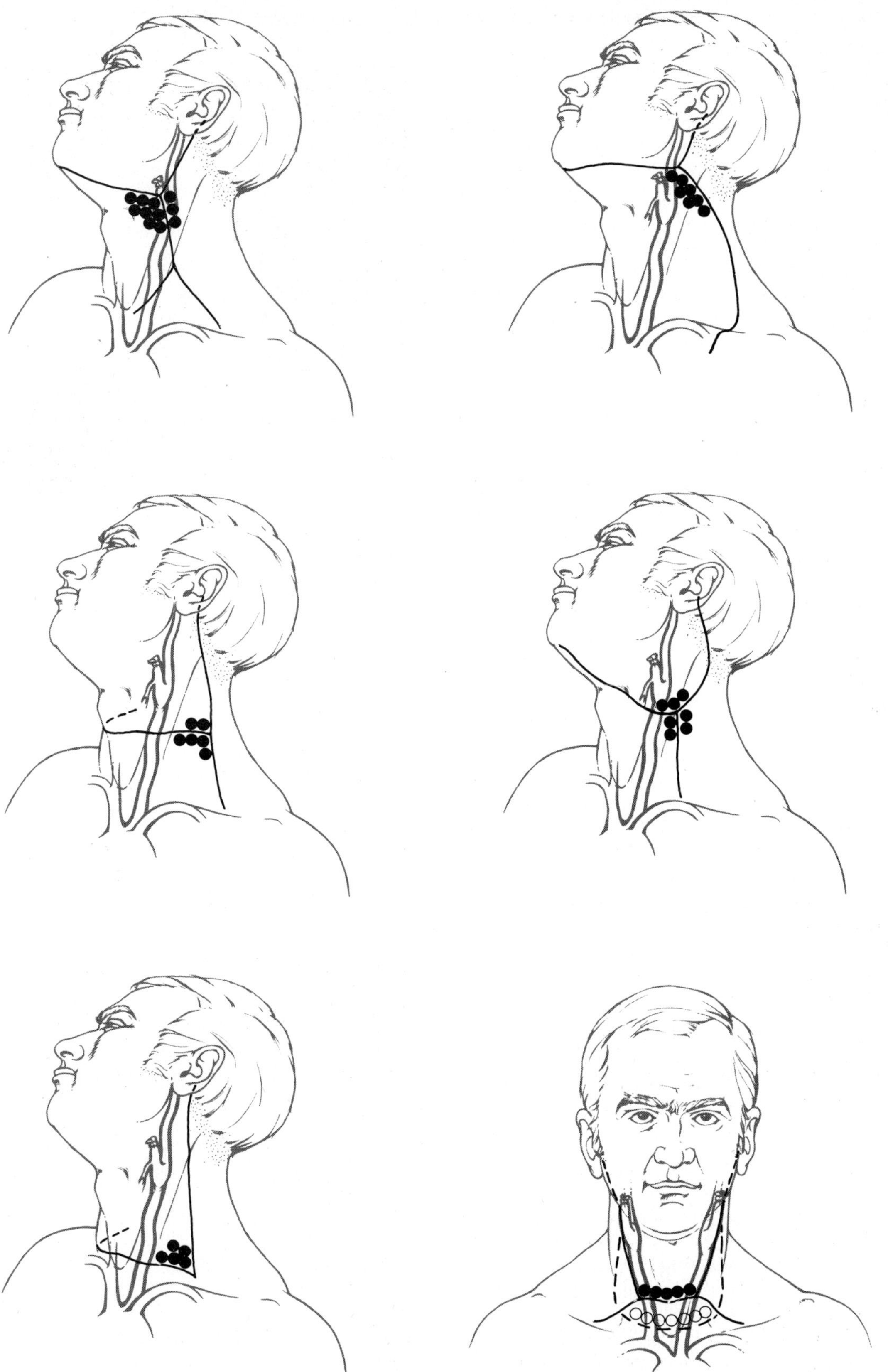

**Figure 26–1** Area of potential flap necrosis with different neck incisions.

does not fit the urgency of the treatment program; causes edema and fibrosis in the flap, thus reducing its length and viability; increases the number of operations; and extends the morbidity. A nondelayed transfer of a regional flap in this area, using single or multiple flaps when necessary to do this in a one-stage procedure, is therefore preferred in over 95 per cent of the cases. The fundamental concept for 30 years has been nondelay in transfer of the regional flap in head and neck surgery.

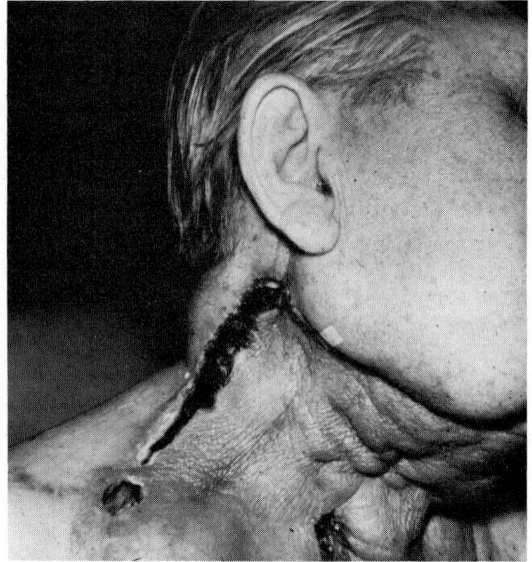

**Figure 26–2** This patient underwent laryngectomy and radical neck dissection using the large lateral cervical flap. There has been induration and contraction in the submental area and anterior cervical portion of the flap and a dry eschar along the posterior lateral border of the flap. This eschar is due to ischemia of this portion of the flap. Although the patient never developed a fistula, the anterior border of the flap had been under considerable biologic stress, and this most likely reflected itself in the lateral posterior border. The position of this eschar does not compromise the carotid artery in any manner, and it healed over an interval of three or four weeks by secondary intention.

## ETIOLOGY OF COMPLICATIONS

The basic etiologic factors in flap complications relate to necrosis of the flap due to ischemia and to loss of the flap secondary to infection. Ischemia is by far the most common cause. It is manifested by the loss of a small area of the tip or the catastrophic loss of a major portion of the flap.

### *Planning*

The most important aspect of flap transfer is the strategy of the plan and the design to carry it out. These must be conceived and executed within the limits of strict criteria that will establish its viability. If the wrong plan is ordained and the wrong design employed, the flap will fail. On the other hand, the perimeter of safety for survival of these flaps is variable to a certain degree, and there may be several different flaps in the region that are available to do the job. The surgeon should not be frozen into the position of believing that he can use only one flap but should carefully evaluate all possibilities.

### *Nutritional Status of Patient and Flap*

The nutritional status of the patient has a direct relation to the strength of the flap. Cachexia, wasting, diabetes, arteriosclerosis and poor general health all detract from the possibility of using a flap and reduce its chances of survival. It is important to also appreciate that each flap is maintained by an individual system of nutrient vessels that support the different regions with patterns of superficial and deep axial and perforating vessels.[11, 12, 29, 32, 35, 36, 37] These specific channels of nourishment are the keys that control the design and the viability of the flap. The strongest flaps contain a primary axial artery with numerous perforating regional connections. The weakest flaps are supported only by perforating cutaneous vessels. Some flaps are a combination of these two vascular systems. A thorough understanding of these nutritional factors creates and determines the possibilities for flap transfer.

### *Infection and Hematoma*

Regional flaps rarely die from infection. When a flap is moved into a fresh external wound or a properly prepared granulating bed, infection *de novo* is not to be expect-

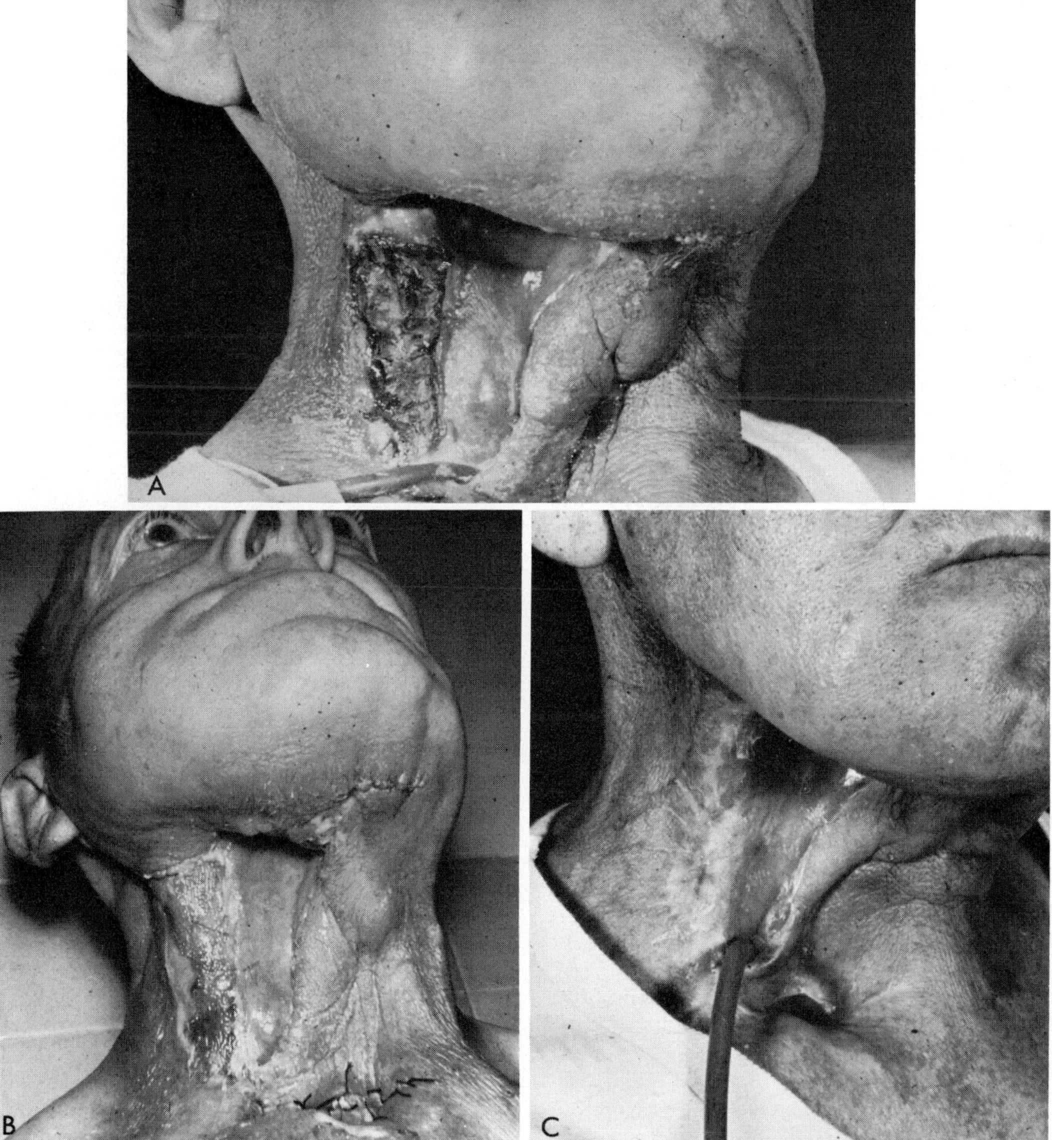

**Figure 26–3** *A,* Necrosis of the large portion of the posterior cervical flap, using Y incision for total laryngectomy, neck dissection and partial pharyngectomy. A large stoma was intentionally created to control the wound. The necrosis of the posterior flap is due to ischemia. *B,* The carotid artery system was protected by a levator scapulae muscle flap. The eschar has been removed, and it proved to be superficial. The carotid artery is not compromised. *C,* This wound has healed by secondary intention in an interval of four weeks. The large stoma was closed by the use of mucosa and regional tissue for the internal lining and a regional chest flap for external resurfacing.

ed. All tissue beds are potentially contaminated in composite resections that include oral and pharyngeal mucosa. There is a mixed bag of organisms, including *Straphyloccoccus, Streptococcus, Escherichia coli, Pseudomonas,* and occasional anaerobe, spirochete and fungiform organisms. They can necrose all or part of the flap. It is imperative that the mucous membrane repair be "spit-tight," that hemostasis be absolute, that the wound have adequate drainage and that the patient be covered with antibiotics. If this prophylactic regime should fail and the flap becomes infected and necrotic, an active debridement is indicated, with externalization of the wound, culture for specific organism identification and aggressive conservative management, with hourly changes of saline dressings in order to prepare the bed for either free skin grafting or another flap.

Hemorrhage is uncommon when hemostasis and postoperative drainage of the wound are properly maintained. Gall, Sessions and Ogura (1977)[15] reported an overall incidence of hematoma of 1 per cent in major surgical procedures in the area of the head and neck. It is imperative to recognize this complication without delay by assessing the amount of bloody drainage, inspecting the wound and evaluating the hematocrit levels. Pressure from a large hematoma will disrupt the wound and ultimately kill the flap. Hematomas should be immediately evacuated in the operating room. Wound inspection usually does not reveal a single bleeder but a more diffuse pattern of bleeding. The clots are removed, the wound flushed, the bleeding meticulously controlled and the flaps repositioned with adequate drainage.

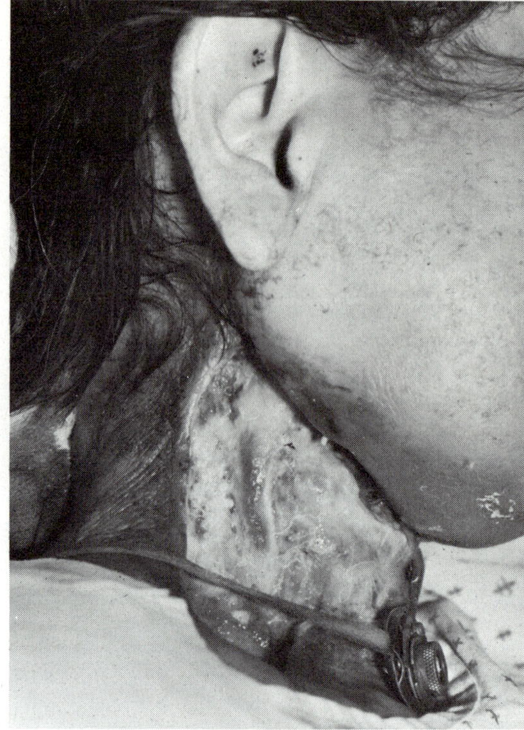

**Figure 26–4** Postoperative slough of entire neck requiring carotid artery resection following 11,000 rads preoperatively. Patient has had an open wound for six months. It will eventually require flap transposition.

### *Irradiation*

It is well established and well recognized that irradiation has a harmful effect on tissue and that this is apparent as early as four to six weeks after the beginning of the irradiation.[4, 5, 33] It increases in intensity over the following months and years. It consists of a graduated destruction and diminution of all of the tissue elements, with a reduction in their volume, quality and chemical and physiological capabilities. In a skin flap, this means a reduction in the vascular network, increased fibrosis and, consequently, a weaker flap. The subdermal vascular plexus is particularly vulnerable to the effects of irradiation. It is obvious that the use of this type of tissue for flap transfer has a built-in hazard of failure and that the surgeon should consider other regional, nonirradiated tissues. This is, of course, impractical in certain conditions involving incisions or flaps in the cervical area that have had previous irradiation for cancer of the larynx, pharynx or tongue. Under these circumstances, the flaps are reduced in size and the incisions comply with this reduced viability. Although it would be ideal to transfer an irradiated flap within four to six weeks of the beginning of irradiation, this is not practical because the tissue is, at that time, at the peak of irradiation reaction. Waiting for this to subside leads into the ascending changes in fibrosis, atrophy and reduced vascularity. This deleterious effect exists in direct proportion to the dose, size of the irradiation port, level of penetration and its time interval. It is obvious that heavily irradiated tissues are not satisfactory for flap transfer and that any surgical involvement with this type of tissue must be circumspect and modified to comply with these hazards.

### *Mechanical Factors and Suturing*

The mechanical factors that relate to the flap placement may determine its fate. Ideally, the flap should be rotated in a graceful manner and fit the deficient area amply. Precautions are taken against stretching the flap by preliminary proper design and measurements. It is often possible to gain a few extra centimeters of relaxation if the flap is short by bending or flexing the recipient area or by elevating the base of the donor region. These facilities are available in the movement of the neck and shoulders. Kinking and torsion are caused by deep recesses, prominent ledges, twisting and severe rotation. These impediments should be relieved by adjusting the base of the flap or the wound, by augmenting the area or by the use of skin grafts or additional flaps. Strong pressure should never be applied to a flap, as it will obstruct the blood components and kill the flap. It is also important that the base of the flap itself be free of this pressure, since this is the source of the blood supply and blood drainage. Hemovac drainage has eliminated the necessity for a pressure dressing over the flap and assists in coapting the flap to the recipient bed. Gravity is an important mechanical factor, in that large flaps are weighty and may cause excessive stress on the suture line when the patient is in the upright position. This pull can be eliminated by neutralizing the effects of gravity by keeping the patient prone during the early healing process. Gravity, on the other hand, may have a favorable effect on the venous and lymph drainage of a flap when the base is dependent. This reduces congestion, thickening and fibrosis and should be incorporated in the original plan for the flap.

These large flaps are sutured into their new beds with #3-0 chromic catgut or #5-0 Dexon Vicryl in the deep fascia and subdermis. The skin is usually closed with #5-0 Dermalon. The flaps and the entire adjacent area are further secured by stripping with one-half or one inch SteriStrips. A large, soft, bulky dressing is then added in order to support the flap. The area is immobilized, or kept quiet, during the first three days of the healing process.

## SIGNS OF POSSIBLE FAILURE

### *Immediate Subjective and Objective Signs*

There has been considerable clinical effort and scientific experimentation to establish a judgment that will permit a regional flap to be transposed with safety. Many of the tests have been ingenious, and although each presents a certain aspect of the circulatory phenomenon, not one presents the total physiological picture, and they are therefore only relative levels of security. They measure heat, gas content, pH, metabolic activity, light, absorptive capacity, color changes to various injected dye substances, intraflap blood pressures and angiographic studies in the flap and flap clearance of radioactive isotopes.[1, 2, 3, 7, 10, 13, 14, 16, 19, 20, 21] Some of these tests are time-consuming and require specialized equipment, and this has been a deterrent to their general adoption. Perhaps the most popular test is the injection of fluorescein dye and examination of the flap under Wood's light.

The vast majority of regional flaps in the area of the head and neck have established their reliability on the basis of substantial clinical trials. They are, consequently, not investigated preoperatively or even at the time of operation but simply elevated and transposed on the basis of experience. If the criteria of design and of craftsmanship are applied, there should be a 95 per cent success rate by this method. When a "standard" flap is elevated, it is inspected for free bleeding at its distal margins. If there is active blood from the subdermal and deep fascial vessels, one can be confident that the flap will survive. If there is only free bleeding from the subdermal plexus, the flap is still classified as a strong flap. This is further supplemented by the normal color of the skin of the flap. Digital pressure on the flap is a gross test for refilling and is reassuring when color returns to normal within five seconds. If the flap is white, with no free bleeding, cool to touch or does not blanch upon pressure, its arterial circulation is inadequate and one can assume that all or part of the flap will necrose. It is not logical, therefore, to transfer this type of flap. This is the type of flap one might test with fluorescein injection for additional information before establishing a definitive plan. If it does not improve spontaneously after waiting an interval of 15 minutes, it should be returned to its original bed or only the healthy part of it should be used. A new solution should then be developed immediately for resurfacing the wound. This is accomplished by shortening the original flap, selecting a new flap or complementing the technique with the use of free skin grafts. The abundance of available tissue about the area of the head and neck and the variety of flaps that can be developed permit an immediate solution to this rare problem of flap failure.

Delayed failure is classified as the phenomenon that appears one to seven days after transfer in what seemed to be a successful operation. The causes for delayed failure may be readily apparent or remain obscure. The alterations in sympathetic control of the blood vessels in the flap, the role played by the microcirculation in the flap and the effect of arteriovenous shunting are still not perfectly understood. Most of the obvious causes appear to be associated with subacute infection, the development of fistulas, irradiation endarteritis and poor tissue bed. All of these factors interfere with the adjustments of the internal circulation of the flap, fail to support the early anastomosis of the microcirculation of the flap with its new tissue bed or, specifically, destroy the circulating apparatus. This process establishes its own line of demarcation and viability.

## SALVAGE

When the blood supply to a flap is intrinsically inadequate, there is no known method of making it adequate. When this blood supply becomes inadequate as a result of external mechanical abnormalities, this can be improved and, in many instances, reversed if carried out expeditiously. When the blood supply is made inadequate by a biologic process, it usually cannot be reversed quickly enough to save the entire flap. All flaps will tolerate relative ischemia for several hours, but any procedure reducing oxygenation should be corrected as quickly as possible. In a normal tissue bed, the ingrowing capillaries will assist in supporting a transposed flap within five days. This important increment of assistance emphasizes the advantages of a healthy recipient bed.

There are marginal degrees of ischemia that may be assisted by cooling the flap or by exposing it to hyperbaric oxygen. This may prolong the viability of the flap or reverse a localized area of ischemia. Vasodilators, gravitational position, induced hypertension and Dextran have not significantly improved the condition of the flap.[18, 22, 30, 34] If the flap is deteriorating, if it is performing a service, such as holding the wound together, and if it is not infected, it should remain in its position until its local value to the wound has accomplished its purpose and a line of demarcation has been established. It is then debrided and the area resurfaced with a skin graft or another flap. If a necrotizing flap covers the carotid artery, it should be debrided immediately, the wound placed under aggressive medical management in preparation for resurfacing. In only rare instances can the flap be shortened and advanced. The loss of minimal areas about the periphery of the flap is not significant and they are permitted to heal by secondary intention. It probably will never be possible to guarantee the viability of every flap, regardless of the tests devised to evaluate them. The only meaningful clinical test in flap transfer is its survival, and a thorough knowledge of the empiric value of the different flaps in the area of the head and neck is the best prophylaxis against complications.

# Skin Grafting Complications

The basic principles governing skin grafts in all areas of the head and neck, whether they relate to dressing primary wounds in the oral cavity, in the pharynx, on skin surfaces of the head and neck region or in donor areas of large regional flaps, are the fundamental criteria that favor a "take" of the graft, good color match, minimum contraction and good serviceability.

## INTRODUCTION

1. All large grafts should be "pie-crusted" in order to permit the escape of serum and blood. These perforations are put in critical positions in the graft, preferably close to a valley or an abutment.
2. Large grafts are fixed in their recipient bed with a series of accurately positioned atraumatic #5-0 nylon sutures.
3. Each graft is supported by a bolus dressing with overties.
4. The dressing is moist, permitting good molding and firm pressure and creating an osmotic mechanism at the site of the small perforations.
5. The region to be grafted is immobilized as much as possible by the use of a sling, nasogastric feeding tube, a bulky supportive dressing and specific instructions to the patient not to move.

If the surgical plan includes free skin grafting, it is wise to take this step in a clean field at the beginning of the operation, so that the possibility of contamination by cancer cell seeding may be avoided. When grafts are taken after ablation, there is always the possibility of seeding, in spite of careful preparation, changing of gloves, and the use of a clean tray. This author has seen two instances of seeding — one was a squamous cell cancer in the anterior chest that invaded the area of a deltopectoral flap and another was a melanoma at the donor area of a skin graft from the lateral thigh.

The complications that befall free skin grafts are (1) loss of the implant, (2) contracture, (3) hypertrophied scar, (4) pigmentation, (5) collections under the graft and (6) unexpected hair growth.

## LOSS OF THE GRAFT

This may be precipitated by a collection of serum or blood underneath the graft, infection or a poorly nourishing tissue bed. Immobilization of the region, "pie-crusting" of the graft, absolute hemostasis, obtaining a satisfactory tissue bed and using appropriate antibiotics and a pressure dressing are the best prophylactics. A collection of serum or blood underneath the graft may be aspirated or expressed, and the graft may still "take" if it is no more than five days old and there is no infection. In a severe loss of the graft, the deficit can usually be recouped by regrafting.

## CONTRACTURE OF THE GRAFT

All grafts have an intrinsic tendency to contract spontaneously. Very thin ones do not have this capacity to such a degree and can consequently be laid on the wound without excessive tension. In this instance, the wound itself will contract. The thicker the graft, the greater the amount of intrinsic contraction, particularly in younger individuals. Consequently, more tension must be applied to the suture line in order to approximate the graft to the wound. A moderate amount of tension is desirable. A collection under the graft, undue tension, movement of the muscles under the graft and subclinical inflammation all may contribute to contracture. Gentle massage, heat, the judicious use of steroids and the passage of time will cause some improvement.

Resurfacing any soft tissue in the oral cavity or pharynx or rebuilding any tubular structures with a free skin graft is always followed by contraction. This is of particular significance in the region of the buccal mucosa, pharyngoesophagus and trachea. All skin grafts into the buccal area

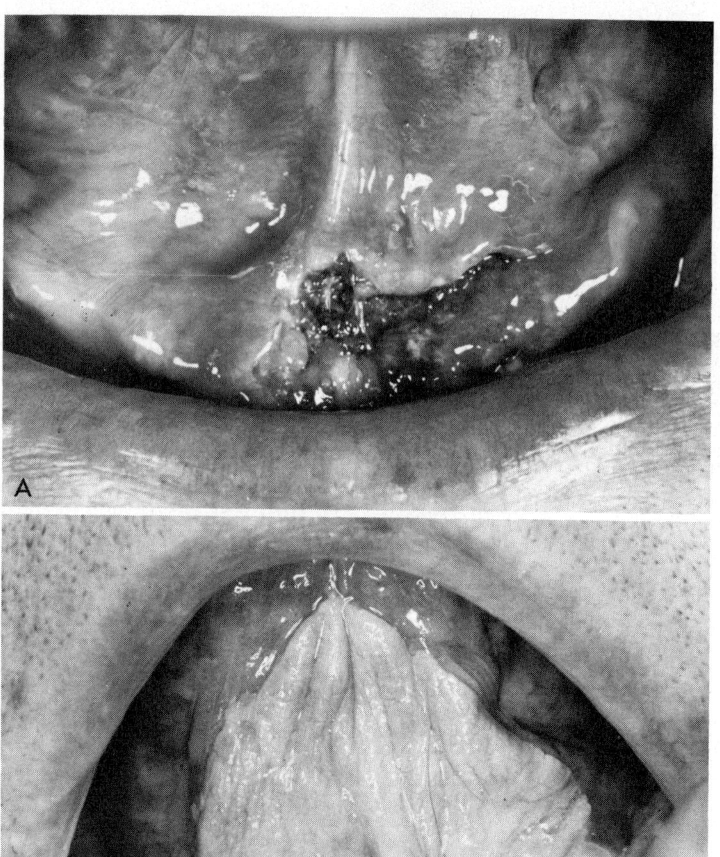


**Figure 26–5** *A,* Squamous cell cancer of the floor of the mouth invading the undersurface of the tongue. *B,* This cancer along with the undersurface of the tongue and floor of the mouth bilaterally and margins of the mandible, sublingual glands and associated muscles is resected and dressed with an epithelial onlay skin graft held in position over a bolus. One can immediately recognize the flexibility, softness and excellent movement of the tongue reaching up to and touching the palate. This technique has proved extremely beneficial in the elimination of contraction and heavy scar formation with resultant fixation of the tongue.

should be overcorrected. The bolus supporting the graft should keep the mouth in an open position so that as the graft heals there will be no tightness immediately after the operation. These grafts must be controlled for at least three months by exercise, massage, opening the mouth and stretching.

Reconstruction of the pharyngoesophagus and trachea with free skin grafts results in contraction unless an indwelling stent is placed in position and remains there for 6 to 12 months. It is recognized that free skin grafting for rehabilitation of these systems is not as desirable as direct approximation or the use of regional pedicle flaps.

Skin grafts placed over osseous surfaces (such as following radical ablation of the sinuses) and over the alveolus of the mandible are not complicated by contraction, since they are stented by their attachment to the bony surfaces on which they grow. A recognized deficiency of skin grafts over bone, however, is the difficulty of getting a "take" and the inability of the graft to support wear and tear.

## HYPERTROPHIED SCAR

This conspicuous complication about the margins of a free skin graft may be precipitated by tension, contraction, torsion, subclinical infection with inflammation, irritating suture material or contraction of the wound. These hypertrophied scars may develop into keloids. They are violescent, red, swollen, thick, tight in the beginning and gradually mature over an interval of one to two years. These scars mature much more slowly in children and teen-agers than in adults. As they mature, they become soft, white, flat or depressed and widened. Bimonthly injections with triamcinolone acetonide (Kenalog or Aristocort) augment the resolution. The scar will ultimately have to be revised. (See Chapter 28.)

## PIGMENTATION

There may be alterations in the color of the skin. An absence of normal pigment produces a white effect, or an increase in the amount of pigment produces a red or brown effect. Although carotene may produce a yellowish tinge to the skin on occasion, the predominant pigment effect comes from the production of melanin. Transplanted skin should not be unduly exposed to the stress of sunburn.

Full thickness skin grafts, particularly those taken from the cervical or postauricular areas, have the best opportunity to produce good color matching. Topical application of hydroquinone may decrease the amount of melanin synthesis. Psoralens have been used successfully in producing pigment in vitiligo and may be considered for treatment in certain deeply pigmented skin grafts. Dermabrasion and cryosurgery will diminish pigmentation. They must be first applied on a trial basis. Injection of pigments by tattooing the skin may increase pigmentation.

## SEBACEOUS MATERIAL

Small collections may develop two or three weeks after a split-thickness skin graft is applied. These result from accumulations of desquamations caused by blocked ducts in the graft. These accumulations will respond when a small excision is made over the cyst and its contents are expressed.

## HAIR GROWTH

A curious phenomenon is the sight of increased hair growth in a free split-skin graft. The stimulation process associated with the survival of the graft also affects the hair follicles in certain instances so that hair growth may be more conspicuous several months after the grafting than it was at the original site. One would not expect hair regrowth in medium or thin skin grafts because the follicle would not have been transplanted. Hair growth does not require treatment.

## Bibliography


1. Barron, J. N.: The congestion test. Br. J. Plast. Surg., *8*:114, 1955.
2. Barron, J. N., Veall, N., and Arnott, D. G.: The measurement of the local clearance of radioactive sodium in tubed skin pedicles. Br. J. Plast. Surg., *4*:16, 1951.
3. Ben-Hur, N., Mahler, Y., Shulman, J., et al.: A study of the peripheral blood flow in skin tubed flaps by photoconductive plethysmography. Isr. J. Med. Sci., *2*:218, 1966.
4. Berry, R. J., Wiernik, G., and Patterson, T. J. S.: Dose-response relationships for early and mid-term reactions in the skin of pigs exposed to 250 kVp x-rays in courses of 1, 6 or 30 fractions. Br. J. Radiol., *45*:793, 1972.
5. Berry, R. J., Wiernik, G., Patterson, T. J. S., et al.: Excess late subcutaneous fibrosis after irradiation of pig skin, consequent upon the application of the NSD formula. Br. J. Radiol., *47*:277, 1974.
6. Biller, H. F.: Pedicled flaps: An experimental and clinical study. Laryngoscope, *82*:1831, 1972.
7. Broadbent, T. R., Masters, F. W., and Pickrell, K. L.: A new compression clamp to test and occlude the circulation in pedicle flaps. Plast. Reconstr. Surg., *12*:187, 1953.
8. Brown, W. F., Litzow, T. J., Anderson, J. A., et al.: An experimental method of studying blood flow in canine bipedicle tube flaps. Mayo Clin. Proc., *44*:742, 1969.
9. Climo, S.: Dermal bleeding and the delay operation. Plast. Reconstr. Surg., *8*:59, 1951.
10. Conway, H., Stark, R. B., and Joslin, D.: Cutaneous histamine reaction as a test of circulatory efficiency of tubed pedicles and flaps. Surg. Gynecol. Obstet., *93*:185, 1951.
11. Conway, H., Stark, R. B., and Nieto-Cano, G.: The arterial vascularization of pedicles. Plast. Reconstr. Surg., *12*:348, 1953.
12. Creech, B. J., and Miller, S. H.: Evaluation of circulation in skin flaps. *In* Grabb, W. C., and Myers, M. B. (eds.): Skin Flaps. Boston, Little, Brown and Company, 1975, p. 21.

13. Creech, B. J., and Thorne, F.: The pocket photoplethysmograph. Plast. Reconstr. Surg., *49*:380, 1972.
14. Dingwall, J. A., and Lord, J. W.: The fluorescein test in the management of tubed (pedicle) flaps. Bull. Johns Hopkins Hosp., *73*:129, 1943.
15. Gall, A. M., Sessions, D. G., and Ogura, J. H.: Complications following surgery for cancer of the larynx and hypopharynx. Cancer, *39*:624, 1977.
16. Glinz, W., and Clodius, L.: Measurement of tissue pH for viability in pedicle flaps: Experimental studies in pigs. Br. J. Plast. Surg., *25*:111, 1972.
17. Grabb, W. C., and Myers, M. B. (eds.): Skin Flaps. Boston, Little, Brown and Company, 1975.
18. Grabb, W. C., and O'Neal, R. M.: The effect of low molecular weight dextran on the survival of experimental skin flaps. Plast. Reconstr. Surg., *37*:406, 1963.
19. Guthrie, R. H., Goulian, D., and Cucin, R. L.: Predicting the extent of viability in flaps by measurement of gas tensions using a mass spectrometer. Plast. Reconstr. Surg., *50*:385, 1972.
20. Hoehn, R., and Binkert, B.: Cholesteric liquid crystals: A new visual aid to study of flap circulation. Plast. Reconstr. Surg., *48*:209, 1971.
21. Hynes, W.: A simple method of estimating blood flow with special reference to the circulation in pedicle skin flaps and tubes. Br. J. Plast. Surg., *1*:159, 1948.
22. Kernahan, D. A., Zingg, W., and Kay, C. W.: The effect of hyperbaric oxygen on the survival of experimental skin flaps. Plast. Reconstr. Surg., *36*:19, 1966.
23. Lange, K., and Boyd, L. J.: The use of fluorescein to determine the adequacy of the circulation. Med. Clin. North Am., *26*:943, 1942.
24. McFarlane, R. M., Heagy, F. C., Rodin, A., et al.: A study of the delay phenomenon in experimental pedicle flaps. Plast. Reconstr. Surg., *35*:245, 1965.
25. Milton, S. H.: The effects of "delay" on the survival of experimental pedicled skin flaps. Br. J. Plast. Surg., *22*:244, 1969.
26. Milton, S. H.: Experimental studies on island flaps. II. Ischemia and delay. Plast. Reconstr. Surg., *49*:444, 1972.
27. Muir, I. F. K., Fox, R. H., Stranc, W. E., et al.: The measurement of blood flow by a photoelectric technique and its application to the management of tubed skin pedicles. Br. J. Plast. Surg., *21*:14, 1968.
28. Myers, M. B.: Attempts to augment survival in skin flaps — mechanism of the delay phenomenon. *In* Grabb, W. C., and Myers, M. B. (eds.): Skin Flaps. Boston, Little, Brown and Company, 1975, p. 65.
29. Myers, M. B., and Cherry, G.: Causes of necrosis in pedicle flaps. Plast. Reconstr. Surg., *42*:43, 1968.
30. Myers, M. B., and Cherry, G.: The blood pressure in tubed pedicles. Plast. Reconstr. Surg., *38*:49, 1966.
31. Myers, M. B., Cherry, G., and Milton, S.: Tissue gas levels as an index of the adequacy of circulation: The relation between ischemia and the development of collateral circulation (delay phenomenon). Surgery, *71*:15, 1972.
32. Patterson, T. J. S., and Milton, S. H.: Study of the circulation in experimental skin flaps using an intra-vital dye. *Bibl. Anat., 9*:501, 1967.
33. Patterson, T. J. S., Berry, R. J., Hopewell, J. W., et al.: The effect of X-radiation on the survival of experimental skin flaps. *In* Grabb, W. C., and Myers, M. B. (eds.): Skin Flaps. Boston, Little, Brown and Company, 1975, p. 39.
34. Reinisch, J., and Myers, M. B.: Effect of local anesthetics and epinephrine on survival of experimental flaps. Plast. Reconstr. Surg., *54*:324, 1974.
35. Schnur, P., Simons, J. N., and Tauxe, W. N.: Circulation of pedicle flaps studied by tissue clearance of $^{99m}$Tc-Pertechnetate. Surg. Forum, *20*:513, 1969.
36. Tauxe, W., Simons, J., Lipscombe, P., et al.: Determination of vascular status of pedicle skin flaps by use of radioactive Pertechnetate (99m Tc). Surg. Gynecol. Obstet., *130*:87, 1970.
37. Teich-Alasia, S.: A study of the vascularization of pedicle flaps using Disulphine Blue. Br. J. Plast. Surg., *24*:282, 1971.
38. Thorne, F. L., Georgiade, N. G., and Mladick, R.: The use of thermography in determining viability of pedicle flaps. Arch. Surg., *99*:97, 1969.

# 27 COMPLICATIONS IN MICROSURGERY IN THE HEAD AND NECK

*William R. Panje*
*Charles J. Krause*

The operating microscope was introduced more than fifty years ago and was used by Professor Carl Nylen of Sweden for middle ear operations. Modern contributions to the operating microscope by Zeiss in the 50's have made possible the emergence of sophisticated new techniques in otology, ophthalmology, neurosurgery, vascular surgery and plastic and reconstructive surgery.[30, 40]

In 1960, Jacobsen and Suarez[21] reported on the value of using an operating microscope when making small vessel repairs. The subsequent development of specialized microinstrumentation and refinement of techniques in the repair of vessels 1 to 2 mm. in diameter have allowed replantation of digits and extremities, revascularization of the heart and central nervous system and the one-stage transposition of skin flaps to distant sites on the body.

The transplantation of a skin flap utilizing transection and reanastomosis of its vessels at the recipient site was first performed in September, 1972.[16] Other case reports soon followed.[5, 33] Since then, flaps have been utilized in the closure and reconstruction of traumatic defects, resurfacing of scarred areas following burns, closure of fistulas and repair of congenital defects and in reconstruction following ablative cancer operations. Microvascularized transplants of bone, muscle and skin flaps with sensory innervation are now being reported.[6, 18, 41] Two recently reported series of free flaps revealed an overall complete success rate approaching 80 per cent. The larger series by Harii and Ohmori[15] included 94 cases, and the other by Serafin[39] included 35 cases.

As expertise in microscopic anastomoses of small vessels and nerves has developed, a better understanding has been gained of the nature and causes of complications associated with these procedures. Because of the dimensions of the structures and techniques involved, allowable margin for error is extremely small and technical expertise is crucial. The purpose of this chapter is to deal with complications in the microsurgical repair of vessels and nerves. Etiology, prevention and treatment of these complications will be discussed, expressing the opinion of the authors. The first part of the chapter will pertain mainly to microvascular anastomoses and free flap reconstruction in the head and neck. The second part will deal with nerve anastomoses.

## COMPLICATIONS OF MICROVASCULAR ANASTOMOSIS

### Intraoperative Complications

#### *General Factors*

Advancing age and disease states such as arteriosclerosis and diabetes predispose to thrombosis at the site of small vessel anastomoses owing to thickening and an increased friability of the small vessel walls. In addition, polycythemia, blood coagulopathies and collagen vascular disorders appear to increase the chance of thrombosis. One should avoid microvessel anastomosis if these conditions exist.

Free flaps have been utilized in patients ranging from 18 months to 70 years of age.[14, 25] In younger patients, however, the smaller vessel size may increase the technical difficulty of vascular anastomosis, and in elderly patients, vessel wall deterioration is commonly found.

Obesity has been a contributing factor to free flap complications, particularly with groin flaps (Fig. 27–1). The large amount of subcutaneous fat interferes with placement at the recipient bed, especially in certain complex anatomic sites in the head and neck. The flap may be defatted at the time of transfer, but extensive removal of fat increases the risk of injury to the vascular pedicle. We recommend seeking another flap alternative rather than utilizing a "fat flap."

It has been generally assumed that irradiation of small vessels would lead to a high failure rate at the anastomosis. This concept was based upon histopathologic evidence of changes induced in small vessel walls subjected to high-energy irradiation. Although the endothelium tolerates the irradiation quite well, the media is markedly damaged, with proliferation of fibrous tissue and subsequent arteriosclerosis. Baker, Krause and Panje[2] have shown that in rats receiving preoperative irradiation in dosages comparable to that delivered to humans with cancer, no increase in thrombus formation occurred in the first four weeks after anastomosis of blood vessels 1 to 1.5 mm. in diameter. Panje, Bardach and Krause[36] have demonstrated in the human that free flap transpositions are possible despite preoperative or postoperative irradiation to the recipient vessel sites.

### *Selection for Appropriate Donor Site*

Just as a number of regional vascular flaps have been described for closing head and neck defects, there have now also been several acceptable donor sites for free flaps described. The scalp, pectoral, groin and dorsalis pedis areas are the most commonly used. Essential to the design of a free flap is the existence of direct cutaneous arterial and venous networks. Examples of sites where such networks have been described include the following: scalp, temporal artery and vein; pectoral, internal mammary artery and vein perforators; groin, superficial external iliac artery and vein; dorsum of foot, dorsalis pedis artery and its venae comitantes; postauricular, postauricular artery and veins. Other direct arterialized flap sites such as subaxillary and lateral femoral cutaneous have been described but have been used infrequently. (Fig. 27–2)

The scalp flap contains relatively thin hair-bearing skin and has a long vascular pedicle with arterial vessel sizes usually approaching 2 to 2.5 mm. in diameter. This flap is primarily used to cover hair-bearing areas.

The pectoral flap is relatively thin and pliable, non-hair-bearing in the female, and possesses veins with relatively large diame-

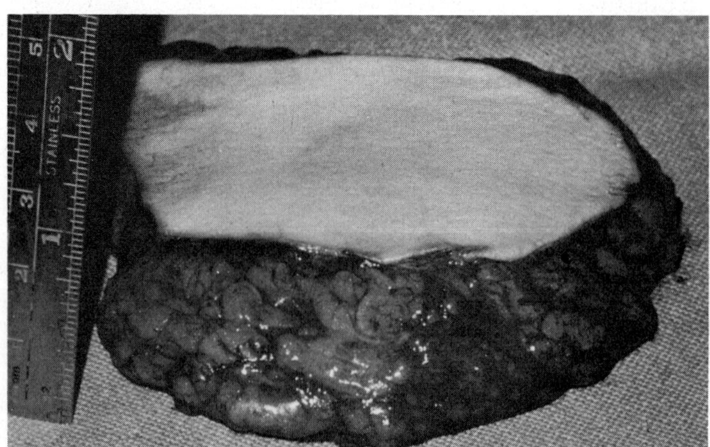


**Figure 27–1** Free groin flap demonstrating excessive subcutaneous fat, which may be troublesome in the obese patient.

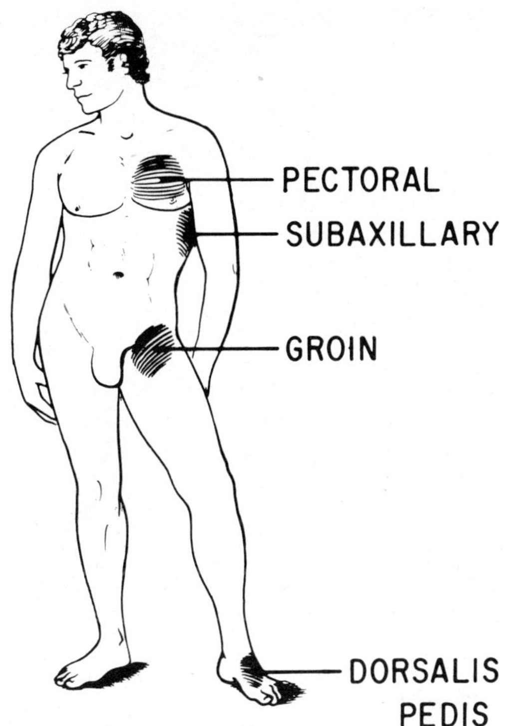


**Figure 27–2** Some of the free flap sites that have been described.

ters (sometimes 5 to 7 mm.). The vascular pedicle is quite short, however. The pectoral flap is an alternative to the groin flap in obese people and is relatively easy to dissect. Color match to facial skin is good.

The groin flap has been the mainstay of free flap reconstruction to date. This flap may be thick at times, but large areas of tissue can be developed with a vessel diameter size usually greater than 1.5 mm. There is minimal secondary deformity of the site since it can usually be closed primarily. There have been no problems encountered with lymphatic drainage from the groin area postoperatively.

The dorsalis pedis flap is a thin flap with minimal hair coverage containing a sizeable vascular pedicle. It is relatively difficult to dissect, however. The flap is usually thin in obese people. The superficial peroneal nerve innervates the skin of this flap and may be used as a neurovascular free flap. This flap should not be utilized if posterior tibial artery pulsation is absent. Morbidity on the dorsum of the foot may be encountered postoperatively since the area is usually covered with a split thickness skin graft.

The postauricular flap is thin and encompasses a small area. This flap has been used successfully by Fujino. The vascular pedicle is relatively difficult to dissect, however, because of a lack of predictable location of the feeding vessels.

### *Technical Factors*

No single factor is so important to the success of microvascular anastomosis as is the technical expertise of the surgeon. Many hours of practice on animals are necessary before consistently high patency rates in doing 1 mm. diameter vessels may be attained. Even then, the surgeon must continue to practice this technique regularly. There is no substitute for well-honed technical expertise by the surgeon.

An array of fine microsurgical instruments that allow precise approximation of vessel walls with minimal trauma to the tissues (Fig. 27–3) has been developed for use in small vessel anastomosis. The surgeon should have a selection of specially designed instruments available to him both for practice and for use in the clinical setting.[37]

Anastomosis of vessels that are of widely disparate dimensions may contribute to thrombus formation. If the two vessels vary more than 50 per cent in diameter, the smaller should be opened in a fish-mouth fashion or cut on a diagonal to increase its circumference. This prevents undue constriction at the anastomotic site and makes for an easier anastomosis. If at all possible, however, one should avoid this necessity by selecting recipient vessels similar in size to those at the donor site. If appropriately sized vessels are not available at the donor site, one might consider the use of vein grafts or end-to-side anastomoses. O'Brien's group has reported the usefulness of vein and arterial grafts as interposition conduits.[12] End-to-side anastomoses have also been employed with varying degrees of success.

When performing the anastomosis, careful surgical technique is of utmost importance. The adventitia should be stripped back from the cut ends of the vessels so as to prevent inversion of adventitia into the

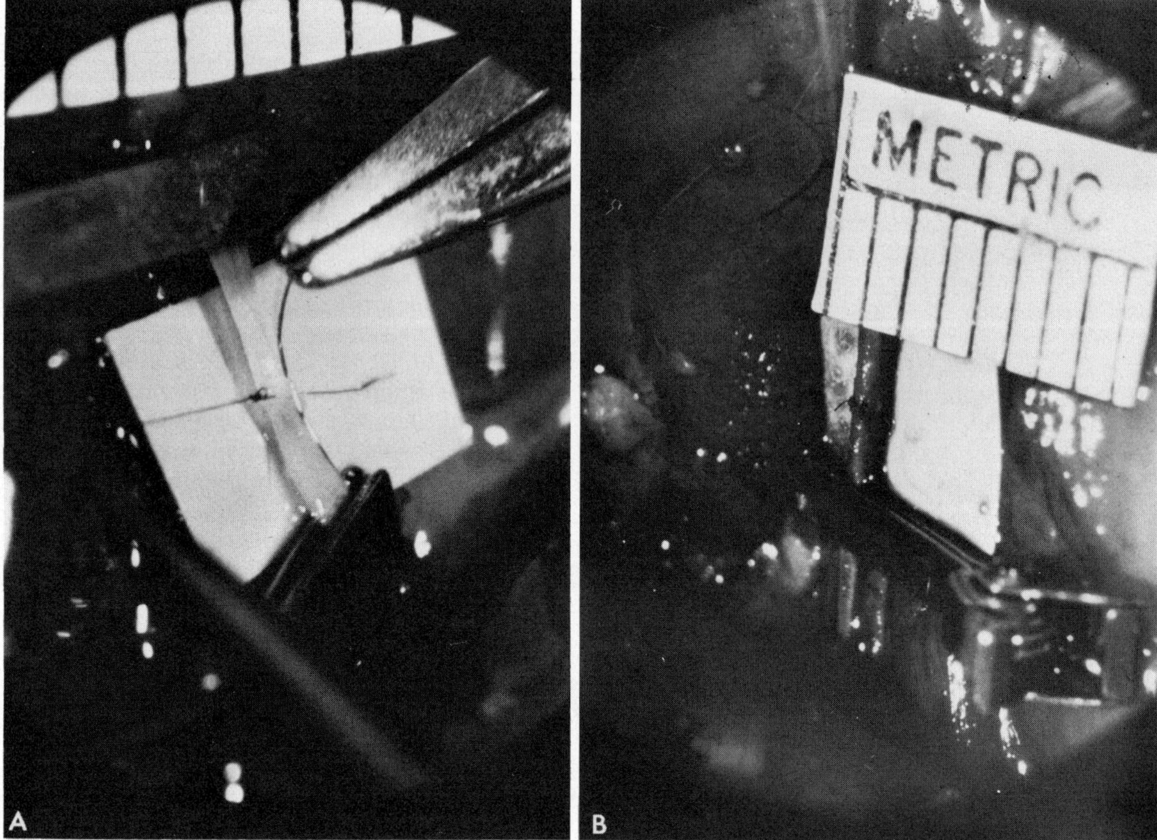


**Figure 27–3** Photograph illustrating the anastomosis of a 1 mm. diameter vessel. *A*, Placement of #10–0 suture. *B*, Completed anastomosis with proximal vascular clip still in position.

lumen. Adventitia has been demonstrated to be extremely thrombogenic to platelets and may cause thrombosis at the anastomotic site. Excessive stripping may lead to vessel wall necrosis, however, so this step should be done carefully and atraumatically.

The anastomosis should be performed with evenly spaced interrupted sutures. Special #10–0 or #11–0 nylon suture material with a fine curved needle swadged on is commercially available. Two sutures are placed top and bottom to be used for manipulation of the vessel during anastomosis. The vessel is then rolled over, and the posterior wall is closed with interrupted sutures. The vessel is then rotated again to facilitate closure of the anterior wall. Vessels with diameters of 1 mm. should have 8 to 10 sutures placed so that no gaps will occur in the anastomotic site to stimulate thrombus formation. A running closure should be avoided in vessels of this size, since some degree of narrowing may occur.

Care must be taken to avoid any tension, torsion or kinking at the site of anastomosis. To this end, the flap should be sutured into position within the recipient site before beginning the anastomosis. The surgeon may then mobilize the recipient vessels or use an interposition vein graft if necessary to avoid tension.

Excessive movement of the part being restored, which may result in motion at the anastomotic site, should be avoided. Immobilization of tissues about the site may be necessary during the postoperative period.

Unlike organ or limb transplantation, the use of perfusates such as the balanced mediums used in kidney transplants or heparinized saline has proved to be of little value in preventing thrombus formation in free cutaneous flaps.[13] Blood tends only to sludge within the untraumatized microcirculation rather than to clot.[26] Heparinized saline, however, should be used to irrigate clotted debris from the cut vessel ends at the time of anastomosis. Introduction of cannulas into the small vessels and high perfusion pressures may cause damage to vessel endothelium and result in thrombosis due to the exposure of underlying collagen and subsequent platelet aggregation.

Systemic anticoagulation does not appear to be warranted in flap transfers utilizing normal vessels.[17, 19, 34] When vessel anastomosis has been traumatic or when partially diseased vessels are joined together, however, the judicious use of anticoagulants may improve patency rates. Anticoagulants that affect platelet adhesiveness, such as aspirin, dipyridamole and dextran, appear to be the best for this purpose. Heparin, which mainly inhibits thromboplastin generation, has been demonstrated to have some clinical efficacy, however.

A problem most frequently encountered when anticoagulants have been used is the formation of a hematoma beneath the flap. This is particularly true in the head and neck, where large, irregular raw surface areas frequently exist following cancer resection. We have successfully utilized suction drainage to avoid hematoma formation in anticoagulated as well as nonanticoagulated patients.

Thurston and his associates[42] have shown that clamping of small vessels with standard microvascular clips may lead to endothelial slough and necrosis of the media at the site of clamp placement. Later, fusiform dilatation of the vessel may occur at that site, resulting in turbulence and thrombus formation. Therefore, it is best to use Heifitz microvascular clips only on the recipient vessels during the anastomosis and thus decrease the amount of small vessel trauma. An adjustable microvascular clamp has recently been developed that exerts minimal occluding pressure on the vessel walls.

### *Vasospasm*

Small vessel spasm is a perplexing problem that is poorly understood at present. It is known that spasm may be the result of excessive intraoperative manipulation of the cut vessels, exposure of the extraluminal vessel surface to fresh blood, desiccation of the vessel or exposure to cold. Therefore, the cut vessels should be handled gently, and the surgical field should be kept free of blood. The cut vessel tips should be gently irrigated with heparinized saline (10 U. per cc.) before beginning the anastomosis. During the suturing process, the exposed vessels should be frequently wetted (every 5 minutes) with warmed (38° C.) heparinized saline to avoid drying and cooling.

When the spasm is the result of tension across the anastomosis, it can be relieved only by reducing the tension. This may be accomplished by repositioning the flap, removing retention sutures or mobilizing recipient and donor vessels in some instances, but if tension remains, a vein graft should be interposed within the anastomosis. By interposing a vein graft, one can frequently avoid the need for flap repositioning and possible flap or recipient vessel damage that may occur during mobilization.[35] The vein graft has worked best in our hands when used for the arterial side of the anastomosis. Extremity veins appear to be more suitable as interposition grafts than head and neck veins because of their thicker walls and lack of distensibility. It is important to remember to reverse the vessel ends when using veins for an interposition graft so that the valves do not cause interference with blood flow.

Once blood flow has been established across the anastomosis, vasospasm may develop simply from the presence of fresh blood in the field or from the washout of metabolic by-products associated with flap ischemia. The direct application of vasodilator substances, such as magnesium sulfate, papaverine 0.25 per cent, lidocaine 2 per cent or warmed normal saline, to the repaired vessels has been used with some success.[3, 29]

The use of systemic vasodilator therapy postoperatively in cases of compromised flap circulation appears to be of little value. Chlorpromazine, tolazoline hydrochloride (Priscoline), papaverine and lidocaine (Xylocaine) have all been used but with little firm evidence of efficacy. The use of systemic vasodilators will probably remain controversial until the mechanism of obstruction and the physiology of flap circulation are better understood.

### *Detection of Thrombosis*

Acland[1] described simple signs by which a surgeon could detect success or failure of an anastomosis by direct inspection through the operating microscope. In arteries, the signs concern the way in which the vessel pulsates. Blockage of an arterial anastomosis is indicated by forward longitudinal pulsation at the anastomotic site. Patency is indicated by expansile pulsation or wriggling distal to the anastomosis. Venous anastomotic failure is suggested by pressure distension of flap veins and collapse of the recipient veins. Stroking the vessel distal to the anastomosis and noting the direction of blood flow as the vein refills may also be used as an indicator of venous patency.

Although these techniques are helpful, they do not allow assessment of the quality of the anastomosis, nor do they allow one to follow the anastomosis postoperatively. Ultrasound analysis provides a tangible way to assess blood flow through the anastomosis both intraoperatively and postoperatively.[23, 43] An electrocardiographic recorder may be attached to the Doppler ultrasound flowmeter and thus provide a tracing of the blood flow. By placing the probe over the repaired artery, one can detect the development of a thrombus when a decrease in blood flow velocity and increase in turbulence is noted. When blood flow through the anastomosis ceases, this may be detected as well. An absence of fluctuation in venous flow synchronous with respirations indicates venous obstruction. The location of vessel anastomoses should be marked on the skin surface at the time of the operation so that subsequent Doppler recordings will all be made at exactly the same site.

Blood flow across the anastomosis should be carefully monitored for at least 45 minutes in the operating room and every two hours during the first 72 hours postoperatively. If any indication of thrombus formation develops, the patient should be returned to the operating room immediately and the anastomosis revised.

Other means of assessing flap circulation postoperatively include color, capillary refill, temperature and turgor. These techniques are not easily quantified and should be performed by a single individual during the observation period.

Flap color can be deceiving at times, especially if viewed within the oral cavity, where a strikingly pale appearing flap is usually normal. Free flaps, in general, are rather pale when compared to the surrounding tissues in the early postoperative days. The appearance of a pinkish-red flap should alert one to early venous thrombosis. As venous thrombosis proceeds, the flap will take on a violaceous-blue color. If the flap is punctured, rapid leakage of dark blood will occur (Fig. 27–4). Arterial thrombosis results in a white flap that lacks turgor.

Capillary refill is tested by applying the index finger to the flap for 30 seconds and then withdrawing the finger with constant observation of the test site, in natural light if possible. Brisk refill usually indicates a healthy flap, although the same finding can be seen in early flap vein thrombosis or simultaneous arterial and venous occlusion. Slow refill usually indicates a deteriorating arterial anastomosis or capillary vasoconstriction.

Flap temperature has not been reliable as a single test in assessing flap viability. A warm flap can mean adequate circulation, body temperature conduction through a nonviable flap or early infection. A cold flap means reduced blood flow into the flap. Temperature studies done on pedicle flaps have also been unreliable as a predictor of flap survival.[44]

Tissue turgor of the microvascularized replant has been useful at times in differentiating venous from arterial thrombosis. The flap will feel thick and tense when venous thrombosis occurs with an intact arterial supply. In the reverse situation, the dearterialized flap will feel "empty." A normal flap will feel doughy and spring back on release of pressure.

The combined, rather than individual, use of these clinical parameters has proved to be most reliable for us in assessing flap viability. In any event, one must remember that the flap is in a dynamic vascular state, and what has been described represents only one point in time. The importance of close observation of the newly replanted microvascularized flap cannot be overempha-

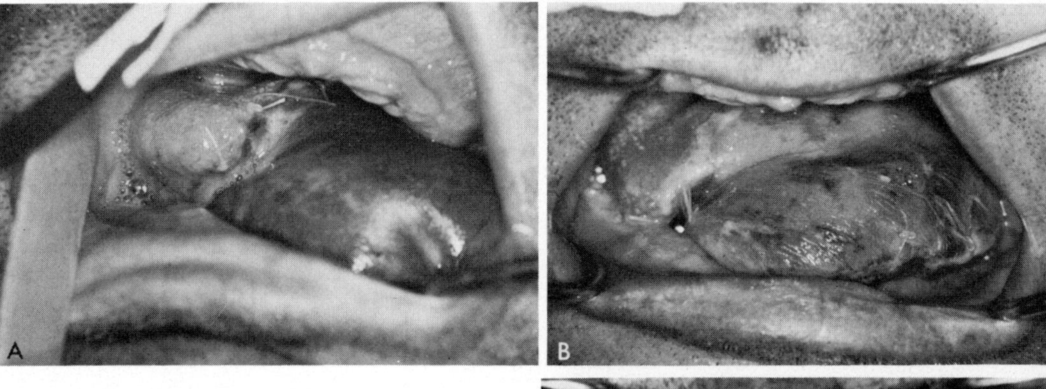

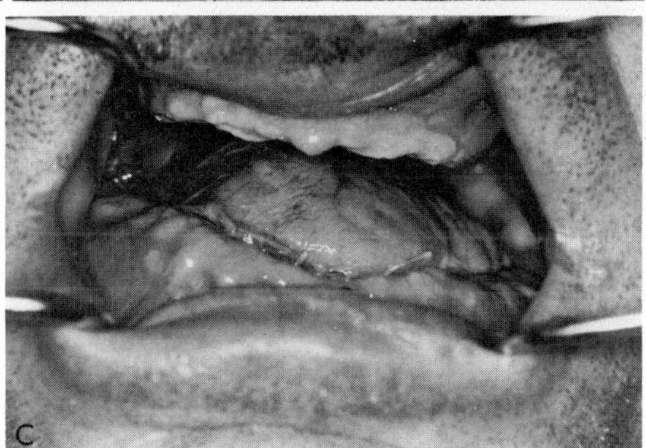

**Figure 27–4** Intraoral photograph illustrating a free groin flap used for reconstruction following near total glossectomy. *A,* Marked venous congestion and swelling 12 hours postoperative. *B,* Diminished congestion at 36 hours postoperative following administration of diuretics. (Note epidermolysis.) *C,* Complete flap survival at two months postoperative. (Note hair growth.)

sized, since the possibility exists that the impending flap death may be prevented with a revision of the thrombosed anastomosis.

### *Revision Anastomosis*

The most common cause for failure is thrombosis at the anastomotic site. This has usually resulted from faulty surgical technique, such as tying sutures too tightly, inverting adventitia into the anastomosis or traumatizing the vessel tips excessively. The anastomotic site should be excised back to normal vessel without clot, since thrombus adheres to small tears in endothelium and when pulled or vigorously irrigated from the vessel's lumen, additional exposure of subendothelial collagen may develop. When a significant length of vessel must be removed, a vein or arterial interposition graft should be inserted to avoid tension.

### *Lack of Recipient Vessel*

One drawback that has been mentioned in free flap utilization in the head and neck cancer patient is the lack of appropriate recipient vessels that may occur after a radical neck dissection or carotid artery sacrifice. When contemplating free flap reconstruction following a radical neck dissection, one should attempt to save the anterior jugular vein to provide venous drainage. If the anterior jugular vein is sacrificed, a vein or arterial graft can be used to reach a suitable neck vein. If no other alternative is available, an end-to-side anastomosis into the remaining lower stump of the internal jugular vein may be used.

Usually, some portions of the external carotid arterial system are left intact and provide numerous vessels for anastomosis. Depending upon the availability of carotid artery branches in the area of reconstruction, a vein graft can be utilized to perform an end-to-end or end-to-side anastomosis with a branch at some distance.

### *Ischemia Time*

Prolonged free flap ischemia time (more than 6 hours in the human) may have an adverse effect on flap survival. An experimental study has demonstrated varying degrees of endothelial slough following prolonged ischemia times.[20] The endothelial slough allows exposure of collagen with subsequent platelet thrombosis. Skin flaps in rats demonstrated considerable necrosis after only six hours of arterial occlusion.[39] Our laboratory results corroborate this finding. Although good blood flow may be initially established in a flap with prolonged ischemia, the free flap will usually swell excessively and may proceed to circulatory occlusion secondary to vasospasm or clotting. This vasospasm may be caused by exposure to high concentrations of metabolic byproducts that have collected within the flap during the ischemia time. To avoid prolonged ischemia, the vascular pedicle should be left intact until the surgeon is ready to transfer it. The recipient site must be completely readied with special attention to preparation of the recipient vessels before detaching the donor flap.

### *Flap Perfusion*

The flap should not be perfused during transfer. Introduction of a cannula or uncontrolled perfusion pressure within a small vessel lumen causes endothelial damage and may result in subsequent thrombosis. In contradistinction to cutaneous flaps, however, composite free grafts consisting of bone, muscle and skin appear to warrant perfusion before replantation.

### *Flap Edema*

Because in a free cutaneous flap no skin pedicle remains to provide lymph drainage, some postoperative edema usually occurs. This edema usually develops within the first 12 hours after a successful anastomosis, reaches a peak in 48 to 72 hours and then gradually subsides over the next 48 hours. Flap edema appears to be more pronounced when only a single venous anastomosis is done, especially when the vein is less than twice the diameter of the flap's artery. If the flap is perfused during transfer, severe edema will usually result and be refractory to medical or surgical management. Emphasis should be placed on positioning the patient in a semi-sitting position postoperatively and on careful control of fluid intake and output.

### *Infection*

Infection has not been a problem as long as an adequate blood flow into the flap has been maintained, even when the flap is placed within an irradiated oral cavity.[38] We have utilized cephalosporin (Keflin) as a prophylactic antibiotic in all intraoral cases. Other microvascular surgeons report frequently using prophylactic antibiotics in free flap reconstruction. Our only infections have been in flaps with marginal blood supply. Finseth, Kavarana and Antia noted that infection and partial loss were a common problem when free flaps were used close to the oral cavity.[10]

### *Exposure of Anastomosis*

Head and neck surgeons recognize that carotid artery exposure can lead to disaster from thrombosis or rupture of this great vessel. Similar complications can occur to a free flap vascular pedicle. Thus, if the vascular pedicle becomes exposed, one should attempt to cover the vessels with another skin flap and redirect saliva flow away from the anastomosis by the use of drains or controlled fistulization.

### *Free Flap Necrosis*

As in nearly all operations, alternatives exist preoperatively, intraoperatively and postoperatively. If a free flap replant is to be done, one should discuss with the patient the advantages of using this specific type of flap as well as the drawbacks that have been discussed in earlier papers.[32] The patient should also be warned that if the free flap fails either intraoperatively or postoperatively, another flap will, in most circumstances, be needed. An alternative should always be planned when using a free flap in reconstruction. Unlike pedicle flaps, which may take several days to demonstrate failure, a free flap usually exhibits its trend to failure within hours.

In the very early postoperative period (0 to 96 hours), if thrombosis or vasospasm is encountered and blood flow is not re-established to the flap in four to six hours or if revision anastomosis is not successful, then one should consider replacement of the free flap with an alternative pedical flap. This tact is strongly encouraged if carotid artery, bare bone or irradiated tissue bed needs coverage. Repeated replantation of another microvascularized flap when the initial free flap has failed is discouraged. Usually, placement of the second free flap will be more difficult technically, and chances of an unfavorable result due to recipient site infection are great.

If blood flow can be maintained through a patent anastomosis for at least four days, then in most cases neovascularity will have occurred and only partial free flap necrosis will occur. The neovascularity occurs in a centripetal pattern; thus, if a late anastomotic revision is undertaken (3 to 4 days postoperatively), one should incise down over the anastomosis and not disturb the periphery of the flap. This time period of neovascularity does not appear to occur with free flaps utilized in an irradiated field. We, as well as Kaplan, Buncke and Murray, have reported complete free flap loss at approximately two weeks postoperatively when irradiation was used preoperatively, despite having evidence of a patent anastomosis up until that time.[22]

### *Free Flap Partial Necrosis*

As many as 15 to 20 per cent of replanted microvascular flaps may be expected to undergo partial necrosis. Usually this occurs as a result of a faulty anastomosis with partial or complete occlusion developing later (after four days) postoperatively. The skin surface is usually lost, with only peripheral islands of skin remaining. The subcutaneous tissues of the flap usually remain viable and develop exuberant granulation tissue, which can be easily skin grafted. Autoepithelialization will usually occur if left ungrafted. In this instance, one may anticipate 30 to 50 per cent shrinkage of the original flap area. In our cases of partial flap loss, further reconstruction was not needed.

## NERVE ANASTOMOSES

Although the pathophysiology is quite different, complications of microsurgical anastomoses of peripheral nerves occur for many of the same reasons discussed for vascular anastomoses. In nerve anastomoses, limitation of transmission occurs because of a proliferation of fibrous tissue within the anastomotic site either misdirecting or preventing axonal regeneration. The surgeon may prevent much of this fibrous tissue ingrowth by utilizing very careful technique, but a certain degree of axonal misdirection always occurs and return of function is never complete. The goal, therefore, is to achieve a level of function that approximates that of the normal state.

Nowhere in the practice of surgery is the axiom that "it is far better to prevent a complication than to treat one" more appropriate than in the performance of nerve anastomoses. Because it takes 9 to 18 months for function across the anastomosis to be demonstrable, complications may not be apparent until it is too late to correct them optimally. To that end, each of the following considerations is important and must be carefully observed when performing a nerve anastomosis: (1) use of atraumatic technique; (2) avoidance of tension, torsion and kinking of the anastomosis; (3) debridement of heavily traumatized nerve; (4) removal of epineurium from nerve ends; (5) use of as few sutures as possible; (6) avoidance of a tight cuff about the anastomosis; and (7) performance of the anastomosis at the optimal time. We will deal with each of these considerations in some detail.

### *Use Atraumatic Technique*

Under 10× magnification, one may readily excise heavily traumatized nerve, excise epineurium from the nerve end and approximate groups of fasciculi with a minimal amount of trauma to the perineurium. Unless the surgeon is called upon to perform microanastomoses in the operating room at frequent intervals, he should practice the techniques regularly in laboratory animals. As in other aspects of surgery that demand attention to fine detail, constant practice will provide handsome rewards in the form of improved functional results.

### *Avoid Tension at the Anastomosis*

The single most important factor in obtaining a satisfactory result is the avoidance of tension at the anastomosis. When tension is present across the anastomosis, separation of the cut ends inevitably develops and results in an excessive proliferation of fibrous tissue. Although linear tension is the most common problem, torsion at the anastomosis will give a similarly poor result. Whenever a portion of the nerve has been lost or has required excision, either the remaining nerve should be rerouted or a segment of nerve at least 3 mm. longer than the resulting defect should be inserted as a cable graft so as to avoid any tension across the anastomosis.

### *Debridement of Traumatized Nerve Ends*

Unless the nerve has been transected by a surgical instrument, disruption of normal fascicular architecture will have occurred for a considerable distance proximal and distal to the injury site. The mesenchymal scar that develops within these traumatized segments is for the most part not aligned longitudinally and will result in neuroma formation. The injured portions of the nerve should be excised proximally and distally until a normal fascicular pattern is observed. When delayed anastomosis is being performed, a well established neuroma will always be present. Each fascicle should be carefully transected just before it enters this fibrous tissue. Sharp transection of the nerve with minimal trauma is best accomplished with a splinter of Teflon-coated razor blade[27] in a plane perpendicular to the axis of the nerve. Bundles of fascicles may then be matched and accurately approximated.

### *Removal of Epineurium from Nerve Ends*

The proliferation of connective tissue that impairs axonal regeneration across a nerve anastomosis has been shown experimentally by Millesi, Meissal and Berger to derive primarily from the epineurium.[28] By carefully excising the epineurium under microscopic magnification for a distance of 5 to 10 mm. back from each cut end of the nerve, axonal regeneration across the anastomosis occurs before the fibrous tissue has an opportunity to grow up to and between the nerve ends. In addition, this technique allows very precise approximation of individual bundles of fascicles, further limiting axonal misdirection.

### *Use Fine Suture Material and as Few Sutures as Possible*

The sutures themselves, so essential in stablizing the cut ends of the nerve, produce a degree of connective tissue proliferation that retards axonal regeneration. Therefore, very fine, nonreactive suture material should be used, and only as many sutures should be placed as absolutely necessary to approximate fascicular bundles. Usually only one suture is required in the perineurium of each group of fasciculi when there is no tension across the anastomosis. The #10–0 monofilament nylon suture material developed for microvascular anastomoses works nicely. Nonsuture techniques utilizing adhesives have been reported by some surgeons,[9] and the use of tissue adhesives to further stabilize anastomoses has been advocated by others.[11] Thus far, experience with the use of tissue adhesive in nerve anastomoses has been too limited to adequately assess its effectiveness.

### *Avoid a Tight Cuff about the Anastomosis*

For many years, surgeons advocated the use of vein or synthetic cuffs about the anastomotic site in hopes of further assuring the proper alignment of nerve segments and preventing ingrowth of connective tissue. These cuffs may themselves stimulate greater proliferation of fibrous tissue between the nerve segments, however. In addition, the nerve ends may swell to three times their normal size,[8] and unless the cuff is large enough to accommodate this increased size, necrosis and stenosis at the repair may occur. Therefore, if cuffs are to be used, be certain their lumen size is at least three times the nerve diameter. In most instances, however, careful anastomosis of fascicle bundles without tension makes the use of cuffs unnecessary.

***Perform Anastomosis at an Optimum Time***

There is a great deal of controversy today with regard to when is the optimum time for nerve anastomosis. When deciding upon an

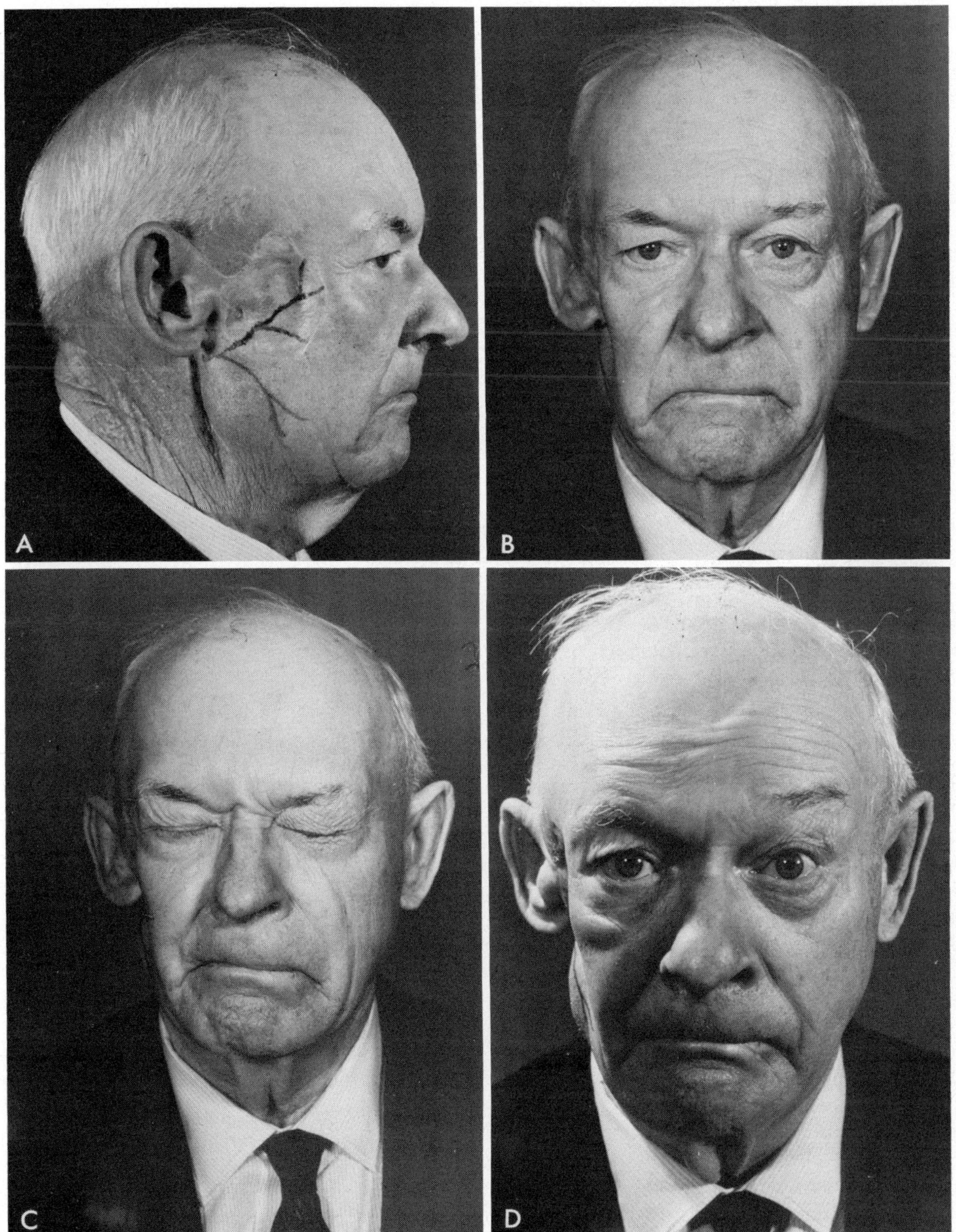


**Figure 27–5** 80-year-old man, 28 months following greater auricular nerve graft to right facial nerve. *A,* Position of nerve indicated beneath split thickness skin graft. *B,* Patient in repose. *C,* Patient in grimace. *D,* Patient demonstrates regeneration to forehead. (Courtesy of Dr. Brian McCabe, University of Iowa, Iowa City, Iowa.)

optimum time for a particular patient, several considerations are important. For instance, difficulty in identifying distal ends of motor nerves after degeneration has occurred and avoidance of nerve retraction favors early primary anastomosis. On the other hand, the pathophysiologic mechanisms of nerve regeneration, difficulty in determining extent of nerve debridement needed and the presence of a dirty wound favor delayed primary anastomosis.

#### EARLY PRIMARY ANASTOMOSIS

In the 72 hours following motor nerve transections, the distal segments may be depolarized using a nerve stimulator, making their identification very easy. For this reason, the distal segments of motor nerves should always be identified within 72 hours of injury whenever possible. Most surgeons would proceed with anastomosis at that time, particularly if the wound about the nerve injury requires approximation (Fig. 27–5).

#### DELAYED PRIMARY ANASTOMOSIS

During the first 7 to 14 days following nerve transection, wallerian degeneration occurs proximally at least as far as the last node of Ranvier. Then a period of increased metabolism in the nerve cell and active axonal budding occurs. If repair of the severed nerve is carried out at 14 to 21 days following transection, the axon end pushes across the anastomosis almost immediately,[8] before there is time for ingrowth of connective tissue between the nerve ends to block it. This usually results in less axonal misdirection across the anastomosis and a greater degree of nerve function than with primary anastomosis.[24, 45]

#### DELAYED ANASTOMOSIS

As time goes by, the neurilemmal sheaths in the distal segment of a transected nèrve gradually shrink until little room remains for axonal regeneration should anastomosis be carried out. Therefore, results from delayed anastomoses are rarely as good as those from earlier repair. Some return has been reported even after several years,[4] however, and should be attempted whenever possible.

### *Revision of Anastomosis*

If trauma or stretching across the anastomosis should occur in the early postoperative period, the anastomotic site should be inspected immediately. When trauma occurs after 6 to 12 weeks, the chance of disruption occurring at the anastomosis is much less than in the early postoperative period. A decision regarding whether to explore the anastomosis will depend on an evaluation of the degree of force exerted upon the nerve, the time elapsed since surgery and the vulnerability of the nerve in the area traumatized.

A much more difficult decision must be made when no return of function is demonstrable after 12 to 18 months. When the surgeon is satisfied with the technique utilized and no significant trauma has occurred to the anastomosis, it is best to wait a full 12 months for evidence of regeneration. If the nerve branch demonstrates no evidence of regeneration on electromyography at 12 months, the nerve should be explored for evidence of neuroma formation or disruption. When either is found, the area should be excised and replaced with a cable graft or an alternative method of reanimation should be utilized.

## Bibliography

1. Acland, R.: Signs of patency in small vessel anastomosis. Surgery, *72*:744–748, 1972.
2. Baker, S., Krause, C. J., and Panje, W. R.: Radiation effects on microvascular anastomosis. Arch. Otolaryngol., *104*:103–107, 1978.
3. Buncke, H. J., and Schulz, W. P.: Experimental digital amputation and reimplantation. Plast. Reconstr. Surg., *36*:62, 1965.
4. Conley, J., Hamaker, R. C., and Donnenfeld, H.: Long-standing facial paralysis rehabilitation. Laryngoscope, *84*:2155–2162, 1974.
5. Daniel, R. K., and Taylor, G. I.: Distant transfer of an island flap by microvascular anastomoses. Plast. Reconstr. Surg., *52*:111–117, 1973.
6. Daniel, R. K., Terzis, J., and Midgley, R.: Restoration of sensation to an anesthetic hand by a free neurovascular flap from the foot. Plast. Reconstr. Surg., *57*:275–280, 1976.
7. Daniller, A. I., and Strauch, B. (eds.): International Symposium on Microsurgery. Vol 14. St. Louis, The C. V. Mosby Company, 1976.
8. Ducker, T. B., Kempe, L. B., and Hayes, G. J.: The metabolic background for peripheral nerve surgery. J. Neurosurgery, *30*:270–280, 1969.
9. Freeman, B. S., Perry, J., and Brown, D.: Experimental study of adhesive surgical tape for

nerve anastomosis. Plast. Reconstr. Surg., *43*:174–179, 1969.
10. Finseth, F., Kavarana, N., and Antia, N.: Complications of free flap transfers to the mouth region. Plast. Reconstr. Surg., *56*:652–653, 1975.
11. Fisch, U.: Facial nerve grafting. Otolaryngol. Clin. North Am., *7*:517–529, 1974.
12. Fujikawa, S., and O'Brien, B. M.: An experimental evaluation of microvenous grafts. Br. J. Plast. Surg., *28*:244–246, 1975.
13. Harashima, T., and Buncke, H. J.: Study of washout solutions for microvascular replantation and transplantation. Plast. Reconstr. Surg., *56*:542–548, 1975.
14. Harii, K., and Ohmori, K.: Free groin flaps in children. Plast. Reconstr. Surg., *55*:588–592, 1975.
15. Harii, K., and Ohmori, K.: Free skin flap transfer. Clin. Plast. Surg., *3*:111–127, 1976.
16. Harii, K., Ohmori, K., and Ohmori, S.: Hair transplantation with free scalp flaps. Plast. Reconstr. Surg., *53*:410–413, 1974.
17. Harii, K., Ohmori, J., and Ohmori, S.: Free deltopectoral skin flaps. Br. J. Plast. Surg., *27*:231–239, 1974.
18. Harii, K., Ohmori, K., and Sekiguchi, J.: The free musculocutaneous flap. Plast. Reconstr. Surg., *57*:294–303, 1976.
19. Hayhurst, J. W., and O'Brien, B.: An experimental study of microvascular technique, patency rates, and related factors. Br. J. Plast. Surg., *28*:128–132, 1975.
20. Hayhurst, J. W., O'Brien, B. F., Ishida, H., et al.: Experimental digital replantation after prolonged cooling. Hand, *6*:134–141, 1974.
21. Jacobson, J. H., and Suarez, E. L.: Microsurgery in the anastomosis of small vessels. Surg. Forum, *11*:243–245, 1960.
22. Kaplan, E. N., Buncke, H. J., and Murray, D. E.: Distant transfer of cutaneous island flaps in humans by microvascular anastomoses. Plast. Reconstr. Surg., *52*:301–305, 1973.
23. Karkowski, J., and Buncke, H. J.: A simplified technique for free transfer of groin flaps by use of a Doppler probe. Plast. Reconstr. Surg., *55*:682–686, 1975.
24. Kleinert, H. E., and Griffin, J. M.: Technique of nerve anastomosis. Orthopedic Clin. North Am., *4*:907–915, 1973.
25. Lendvay, P. G.: Third International Symposium on Microsurgery, East Grinstead, 1975.
26. Maggio, E.: Pathologic variables of microhemocirculation. *In* Microhemocirculation. Springfield, Charles C Thomas, 1965, pp. 95–118.
27. McCabe, B. F.: Facial nerve grafting. Plast. Reconstr. Surg., *45*:70–75, 1970.
28. Millesi, H., Meissl, G., and Berger, A.: The interfascicular nerve grafting of the median and ulnar nerves. J. Bone Joint Surg., *54A*:727–750, 1972.
29. Nomato, H., Buncke, H. J., and Chater, N. L.: Improved patency rate in microvascular surgery when using magnesium sulfate and a silicone rubber vascular cuff. Plast. Reconstr. Surg., *54*:157–160, 1974.
30. Nylen, C. O.: The otomicroscope and microsurgery 1921–71. Acta Otolaryngol., *73*:453–454, 1972.
31. O'Brien, B. M.: Microvascular Reconstructive Surgery. Churchill Livingstone, Inc., Edinburgh, 1976.
32. O'Brien, B. M., and Hayhurst, J. W.: The principles and techniques of microvascular surgery, *In* Converse, J. M. (ed.): Reconstructive Plastic Surgery. Philadelphia, W. B. Saunders Company, 1976.
33. O'Brien, B. M., MacLeod, A. M., Hayhurst, J. W., et al.: Successful transfer of a large island flap from the groin to the foot by microvascular anastomoses. Plast. Reconstr. Surg., *52*:271–278, 1973.
34. O'Brien, B., Morrison, W. A., Ishida, H., et al.: Free flap transfers with microvascular anastomoses. Br. J. Plast. Surg., *27*:220–230, 1974.
35. O'Brien, B. M., Sharzer, L. A., and MacLeod, A. M.: Clinical experience in microvascular free flap transfer. In Symposium on Microsurgery. Daniller, A. I., and Strauch, B. (eds.): Vol. 14. St. Louis, The C. V. Mosby Co., 1976.
36. Panje, W. R., Bardach, J., and Krause, C. J.: Reconstruction of the oral cavity with a free flap. Plast. Reconstr. Surg., *58*:415–418, 1976.
37. Panje, W. R., Krause, C. J., and Bardach, J.: Microsurgical techniques in free flap reconstruction. Laryngoscope, *87*:692–698, 1977.
38. Panje, W. R., Krause, C. J., Bardach, J., et al.: Reconstruction of intraoral defects with the free groin flap. Arch. Otolaryngol., *103:78*–83, 1977.
39. Serafin, D., Shearin, J. C., and Georgiade, N.: The vascularization of free flaps. Plast. Reconstr. Surg., *60*:233–241, 1977.
40. Smith, J. W.: Microsurgery: review of the literature and discussion of microtechniques. Plast. Reconstr. Surg., *37*:227–245, 1966.
41. Taylor, G. I., Miller, G. D. H., and Ham, F. J.: The free vascularized bone graft. Plast. Reconstr. Surg., *55*:533–544, 1975.
42. Thurston, J. B., Buncke, H. J., Chater, N. C., et al.: A scanning electron microscopy study of micro-arterial damage and repair. Plast. Reconstr. Surg., *57*:197–203, 1976.
43. Van Beek, A. L., Link, W. J., Bennett, J. E., et al.: Ultrasound evaluation of microanastomosis. Arch. Surg., *110*:945–949, 1975.
44. Winston, J., Manalo, P. H., Barsky, A. J.: Studies on the circulation of tubed flaps. Plast. Reconstr. Surg., *28*:619, 1961.
45. Yahr, M. D., and Beebe, G. W.: Recovery of motor function. *In* Woodhall, B., and Beebe, G. W. (eds.): Peripheral Nerve Regeneration. Washington, D. C., U. S. Government Printing Office, 1956 pp. 71–97.

# TREATMENT OF SCARS

# 28

*Richard C. Webster*
*Terence M. Davidson*
*Richard C. Smith*

## INTRODUCTION

Every surgeon deals regularly with healing tissue and scar. Some scars represent normal healing of traumatic or surgical wounds and are cosmetically and functionally acceptable; some represent abnormal healing. Before attempting scar revision the surgeon should be aware of recent thinking regarding both normal and abnormal wound healing, particularly that having to do with skin.

In this chapter, the normal healing of skin is discussed briefly. A description of some of the most important factors affecting wound healing will then be given. The subject of hypertrophic scars and keloids will be discussed next. Finally, selected techniques of scar treatment will be presented.

## WOUND HEALING

For purposes of discussion, normal wound healing in skin is divided into epidermal and dermal healing. Although they occur simultaneously and depend on each other, they are distinctly different and will be described separately.

Epidermal healing refers only to the covering or closure of the wound with epidermis and the final maturation and thickening of this layer. In a wide wound not extending completely through the dermis, such as a split thickness skin graft donor site or second degree burn, a multitude of epithelial islands are left alive, separated and supported by deeper dermis. Epithelial migration over the exposed dermis occurs outward radially from these points. Usually, an intact epithelial covering will grow within 24 to 72 hours. A wound with subcutaneous tissues exposed and with dermal and epithelial edges widely separated is covered by epithelial growth occurring inward over the exposed mesodermal tissues from the epithelial edges. Epithelial covering will be complete as early as 48 to 72 hours after wound occurrence in a well approximated incision; it may take weeks to years in an infected ulcer; or it may never occur if certain conditions are present.

In the typical partial thickness incised wound involving skin left exposed to the air, bleeding soon ceases, a fibrinous clot crusts over the wound, an acute inflammatory process begins promptly and continues until healing is nearly complete and epithelial migration begins from bordering epithelial elements. Over the next several weeks, after epithelial coverage, the epithelium thickens and matures. Concomitantly, the underlying dermis reorganizes and provides a rich blood supply. The initial crust is shed in 5 to 21 days.

In an uninfected covered or "wet" partial thickness incised wound, epithelial migration often occurs quickly, since it need not burrow underneath a crust forming between and separating the wound edges. This phenomenon has been demonstrated by a number of investigators in both animals and humans. One of the clearest demonstrations is reported by Rovee and his associates.[37] On human skin, 0.3 mm. deep incisions were made and covered with Saran Wrap to give an occluded or "wet" dressing or left open to the air. Biopsies of the healing areas were taken daily. As is seen in Figure 28–1, the dry wounds required that the advancing epithelium burrow underneath crusts, as contrasted to the wet

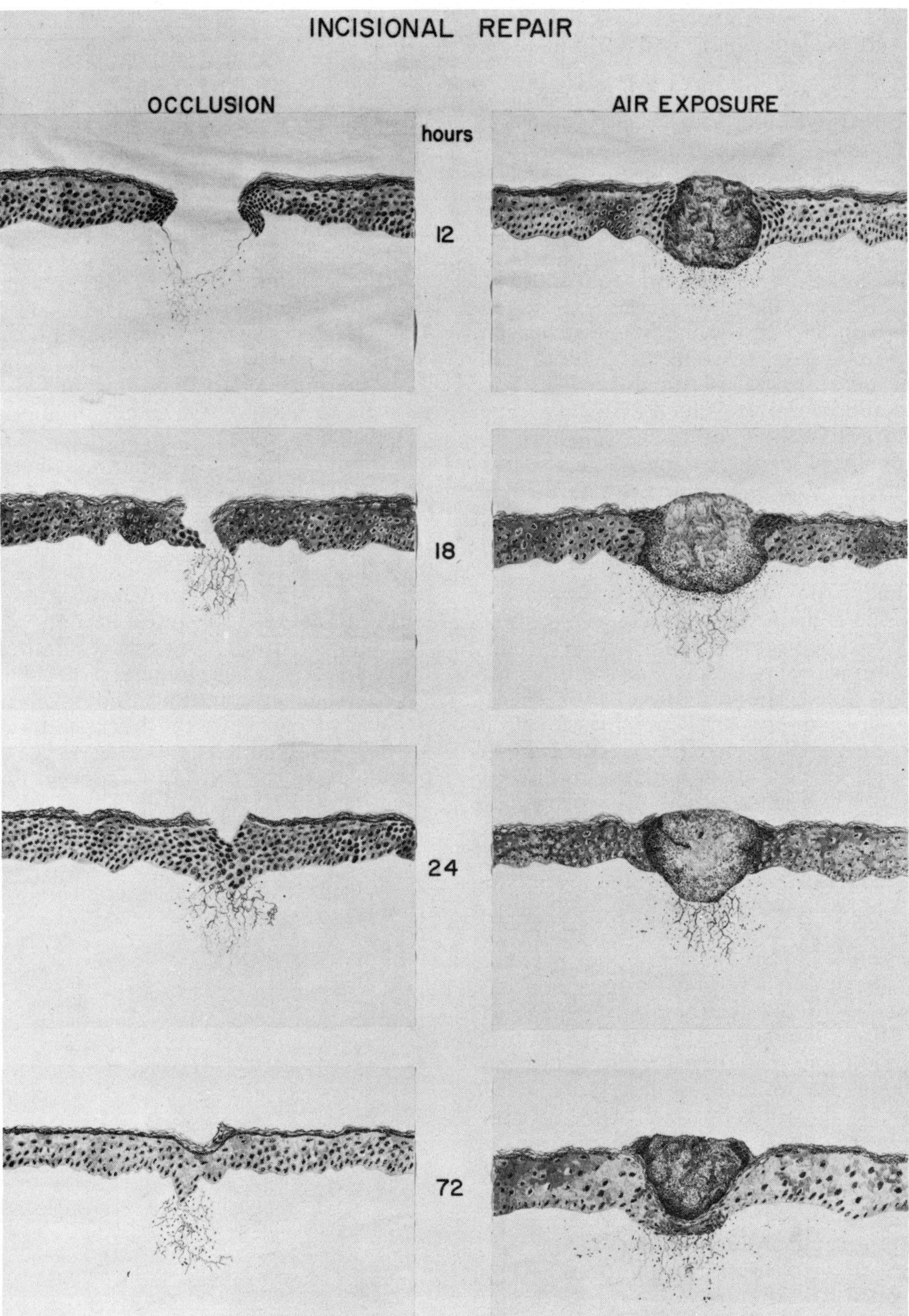


**Figure 28–1** Incisions through epidermis and superficial dermis. Epithelial healing under occlusive dressings contrasted with that in wounds exposed to air. (From Rovee, D. T., et al., Effect of local wound environment in epidermal healing. *In* Maibach, H. I., and Rovee, D. T. [eds.]: Epidermal Wound Healing. Copyright © 1972 by Year Book Medical Publishers Inc., Chicago. Used by permission.)

wounds, in which the epithelium grew straight across the incisions. The wet wounds healed sooner and without initial depressions.

This finding in wounds made by incising only through epithelium and superficial dermis cannot be applied necessarily to all partial thickness wounds, however. For example, our observations made on second degree burns, split thickness skin graft donor sites and dermabrasion cases revealed more predictable and rapid epithelial closure when the wound was exposed to light and air at room temperature than when occlusive dressings (tantalum foil, gold foil, silver foil, plastic sheeting, rubber dam and so on) prevented exudate escape, water evaporation and scab formation. Retardation of epithelial ingrowth also was noted over granulating surfaces in third degree burns and other large granulating wounds in many cases as compared with exposure treatment.

One of the disadvantages of an occlusive dressing is the increased incidence of infection as compared with that when the wound is left exposed to the air. Many authors recommend regular changing of bulky dressings or semi-occlusive dressings, such as Steri-Strips. This changing of dressings is thought to allow enough drying to discourage infection while providing a sufficiently moist wound to allow rapid epithelial covering.

Much effort has been devoted to studying dermal healing. As in so many fields, much remains to be understood. For a fuller description of the basic aspects of dermal healing, the reader is referred to pertinent reviews.[33, 1, 32, 12] Most authors agree that there are three somewhat different phases of wound healing, but these are given a variety of names. We find it most descriptive to call these (1) the inflammatory phase, (2) the fibroblastic phase and (3) the maturation phase. It is important to realize that these phases overlap each other; there is no clear-cut end to any of the three.

The inflammatory phase begins immediately with the onset of the wound. Blood clot is formed, and the raw edges of the wound ooze a fibrinous exudate. A host of local factors, such as histamine release, incite the influx of polymorphonuclear leukocytes. These immediately begin cleaning the wound. Some authors feel that this is a necessary precursor for the fibroblastic phase; others feel that it is not a necessity. The inflammatory phase lasts about one week in a clean wound. Beginning on the second day, fibroblasts are found growing into the wound along the fibrin strands. This fibroblastic activity increases rapidly for the first week and then subsides over the ensuing week or two. Concomitantly with fibroblastic ingrowth, but slightly delayed, collagen is produced within the fibroblast and begins to be deposited in the wound. The final phase, which really does not begin for one to two weeks is the maturation of this collagen. This maturation normally extends for six months to several years and, in abnormal cases such as keloid formers, may continue even longer. During this phase, collagen is reabsorbed and reproduced in such a way as to constantly strengthen the wound. This process of wound strengthening extends over time (Fig. 28–2). The entire subject of tensile strength in wound healing is complex, and the reader is referred to the article by Heughan and Hunt[21] and another by Forrester.[18] The biochemistry of collagen, so important in wound healing, involves sophisticated concepts; the interested reader again is referred to reviews[1, 12, 32, 33] and, in particular, to the work of Grant and Prockop.[19]

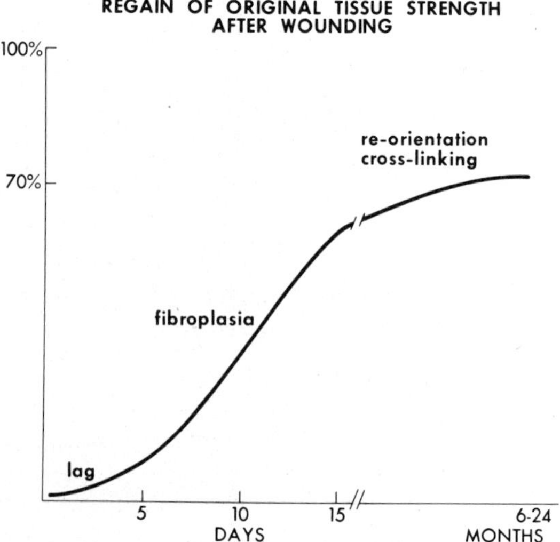


**Figure 28–2** See text. (From Heughan, C., and Hunt, T. K.: Some aspects of wound healing research. Can. J. Surg., *18*:118, 1975. Used by permission.)

## FACTORS AFFECTING WOUND HEALING

There are a host of factors capable of modifying the normal healing process. Some are listed in Figure 28–3 and will be discussed next.

Ascorbic acid (vitamin C) has been known to affect wound healing for years. Surgeons of the past knew all too well that a patient with scurvy healed incisions very poorly. Ascorbic acid is needed in the synthesis of collagen. Proline hydroxylation, which is one of the rate limiting steps in collagen synthesis, is governed by the enzyme prolyl hydroxylase. This enzyme requires four co-factors: ascorbic acid, molecular oxygen, iron and alpha ketoglutarate. Without them, collagen is not produced, and, when they are deficient, it is produced slowly. Dunphy, Udupa and Edwards[13] contrasted wound healing in guinea pigs on normal and deficient ascorbic acid diets. They found that the wounds acted identically except that there was less collagen production, and, consequently, the wounds did not mature in the ascorbic acid–deficient animals. This finding could be reversed almost immediately with the addition of ascorbic acid to the deficient guinea pigs' diet. They found no evidence that excessive ascorbic acid intake improves or facilitates normal wound healing but an excess within reasonable limits (up to 1000 mg./day by mouth) will not retard healing.

Almost all physicians have had to deal with the slowly healing patient on systemic steroids. Many plastic surgeons use steroids to inhibit excessive scar formation. The steroids most studied are the glucocorticoids, particularly cortisone and its close relatives. The question is not do glucocorticoids inhibit wound healing, but how much and why. Sandberg[38] showed that glucocorticoids inhibit wound healing most when given early in the healing process and that they did not affect healing as significantly after the inflammatory phase of healing was over. Ehrlich, Tarver and Hunt[16] studied the effects of the glucocorticoids on wound healing in rats and concluded that they decreased inflammation and fibroplasia and slowed normal healing. It seems evident to us that systemic or local steroids inhibit wound healing most in its early phases, but

FACTORS AFFECTING WOUND HEALING

1. Ascorbic acid
2. Steroids
3. Vitamin A
4. Protein deficiency
5. Zinc
6. Oxygen
7. Infection
8. Drugs
9. Sutures
10. Patient Age
11. Surgical technique

**Figure 28–3** See text.

we know that they are capable of shrinking even fairly mature hypertrophic scars and keloids if given in repeatedly adequate dosages. Lenco, McKnight and MacDonald[31] studied several steroids and their effects on wound contracture in rabbits. Large daily parenteral doses of cortisone acetate, methylprednisolone and medroxyprogesterone prolonged wound healing, slowed the rate of contracture and decreased the total contracture. Cortisone acetate alone inhibited epithelialization.

Interesting data came from research on the effects of vitamin A in restoring normal wound healing in rats on glucocorticoid therapy. Ehrlich and Hunt[15] showed that vitamin A given concurrently with glucocorticoids reverses the inhibitory effects of the steroids as measured by tensile strength of the wounds. Lately, Ehrlich, Tarver and Hunt[16] reported that vitamin A given early with glucocorticoid therapy restores the inflammatory process and stimulates fibroplasia. Heughan and Hunt[21] feel that cortisone decreases healing in the first five days by acting on the lysosomal membrane during the inflammatory phase. This action is prevented by administration of vitamin A during these first five days. Hunt stated in this paper that he had collected 50 patients in whom this finding had been verified.

In summary, glucocorticoids do inhibit wound healing predominantly during the early phases, especially the inflammatory phase. Vitamin A administered concomitantly will reverse this phenomenon in animals and appears to do the same in humans. The final answer will require further scientific experience and verification. If such verification comes and if a 5- to 7-day course of moderate doses of vitamin A is found not to diminish the effects of glucocorticoids for which they are being used, then it would seem prudent to administer this to the healing patient required to be on steroid therapy. We are seeking to verify this finding on appropriate cases at present.

Malnutrition may delay wound healing by many means. One of these is actual hypoproteinemia, which results in a decrease or a failure of collagen formation. In test animals on controlled protein starvation diets, collagen synthesis can be returned to normal by the addition of methionine and cysteine. Hunt[24] felt that humans on a starvation diet would have to lose as much as 20 per cent of their body weight before wound healing would be retarded.

There are dietary deficiencies other than vitamins and protein that will delay wound healing. One of these is mineral deficiency. Pories and his coworkers[34] noted that animals on zinc-deficient diets formed skin ulcers and were generally poor wound healers. They gave patients zinc sulfate orally and felt that those undergoing excision of pilonidal cysts healed faster if they received supplemental zinc than those not given it. Hsu and Hsu[23] monitored wound healing by the uptake of $^3$H thymidine in rats. They found that animals deficient in zinc had decreased epithelial growth. Rahmat, Norman and Smith[35] concur that rats fed zinc-deficient diets have impaired wound healing as measured by the rate of epithelialization and by the tensile strength of the wound. Elias and Chvapul[17] reported the same finding; rats fed deficient zinc diets did not heal normally. They also found that more than a normal intake of zinc does not accelerate wound healing, however. They conclude that supplemental zinc may benefit the chronically ill or malnourished but is of no benefit in normal healthy patients. Although there has been much talk in some surgical specialties about supplemental zinc, it remains to be shown that it will alter wound healing for the better in normal patients.

Oxygen tension abnormalities measured at the site of healing change the rate of healing by affecting wound metabolism and collagen synthesis. Prolyl hydroxylase requires molecular oxygen as a cofactor. Decreased oxygen concentration would be expected to decrease collagen synthesis, and, in fact, it does. Hunt and Pai[25] showed in rabbits that decreasing the ambient oxygen tension diminished the synthesis of collagen and conversely that increasing the ambient oxygen pressure increased the rate of collagen synthesis. Sophisticated experiments have correlated wound healing with available oxygen in the fluids of the wound. Even epithelialization can be altered by changing the oxygen tension in the air contacting the epithelium. Anemia has been thought to inhibit wound healing by decreasing local oxygen concentration, but, in studies to date, normovolemic anemia down to a hematocrit of 20 per cent has not altered the local oxygen concentrations and has not interfered with wound healing in incised wounds.[20]

Infection is a well known antagonist of healing. Obviously, with massive local infection, tissue is lost, sutures dissolve or are extruded and the wound dehisces. Even a low-grade infection, local, elsewhere or systemic, may exert its effects by interfering with the inflammatory phase of healing. If in the wound itself, infection also consumes oxygen locally and thereby retards healing. Much of this work has been done in rats, in which de Haan, Ellis and Willis[11] have shown that even distant sterile inflammations or a transient bacteremia have a marked effect on the early healing of skin and muscle. They demonstrated in these cases that this effect was not related to lower plasma proteins.

Several classes of drugs will retard wound healing. The effects of glucocorticoids have been discussed. Among others are certain of the anticancer drugs that exert effects on DNA and RNA and hence on protein synthesis and wound healing.

Suture material may affect healing by causing a local inflammatory response or by actually squeezing the tissues, thereby decreasing blood flow and oxygenation. Brunius[3] studied wound healing in rats and found that taped wounds healed better than sutured wounds and that wounds sutured for a short time healed better than those sutured for a longer period. Conolly and his associates[7] compared cosmesis in abdominal wounds closed with tapes or sutures. If bleeding was stopped and dead space was eliminated by closure of muscular and subcutaneous layers, taped wounds resulted in better appearing closures than those in which skin was sutured as well. Crikelair[9] investigated suture marks on pig skin and reported that tension, keloid formation and stitch abscesses increased suture marks. Needle size and even suture size did not, under the conditions of his experiment. Our experience would indicate that the degree of constriction of the tissues enclosed in the loop of the suture has more to do with leaving permanent suture marks than other factors. A tightly constricting suture will kill tissue quickly and, if the suture extends far enough from the wound edge and is large enough, a visible scar produced by the suture will result. Larger sutures are likely to be applied further out from the wound edges and to be tied tighter than finer sutures. In general, this is what does happen and why, in practice, they are likely to leave more visible suture marks. Of course, some materials left in longer than needed will produce suture marks as inflammation and infection develop from their continued presence. In general, monofilament metallic and plastic sutures employed today produce less reaction than braided suture materials and those made from historically useful natural fibers such as cotton and silk.

Older patients heal more slowly and usually with a finer scar than do children. Medical diseases such as diabetes and arterial vascular disease interfere significantly with, and may even prevent, wound healing. Surgical technique is an important variable. Crushing tissue, excessive cauterization and drying of tissue all set back normal wound healing. Excessive tension requires tighter sutures or more of them. The surgeon's choice here can produce or prevent suture marks.

## KELOIDS AND HYPERTROPHIC SCARS

Keloids and hypertrophic scars represent overactive scar production. Ketchum, Cohen and Masters[27] define hypertrophic scars as those overgrown scars confined to the original wound and keloids as those growing beyond the original wound into normal surrounding tissues. Usually, there is a balance between collagen synthesis and reabsorption. This may be called remodelling; in patients forming overgrowth of scars, the remodelling balance is upset. Collagen production has been reported to be 20 times higher in hypertrophic scarring than in the usual wound. Collagen breakdown is normal, but production is in excess. Increased wound closure tension predisposes to scar overgrowth and widening. Young people are more likely to form exuberant scar than are older people.

No one really knows the cause of keloid. There is a familial predisposition. The darker races show a 5 to 15 times greater incidence of keloid than do the lighter races.[27] This may be related to melanocyte stimulating hormone (MSH) production, according to the same authors. Ramakrishnan, Thomas and Sundararajan[36] report on 1000 patients from South India with keloids. There were 525 males and 475 females in their series. The majority of patients were from 11 to 30 years of age. Most of the keloids resulted from trauma or surgical incisions, but 114 patients reported no preceding trauma. These were called spontaneous keloid formers. The keloids were located as shown in Figure 28–4. Another excellent review of 800 Sudanese patients with keloids is reported by Crockett.[10] Blackburn and Cosman[2] examined the histologic appearances of keloids versus hypertrophic scars. One hundred sixty-three le-

ANATOMICAL DISTRIBUTION OF 1000 KELOIDS

Ramakrishnan et al[26]

| Location | Number | Location | Number |
|---|---|---|---|
| Presternal | 336 | Face and neck | 60 |
| Deltoid | 170 | Breasts and chest wall | 49 |
| Upper limbs | 126 | Penis and scrotum | 0 |
| Lower limbs | 104 | Sole of foot | 0 |
| Pinna and earlobes | 88 | Palm of hand | 0 |
| Other locations | 67 | | |

**Figure 28–4** See text.

sions were examined and a clinical diagnosis was made. They were able to correlate the histology with the clinical diagnosis in all but eight cases and felt that this was of clinical importance in predicting recurrence after excisional therapy. Kischer[30] examined normal and hypertrophic scars with the electron microscope and reported that the collagen was more tightly bound in the hypertrophic scar. Craig, Schofield and Jackson[8] measured the rate of synthesis of collagen by uptake of $^{14}C$ proline into hydroxyproline and found the uptake greater in keloids than in hypertrophic scar. Normal scar had the lowest uptake. Cohen and his associates,[4, 5, 6] utilizing proline hydroxylase activity as a measure of collagen synthesis, found that the greatest collagen synthesis was in keloids followed by hypertrophic scar. Skin and normal scar had the lowest levels of synthesis. They then examined the concentrations of histamine in these scars and found it highest in keloids and lowest in normal scars, with hypertrophic scar concentrations in between. They felt that this accounted for itching in keloids and hypertrophic scars, this itching being diminished with antihistamines. Then they examined changes in collagen synthesis following intralesional use of triamcinolone. Collagen synthesis decreased with the use of systemic steroids but not with intralesional triamcinolone, despite the fact that the keloids themselves diminished with intralesional steroid usage.

The treatment of keloids is not always successful but, if properly performed, will help most patients. Several modes of therapy are available. These include intralesional steroids, surgical resection with a low tension closure (utilizing skin grafts, if needed to keep the tension low) and radiation therapy. Ketchum and his coworkers[29] treated 195 scars, of which 22 were keloids, 29 were burns and the rest were hypertrophic scars. They found that 92 per cent of these scars showed marked regression within three weeks of intralesional injection of triamcinolone acetonide (Kenalog). They noted occasional atrophy and depigmentation, but these corrected themselves with time. Vallis[40] treated 28 cases of hypertrophic scars and keloids with intralesional triamcinolone acetonide and felt that the Dermo-Jet worked as well as needle injection. Singleton and Gross[9] treated 51 earlobe lesions, all in blacks, by excision and intralesional steroids given monthly for 12 months. Eighty-two per cent had acceptable results. Ketchum, Robinson and Masters[28] in 1971 gave a follow-up report on 500 cases of hypertrophic scars and keloids. On the trunk and extremities, they injected only triamcinolone for small lesions and treated larger lesions with excision, split thickness grafts and postoperative injections of triamcinolone. They made a point of using thin grafts 8 to 10/1000 of an inch in thickness. On the face, they usually excised the scar and then injected. They used a maximum of 120 mg. per month of triamcinolone in adults, 80 mg. per month for children 6 to 10 years of age and 40 mg. per month for children 1 to 5 years of age. Jaworski[26] treated 60 children with hypertrophic scars and keloids using weekly injections of triamcinolone for three weeks. They reported no systemic effects and moderate to good improvement in over half the cases. They also found that if the scars were going to respond they did so within the three-week period.

Hintz[22] treated 251 patients with radiation therapy over a 13-year period. Fifty-three patients were available for follow-up. All the lesions were keloids and rereceived 300 rads per treatment daily for 7 to 12 days for a total dose of 1500 to 1800 rads. He reported an overall success rate of 72 per cent. Edsmyr and associates[14] reported on the treatment of keloids in East Africa. Six having no treatment progressively worsened; 12 had excision alone; and all had recurrence within 12 months. One-hundred three had excision plus radiation therapy. Radiation doses varied from 800 rads in one day to 2400 rads in four days. Eighty per cent had no recurrence in 2 to 12 or more months. Seventeen patients had radiation alone. Two had regression of their lesions and 14 had some improvement. His recommendation was surgical excision plus 1200 rads in a single dose.

Our treatment of keloids and hypertrophic scarring will be discussed in the next section.

## SELECTED TECHNIQUES OF SCAR TREATMENT

This chapter is not the place to discuss the details of elective incision-making so that subsequent scarring will be as inconspicuous as possible and impede function as little as possible. Suffice it to say here that every surgeon, certainly those working in the head and neck, should become aware of the factors producing inconspicuous scarring. Among these are (1) making incisions away from the front of the face when feasible; (2) making them as short as they can be and still allow exposure; (3) placing them in gravitational, expression or aging lines or creases, if these are available close by; (4) using junctions of one cosmetic or aesthetic landmark with another when creases are not available; (5) hiding them in a cavity or placing them so that they will be covered by normal hair growth and styling; and (6) knowing how to break incision lines that must be made in unfavorable positions and with unfavorable lengths into shorter segments, parts of which run in favorable directions. It is better by far to prevent conspicuous scarring than to have to treat it.

Whenever possible, mucous membrane or skin closures should be effected primarily to avoid exposed granulating wounds with their build-up of fibrous tissue and subsequent contracture. Even with early primary surface closure, certain wounds, such as those encountered in cavity or inlay skin grafting, may have to be splinted with stents or other devices for as long as six months or until the contractile phase is finished. Dead space must be eliminated by deep closures of severed muscle and other structures with combinations of sutures and pressure applied by dressings and splints. More sutures, however, than needed for dead space elimination and diminution of tension should not be used. Factors, which were discussed previously, that helped in getting early normal wound healing should be employed, and those hindering normal healing should be eliminated or diminished when possible.

It is impossible to go into detail concerning the treatment of all wounds made by surgeons in their work on the head and neck, all soft tissue injuries that can occur in these areas and all scars that might be considered complications of surgery, disease or injury. We shall devote the rest of this chapter to cosmetic concepts involved in scar camouflaging, whatever might be the cause of the conspicuous scarring. At the onset, it should be said that factors producing the complication of undue scarring should be eliminated or diminished when possible and that enough time should elapse before corrective surgery is started so that tissues are vascular and pliable enough to allow appropriate treatment. If surface coverings are inadequate, they must be supplemented or replaced with resurfacing techniques using grafts or flaps of mucous membrane or skin. Vascular tissue must be provided for appropriate work on underlying structures, such as nerve and skeletal tissues, if such work is to have a good chance of succeeding. Thus, radiated tissues or dense fibrous tissues with poor blood supply may need replacement with healthier tissues from adjacent or distant areas. Compliance with these surgical fundamentals then can be followed by definitive work on deforming surface scarring.

Almost every experienced surgeon has seen certain incisions that should heal with narrow inconspicuous scars at the surface overgrow in width and height, even when no skin was excised and the closure took place with essentially no tension. If such an incision is long enough and runs in an unfavorable direction so that it is constantly being stretched and compressed along its length (vertical scar in midline of neck or one radiating out from free border of lid or lip), merely breaking the linear scar into a zigzag one with Z-plasties, running W-plasties or geometric broken line closures may end the tendency toward hypertrophy and widening. Some scars, however, treated with one of these techniques, and some running in relatively favorable directions will overgrow and widen. Prudence may be the better part of valor here; it may be advisable to put off revisional work until a young patient is considerably older. If such a scar, with or without treatment, reaches an end point in its elevating and widening, then softens and flattens but does not get narrower, it may be found helpful to use the technique of extreme eversion to achieve narrowing. In this approach, undermining is carried out, separating deeper fat from superficial fat for a distance sufficient to allow up to a 2 cm. overlap of the edges of skin. Enough permanent white sutures are then applied to superficial fat and dermis from below to produce up to a 1 cm. elevation of the skin edges when these sutures

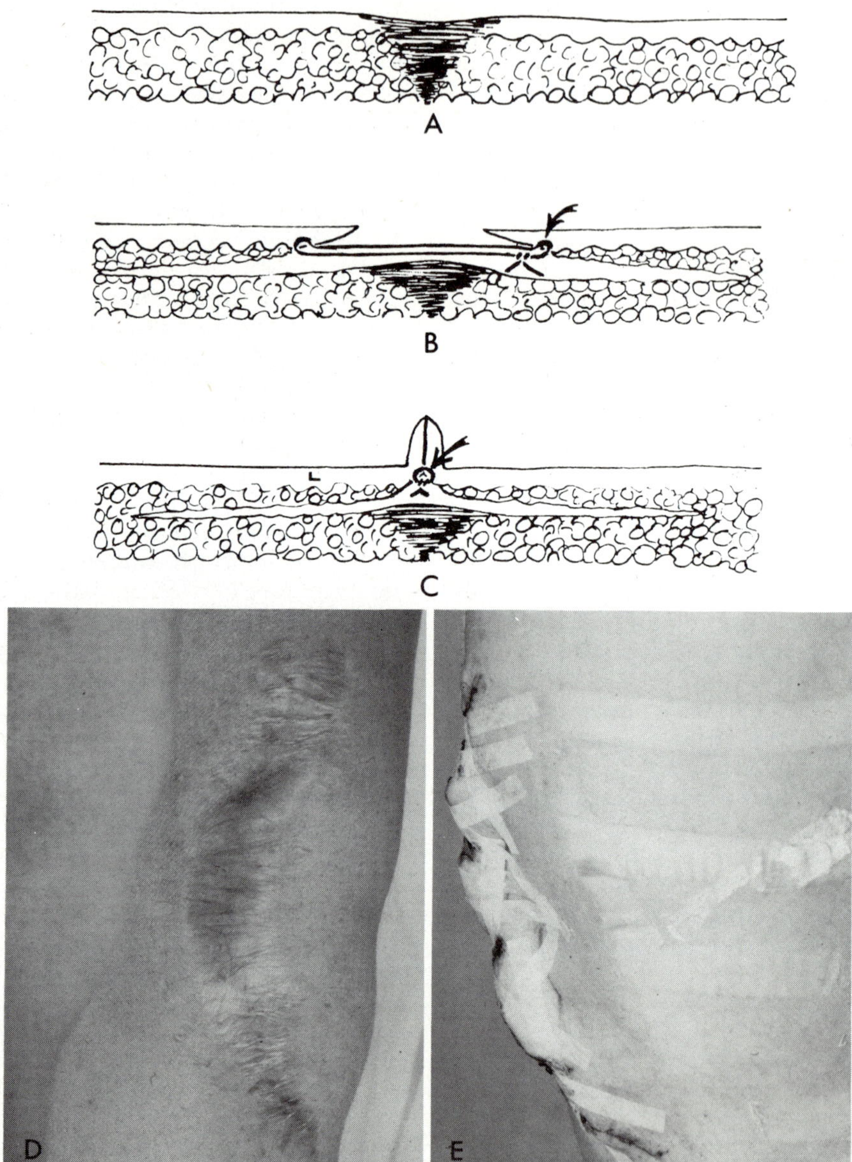


**Figure 28–5** Extreme eversion. *A*, Cross section of skin and fat showing wide mature scar. *B*, Scar epithelium and superficial fibrous tissue excised, deep scar left in place, wound edges undermined and permanent white suture applied as shown (arrow) to draw dermis to dermis about 1 cm. from wound edges. *C*, Extreme eversion produced by tying suture shown in *B* (arrow). *D*, Wide scar, anteromedial aspect left knee following orthopedic procedures to knee. *E*, Anterolateral view shortly after multiple Z-plasty and extreme everting revision. Note dimpling, indentations from crossbars of the Z-plasties and taping designed not to flatten everted edges.

are tied (Fig. 28–5). Dimpling should be slight but will be noticed from the outside as a result of pulls exerted on the underside of the dermis by each of these everting sutures. At present, we use #5-0 white Tevdek for this purpose. Epithelial and superficial dermal edges are approximated with #6-0 catgut, as will be described later, but any taping and dressing used must be applied so as not to squeeze the everted edges downward toward the level of the normal surrounding skin. Though this wound is unsightly at first (the patient and relatives must be warned about its early appearance), the everting sutures must pull out and the mountainous ridge must flatten before the surface scar can widen appreciably, unless the patient forms a real keloid. We predicate the amount of eversion and the number of everting sutures according to the width of the scar before this procedure; and we try to apply enough sutures so that almost six months must go by before eversion has ended and the surface scar can widen. Fortunately, this approach is not required frequently in facial work. It is needed more often in the neck and far more often than that in extremity work.

If the patient is a true keloid former (and we must admit that, despite histologic tests alleged to be of help in differentiating between hypertrophied scar and keloid, our practical diagnosis is made on the basis of history, location and examination), then, until we know that we can control the keloidal tendency, we dare not attempt revisional work of an aesthetic nature. Many years ago we used several classic treatments for keloid, the most helpful of which was radiation therapy. Use of the Dermo-Jet and intralesional steroids has replaced radiation in our treatment of keloids. Dermo-Jet injections with triamcinolone acetonide (Kenalog) or triamcinolone diacetate (Aristocort) have allowed us to stop active expansion of keloid into surrounding tissues, diminished the redness, induration and discomfort in the keloid itself and, in fact (despite reports of some others to the contrary), allowed us to shrink and flatten many elevated and old hypertrophied scars or keloids (Fig. 28–6). When we have noted softening, loss of redness and cessation of spread into surrounding tissues, we have felt it safe to excise those keloids that must be excised to allow narrowing of the scar. Approximately 10 to 14 days after such excision, leaving a millimeter or less of keloid at the edges, into which we apply a minimal number of #6-0 catgut sutures, we inject intralesional steroids with the Dermo-Jet. Repetitive injecting is carried out as long as there is a tendency toward overgrowth of scar. Frequency of injection and dosage are regulated downward at the first sign of atrophy or the treatment is stopped completely. If scar overgrowth begins again eventually, treatment is started again.

One of the complications of overgrowth of scar particularly bothersome and fairly frequent is supratip thickening or bulging occurring after some rhinoplasties. When this fullness or convexity first manifests itself, we inject triamcinolone acetonide (Kenalog) or triamcinolone diacetate (Aristocort) in the midline just above the tip in the center of the convexity (Fig. 28–6). If the patient is dark-haired, dark-skinned and of Mediterranean or Negroid extraction, we start right away with the triamcinolone acetonide (Kenalog), using 1/10 of a cc., the amount delivered with one standard Dermo-Jet injection. Kenalog has a more profound effect on subcutaneous scarring but also may produce more atrophy than does the Aristocort. The latter is used in patients of other extractions. One week to two weeks later, the injection is repeated if there has been no improvement. If the scarring has increased, the dosage is doubled or tripled, or, if Aristocort was used at first, we may shift to Kenalog. This routine is repeated every two to three weeks until the patient shows no signs of overgrowth of the subcutaneous supratip scarring. When extensive work has been done in the nasofrontal angle region and when hard scar is forming there beneath the skin, we use the same treatment on that subcutaneous scar mass.

It should be mentioned here that webs produced by scar contraction are generally treated by Z-plasties or transposition, rotation or advancement of local flaps into incisions made relaxing the web contractures. If the contractures are not narrow weblike ones, relaxing incisions must be made through scar to underlying vascular tissues, and the defects thus produced usually are resurfaced with split or full thickness skin

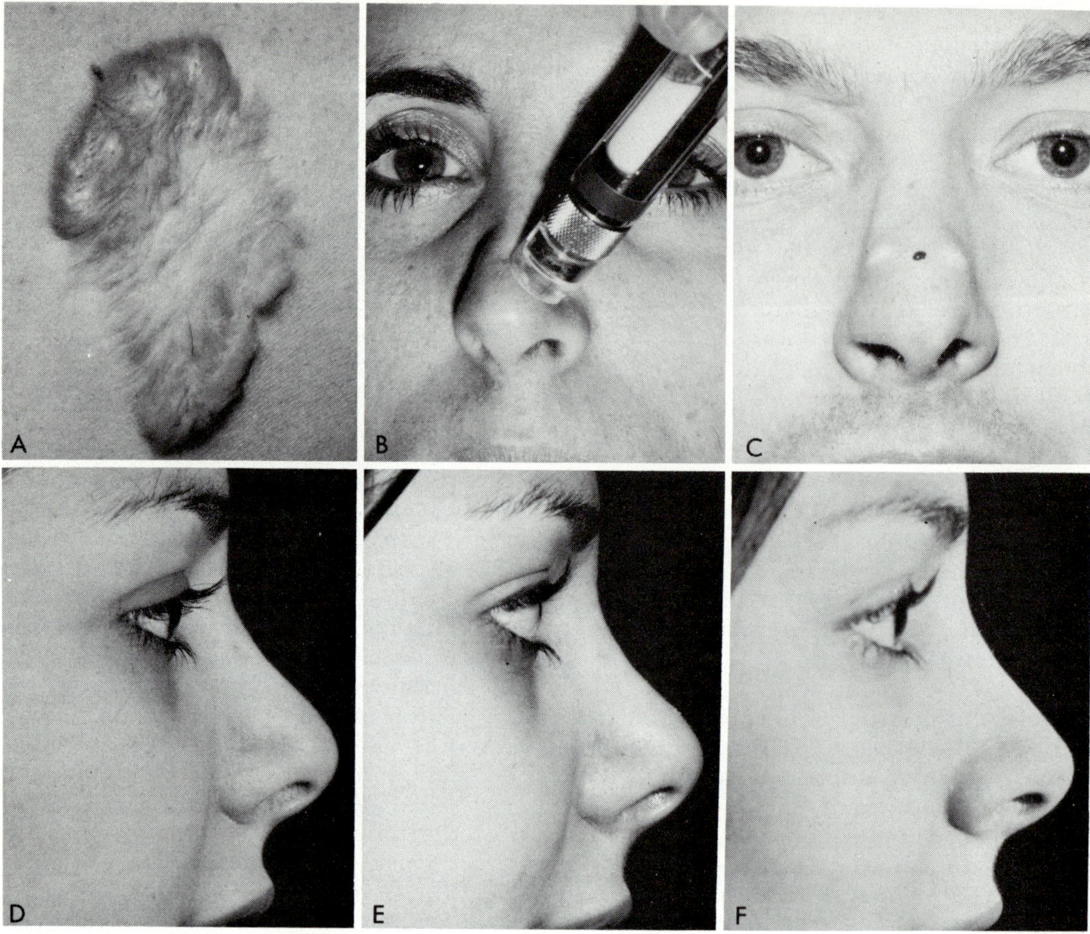


**Figure 28–6** Intralesional corticosteroid treatment of keloid and hypertrophic scarring. *A*, Old keloid of shoulder. Three stages of treatment shown. Central third treated first and most often, lower third second and fewer times and upper third treatment last and just beginning. Note 4/10 cc. Kenalog injected (4 places) with Dermo-Jet on this visit. *B*, Supratip fullness being treated with Dermo-Jet. *C*, Patient requiring three injections of 1/10 cc. each injection. *D*, Supratip convexity beginning shortly after surgery. *E*, Dermo-Jet injection (1/10 cc.). *F*, One week after *D*.

grafts. Obviously, restoration of function takes precedence over cosmesis ordinarily, although it frequently is possible to strive for both goals in the same treatment.

The rest of this discussion of our treatment of scarring will apply to the patient who does not show signs of abnormal overgrowth of scar. How do we make conspicuous scars less visible? To be inconspicuous, a scar should be (1) narrow; (2) level with surrounding surfaces, which themselves should exhibit no abnormal elevations or depressions; (3) such as to permit normal mobility of structures without producing abnormal displacement of aesthetic landmarks or contour deformities during motion of the involved areas; (4) short or broken into short lengths with as many portions placed in facial grooves or landmark junctions or running in as favorable a combination of directions as can be achieved for the involved location; and (5) one in which the short portions surgically produced should meet at angles of 90° or less. It is true that some scar lines considerably longer than 2 cm. and not located precisely in facial grooves or exactly at the junctions of one landmark with another can be inconspicuous without any angulations, particularly if exquisite plastic surgical techniques have been used in deep and superficial approximation and if much time has elapsed after the closure. When such techniques have been used and the scar widens, elevates as it runs across a concavity, indents as it crosses over a convexity, is surrounded by a more or less regular linear area of diminished beard growth or increased vascularity or interferes with normal facial mobility because of inability to stretch and contract as do the normal surrounding tissues, then the use of broken line scar revisional techniques may prove helpful. These will be discussed in more detail later.

Let us mention here that meticulous scar revisional work ordinarily should not be done if underlying structures must be treated or reconstituted or if gross depressions or elevations or excesses (Fig. 28–7) involving these underlying structures are present. It often is possible to do definitive work on underlying areas and then in the same operation to begin meticulous scar revisional work, but it is foolish to do the latter before work on the foundation is completed. Until such work is completed, aside from providing vascular, healthy coverage for the underlying surgery, final scar revisional work should not be undertaken.

A scar line wider than 1/2 to 1 mm. may

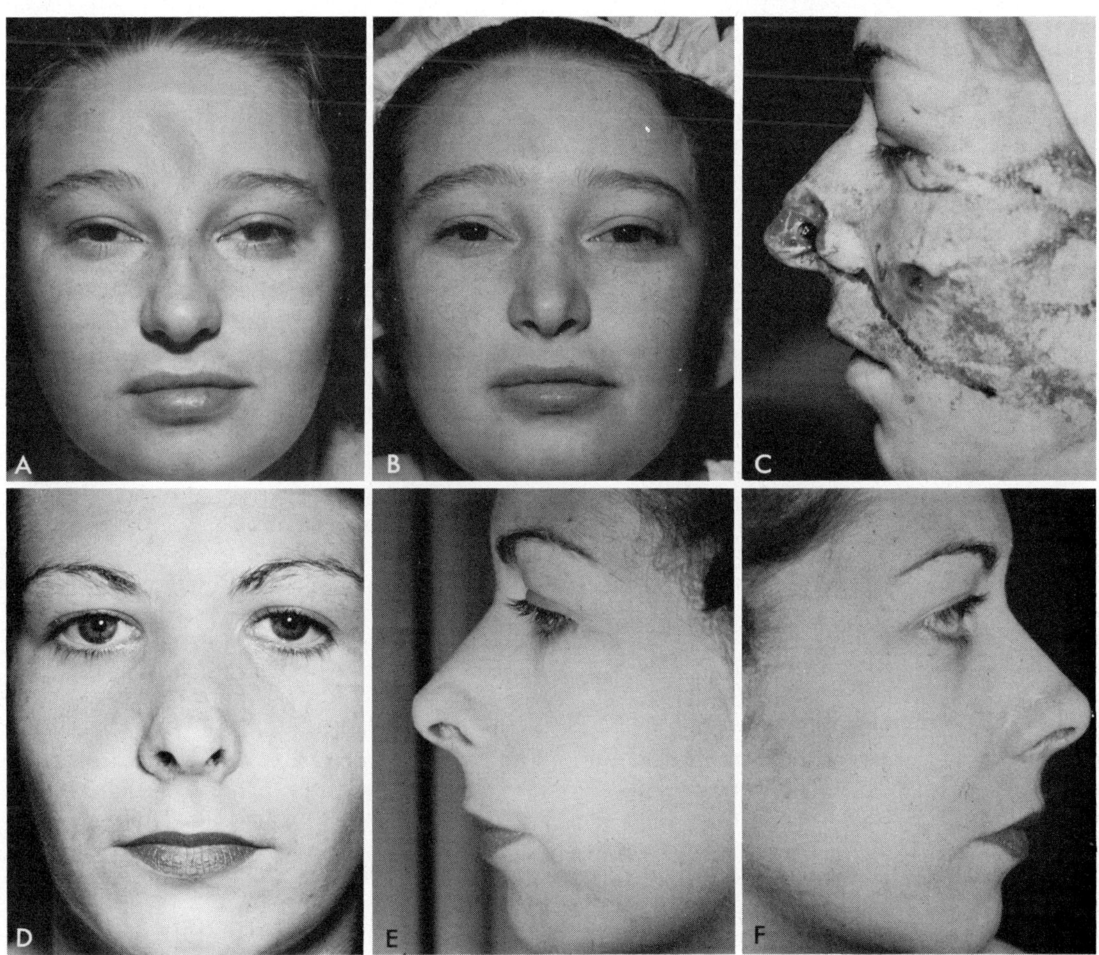


**Figure 28–7** Treatment of underlying tissue deficits or excesses. *A,* Oblique scar of forehead with skull defect to dura. *B,* Carved silicone rubber implant corrects skull defect. Geometric broken line closure then performed to finish first procedure. In hospital here for abrasive surgical completion of revision. *C,* Through and through loss of left side of tip and ala. Bony and cartilaginous excess above. Cheek avulsion and laceration. *D,* Early running W-plasty revision of cheek scarring (1951). Hump removal and superior rotation of tip allowed relative excess of skin from above (where hump had been) to be used for flap repair of tip and ala below. *E,* Wearing makeup. *F,* No makeup; note scar positioned at junction of tip and alar lobule with lateral nasal wall above. Flap from this right side has been moved to help cover left side defect.

be more visible than it has to be. Definitely, most scars wider than 1 mm. lend themselves to improvement by excision of the scar, closure of dermal and epithelial edges with fine sutures and antitension taping for up to six months following the revision. In the past, we employed interrupted white or colorless permanent sutures or continuous intradermal pull-out sutures for deep dermal approximation, using fine monofilament nylon interrupted sutures for superficial dermal and epithelial closure. For over 10 years, we have used #6-0 chromic catgut as a replacement for the fine nylon formerly employed for superficial dermal and epithelial approximation. As described previously,[41-45, 47] bites of 1 mm. or less are taken in the edges with this catgut. Ordinarily, it dissolves in three to seven days, so it is important that the edges be splinted together with antitension taping applied at surgery. The publications and videotapes just mentioned show examples of these catgut closures and illustrate variations in the techniques used over the years. Not just any #6-0 catgut will do for these purposes. The catgut must dissolve quickly, before much inflammatory reaction can build up around it. It must hold the two edges on the same level long enough so that the antitension taping does not fold or move one edge inward in relation to the other. Davis and Geck #6-0 mild chromic catgut works well in these applications and Ethicon has produced two #6-0 catguts with satisfactory rates of dissolution. No others tested work as well. Generally, careful removal of the antitension taping applied at surgery, always pulling toward incision edges, can be effected on the fourth to sixth postoperative day. Most of the catgut stuck to the tapes comes away with them, the portions in skin having been digested to the point of dissolution of continuity. The process of suture and tape removal, therefore, is essentially as painless as the removal of the tape itself. Rarely, with the tiny bites mentioned, do visible suture marks show and almost never do suture tracts lined with epithelium occur. The enormous advantage of the fine catgut closures mentioned is that we do not have to remove sutures from lodgement in skin, as permanent sutures must be removed, at the office. Although the time saved is convenient for us, the lack of pain, apprehension and possible wound separation in a struggling patient is of paramount importance to the patient.

Some scars are so wide that they cannot be narrowed in one session. Some are positioned far enough away from the junction of one landmark with another so that they cannot be moved to the junction in one procedure. It is here that the technique of multiple or *serial excision* (Fig. 28–8) often is called upon. Unscarred skin and immediately subjacent fat can be separated from deeper attachments by undermining and then pulled over the widely scarred area, often toward its center. At the limit of stretch of the normal skin flap advanced over the scar, the overlapped part of the scar is excised and the flap is sutured in place. We usually leave about 4 mm. of scar on the edge of the flap in the early stages of serial excision. Into this already scarred margin go the skin sutures of #4-0 nylon, joining this scarred edge to the edge of the scar still remaining. Six weeks to six months later, the procedure can be repeated and it will be found that the flap can be stretched still further, allowing more of the remaining scar to be removed. In the final stage of serial excision, the 4 mm. scar border is excised and our regular suture technique is used. All surgeons have seen slowly growing tumors beneath the skin exhibit the capacity to stretch the skin enormously over a period of time. Obstetricians observe this phenomenon constantly. Serial excision is merely surgical extension of these observations. With it, very large benign lesions or areas of scarring can be narrowed or moved to areas where one aesthetic landmark meets another. In serial excision, one must be aware of pulls put upon distant structures and should remember that underlying structures such as bone may be influenced and their shapes modified in the still growing patient.

Once the scar is narrow enough, the surgeon must determine whether or not it should be broken into shorter segments, some of which run in favorable directions. There are three main techniques used for this purpose.

*Transposition flap* maneuvers, including *Z-plasties,* may be used to draw adjacent tissues across a scarline. The tissue interposed in-

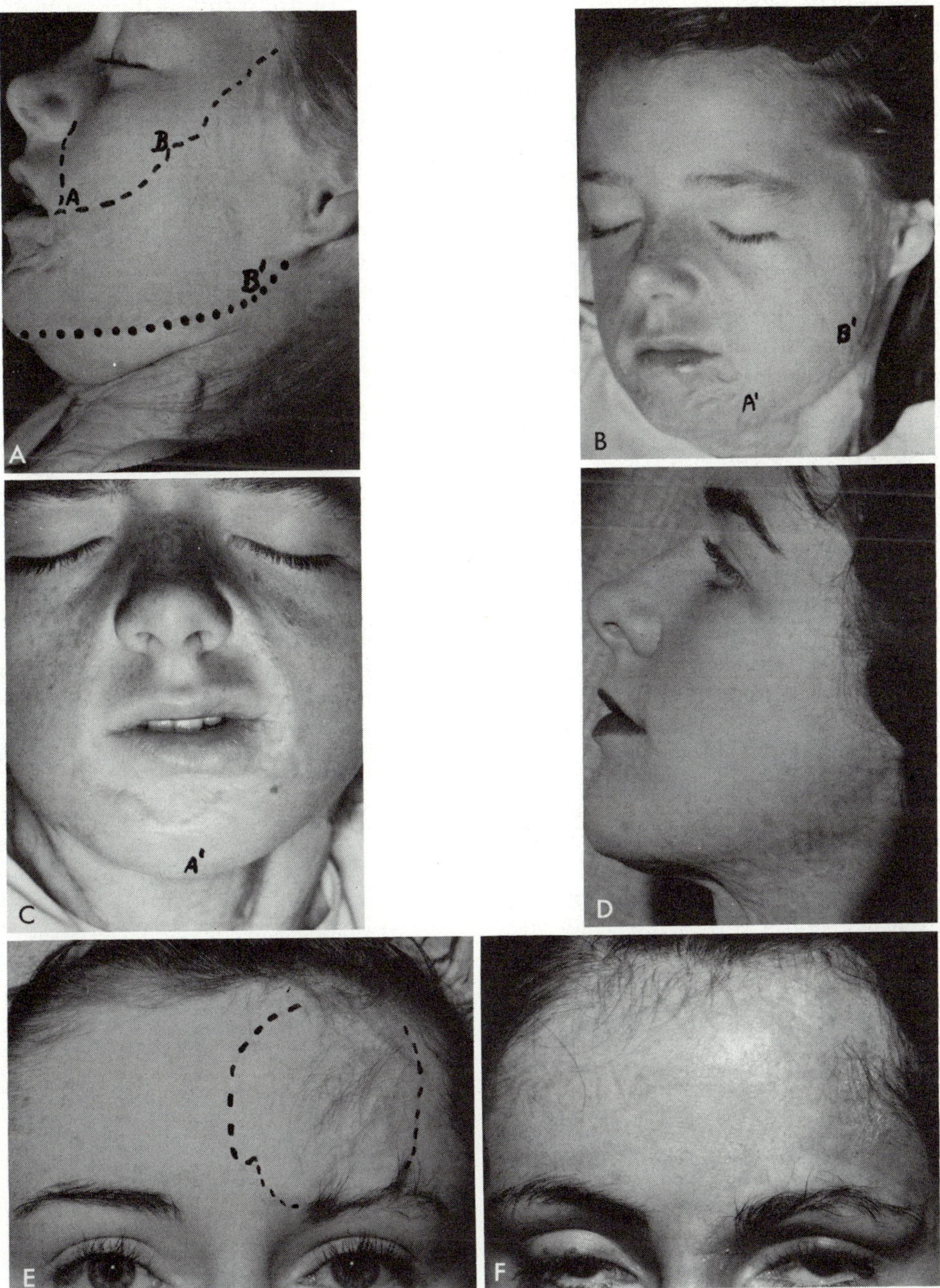


**Figure 28–8** Serial excision. *A,* Burn scar and skin graft of cheek and chin to be resurfaced with good facial skin shown above dashed line. B will be moved to B¹; A will go to midline of chin at junction with submental region. Several steps three to six months apart required. *B,* Triangular flap being stretched to replace old scar and graft. *C,* A has moved to A¹ to meet its counterpart from opposite side. *D,* Facial skin coverage now almost entirely from cheek flap shown above dashed line in *A. E,* Unsightly skin graft on forehead. Dashes indicate its extent. *F,* Most of graft removed in serial excision; even forehead tissues can be stretched over a period of time.

creases the distance between two points at the ends of the former scar line and, if the interposed flap or flaps are short and narrow enough, may make the long unfavorable scar less conspicuous. If the long scar runs in such a direction that repetitive required motions stretch and compress it along its length, it is likely to overgrow in height and width and ultimately to contract along its length. It tends to remain unstable, indurated and reddened, and the patient may be bothered by itching, burning, stinging and tenderness. The mere process of narrowing this kind of scar may require interruption of the scar along its length by grafting or transposition flap maneuvers so that the necessary motions change angles in an accordion pleat-like arrangement of the scarline rather than stretch and compress a long straight mass of scar tissue. Long scars tend to contract along their lengths, pulling more mobile landmarks or tissue toward the less mobile ones, indenting a convex surface and producing an elevated ridge of linear scar when running across a concavity. Z-plasties and other transposition flaps or grafts are used to prevent or correct these effects. Even small Z-plasties or transposition flaps tend to produce a tight line at the junction of the two transposed flaps, that is, tension along the line now crossing the original direction of the long scar being worked upon.

The crossbars just mentioned may be hidden well in certain cases when they are placed in a normal facial groove such as the alar-labial groove, the buccolabial groove, or the mentolabial groove. If they must be placed in a convex area instead of in a normal groove, then they will tend to produce an indentation of the convex surface (Fig. 28–9). We used ever-smaller Z-plasty flaps that we called "Cosmetic Z-plasties" to produce sharply angulated incision line lengths for aesthetic improvement of certain scars until 1947.[41, 46] Flaps interposed across the scarline increase the distance between the two points mentioned on that line by compressing or pushing them apart. This is manifested by a small elevation on either side of the crossbar. The crossbar itself tends to cut into or indent the convex surface. The equivalent of two rounded or ridged mountains on either side of a linear valley is produced. Shadows and highlights tend to make these little deformities more visible than they should be. Moreover, our ultimate step in camouflaging scars is that of shave excising or abrading to get a smooth surface without mountains and valleys. If the top of the elevation is a millimeter or more above the depth of the valley, shave excising or dermabrading 1 mm. or more of epithelium and dermis is likely to leave easily perceived sequelae, including enlarged pores, hypopigmentation and telangiectatic changes.

In 1947,[41, 46] it had become apparent that another approach was needed. We wanted zigzag closures without repetitive depressions and elevations produced along the length of the scar. We began excising small triangles of normal skin and fat on either side of the scarline, these triangular exci-

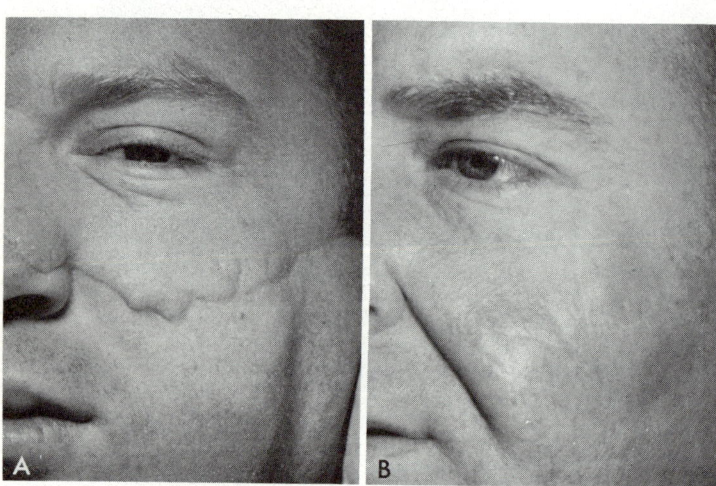


**Figure 28–9** Cosmetic Z-plasties. *A,* Scar from windshield accident. *B,* Crossbars of Z-plasties have "dug in" to extent that even with shave excision and abrasion deep enough to produce visible vascular and other changes in the convexities of the cheek and the Z-plasty flaps, we have not been able to get acceptably flat or smooth surfaces. Shadows and highlights result.

sions being arranged to produce triangular flaps that would fit into appropriate triangular defects on the opposite side. Undermining beyond the bases of these flaps produced two large advancement flaps, each one with sawtooth edges. We called these "advancement flaps with serrated edges" and the closures produced by their use *"zigzag closures."* We used and taught these techniques, now called *"running W-plasties"* (Fig. 28–10), for several years to the exclusion of most other approaches and still use them in certain cases. They had the advantage of not producing elevations and depressions with disparities in surface levels of 1 mm. or greater. Also, two points along a contracted linear scar separated by excision of the contraction were not pulled together toward each other by scar contraction after zigzag closure as much as in a scar excision with repair in an uninterrupted linear fashion. What happened in the contractile phase was that the angles of the running W-plasty tended to become slightly more obtuse. If still greater separation of two points at the ends of a linear scar was needed, we either added one or more small Z-plasties to the zigzag revision or carried small incisions outward from the apices of the triangular defects, into which the tips of the triangular flaps from the other were advanced (Fig. 28–10). This advancement into the linear

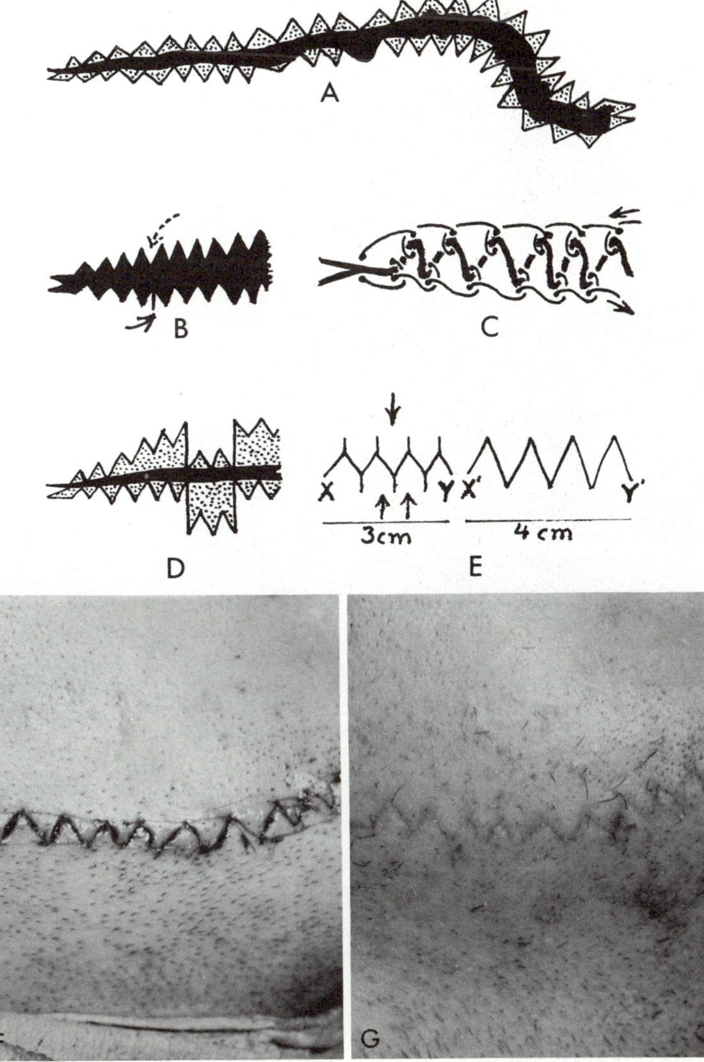


**Figure 28–10** Running W-plasty. *A,* Black shows scar to be excised. Stippled areas show triangular pieces of unscarred skin and fat to be removed to produce advancement flaps with serrated edges. Note M-plasties at each end used to avoid undue extension of incisions. *B,* Correcting error in planning. One triangular flap too many will go into slit defect on other side made for its reception (arrows). *C,* Continuous locking #6-0 catgut suture locks tips of flaps into corners of defects. *D,* Attempts to lessen predictability of pattern by greater excisions and irregular offsets produce wider defects leading to greater wound closure tension. *E,* Small slits made at ends of defects so that Y to V wedging effects can be produced will lengthen the distance between two points along the scar. Depressions and elevations produced limit this technique to short parts of a long scar revision, however. *F,* Suturing detail shown. Note fine catgut going down one side and up the other. Taping further joins the edges. *G,* Same area two weeks later. Observe regularity of pattern.

A

B

C

OR

D

OR

E

OR

INFINITE CHOICE

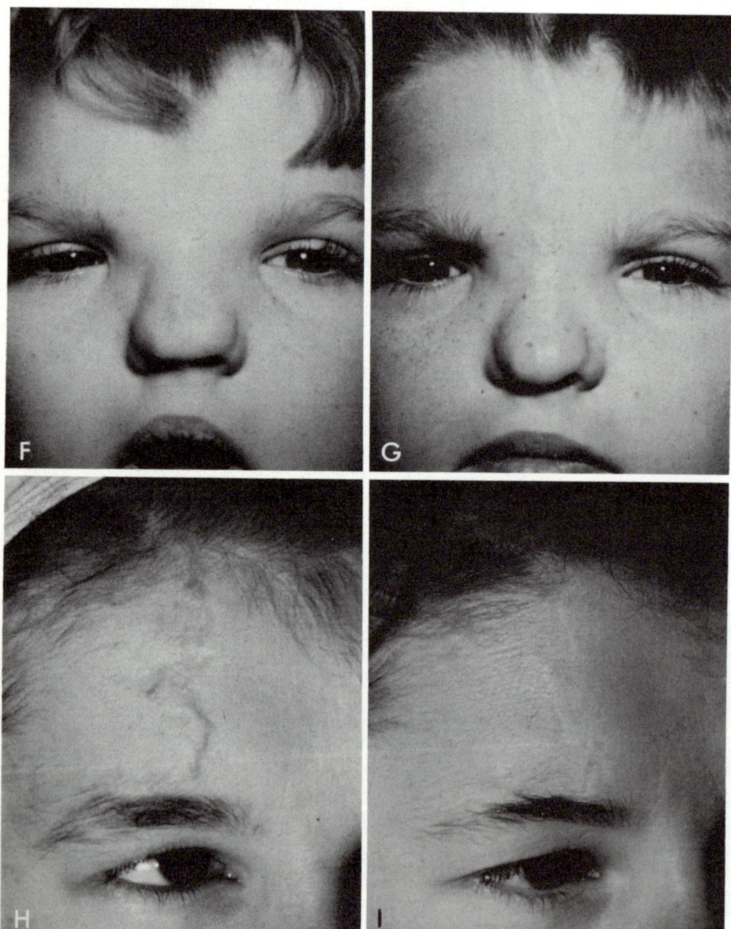


**Figure 28–11** Predictability of running W-plasty versus geometric broken line closures and lengths of segments of these revisional techniques. *A,* Running W-plasty. If the observer perceives two or more triangles in the row (solid line), he is likely to predict accurately where others will be (dashed line). *B, C, D* and *E,* Geometric broken line closure. Perception of part or all of the solid line does not allow accurate prediction of the rest of the closure (dashed lines). *F,* Hypertelorism, preoperative. *G,* Modified running W-plasty on forehead more visible than geometric broken line closure portion below. *H,* Forehead scar. *I,* Linear segments much too long; 6 mm. lengths or less would be more appropriate.

defects, of course, produced elements of compression, since each triangular flap, instead of merely fitting into a similar sized triangular defect, now was wedged between the edges of the skin separated by these small additional incisions. The reader can imitate this effect by putting his fingertips together and then sliding the fingers of one hand between the fingers of the other. The index fingers will be spread farther from the little fingers than they were before the advancement. In essence and in plastic surgical terms, this maneuver, superimposed on simple zigzag closure, is the equivalent of multiple tiny *Y-V maneuvers.* Running W-plasties have the advantage of relatively simple and quick planning and tailoring and are almost a necessity in dealing with curved portions of long linear scars, if it is elected to revise such a scar with broken line techniques. It is far easier to fit a narrow triangular flap into a wider triangular defect and close the wound by simple changes in the angulation at the apices than it is to fit a narrow rectangular flap into a wide rectangular defect.

One disadvantage of the running W-plasty approach caused us to keep looking for a better fundamental technique. This was the regularity of the patterning. The observer's eye and brain, perceiving two triangle tips, could predict much of the rest of the pattern and could "read" the scar more easily than if deliberate "randoming" was used. If the surgeon was willing to go farther out from the edges of the linear scar on either side, he could make short and long triangles and thus achieve some aspects of randomization, but then the edges had to be brought together under more tension. Even with antitension taping, this tended to result in a wider scarline ultimately.

We decided to try varying combinations of triangles, rectangles and squares. For want of a better term, we called this approach "*geometric broken line closure.*"[41] By varying the widths and lengths of the geometric shapes as well as the order in which the three shapes themselves were used, a random arrangement could be produced so that, even if the observer's perceiving eye and brain saw two parts of the final scar, it would be almost impossible to predict exactly where the scar line might be somewhere else along its length (Fig. 28–11). Although the eye might travel a short distance along the scar line, it would soon come to an acute angulation and tend to hurtle out into adjacent nonscarred skin. We had already observed that flaps with edges longer than 6 mm. tended to be more conspicuous on most parts of the face than ones with shorter edges. In some areas, such as the philtral region, best results were achieved with the segments being as short as 2 mm. These observations were found to apply to geometric broken line closures as well as to running W-plasties.

If the long scar already runs in a favorable direction but not in an aesthetic landmark junction or in a groove or crease, it may be wise merely to revise it by meticulous layered closure followed by appropriate splinting. The next step in complexity of repair would be to break its length with one or two small Z-plasties, resorting to running W-plasty or geometric broken line closures only when the simpler techniques do not produce the desired result. If the original long scar runs in an unfavorable direction, the crossbars produced in geometric broken line closures should be planned so that they run in the most favorable direction. The parts still left running in the unfavorable direction are short, vary in length and are separated by up to 6 mm. of normal nonscarred skin (Fig. 28–12). In the planning of a running W-plasty or geometric broken line closure, to avoid extending the excision beyond the length of the scar being improved, the M-plasty technique (Figs. 28–10 and 28–12) is of value. Thus, two angles of approximately 30° are provided at the end of the excision to avoid excising far beyond the end of the scar to get one 30° angle. This technique tends to prevent a protrusion of more than 1 mm. at the end of the scar when the flaps are advanced in the closure. Despite the most careful planning, it is possible at the end of trimming to have, for example, 13 flaps on one side and only 12 defects on the other. Conversion of one rectangular or square flap into a triangle and a slit made opposite it for its reception on the other side will save the day (Fig. 28–12). Actual planning of one of these closures is shown in Figure 28–13.

In excising the old scar, it is not advisable to dissect out all of the deep scar if this fibrous tissue is stable, not limiting motion

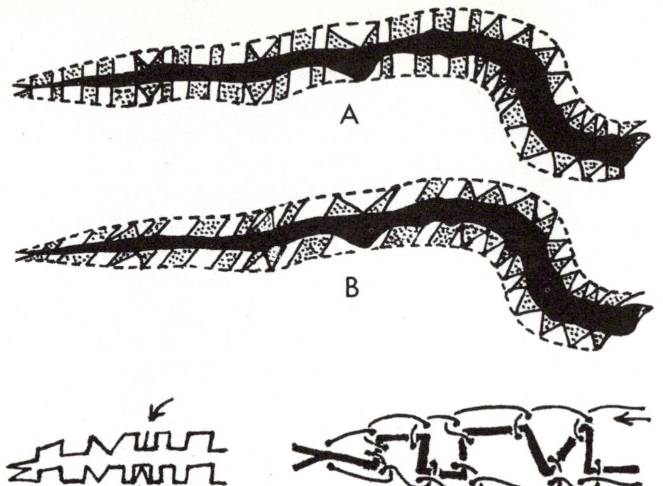


**Figure 28–12** Geometric broken line closures. *A* and *B*, Planning. In one case, the favorable incision direction is at right angles to the long part of the scar; in the second, oblique to it. Dashed lines indicate where bases of flaps and ends of defects are to be. Stippling shows areas to be excised to tailor the two sides of the wound. Note running W-plasty used where curved scar would lead to wound edges of quite different lengths on opposing sides. Observe M-plasties. *C*, Correction of improper planning by conversion of rectangle into triangular shape to fit into slit made in rectangular portion on other side of wound (arrows). *D*, Suturing detail.

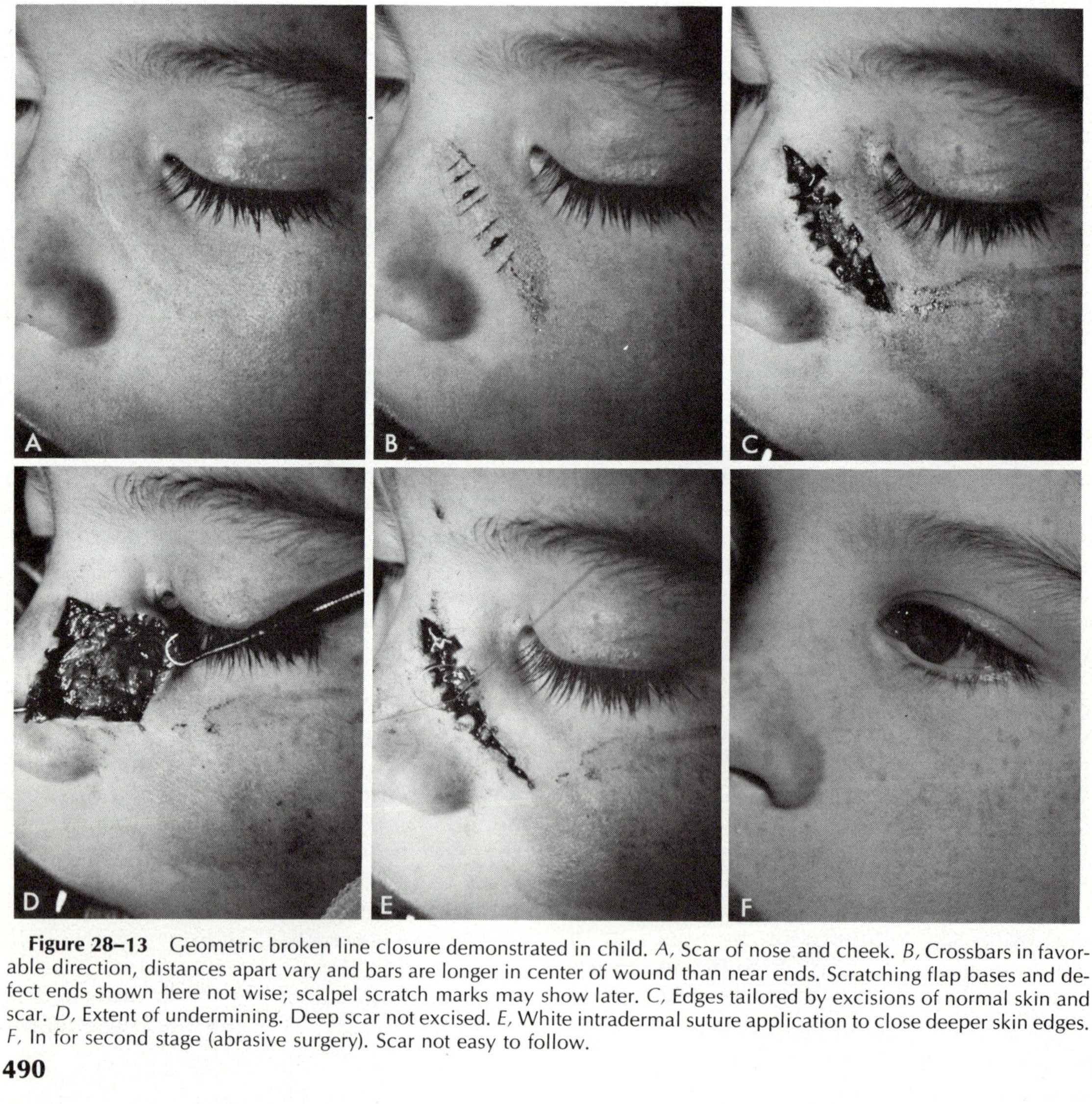

**Figure 28–13** Geometric broken line closure demonstrated in child. *A*, Scar of nose and cheek. *B*, Crossbars in favorable direction, distances apart vary and bars are longer in center of wound than near ends. Scratching flap bases and defect ends shown here not wise; scalpel scratch marks may show later. *C*, Edges tailored by excisions of normal skin and scar. *D*, Extent of undermining. Deep scar not excised. *E*, White intradermal suture application to close deeper skin edges. *F*, In for second stage (abrasive surgery). Scar not easy to follow.

and not producing deformity by its bulk and if its removal would in any way jeopardize deeper or surrounding structures. Stable scar can act as an excellent filler. After undermining far enough away from the old scar so that the flaps can be brought together under reasonable tension without having to compress unduly the underlying tissues from which they have been separated in the undermining, and after getting good hemostasis, closure can begin. In rare cases, it may be advisable to put permanent plicating sutures in the underlying tissue to help take tension off the closure of the flaps themselves. For this purpose and for deep dermal closure, we presently use #5-0 white Tevdek. Enough of these are applied in the deep dermal closures so that the epithelial edges of the triangular or rectangular flaps are almost in contact with their counterpart defects all along the length of the wound. These are applied so that the knots face away from the epithelial surface. A continuous, locked, #6-0 catgut suture (mentioned earlier) is used for superficial dermal and epithelial closure. Generally, except at the extremities of the incisions, this catgut stitch catches only the tips of the flaps. Time is saved and flap tips stay better in the angles of the defects made for their reception if the continuous locked stitch goes down one side from end to end and then back on the other side to the beginning, rather than attempting again and again to cross over the incision line. The latter would unlock the loops holding the tips of the flaps in place. This recommended closure leaves little gaps at crossbars and along the edges of the rectangular flaps and defects but not where tips of flaps meet angles of defects. These gaps are closed with antitension taping. We have used Ethistrips and Steri-Strips for this final approximating and for postoperative splinting of the wound. Suturing and taping details are shown in Figure 28–14.

Over the years, a fair number of patients

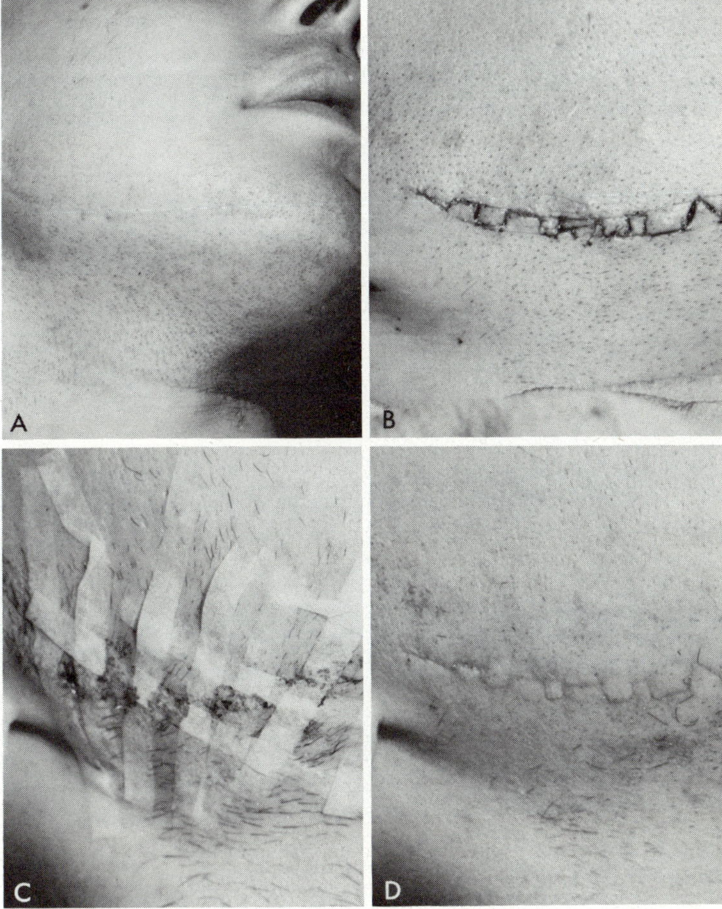


**Figure 28–14** Geometric broken line closure: taping and suturing details. *A,* Old scar revised in linear fashion several times previously. *B,* Continuous #6-0 catgut locking suture running down one side and up the other joins two tips of each rectangular flap to the opposing corners. *C,* Antitension taping applied at surgery shown six days later. *D,* Same wound two weeks postoperative.

have required only geometric broken line closure without further steps in revision (Fig. 28–15). The same remark applies to running W-plasties. In each, however, the incision line surrounding the small flap may indent slightly and the flaps themselves may mound outward or protrude slightly. These slight level discrepancies, if sufficient to catch highlights and produce shadows, require a second stage (to be mentioned in a few moments) if the most professional cosmetic result is to be achieved.

Geometric broken line closures have some disadvantages. The planning must be precise. It and trimming are even more time-consuming than they are for the running W-plasty, which itself takes appreciably more time than does a straight linear closure. Curved portions of a long scar are more easily handled with the running W-plasty than with geometric broken line closure. If the scarline itself widens or overgrows more than 1/2 to 1 mm. or gets infected, the final scar from any broken line closure may be more visible than a linear scar might be. Rarely should they be used in closing lacerations in a primary maneuver, and they certainly should not be used when the patient's general condition or other injuries preclude investment of the extra time required for their execution.

Assuming that (1) the steps taken in the first stage revision and the taping carried out at home with flesh colored Micropore tape until the scar shows no evidence of further widening have produced a truly narrow scar line and (2) the slight elevations and depressions mentioned a few moments ago have reached the stage of showing no further spontaneous flattening after the taping has ended (often up to six months to over a year after surgery), then the second step is performed. This consists of one or more of three maneuvers with a possible fourth approach being occasionally used. The goal is to take down the protrusions, elevate the depressions and to make slightly elevated edges less easily discernable. Shave excision and abrasion (Fig. 28–16) are used for treating the protrusions involving the unscarred skin adjacent to the depressed scarline. It should be emphasized that neither of these modalities are very useful for permanently eliminating protrusions of scar itself; they are used on normal but relatively elevated epithelial and superficial dermal elements. If just a few elevations require treatment, we often use razor blade shave excision and scalpel abrasion to get rid of the carving marks left when the razor blade shave excision is finished. If many protrusions are present, we usually freeze the protrusions and use mechanical dermabrasive equipment. In the past, for elevating depressions, we tried injectable silicone, Gelfoam, fibrin foam, tiny strips of dermis and thin strips of stable scar from which all epithelium had been removed. The injectable silicone did not work well for this purpose. It was difficult to confine it to the area just beneath the indented scar, and in a few cases, we noted slightly more protrusion of the already elevated areas adjacent to the scar line itself. Although we found it of

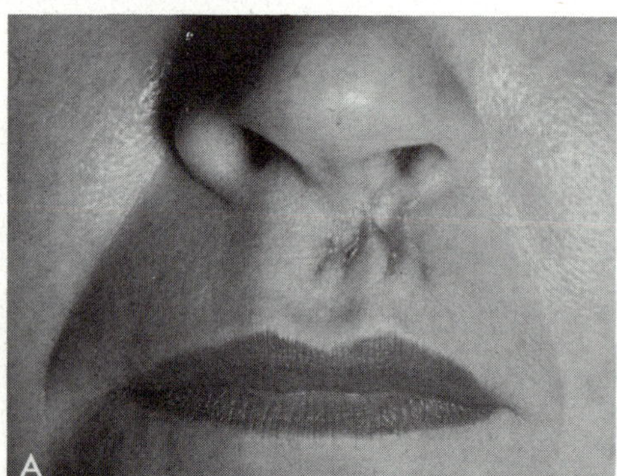


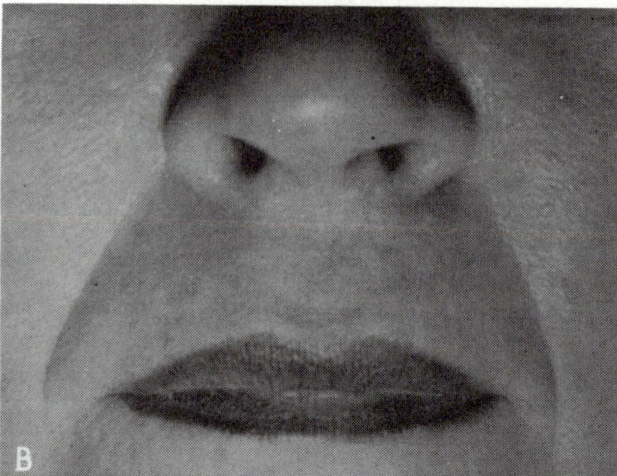


**Figure 28–15** Conspicuous scarring and traumatic tattoo of lip. One stage geometric broken line closure. *A*, Preoperative. *B*, Three months later.

great value in elevating broad areas of depression, for this specific purpose of elevating narrow depressed scars it was not as useful as the other modalities just mentioned. Of these, the more useful and permanent were those using the patient's own dermis or stable scar. Slight but sharp edges of normal skin slightly elevated above a depressed scar may be made less discernable by cross-hatching (Fig. 28–16). Here, incisions less then 1 mm. apart are made in at least four directions across the depression and the elevations adjacent to it. They must not be made all the way through the dermis. If they do go through dermis, they are likely to produce permanently visible scarring. If, as recommended, they go less than a millimeter into dermis, the fibrous tissue that forms along each length ultimately contracts and seems to slightly elevate the valley and to pull down the "cliff top" on either side of the valley or "gulch." In addition, the cross-hatching tends to break up the linearity of the elevated edge.

With the techniques mentioned, Z-plasty or local transposition flaps, running W-plasties and geometric broken line closures, often used in combinations, and with the adjunctive secondary maneuvers of filling, shave excision, dermabrasion and cross-hatching, when these are known to be indicated, we have been able to improve over

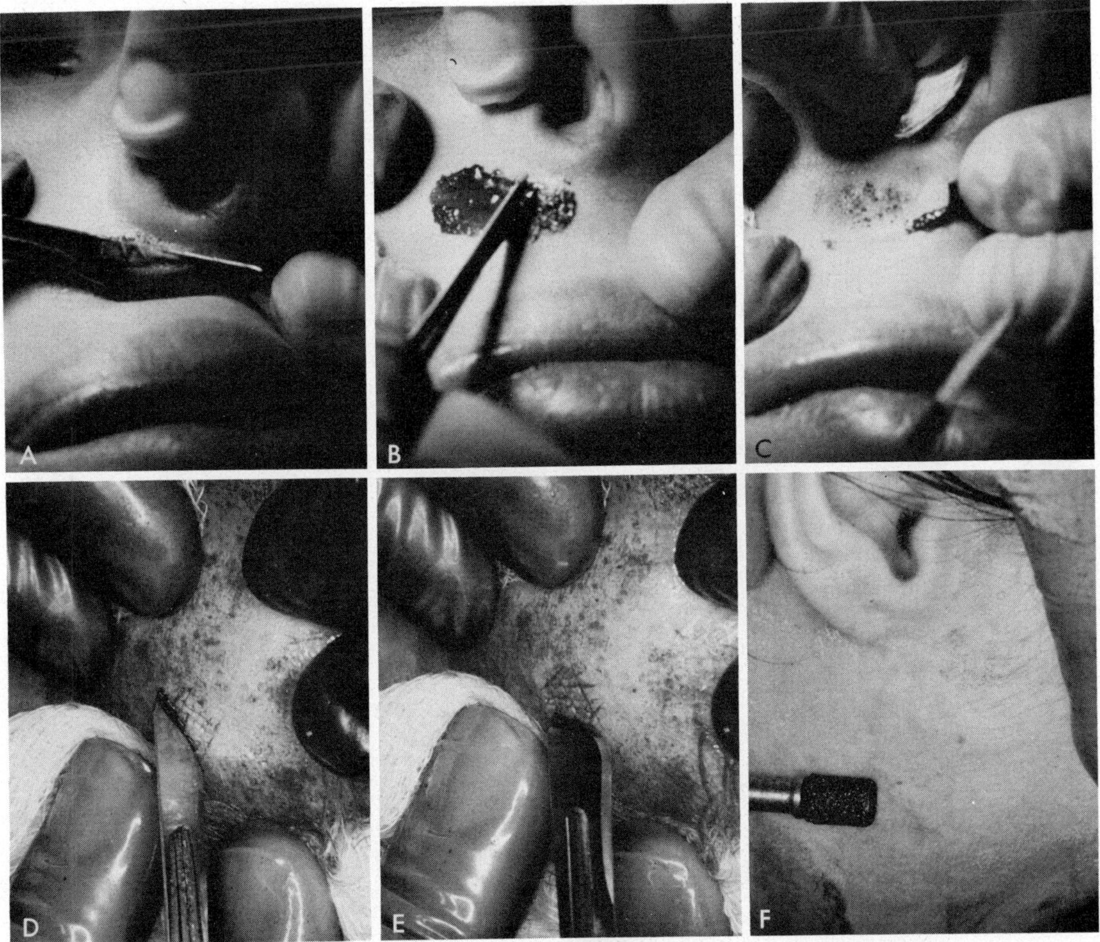


**Figure 28–16** Shave excision, abrasive surgery and cross-hatching. *A,* Elevations adjacent to upper lip being shaved off with razor blade in curved hemostat. *B,* Scalpel abrasion for removal of shave excision carving marks. Skin tensed while curved scalpel blade scrapes rapidly from side to side. *C,* Flat surface produced. *D,* Cross-hatching around punched out cheek scar. Do not incise through dermis into fat. *E,* Incisions made in four directions. *F,* Larger areas requiring abrasion are frozen and dermabraded with rapidly revolving equipment.

the years many scars not handled well by other techniques (Figs. 28–17 and 28–18). The head and neck surgeon should realize, as should all others, that no technique available today will produce a scar as good as no scar at all. He should become comfortable in working with scars that come to him or that he must produce in order to get his other work done, however. Obviously, it is hazardous to say that "there will not be any scar," and it is scientifically and ethically improper to tell a patient that there is any certainty that a scar will be inconspicuous. It *is* safe to say that most scars can be made relatively inconspicuous. Without question many patients are walking around today with scars far more visible than they need to be, often because they and their surgeons do not know that anything can be done to make them cosmetically more acceptable. Learning what can be done is worthwhile, but much more important is the surgical goal of getting to live comfortably with scarring. Our hope is that this chapter will help the surgeon do just that.

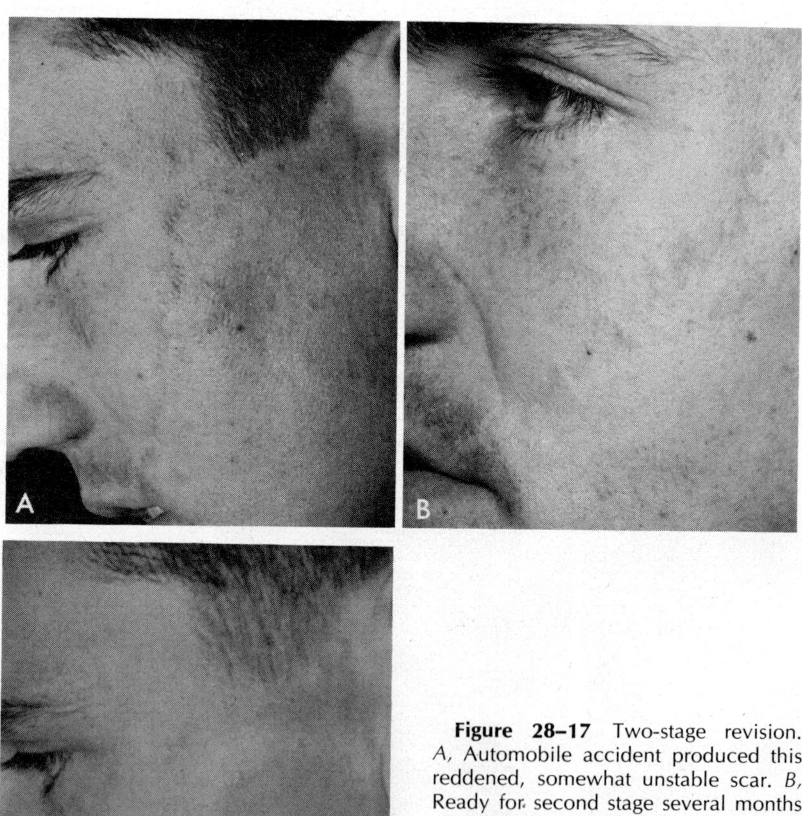


**Figure 28–17** Two-stage revision. *A,* Automobile accident produced this reddened, somewhat unstable scar. *B,* Ready for second stage several months after geometric broken line closure revision. *C,* Several years after two stage revision. Shave excisional and abrasive surgery done in second step.

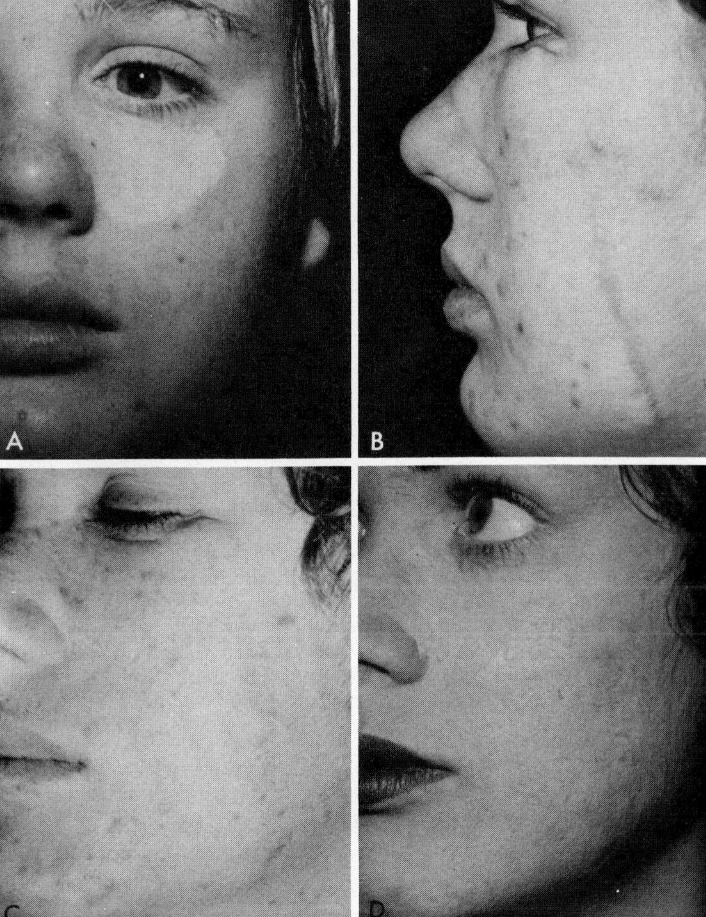


**Figure 28–18** Improvement of surgical scarring. *A,* Many years after skin graft replacement of nevus. *B,* Long cheek flap transposed for replacement of graft. *C,* Junction of flap with cheek and flap donor scar improved with geometric broken line closures. No makeup. *D,* After shave excisional, abrasive and cross-hatching techniques employed. Makeup hides acne and freckles but not contour irregularities. Slight ones still visible could be improved further with freezing and dermabrasion but patient declined this last step.

## Bibliography


1. Artz, C. P., and Hardy, J. D.: Management of Surgical Complications. 3rd ed. Philadelphia, W. B. Saunders Co., 1975.
2. Blackburn, W. R., and Cosman, B.: Histologic basis of keloid and hypertrophic scar differentiation. Arch. Pathol., *82*:65, 1966.
3. Brunius, U.: Wound healing impairment from sutures. Acta Chir. Scand. Suppl. 395, 1968.
4. Cohen, I. K., Beaver, M. A., Horakova, Z., et al.: Histamine and collagen synthesis in keloid and hypertrophic scars. Surg. Forum, *23*:509, 1972.
5. Cohen, I. K., and Keiser, H. R.: Collagen synthesis in keloid and hypertrophic scar following intralesional use of triamcinolone. Surg. Forum, *23*:521, 1973.
6. Cohen, I. K., Keiser, H. R., and Sjoerdsma, A.: Collagen synthesis in human keloid and hypertrophic scar. Surg. Forum, *22*:488, 1971.
7. Conolly, W. B., Hunt, T. K., Zederfeldt, B., et al.: Clinical comparison of surgical wounds closed by suture and adhesive tapes. Am. J. Surg., *117*:318, 1969.
8. Craig, R. D. P., Schofield, J. D., and Jackson, S. S.: Collagen biosynthesis in normal human skin, normal and hypertrophic scar, and keloid. Eur. J. Clin. Invest., *5*:69, 1975.
9. Crikelair, G. F.: Skin suture marks. Am. J. Surg., *96*:631, 1958.
10. Crockett, D. J.: Regional keloid susceptibility. Br. J. Plast. Surg., *17*:245, 1964.
11. de Hann, B. B., Ellis, H., and Wills, M; The role of infection on wound healing. Surg. Gynecol. Obstet., *138*:695, 1974.
12. Dingman, R.: Factors of clinical significance affecting wound healing. Laryngoscope, *83*:1540, 1973.
13. Dunphy, J. E., Udupa, K. N., and Edwards, L. C.: Wound healing. A new perspective with particular reference to ascorbic acid deficiency. Ann. Surg., *144*:304, 1956.

14. Edsmyr, F., Larsson, L. G., Onyango, J., et al.: Radiation therapy in the treatment of keloids in East Africa. Acta Radiol. [Ther.] (Stockh), *13*:102, 1974.
15. Ehrlich, H. P., and Hunt, T. K.: Effects of cortisone and Vitamin A on wound healing. Ann. Surg., *167*:334, 1968.
16. Ehrlich, H. P., Tarver, H., and Hunt, T. K.: Effects of Vitamin A and glucocorticoids upon inflammation and collagen synthesis. Ann. Surg., *177*:222, 1973.
17. Elias, S., and Chvapul, M.: Zinc in wound healing in normal and chronically ill rats. J. Surg. Res., *15*:59, 1973.
18. Forrester, J. C.: Mechanical, biochemical and architectural features of surgical repair. Adv. Biol. Med. Physics, *14*:1, 1973.
19. Grant, M. E., and Prockop, D. J.: Biosynthesis of collagen. N. Engl. J. Med., *286*:194, 242, 291, 1972.
20. Heughan, C., Chir, B., Grislis, G., et al.: The effect of anemia on wound healing. Ann. Surg., *179*:163, 1974.
21. Heughan, C., and Hunt, T. K.: Some aspects of wound healing research. Can. J. Surg., *18*:118, 1975.
22. Hintz, B. L.: Radiotherapy for keloids. J. Nat. Med. Assoc., *65*:71, 1973.
23. Hsu, T. H. S., and Hsu, J. H.: Wound repair. An autoradiographic study with $^3$H thymidine incorporation. Proc. Soc. Exp. Biol. Med., *140*:157, 1972.
24. Hunt, T. K.: Diagnosis and treatment of wound failure. Adv. Surg., *8*:287, 1974.
25. Hunt, T. K.: and Pai, M. P.: Effect of varying ambient oxygen tensions on wound metabolism and collagen synthesis. Surg. Gynecol. Obstet., *135*:561, 1972.
26. Jaworski, S.: Kenacort A in the treatment of hypertrophic scars and keloids in children. Acta Chir. Plast., *15*:206, 1973.
27. Ketchum, D., Cohen, I. K., and Masters, F. W.: Hypertrophic scars and keloids. Plast. Reconstr. Surg., *53*:140, 1974.
28. Ketchum, L. D., Robinson, D. W., and Masters, F. W.: Follow-up on treatment of hypertrophic scars and keloids with triamcinolone. Plast. Reconstr. Surg., *48*:256, 1971.
29. Ketchum, L. D., Smith, J., Robinson, D. W., et al.: The treatment of hypertrophic scar, keloid and scar contracture by triamcinolone acetonide. Plast. Reconstr. Surg., *38*:209, 1966.
30. Kischer, C. W.: Collagen and dermal patterns in the hypertrophic scar. Anat. Record, *179*:137, 1974.
31. Lenco, W., McKnight, M., and MacDonald, A. J.: Effects of cortisone acetate, methylprednisolone and medroxyprogesterone on wound contracture in rabbits. Ann. Surg., *81*:67, 1975.
32. Menaker, L.: Biologic Basis of Wound Healing. New York, Harper and Row, 1975.
33. Peacock, E. E., and Van Winkle, W.: Surgery and Biology of Wound Repair. Philadelphia, W. B. Saunders Co., Philadelphia, 1970.
34. Pories, W. J., Henzel, J. H., Rob, C. G., et al.: Acceleration of healing with zinc sulfate. Ann. Surg., *165*:432, 1967.
35. Rahmat, A., Norman, J. N., and Smith, G.: The effect of zinc deficiency on wound healing. Br. J. Surg., *61*:271, 1974.
36. Ramakrishnan, K. M., Thomas, K. P., and Sundararajan, C. R.: Study of 1000 patients with keloids in South India. Plast. Reconstr. Surg., *53*:276, 1974.
37. Rovee, D. T., Kurowsky, C. A., Labun, J., et al.: Effect of local wound environment on epidermal healing. *In* Maibach, H. I., and Rovee, D. T. (eds.): Epidermal Wound Healing. Chicago, Yearbook Medical Publishing Co., 1972, pp. 159–181.
38. Sandberg, N.: Relationship between cortisone and wound healing in rats. Acta Chir. Scand., *127*:466, 1964.
39. Singleton, M. A., and Gross, C. W.: Management of keloids by surgical excision and local injections of steroids. South. Med., J., *64*:1377, 1971.
40. Vallis, C. P.: Intralesional injection of keloids and hypertrophic scars with the Dermo-Jet. Plast. Reconstr. Surg., *40*:255, 1967.
41. Webster, R. C.: Cosmetic concepts in scar camouflaging serial excision and broken line techniques. Trans. Am. Acad. Ophthalmol. Otol., *73*:256, 1969.
42. Webster, R. C.: Revisional rhinoplasty. Otol. Clin. North Am., *8*:753–782, 1975.
43. Webster, R. C.: Implants and grafts above and below periosteum in chin augmentation. The International Microform Journal of Aesthetic Plastic Surgery. 1976.B.
44. Webster, R. C.: Instrument techniques in soft tissue surgery. Video Medical Education Systems. St. 101.
45. Webster, R. C.: Surgical scar camouflage. Video Medical Education Systems. St. 102.
46. Webster, R. C., and Coffey, R. J.: Cosmetic concepts in scar camouflaging. Excerpta Medica International Congress Series No. 58, excerpt 143, 1963.
47. Webster, R. C., Davidson, T. M., and Nahum, A. M.: San Diego Classics in Soft Tissue and Cosmetic Surgery. Tapes 1–20. Distributed by The American Academy of Facial Plastic and Reconstructive Surgery.

# INDEX

*Note:* Page numbers in *italics* refer to illustrations. Page numbers followed by (t) refer to tables.